Adolescent Drug Use: Recent Patterns and Consequences

Adolescent Drug Use: Recent Patterns and Consequences

Edited by Nicholas Walker

STATES
ACADEMIC PRESS
www.statesacademicpress.com

States Academic Press,
109 South 5th Street,
Brooklyn, NY 11249, USA

Visit us on the World Wide Web at:
www.statesacademicpress.com

ISBN: 978-1-63989-016-3

Cataloging-in-Publication Data

Adolescent drug use : recent patterns and consequences / edited by Nicholas Walker.
p. cm.
Includes bibliographical references and index.
ISBN 978-1-63989-016-3
1. Teenagers--Drug use. 2. Youth--Drug use. 3. Drug abuse. I. Walker, Nicholas.

RJ506.D78 A26 2022
616.860 083 5--dc23

Table of Contents

Preface

The period of transition from childhood to adulthood is called adolescence. It is accompanied by various psychological and physical changes in an individual. In terms of behavior, the probability of adolescents making rash and impulsive decisions is high. Therefore, it has been noted that drug use begins during adolescence and is connected to later problems with drug addiction related disorders. The usage of drugs during this sensitive period can have a negative effect on the neurological development which takes place during this period. This in turn can lead to long-term cognitive and emotional deficits. Some of the substances commonly abused by adolescents are cannabis, alcohol and tobacco. This book unfolds the innovative aspects of research on adolescent drug use which will be crucial for the progress of this field in the future. Also included herein is a detailed explanation of the recent patterns and consequences which have been observed. The extensive content of this book provides the readers with a thorough understanding of the subject.

The information shared in this book is based on empirical researches made by veterans in this field of study. The elaborative information provided in this book will help the readers further their scope of knowledge leading to advancements in this field.

Finally, I would like to thank my fellow researchers who gave constructive feedback and my family members who supported me at every step of my research.

Editor

Preface

1

Adolescent Alcohol Use in Spain: Connections with Friends, School, and Other Delinquent Behaviors

*Lisa D. Goldberg-Looney[1], Miriam Sánchez-SanSegundo[2], Rosario Ferrer-Cascales[2], Natalia Albaladejo-Blazquez[2] and Paul B. Perrin[1]**

[1] Department of Psychology, Virginia Commonwealth University, Richmond, Virginia, USA, [2] Department of Health Psychology, University of Alicante, Alicante, Spain

Edited by:
Gianluca Castelnuovo, Università Cattolica del Sacro Cuore, Italy

Reviewed by:
Michelle Dow Keawphalouk, Harvard and Massachusetts Institute of Technology, USA
Roberto Cattivelli, Istituto di Ricovero e Cura a Carattere Scientifico, Italy

***Correspondence:**
Paul B. Perrin
pperrin@vcu.edu

This study examined the connections between adolescent alcohol use in Alicante, Spain and variables reflecting adolescents' academic problems, potentially delinquent behaviors, friends' alcohol consumption, and friendship quality. Information about alcohol use and a number of school and social variables was collected from adolescent students ($N = 567$) who completed the National Students School-Based Drug Survey in a classroom setting. Results suggested that gender was not significantly associated with alcohol use, although alcohol use increased with age and was more likely for adolescents enrolled in public schools compared to private. After controlling for age and type of school (public vs. private), academic problems explained 5.1% of the variance in adolescents' alcohol use, potentially delinquent behaviors explained 29.0%, friends' alcohol use 16.8%, and friendship quality 1.6%. When all unique predictors from these four models were included in a comprehensive model, they explained 32.3% of the variance in adolescents' alcohol use. In this final model, getting expelled, participating in a fight, going out at night, the hour at which one returns, and the number of friends who have consumed alcohol were uniquely and positively associated with adolescents' alcohol use. These results provide important information about multi-system influences on adolescent alcohol use in Alicante, Spain and suggest potential areas of focus for intervention research.

Keywords: adolescent alcohol use, delinquent behaviors, friendship quality, intervention/prevention, peer influences, Spain

INTRODUCTION

Adolescent alcohol consumption has major health and social implications: 12.8% of male and 8.3% of female deaths among 15–29 year olds in Europe result from alcohol-related accidents, health conditions, and risky behaviors (Rehm et al., 2001). Occasional heavy drinking and intoxication common among young adults and adolescents can lead to accidents, injuries, violence, and alcohol poisoning (Ahlström and Österberg, 2004; Llorens et al., 2011). Adolescent alcohol abuse may also be associated with increased predisposition to drink excessively later in life (Jefferis et al., 2005; Windle et al., 2008) when chronic, heavy drinking has been shown to contribute to health conditions, such as alcohol dependence and liver disease (Ahlström and Österberg, 2004; Room et al., 2005). In addition, alcohol use can lead to relationship issues, legal and financial problems, emotional distress, academic problems, sexual assault, and other risk behaviors (Windle, 2000; Ahlström and Österberg, 2004).

Recent studies have found that adolescent drinking is becoming a particularly large health concern in Spain. Traditionally, alcohol has been consumed by Spanish teenagers regularly at family meals, but this behavior is becoming less frequent and instead is being replaced by social drinking with friends on weekends (Villalbí etal., 2006; Delegacion del Gobierno para el Plan Nacional sobre Drogas, 2010). The Spanish Drug Observatory (Ministerio del Interior, 2012) reports that 41.6% of adolescents ages 14–18 years consume alcohol in public parks and squares on the weekends, causing noise disturbances and leaving large amounts of garbage behind. Nearly 20% of these adolescents become involved in disputes while consuming alcohol, 23.3% ride in cars driven by intoxicated drivers, 5.3% operate vehicles under the influence of alcohol, and 7.0% require medical attention for alcohol-related traffic accidents (Ministerio del Interior, 2012).

Past research has identified several school variables that serve as protective or risk factors for adolescent alcohol use (Bryant et al., 2003; Best et al., 2006; Llorens et al., 2011; Vaughan et al., 2011). School bonding, connectedness, and involvement predict lower alcohol use in adolescents. For example, Chapman et al. (2014) examined Australian high school students and found that school connectedness, which they defined as feeling included, supported, and engaged at school, was associated with lower risk taking behaviors, such as alcohol use, as well as students' willingness to prevent their friends from engaging in risky behaviors. School connectedness has also been associated with students' relationships and behaviors with friends (Batanova and Loukas, 2012), which may indirectly influence alcohol consumption. Guo et al. (2001) found that strong bonding to school predicted lower alcohol use in an ethnically diverse sample of adolescents in the United States. School involvement has been found to be a protective factor against alcohol use in American college students (Vaughan et al., 2011) but has not been studied in Spanish adolescents. Academic achievement and better grades also correlate with less substance use (Bryant et al., 2003; Zhen-Duan and Taylor, 2014), and school enjoyment is a protective factor against substance use (Bryant et al., 2003; Vaughan et al., 2011).

While school connectedness, involvement, academic achievement and academic enjoyment may protect against alcohol use, truancy (Hibell et al., 2004; Mounteney et al., 2010), suspension (Bryant et al., 2003), lower educational aspirations (Best et al., 2006), poor academic performance (Vaughan et al., 2011), and misbehavior at school (Guo et al., 2001) are associated with increased adolescent alcohol use. Bisset et al. (2007) found that among secondary schools in the UK, those with lower rates of academic success and higher rates of truancy also had higher rates of alcohol use. Another study examining 14–16 year old school children in London found that more than two-thirds of the excessive drinkers had repeated truancy (Best et al., 2006). Others have suggested that truants are a "high-risk population" with a range of social, psychological, cognitive and behavioral problems, including underage drinking (Henry, 2007; Mounteney et al., 2010). Truants have been found to begin drinking at a younger age and have a higher frequency of drinking, levels of binge drinking, and instances of being drunk (Mounteney et al., 2010).

Adolescents who abuse alcohol have also been found to be less likely than those who do not to obtain academic success (Ingles et al., 2013). Failing grades are associated with increased alcohol use in the United States, particularly in Latino/a adolescents (Vaughan et al., 2011). In London, excessive drinking has been linked to lower educational aspirations and worsened performance (Best et al., 2006). A study examining high school students in Granada, Spain found an association between increased alcohol intake and the risk of academic failure (Lopez-Frias et al., 2001).

As with school, the literature supports the role of peers in adolescent alcohol use (Zhen-Duan and Taylor, 2014). Drinking has been conceptualized as a social activity and adolescent drinking is in part related to the closeness of their friendships (Niland et al., 2013). Maladaptive behaviors and substance use by friends predict adolescent substance use (Denault and Poulin, 2012). In fact, one study of Latino/a adolescents demonstrated that 46% of the variance in alcohol use was accounted for by peer use (Segura et al., 2003). Additional studies have suggested that the drinking behavior of friends is the most reliable predictor of adolescent alcohol use (Ahlström and Österberg, 2004). Friends' perceptions of and behaviors toward alcohol are associated with adolescents' likelihood of use (Waller et al., 2003), as are adolescents' perceptions of their peers' substance use (Bryant and Zimmerman, 2002).

In addition to influences from the school environment and peer group, alcohol consumption has been linked to several other delinquent behaviors (Guo et al., 2001; Best et al., 2006; Llorens et al., 2011). Guo et al. (2001) prospectively followed children beginning at age ten and examined various factors that were associated with increased risk for alcohol abuse at age 21, finding that problem behaviors and antisocial opportunities and involvement were the most consistent predictors. Excessive drinking has been linked to problem behaviors such as impaired social functioning, fighting, and stealing, with those who report drinking excessively also reporting a higher incidence of these behaviors (Best et al., 2006). Other researchers have found associations between alcohol use and misbehavior at school, sexual activity, criminal offenses, and running away from home (Llorens et al., 2011).

The research literature has shown that multiple factors are associated with adolescent drinking behaviors, which have been increasing in Europe generally (Hibell et al., 2009) but in Spain especially (Villalbí etal., 2006; Delegacion del Gobierno para el Plan Nacional sobre Drogas, 2010). However, much of the current literature on adolescent alcohol use comes from the United States or North America, and while some findings may be consistent across countries, countries often have their own cultural norms that impact drinking behaviors (Ahlström and Österberg, 2004). These norms may interact with peer and school variables to influence alcohol use (Batanova and Loukas, 2012). To address the growing issue of adolescent alcohol consumption in Spain, it is important that research be conducted with Spanish adolescents to determine whether similar predictors of alcohol use are operating in Spain. The purpose of the current study was to examine the associations between academic problems, friends' behaviors, friendship quality, and potentially delinquent social behaviors with alcohol consumption by adolescents in Alicante, Spain. It is hypothesized that academic problems, friends' drinking behaviors, and potentially delinquent behaviors will be associated with increased alcohol consumption, but that friendship quality will serve as a protective factor and be associated with fewer alcoholic drinks consumed.

MATERIALS AND METHODS

Participants

A total of 640 high school students in Alicante, Spain completed the survey. Inclusion criteria for the students were: (1) being present in the classroom on the day of the survey, (2) the ability to read and complete the questionnaires on their own, and (3) having signed informed consent by their parents allowing participation. Participants were retained in the final sample only if they responded to the primary dependent variable assessing alcohol use and had at least 83% complete data for the independent variables outlined below. Missing data were then imputed using mean substitution, which for low levels of missing data, as in the current study with the 83% cutoff, has been shown to be comparable to more complex methods such as multiple imputation (Parent, 2013). The final sample consisted of 567 students (52.2% female) from public (57%) and private schools in Alicante, Spain ranging in age from 14 to 21 years ($M = 16.25$, $SD = 0.81$).

Measures

ESTUDES

The National Students School-Based Drug Survey (ESTUDES) is a self-administered questionnaire of drug use in adolescents. It contains 90 multiple-choice questions grouped into three modules covering the following domains: Basic Questions (drug use, perceived risk, leisure time, access to and availability of drugs, health-related problems, family drug consumption, knowledge and attitudes regarding drug use); Emerging Drugs (perceived risk of and accessibility to new emerging drugs); and Drug-related Problems (problems experienced due to drug use, severity of dependence, and questions regarding substance-use disorders). The present study focused solely on a selection of the Basic Questions contained in the first module measuring alcohol use among students and friends' consumption of alcohol.

KIDSCREEN-52

The Kidscreeen-52 is a 52-item self-administered questionnaire measuring health-related quality of life in children and adolescents. It yields 10 subscales, but the present study included only the Peers and Social Support subscale, which examines adolescents' relationships with friends. Items are scored on a 5-point Likert type scale (1 = never, 2 = seldom, 3 = sometimes, 4 = often, 5 = always). Psychometric properties of the Spanish version of the KIDSCREEN-52 have demonstrated adequate validity, reliability, and cross-cultural comparability (Aymerich et al., 2005).

Alcohol Consumption Item

The primary dependent variable in this study was participants' responses to a single item assessing the number of days alcohol was consumed over the past 30 days ("On how many days have you consumed alcohol during the past 30 days?"). Participants selected responses from the following options: 0, 1, 2, 3, 4–5, 6–9, 10–19, 20–29, or 30 days or more. Past research suggests that single item questionnaires for alcohol use and other risky behaviors are often as accurate and sometimes superior to longer, multi-item screening tools (Smith et al., 2009; Barry et al., 2013; Saitz et al., 2014).

Procedure

The present study was a part of a large-scale study on alcohol abuse funded by the Alicante Municipal Plan on Drug addiction using the National Survey on Drug Use (ESTUDES). As such, the measures were preselected. Students completed the survey as part of an annual nationwide review conducted by the Spanish Drug Observatory for Control and Prevention (DGPNSD), a government organization that provides coordination and technical support for the development of policies and programs on adolescent substance use in Spain. This was performed in a geographic region in the east of Spain with a population of 334,000 people. The study was approved by the University of Alicante (AYTOALICANTE3-13I), and parents provided consent to the participation of their children prior to data collection.

Students 14–21 years old from public and private secondary schools were selected using a stratified random cluster sampling in two stages. In the first stage, all schools were randomly selected with a probability of being selected proportional to the sample size. In the second stage, classes were systematically randomly selected within each school using an enumeration procedure. Students who were present on the day of data collection and who agreed to participate completed the questionnaire anonymously. Data were collected by research assistants during the second and third trimester of the 2013/2014 academic year and lasted from 60 to 90 min.

Statistical Analyses

A correlation matrix was created to determine which demographic variables were associated with the primary outcome variable, number of days over the past 30 days that alcohol was consumed. Any demographics with significant associations with alcohol consumption were then entered as predictors in Step 1 in each regression in a series of five regressions, which all had the same dependent variable of alcohol consumption. These five regressions included the following categories of predictor variables in Step 2, respectively: (1) academic problems, (2) potentially delinquent behaviors, (3) friends' alcohol consumption, (4) friendship quality, and (5) all significant predictors from the previous four regressions. The statistical design (hierarchical regression) was chosen in order to understand the associations between adolescent alcohol use and various demographic, social, and academic variables. Using several step-wise models allowed us to control for demographic variables and isolate the unique predictors of the dependent variable.

RESULTS

Correlations between Demographics and Alcohol Consumption

Bivariate correlations were calculated to examine the relationships between the demographic variables of age, gender, and type of school (public versus private) with the criterion variable in the successive regression analyses, number of days alcohol was consumed over the past 30 days (**Table 1**). Age and type of school were significantly correlated with alcohol consumption such that alcohol consumption increased with age and was less likely for adolescents enrolled in private schools. Gender was not significantly correlated with alcohol consumption and was excluded from all further analyses. Additional correlation coefficients were calculated indexing the relationships between all other predictor variables in the current study and alcohol consumption (**Table 1**).

Academic Problems

The first hierarchical multiple regression tested the hypothesis that academic problems would be positively associated with the number of days in which adolescents consumed alcohol during the past 30 days, after controlling for age and type of school. Age and type of school were entered into the first step of the regression which was statistically significant, $F(2,549) = 18.91$, $p < 0.001$, $R^2 = 0.064$. Age [$\beta = 0.25$, $p < 0.001$] was a unique predictor of alcohol consumption such that older adolescents more frequently consumed alcohol, but type of school was not ($\beta = -0.03$, $p = 0.543$). The second step included the following four academic behavior variables: not completing one's homework, missing class, repeating a course, and being expelled. The addition of this step significantly increased the amount of variance explained in alcohol consumption, $\Delta F(4,545) = 7.82, p < 0.001$, $\Delta R^2 = 0.051$. The overall model with both steps was statistically significant, $F(6,545) = 11.83$, $p < 0.001$, $R^2 = 0.115$. With the addition of the second step, age was no longer a unique predictor ($\beta = 0.07$, $p = 0.369$). Repeating a course ($\beta = 0.19$, $p = 0.007$) and getting expelled ($\beta = 0.16$, $p < 0.001$) were significantly associated with higher alcohol consumption. No other academic problems were significant unique predictors (all $ps \geq 0.056$).

TABLE 1 | Correlations between alcohol consumption and all predictors.

Predictors	Correlation (*r*) with alcohol consumption
Demographics	
Age	0.25**
Public vs. private school	0.10*
Gender	0.03
Academic Problems	
Normally I do not complete any of my homework.	0.04
Have you repeated a course?	0.30**
Have you missed class in the past 30 days?	0.13**
Have you been expelled in the past 12 months?	0.19**
Potentially delinquent behaviors	
Have you run away from home in the past 12 months?	0.14**
Have you participated in a fight in the past 12 months?	0.26**
Do you go out at night?	0.52**
When do you return when you go out at night?	0.41**
Friends' alcohol consumption	
How many of your friends consumed alcohol in the past 30 days?	0.42**
How many of your friends got drunk in the past 30 days?	0.37**
Friendship quality	
I receive care from my best friend.	0.03
How often do you hang out with your friends?	0.11*
Friends subscale of the KIDSCREEN-52	0.09*

*** Correlation is significant at the 0.01 level (two-tailed). * Correlation is significant at the 0.05 level (two-tailed).*

Potentially Delinquent Behaviors

A second hierarchical multiple regression was run in the same manner as above but substituting four variables indexing potentially delinquent behaviors in the second step: running away from home, participating in a fight, going out at night, and the hour at which one returns home after going out at night. The addition of this step (after step 1 with age and type of school) significantly increased the amount of variance explained in alcohol consumption, $\Delta F(4,545) = 61.12, p < 0.001$, $\Delta R^2 = 0.290$. The overall model with both steps was statistically significant, $F(6,545) = 49.81$, $p < 0.001$, $R^2 = 0.347$. With the addition of the second step, age was no longer a unique predictor ($\beta = 0.07, p = 0.068$). Participating in a fight ($\beta = 0.14, p < 0.001$), going out at night ($\beta = 0.41$, $p < 0.001$), and the hour at which one returns ($\beta = 0.20$, $p < 0.001$) were significantly associated with higher alcohol consumption. Running away from home was not a unique predictor of alcohol consumption ($\beta = 0.03$, $p = 0.353$).

Friends' Alcohol Consumption

A third regression was run in the same manner but substituting in the second step two variables describing friends' alcohol consumption. The addition of the second step significantly increased the amount of variance explained in alcohol consumption, $\Delta F(2,547) = 59.69$, $p < 0.001$, $\Delta R^2 = 0.168$. The overall model with both steps was statistically significant, $F(4,547) = 41.32$, $p < 0.001$, $R^2 = 0.232$. With the addition of the second step, age remained a unique predictor ($\beta = 0.20$, $p < 0.001$). The number of friends who have consumed alcohol in the past 30 days ($\beta = 0.31$, $p < 0.001$) and the number of friends who have been drunk in the past 30 days ($\beta = 0.13$, $p = 0.012$) each uniquely predicted alcohol consumption such that greater number of friends engaging in these behaviors were associated with increased participant alcohol consumption.

Friendship Quality

The fourth hierarchical multiple regression was run in the same manner but substituting three variables related to friendship quality in the second step: receiving care from one's best friend, spending time with one's friends, and the Friends subscale from the KIDSCREEN-52. The addition of this step significantly increased the amount of variance explained in alcohol consumption, $\Delta F(3,546) = 3.11, p = 0.026, \Delta R^2 = 0.016$. The overall model with both steps was statistically significant, $F(5,546) = 9.51$, $p < 0.001$, $R^2 = 0.080$. With the addition of the second step, age remained a unique predictor ($\beta = 0.25$, $p < 0.001$). None of the friendship quality variables were unique predictors of alcohol consumption (all $ps \geq 0.086$).

Combined

A fifth hierarchical regression included only the significant predictors from the previous regressions, with age in the first step and all other previously significant predictors in the second step. The addition of the second step significantly increased the amount of variance explained in alcohol consumption, $\Delta F(7,543) = 40.92$, $p < 0.001$, $\Delta R^2 = 0.323$. The overall model with both steps was statistically significant, $F(8,543) = 42.87$, $p < 0.001$, $R^2 = 0.387$. With the addition of the second step, age was no longer a unique predictor ($\beta = 0.06$, $p = 0.310$). Getting expelled ($\beta = 0.08$, $p = 0.032$), participating in a fight ($\beta = 0.12$, $p = 0.001$), going out at night ($\beta = 0.33$, $p < 0.001$), the hour at which one returns ($\beta = 0.14$, $p < 0.001$), and the number of friends who consumed alcohol in the past 30 days ($\beta = 0.14$, $p = 0.007$) were significant predictors such that these indices of academic problems, potentially delinquent social behaviors, and friends' alcohol consumption were associated with greater alcohol consumption. However, repeating a course and having a greater numbers of friends who got drunk in the past 30 days were not unique predictors of alcohol consumption ($ps > 0.122$).

DISCUSSION

The current study examined the connections between adolescent alcohol use in Alicante, Spain and variables reflecting adolescents' academic problems, potentially delinquent behaviors, friends' alcohol consumption, and friendship quality. After controlling for age and type of school (public vs. private), academic problems explained 5.1% of the variance in adolescents' alcohol use, potentially delinquent behaviors explained 29.0%, friends' alcohol use explained 16.8%, and friendship quality 1.6%. When all unique predictors from these four models were included in a comprehensive model, they explained 32.3% of the variance in adolescents' alcohol use. In this final model, getting expelled, participating in a fight, going out at night, the hour at which one returns, and the number of friends who have consumed alcohol were uniquely and positively associated with adolescents' alcohol use.

Demographics and Alcohol Consumption

Past studies have found mixed results in regards to gender and alcohol use. A review of several nations (i.e., the United States, United Kingdom, and Nordic countries) has found little differences between the genders for alcohol use (Ahlström and Österberg, 2004). Similarly, gender was not significantly correlated with alcohol consumption in the present study. Alcohol use did increase with age, consistent with past findings (Llorens et al., 2011) and was less likely for adolescents enrolled in private schools in the bivariate correlation matrix. However, these effects were no longer significant when entered into the final regression model with other previously significant predictors. Past research has found that type of school did not predict alcohol use (Lopez-Frias et al., 2001), corroborating the small and fleeting effect of school that emerged in the bivariate correlation matrix in the current study.

Academic Problems

It was predicted that academic problems would be positively associated with the number of days on which adolescents consumed alcohol during the past 30 days, after controlling for age and type of school. Getting expelled was significantly associated with higher alcohol consumption, consistent with previous research (Bryant et al., 2003). The literature overwhelmingly suggests that lower educational aspirations (Best et al., 2006), poor academic performance (Vaughan et al., 2011), and academic failure (Lopez-Frias et al., 2001) are associated with increased alcohol use in many nations. In the current study, these constructs were further broken down into the more measurable actions of completing homework and repeating a course. Repeating a course was initially significantly and positively correlated with alcohol use. However, when entered into the final model with all other previously significant predictors, repeating a course no longer uniquely predicted alcohol consumption. Completing one's homework was not associated with drinking behaviors in the present study.

Despite many previous studies demonstrating an association between truancy and alcohol use (Hibell et al., 2004; Best et al., 2006; Bisset et al., 2007; Mounteney et al., 2010), the current study surprisingly did not find that missing class significantly predicted alcohol consumption. Much of the literature suggesting the link between truancy and alcohol use was conducted with non-Spanish samples, perhaps suggesting that Spanish schoolchildren or school systems differ in some way from those in other countries. It is also interesting to note that the non-significant variables in the current study were behaviors (i.e., not attending class and completing homework), whereas the significant predictors of alcohol use were consequences (i.e., having to repeat a course or being expelled).

Potentially Delinquent Behaviors

It was hypothesized that potentially delinquent behaviors would be associated with increased alcohol consumption. Participating in a fight, going out at night, and the hour at which one returns were positively associated with alcohol consumption. Previous research also found that alcohol use was related to fighting (Best et al., 2006; Salas-Wright et al., 2014), going out at night, and returning home late at night (Llorens et al., 2011). However, while past studies have found a relatively strong influence of running away from home on alcohol use (Llorens et al., 2011), the current study did not find that running away from home predicted alcohol consumption.

Friends' Alcohol Consumption

It was also hypothesized that friends' alcohol consumption would be associated with increased participant alcohol use. The number of friends who have consumed alcohol in the past 30 days and the number of friends who have been drunk in the past 30 days each uniquely predicted alcohol consumption such that a greater number of friends engaging in these behaviors was associated with increased participant alcohol consumption. This is consistent with past findings showing that peers' and friends' alcohol use predicts an individual's alcohol consumption, as does an individual's perception of his or her peers' substance use (Bryant and Zimmerman, 2002; Segura et al., 2003; Waller et al., 2003; Denault and Poulin, 2012). However, when both variables were entered into the final regression examining all previously significant predictors, the number of friends who have been drunk in the past 30 days was no longer significant. This suggests that the amount of alcohol consumed by friends may be less important than the fact that friends are drinking at all.

Friendship Quality

The final part of the hypothesis was that higher friendship quality would serve as a protective factor against alcohol use. However, none of the friendship quality variables were unique predictors of alcohol consumption. Perhaps this is because strong friendships can have a positive or negative impact on one's behavior depending on friends' behaviors (i.e., alcohol use). Strong relationships with friends who are a positive influence (i.e., engage in little to no alcohol use) would likely be associated with decreased alcohol use, while strong relationships with individuals who are a negative influence (i.e., engage in delinquent behaviors including consuming alcohol frequently and/or in large quantities) would probably be associated with increased drinking behaviors. Therefore, a potential reason that no effect was found in the current study may be that the effect of friendship quality on drinking behaviors was washed out by participants having friends who were both a positive or negative influence. This is consistent with previous findings that perceived disapproval of substance use by peers inversely predicted alcohol use, while approval and indifference by peers predicted increased use (Mason et al., 2014).

Implications

The present study identified academic and peer influences on alcohol use. Additional studies are needed to support the current findings as well as explore causality. If the current findings are supported in future studies with more thorough implementation of measures and perhaps a larger population of adolescents, and a causal link can be established between the variables examined in the study and adolescent alcohol use, school-based interventions may have promise in reducing adolescent alcohol use. Such interventions could draw on social norms and social influence. Many global regions have had success with school-based programs, such as the School Health and Alcohol Harm Reduction Project (SHAHRP) in Australia (McBride et al., 2004), Project ALERT (Ellickson et al., 2003) and ALERT Plus (Longshore et al., 2007) in the United States, and the Unplugged program (Caria et al., 2011) that was tested in seven European countries including Spain via the EU-Dap (European Drug Abuse Prevention) study.

Expanding the focus of school-based programs to include efforts to retain problematic students instead of expelling them and trainings to help students resolve conflicts verbally instead of through physical violence may be ripe targets for intervention research, as both expulsion and participating in a fight were unique predictors of alcohol consumption in the current study. Additionally, based on the current findings, interventions aimed at helping parents of adolescents limit going out at night, establish and enforce an appropriate curfew, and monitor adolescents' friends' alcohol consumption may similarly yield promise in helping to curb adolescent drinking in Spain. In fact, Project ALERT, which has been recognized as a model program by the Center for Substance Abuse Prevention, combines instruction, interactive question-and-answer sessions, skill-building activities, group activities, and parental involvement (Ellickson et al., 2003). Cultural tailoring of interventions may be particularly relevant in Spain, where traditional alcohol consumption at family meals is being replaced by social drinking with friends on weekends (Villalbí etal., 2006; Delegacion del Gobierno para el Plan Nacional sobre Drogas, 2010), especially in public parks and squares (Ministerio del Interior, 2001).

Limitations and Future Directions

There are several limitations of the current study that point to potential areas for future research. One limitation was that only limited demographic information was collected. Future studies may examine additional variables such as race/ethnicity, gender identity, sexual orientation, and socioeconomic status to see how differences in these domains may affect adolescent alcohol use. A second limitation was that many of the variables assessed in the current analysis were derived from single-item measures because the present study was a part of a large-scale study on alcohol abuse funded by the Alicante Municipal Plan on Drug addiction using the National Survey on Drug Use (ESTUDES). While this common technique in epidemiological research, we recognize that it is not as strong as using validated multi-item measures of the constructs. Future studies may instead use validated scales for each of these variables for more comprehensive information. For instance, the dependent variable—adolescent alcohol use—was measured with a single item. A validated scale such as the Alcohol Use Disorders Identification Test (AUDIT; Babor et al., 1992) could be used in future studies. Nonetheless, this concern can be tempered somewhat as researchers have suggested that single item questionnaires for alcohol use and other risky behaviors are often as accurate and sometimes even better than longer, multi-item screening tools (Smith et al., 2009; Barry et al., 2013; Saitz et al., 2014). For instance, Barry et al. (2013) found that a single item asking how often participants typically "got drunk" demonstrated both concurrent and convergent validity with validated measures such as the AUDIT-C and biological measures such as breath alcohol concentration. Saitz et al. (2014) similarly reported that a single question regarding alcohol use was more accurate than the more complex AUDIT-C.

A third limitation was that the data were self-reported and participants could have understated the alcohol use. This concern is mitigated by the fact that the questionnaires were individually and anonymously completed, minimizing the potential for social desirability in responding to questions about alcohol use. Nonetheless, future studies may benefit from incorporating social desirability scales and having collateral reports to verify the self-reported information.

The data were cross-sectional, and as a result, causation cannot be directly inferred. Although the host of variables examined in this study might cause adolescent alcohol use, so too could the reverse causal direction exist. Future research using cross-lagged panel methodologies could more readily tease apart causality. Finally, future research might evaluate the effectiveness and feasibility of culturally tailored interventions for Spanish adolescents and families that target some of the variables found in this study to be association with adolescent alcohol consumption. However, randomized clinical trials investigating whether these interventions actually reduce alcohol consumption need to be conducted before any implications for policy or systematic adoption of programs occur.

CONCLUSION

The present study provided important information about multi-system influences on adolescent alcohol use in Alicante, Spain and suggested potential areas of focus for intervention research. Getting expelled from school, participating in a fight, going out at night, the hour at which one returns at night, and the number of friends who consumed alcohol in the past 30 days were uniquely associated with increased adolescent alcohol use. Additional research is needed to support these findings as well as determine a causal direction. If these findings are supported, future research may focus on the development and testing of interventions that target students as well as social and parental influences and may have potential to decrease adolescent alcohol use if they encourage school success, academic achievement, school connectedness, healthy friendships, supervised activities in the home, a curfew, and social opportunities without alcohol. However, such assertions await support from future research.

AUTHOR CONTRIBUTIONS

All authors listed, have made substantial, direct and intellectual contribution to the work, and approved it for publication

FUNDING

This study was funded by Concejalía de Acción Social. Plan Municipal sobre Drogodependencia. Ayuntamiento de Alicante, Spain. Delegación del Gobierno para el Plan Nacional sobre Drogas.

REFERENCES

Ahlström, S. K., and Österberg, E. L. (2004). International perspectives on adolescent and young adult drinking. *Alcohol. Res. Health* 28, 258-268.

Aymerich, M., Berra, S., Guillamón, I., Herdman, M., Alonso, J., Ravens-Sieberer, U., et al. (2005). Desarrollo de la versión en español del KIDSCREEN, un cuestionario de calidad de vida para la población infantil y adolescente. *Gac. Sanit.* 19, 93–102. doi: 10.1157/13074363

Babor, T. F., de la Fuente, J. R., Saunders, J., and Grant, M. (1992) *AUDIT: The Alcohol Use Disorders Identification Test: Guidelines for Use in Primary Health Care.* Geneva: World Health Organization.

Barry, A. E., Chaney, B. H., Stellefson, M. L., and Dodd, V. (2013). Validating the ability of a single-item assessing drunkenness to detect hazardous drinking. *Am. J. Drug Alcohol. Abuse* 39, 320–325. doi: 10.3109/00952990.2013.810745

Batanova, M. D., and Loukas, A. (2012). What are the unique and interacting contributions of school and family factors to early adolescents' empathic concern and perspective taking? *J. Youth Adolesc.* 41, 1382–1391. doi: 10.1007/s10964-012-9768-9765

Best, D., Manning, V., Gossop, M., Gross, S., and Strang, J. (2006). Excessive drinking and other problem behaviours among 14-16 year schoolchildren. *Addict. Behav.* 31, 1424–1435. doi: 10.1016/j.addbeh.2005.12.002

Bisset, S., Markham, W. A., and Aveyard, P. (2007). School culture as an influencing factor on youth substance use. *J. Epidemiol. Commun. Health* 61, 485–490. doi: 10.1136/jech.2006.048157

Bryant, A. L., Schulenberg, J. E., O'Malley, P. M., Bachman, J. G., and Johnston, L. D. (2003). How academic achievement, attitudes, and behaviors relate to the course of substance use during adolescence: a 6-year, multiwave national longitudinal study. *J. Res. Adolesc.* 31, 361–397. doi: 10.1111/1532-7795.1303005

Bryant, A. L., and Zimmerman, M. A. (2002). Examining the effects of academic beliefs and behaviors on changes in substance use among urban adolescents. *J. Educ. Psychol.* 94, 621–637. doi: 10.1037/0022-0663.94.3.621

Caria, M. P., Faggiano, F., Bellocco, R., Galanti, M. R., and The EU-Dap Study Group. (2011). Effects of a school-based prevention program on European adolescents' patterns of alcohol use. *J. Adolesc. Health* 48, 182–188. doi: 10.1016/j.jadohealth.2010.06.003

Chapman, R. L., Buckley, L., Reveruzzi, B., and Sheehan, M. (2014). Injury prevention among friends: the benefits of school. *J. Adolesc.* 37, 937–944. doi: 10.1016/j.adolescence.2014.06.009

Delegacion del Gobierno para el Plan Nacional sobre Drogas (2010). Informe (2009) *del Observatorio Español sobre Drogas. Situación y Tendencias de los Problemas de Drogas en España.* Madrid: Ministerio de Sanidad y Política Social.

Denault, A., and Poulin, F. (2012). Peer group deviancy in organized activities and youths' problem behaviours. *Can. J. Behav. Sci.* 44, 83–92. doi: 10.1037/a0025705

Ellickson, P. L., McCaffrey, D. F., Ghosh-Dastidar, B., and Longshore, D. L. (2003). New inroads in preventing adolescent drug use: results from a large-scale trial of Project ALERT in middle schools. *Am. J. Public Health* 93, 1830–1836. doi: 10.2105/AJPH.93.11.1830

Guo, J., Hawkins, J. D., Hill, K. G., and Abbott, R. D. (2001). Childhood and adolescent predictors of alcohol abuse and dependence in young adulthood. *J. Stud. Alcohol.* 62, 754–762. doi: 10.15288/jsa.2001.62.754

Henry, K. L. (2007). Who's skipping school: characteristics of truants in 8th and 10th grade. *J. Sch. Health* 77, 29–35. doi: 10.1111/j.1746-1561.2007.00159.x

Hibell, B., Andersson, B., Bjarnasson, T., Ahlstroöm, S., Balakireva, O., Kokkevi, A., et al. (2004). *Alcohol and other drug use among students in 35 European countries.* The ESPAD Report 2003. Stockholm: The Swedish Council for Information on Alcohol and other Drugs.

Hibell, B., Guttormsson, U., Ahlstrom, S., Balakireva, O., Bjarnason, T., Kokkevi, A., et al. (2009). *Alcohol and Other Drug Use among Students in 35 European Countries.* ESPAD Report 2007. Stockholm: The Swedish Council for Information on Alcohol and Other Drugs.

Ingles, C. J., Torregrosa, M. S., Rodriguez-Marin, J., Garcia del Castillo, J. A., Gazquez, J. J., García-Fernández, J. M., et al. (2013). Alcohol and tobacco use and cognitive-motivational variables in school settings: Effects on academic performance in Spanish adolescents. *Adicciones,* 25, 63–70.

Jefferis, B., Power, C., and Manor, O. (2005). Adolescent level and adult binge drinking in a national birth cohort. *Addiction* 100, 543–549. doi: 10.1111/j.1360-0443.2005.01034.x

Llorens, N., Barrio, G., Sanchez, A., and Suelvas, J. M. (2011). Effects of socialization and family factors on adolescent excessive drinking in Spain. *Prev. Sci.* 12, 150–161. doi: 10.1007/s11121-010-0195-0

Longshore, D., Ellickson, P. L., McCaffrey, D. F,, and St Clair, P. A. (2007). School-based drug prevention among at-risk adolescents: Effects of ALERT Plus. *Health Educ. Behav.* 34, 651–668. doi: 10.1177/1090198106294895

Lopez-Frias, M., De La Fe Fernandez, M., Planells, E., Miranda, M. T., Mataix, J., and Llopis, J. (2001). Alcohol consumption and academic performance in a population of Spanish high school students. *J. Stud. Alcohol.*62, 741–744. doi: 10.15288/jsa.2001.62.741

Mason, M. J., Mennis, J., Linker, J., Bares, C., and Zaharakis, N. (2014). Peer attitudes effects on adolescent substance use: the moderating role of race and gender. *Prev. Sci.* 4, 56–64. doi: 10.1007/s11121-012-0353-7

McBride, N., Farringdon, F., Milford, R., Meuleners, L., and Phillips, M. (2004). Harm minimization in school drug education: final results of the School Health and Alcohol Harm Reduction Project (SHAHRP). *Addiction* 99, 278–291. doi: 10.1111/j.1360-0443.2003.00620.x

Ministerio del Interior (2001). *Secretaria General Técnica. Informe No. 3. Observatorio Español Sobre Drogas.* Report No. 3 Spanish Drug Observatory. Madrid: Ministerio del Interior.

Ministerio del Interior (2012). *Encuesta Estatal sobre Uso de Drogas en Enseñanzas Secundarias.* Madrid: Delegación del Gobierno para el Plan Nacional sobre Drogas.

Mounteney, J., Hauglang, S., and Skutle, A. (2010). Truancy, alcohol use and alcohol-related problems in secondary school pupils in Norway. *Health Educ. Res.* 25, 945–954. doi: 10.1093/her/cyq044

Niland, P., Lyons, A. C., Goodwin, I., and Hutton, F. (2013). "Everyone can loosen up and get a bit of buzz on": Young adults, alcohol and friendship practices. *Int. J. Drug Policy* 24, 530–537. doi: 10.1016/j.drugpo.2013.05.013

Parent, M. C. (2013). Handling item-level missing data: simpler is just as good. *Counsel. Psychol.* 41, 568–600. doi: 10.1177/0011000012445176

Rehm, J., Gmel, G., Room, R., and Frick, U. (2001). Average volume of alcohol consumption, drinking patterns and related burden of mortality in young people in established market economies of Europe. *Eur. Addict. Res.* 7, 148–151. doi: 10.1159/000050732

Room, R., Babor, T., and Rehm, J. (2005). Alcohol and public health. *Lancet* 365, 519–530. doi: 10.1016/S0140-6736(05)70276-2

Saitz, R., Cheng, D. M., Allensworth-Davies, D., Winter, M. R., and Smith, P. C. (2014). The ability of single screening questions for unhealthy alcohol and other drug use to identify substance dependence in primary care. *J. Stud. Alcohol Drugs* 75, 153–157. doi: 10.15288/jsad.2014.75.153

Salas-Wright, C. P., Hernandez, L., Maynard, B. R., Saltzman, L. Y., and Vaughn, M. G. (2014). Alcohol use among Hispanic early adolescents in the United States: an examination of behavioral risk and protective profiles. *Subst. Use Misuse* 49, 864–877. doi: 10.3109/10826084.2014.880725

Segura, Y. L., Page, M. C., Neighbors, B. D., Nichols-Anderson, C., and Gillaspy, S. (2003). The importance of peers in alcohol use among Latino adolescents: the role of alcohol expectancies and acculturation. *J. Ethnicity Subst. Abuse* 2, 31–49. doi: 10.1300/J233v02n03_02

Smith, P. C., Schmidt, S. M., Allensworth-Davies, D., and Saitz, R. (2009). Primary care validation of a single-question alcohol screening test. *J. Gen. Intern. Med.* 7, 783–788. doi: 10.1007/s11606-009-0928-6

Vaughan, E. L., Kratz, L., and d'Argent, J. (2011). Academics and substance use among Latino adolescents: results from a national study. *J. Ethnicity Subst. Abuse* 10, 147–161. doi: 10.1080/15332640.2011.573315

Villalbí, J. R., Rodríguez-Martos, A., Jansá, J. M., and Guix, J. (2006). Policies to reduce harm caused by alcohol use: a public health perspective. *Med. Clín.* 127, 741–743. doi: 10.1157/13095524

Waller, M. A., Okamoto, S. K., Miles, B. W., and Hurdle, D. E. (2003). Resiliency factors related to substance use/ resistance: perceptions of native adolescents of the southwest. *J. Sociol. Soc. Welfare* 30, 79–94.

Windle, M. (2000). Parental, sibling, and peer influences on adolescent substance abuse and alcohol problems. *Appl. Dev. Sci.* 4, 98–110. doi: 10.1207/S1532480XADS0402_5

Windle, M., Spear, L. P., Fuligni, A. J., Angold, A., Brown, J. D., Pine, D., et al. (2008). Transitions into underage and problem drinking: developmental processes and mechanisms between 10 and 15 years of age. *Pediatrics* 121, S273–S289. doi: 10.1542/peds.2007-2243c

Zhen-Duan, J., and Taylor, M. J. (2014). The use of an ecodevelopmental approach to examining substance use among rural and urban Latino/a youth: peer, parental, and school influences. *J. Ethnicity Subst. Abuse* 13, 104–125. doi: 10.1080/15332640.2013.873006

2

Heavy Drinking in College Students is Associated with Accelerated Gray Matter Volumetric Decline over a 2 Year Period

Shashwath A. Meda[1*], *Alecia D. Dager*[1,2], *Keith A. Hawkins*[2], *Howard Tennen*[3], *Sarah Raskin*[4], *Rebecca M. Wood*[5], *Carol S. Austad*[5], *Carolyn R. Fallahi*[5] *and Godfrey D. Pearlson*[1,2,6]

[1] Olin Neuropsychiatry Research Center, Hartford HealthCare Corporation, Hartford, CT, United States, [2] Department of Psychiatry, Yale University, New Haven, CT, United States, [3] Department of Community Medicine, University of Connecticut School of Medicine, Farmington, CT, United States, [4] Department of Psychology and Neurosciences, Trinity College, Hartford, CT, United States, [5] Department of Psychology, Central Connecticut State University, New Britain, CT, United States, [6] Department of Neuroscience, Yale University, New Haven, CT, United States

Edited by:
Mary M. Torregrossa,
University of Pittsburgh, United States

Reviewed by:
Dieter J. Meyerhoff,
University of California, San Francisco,
United States
Zsigmond Tamás Kincses,
University of Szeged, Hungary

***Correspondence:**
Shashwath A. Meda
shashwath.meda@hhchealth.org

Background: Heavy and/or harmful alcohol use while in college is a perennial and significant public health issue. Despite the plethora of cross-sectional research suggesting deleterious effects of alcohol on the brain, there is a lack of literature investigating the longitudinal effects of alcohol consumption on the adolescent brain. We aim to probe the longitudinal effects of college drinking on gray matter change in students during this crucial neurodevelopmental period.

Methods: Data were derived from the longitudinal Brain and Alcohol Research in College Students (BARCS) study of whom a subset underwent brain MRI scans at two time points 24 months apart. Students were young adults with a mean age at baseline of about 18.5 years. Based on drinking metrics assessed at both baseline and followup, subjects were classified as sustained abstainers/light drinkers ($N = 45$) or sustained heavy drinkers ($N = 84$) based on criteria established in prior literature. Gray matter volumetric change (GMV-c) maps were derived using the longitudinal DARTEL pipeline as implemented in SPM12. GMV-c maps were then subjected to a 1-sample and 2-sample *t*-test in SPM12 to determine within- and between-group GMV-c differences in drinking groups. Supplementary between-group differences were also computed at baseline only.

Results: Within-group analysis revealed significant decline in GMV in both groups across the 2 year followup period. However, tissue loss in the sustained heavy drinking group was more significant, larger per region, and more widespread across regions compared to abstainers/light drinkers. Between-group analysis confirmed the above and showed a greater rate of GMV-c in the heavy drinking group in several brain regions encompassing inferior/medial frontal gyrus, parahippocampus, and anterior cingulate. Supplementary analyses suggest that some of the frontal differences existed at baseline and progressively worsened.

Conclusion: Sustained heavy drinking while in college was associated with accelerated GMV decline in brain regions involved with executive functioning, emotional regulation, and memory, which are critical to everyday life functioning. Areas of significant GMV decreases also overlapped largely with brain reward and stress systems implicated in addictive behavior.

Keywords: substance use, college, binge, morphometry, cortical

INTRODUCTION

Alcohol is the most widely used intoxicant among adolescents and young adults, with rates of binge drinking and alcohol use disorders peaking between ages 18 and 25 (SAMHSA, 2016), a period commonly referred to as emerging adulthood (Arnett, 2000). Recent national surveys revealed that 39% of 18–25-year-olds reported past-month binge drinking, compared to 25% of adults ages 26 and older (SAMHSA, 2016). This age range also encompasses the final stages of neuromaturation (Gogtay et al., 2004), which may be negatively affected by heavy alcohol use.

Age-related refinements in brain structure and function continue well into emerging adulthood. Region-specific patterns of cortical thinning and gray matter volume reduction have been identified, with higher order association cortices, including prefrontal and temporal regions, maturing last, and varying by sex (Gogtay et al., 2004). Measureable changes in gray matter volume have been observed over a 6-month period in first-year college students, between fall and spring semesters (Bennett and Baird, 2006). These neuromaturational changes are thought to underlie cognitive improvements throughout this age range. In particular, executive functions, subserved by late-developing frontal lobe regions, show dramatic enhancements in late adolescence and emerging adulthood (Casey et al., 2000).

Several neuroimaging investigations have characterized structural brain differences among adolescent drinkers, yet fewer investigations have focused on emerging adults. Extant research has most consistently implicated frontal lobe abnormalities among adolescent drinkers (Silveri et al., 2016). Cross sectional studies have revealed smaller volumes and thinner cortices among adolescent heavy drinkers, particularly in frontal, temporal, and cingulate regions (De Bellis et al., 2005; Medina et al., 2008; Fein et al., 2013; Whelan et al., 2014), with greater alcohol consumption associated with larger volume reductions (De Bellis et al., 2005). A recent voxel-based morphometry study of young adults ages 22–28 identified less gray matter volume among heavy drinkers in anterior cingulate, orbitofrontal, temporal, and insula cortices (Heikkinen et al., 2017). Longitudinal investigations have examined adolescents both before and after the onset of heavy drinking, and described steeper declines in cortical thickness in prefrontal (Luciana et al., 2013; Squeglia et al., 2015) and temporal (Squeglia et al., 2014, 2015) regions in alcohol initiators. One diffusion tensor imaging study ascertained white matter integrity in binge drinkers and controls during late adolescence, and again 3 years later during emerging adulthood. Lower fractional anisotropy was observed at baseline among binge drinkers throughout widespread brain regions (Jacobus et al., 2009; McQueeny et al., 2009), many of which showed additional decline among those who continued binge drinking during the 3-year follow-up period (Jacobus et al., 2013). However, to our knowledge, this is the first longitudinal study to examine trajectories of gray matter volume development in an attempt to shed more light on implications of continued heavy drinking among emerging adult drinkers.

To delineate the influence of ongoing heavy alcohol use on brain gray matter development in emerging adulthood, we collected structural magnetic resonance imaging (MRI) scans at two time-points in a college cohort, at approximately age 18 and again ~2 years later at age 20. We conducted longitudinal voxel based morphometry (VBM) analyses in individuals who were either abstainers/light drinking controls or heavy drinkers at both time-points (i.e., sustained light use or sustained heavy use). Given that cortical pruning is part of the normal developmental process at this age, we predicted that both groups would show significantly reduced gray matter over time; however, sustained heavy drinkers would show a greater decline in gray matter volume compared to sustained light drinkers, especially in frontal and temporal brain regions.

MATERIALS AND METHODS

Participants

A cohort of first-year students (age range 18–23; mean 18.5 years) was recruited from two local colleges with diverse populations through e-mail, flyers and classroom visits to solicit participation in the Brain and Alcohol Research in College Students (BARCS) study (Ahmadi et al., 2013; Dager et al., 2014; Worhunsky et al., 2016; Meda et al., 2017). The recruitment captured greater than 95% of possible participants. All subjects provided written informed consent to participate in the study. The study was conducted in accordance with the declaration of Helsinki and was approved by institutional review boards at Central Connecticut State University (CCSU), University of Connecticut, Trinity College, Hartford Hospital, and Yale University.

A representative sub-sample of 200 individuals, all free from MRI contraindications, underwent a neuroimaging battery including structural imaging scans at baseline and follow up (24 months apart on average). Participants were divided into two groups at both baseline and 24-month follow-up based on drinking quantity and frequency (also see below section), similar to definitions used in previous studies (Dager et al., 2014; Worhunsky et al., 2016). Heavy drinking was defined as binge drinking ($\geq$4 drinks/occasion for females, $\geq$5 drinks/occasion for males) $\geq$13 of the past 26 weeks, or meeting criteria for alcohol abuse. Light drinking included teetotalers or binge drinking $<$13 of the previous 26 weeks and never meeting criteria for alcohol abuse. The final sample included 139 participants: (i) 55 light drinkers who either abstained or sparingly drank at baseline and follow-up and (ii) 84 heavy drinkers, who drank heavily at baseline and follow-up (Please see **Table 1**). The rest of the participants were excluded from the study due to one of the following reasons (a) not scanned at one of the two time points, (b) scans did not pass quality control at one or both time points (for e.g., excessive motion, bad scan quality, other artifacts etc.) and (c) could not be categorized into one of the above drinking categories at one or both time points and (d) had valid scans at both time points but were neither sustained abstainer/light or heavy drinkers.

Exclusion criteria included current schizophrenia or bipolar disorder, history of seizures or significant head injury, not meeting our criteria for drinking groups (described in the assessments section below), and excessive motion (visual evaluation by imaging expert SAM) during scanning.

Assessments

At both baseline and follow-up, past 6-month alcohol use and abuse diagnosis was assessed using an in-house interview incorporating items from the Semi-Structured Assessment for the Genetics of Alcoholism (SSAGA; Bucholz et al., 1994) and the alcohol use module from the Structured Clinical Interview for the DSM-IV (SCID; First et al., 1994). In addition at baseline, we collected a variety of variables related to psychiatric status and family history of alcoholism (FHA). Students were administered a select section of the Barkley Adult ADHD Rating Scale–IV (BAARS-IV) to assess ADHD symptoms (Barkley et al., 2011). Students were asked to self-report whether they had ever been formally diagnosed with ADHD and whether they were currently receiving treatment for the same. We coded individuals as having a history of ADHD if they responded "yes" to both questions. All participants also received the M.I.N.I. structured psychiatric diagnostic assessment (Sheehan et al., 1998) (https://medical-outcomes.com/). We found three prevalent diagnoses including major depressive disorder (MDD), agoraphobia and panic disorder among our college sample, which were binary coded (yes/no) and used for further analyses. FHA was assessed using the Family History Assessment Module (FHAM) (Rice et al., 1995). Students completed the trait sections of the State Trait Anxiety Index (STAI) questionnaire (Spielberger et al., 1983). A total STAI sum score was calculated, normed based on gender and was used for further analysis. Students were also administered the Beck Depression Inventory (BDI) to assess depressive symptoms at study entry (Beck et al., 1961); all items from the inventory were summed to yield a total score. At each scan time point, participants provided urine toxicology samples for negative screening of commonly abused substances, negative alcohol breathalyzer screens, and negative urine pregnancy screens (females).

Image Acquisition and Processing

Magnetic resonance structural brain images were collected on a Siemens Allegra 3T system (Siemens AG, Erlangen, Germany) located at the Olin Neuropsychiatric Research Center in Hartford, CT. Images were collected using a sagittal T1 MPRAGE sequence with the following parameters TR/TE/TI = 2,300/2.74/900 ms, flip angle = 8°, slab thickness = 176 mm, FOV = 176 × 256 mm, matrix = 176 × 256 × 176, voxel size = 1 mm^3, pixel band-width = 190 Hz, scan time = 10:09.

Computation of Longitudinal Gray Matter Volume (GMV) Change

In order to compute gray matter volume change maps, structural images from each time point were subjected to a technique called symmetric diffeomorphic modeling of longitudinal data, implemented in SPM12 (Ashburner and Ridgway, 2012). The following steps were implemented to derive the volumetric rate of change maps for each subject (1) a mid-point image was estimated by optimally mapping the template with each time point image by means of a groupwise-consistent 3D non-linear image registration technique. A Jacobian difference image was then estimated that records the difference for deformation from the mid-point image to the first scan and this to the second scan. This Jacobian difference map was further divided by the time elapsed between the two scans to derive a rate of change map. (2) the mid-point image was then segmented into their respective GM, WM, and CSF constituents. (3) GM images from step (2) were used to create a study-specific template using DARTEL. (4) The Jacobian rate of difference images from step (1) were multiplied by the GM image from step (2) to derive a GMV rate of change map (GMV-c). (5) The images from step (4) were normalized to MNI space and smoothed with a 6 mm FWHM Gaussian kernel. (6) Images derived from step (5) were then subjected to further statistical analyses as described below.

Statistical Analyses

Continuous demographic variables were compared between groups using an independent sample *t*-test in SPSS v21 (https://www.ibm.com/analytics/us/en/technology/spss/). Categorical variables were examined with a chi-square analysis using the same software.

The GMV-c maps were subjected to a 1-sample *t*-test in SPM12 (separately for light and heavy drinkers) to detect significant within-group decreases or expansions over the 2-year follow-up period on a voxel-by-voxel basis across the whole brain. Further, we carried out a 2-sample *t*-test (adjusted for sex) within the general linear model framework to assess GMV-c differences across light and heavy drinking groups (group by time interaction). Given that alcohol may influence brain changes differentially by sex (Squeglia et al., 2014) supplementary analyses were conducted to look for any possible group-by-sex or group-by-sex-by-time interactions. In addition to the above, to assess if groups differed in GMV at baseline, we conducted a follow-up 2-sample *t*-test adjusted for sex and total intracranial volume using only GMV calculated at the first time point. Although the major aim of the paper was to capture and report longitudinal changes, this explicit baseline analysis provides readers a better understanding of what volumetric changes already existed at baseline and how these brain structures change over time. All the above statistical analyses were conducted using permutation based analyses coupled with corrections for whole brain multiple

TABLE 1 | Demographics and clinical characteristics of drinking groups investigated in the study.

Subject demographics	Sustained light users (Total $N = 55$)		Sustained heavy users (Total $N = 84$)		Statistic	
	Mean	*SD*	Mean	*SD*	*t*	*p*-value
Age at Baseline (years)	18.38	0.59	18.48	0.81	0.16	NS
Baseline State-Trait Anxiety Inventory (STAI)	42.46 ($N = 41$)	10.12	54.42 ($N = 49$)	12.32	−0.78	NS
Baseline Beck Depression Inventory (BDI)	4.12 ($N = 41$)	6.27	5.22 (N =5 1)	5.56	−0.88	NS
Number of Monthly Drinks (Baseline)	2	5	48	48	−7.18	<0.001
Number of Monthly Drinks (Follow up)	3	5	40	42	−6.54	<0.001
Time Elapsed Between Scans (Months)	24.39	5.02	25.2	5.23	−0.90	NS
Baseline Clinical Characteristics	***N***		***N***		**Chi-square**	***p*-value**
GENDER						
Male	22		49		4.47	0.04
Female	33		35			
CIGARETTE SMOKER						
No	38		49		1.51	NS
Yes	3		1			
Missing	14		34			
FAMILY HISTORY FOR ALCOHOLISM						
Negative	28		34		0.03	NS
Positive	13		17			
Missing	14		33			
ADHD						
No	36		47		3.74	NS
Yes	3		0			
Missing	16		37			
MDD (MINI)						
No	54		78		1.97	NS
Yes	1		6			
AGORAPHOBIA (MINI)						
No	54		78		1.97	NS
Yes	1		6			
PANIC DISORDER (MINI)						
No	40		48		0.65	NS
Yes	1		3			
Missing	14		33			

comparisons using the threshold free cluster enhancement technique (TFCE) as implemented in the TFCE toolbox (http://dbm.neuro.uni-jena.de/tfce/). Resulting maps were thresholded at the $p < 0.05$ family wise error (FWE) whole brain corrected level and displayed using the NeuroElf toolbox (http://neuroelf.net/).

RESULTS

Groups did not differ by age, smoking, FHA or any MINI diagnostic status. Groups also had similar scores on the STAI and BDI. However, groups differed by sex (chi-square = 4.47; $p = 0.03$). Complete description of demographics and clinical characteristics of study participants are provided in **Table 1**.

Within-group analysis revealed significant GMV loss in both drinking groups over time (see **Figure 1**). No significant regional expansion of GMV over time was detected in either group. GMV decline in stable light users was mostly localized to inferior/middle temporal and fusiform gyrus. Gray matter decreases in individuals with sustained heavy alcohol use were lager in magnitude, and included the above regions plus several other brain regions including inferior/middle frontal gyrus (I/MFG), anterior cingulate, insula, thalamus, caudate, and parahippocampal gyri. Longitudinal GMV differences assessed across groups (see **Figure 2**) showed the heavy use group to have a significantly increased rate of gray matter decline, primarily in fronto-striatal regions, including inferior/medial frontal, anterior cingulate, parahippocampus, precentral gyrus,

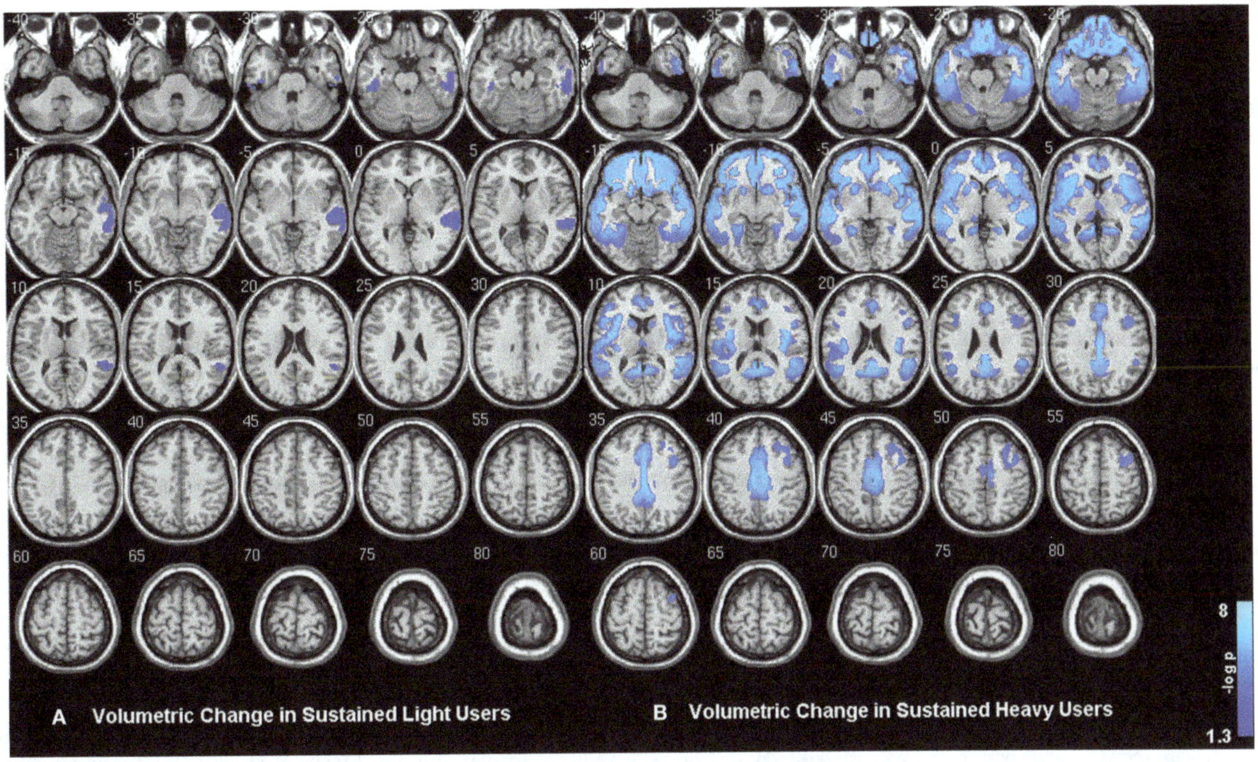

FIGURE 1 | (A) Gray matter volumetric change in sustained abstainers/light and **(B)** sustained heavy users across the two year period. Results are displayed at $p < 0.05$ FWE corrected across the whole brain. Images are on a negative log P scale. Note that both groups only showed significant decline and no expansions.

and insula. A complete description of within-group and between-group results is presented in **Tables 2A,B**. Further, we detected no group-by-sex or group-by-sex-by-time interactions at the whole brain level. Exploratory analysis of between-group baseline differences in GMV revealed significantly decreased GMV in the heavy drinking group in a subset of regions that also showed exaggerated decline across time. Overlap of regions was mainly localized to superior, medial and inferior frontal gyri after correction for multiple comparisons. Regions showing baseline differences are visually represented in **Figure 3**.

DISCUSSION

The present longitudinal study investigated gray matter volume changes over a 2 year period in emerging adult college students who were either sustained light-moderate drinkers or who had continued heavy alcohol use. Consistent with our initial hypotheses, we noted significant brain GMV loss in both groups. However, a direct two group comparison showed a significantly greater rate of loss in students with a sustained pattern of heavy alcohol use over 2 year follow-up. Moreover, this pattern of greater gray matter decline in heavy users occurred largely in regions responsible for emotion, memory, mental flexibility, and decision making, all of which might have a direct impact on student college success (Best et al., 2011).

It is important to recall that cortical pruning and restructuring reflects a normal, beneficial process during adolescence and young adulthood (Gogtay et al., 2004). Although the results noted in abstainers/light drinkers might closely reflect normal developmental processes, the exaggerated GMV-c due to continued heavy drinking would not be fully attributable to such cortical maturation. One possible interpretation could be that alcohol use leads to excess gray matter volume loss similar to that observed in adult alcoholics (Suzuki et al., 2010; Ersche et al., 2013; Sjoerds et al., 2013; Segobin et al., 2014; Droutman et al., 2015). The above hypothesis is supported by animal research that suggests alcohol interferes with neural stem cell proliferation leading to neurodegeneration and changes in brain structure and function (Morris et al., 2010). Animal reports have also shown marked differences in survival of cortical-cells in adolescent animals that were exposed to alcohol compared to controls (Crews et al., 2006; Hansson et al., 2010; Koss et al., 2012). Consistent with the above findings, changes observed in human macro-structural MRI studies such as ours may thus reflect tissue loss or remodeling related to inhibition of cell generation and survival. Preclinical studies also suggest that heavy alcohol intoxication might trigger microglia activation, oxidative stress, and pro-inflammatory changes which in turn leads to neurotoxic degeneration and/or prevents genesis of neurons and glia (Crews and Nixon, 2009; Alfonso-Loeches et al., 2012). Our results are also very consistent with a recent study

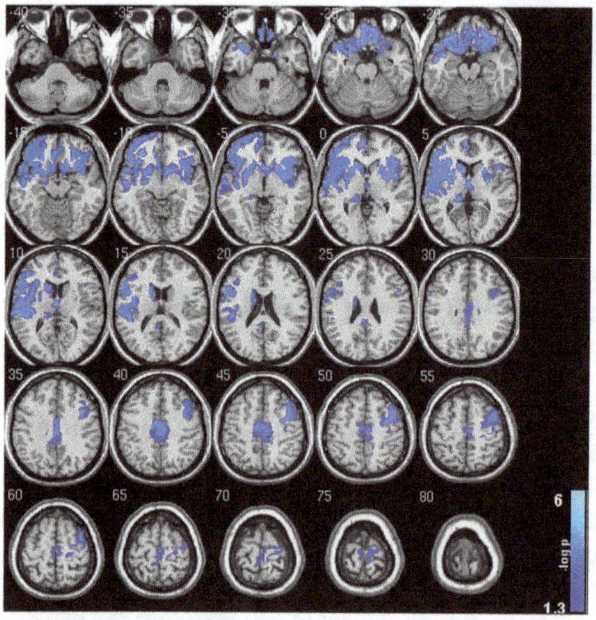

FIGURE 2 | Significant gray matter volumetric change between sustained abstainers/light and sustained heavy user groups across the 2 year period. Note the widespread accelerated GMV decreases in sustained heavy users of alcohol compared to their light user peers. Results are displayed at $p < 0.05$ FWE corrected across the whole brain. Images are on a negative log *P* scale.

that used region of interest based analysis to investigate similar longitudinal gray and white matter changes in adolescents before and after they initiated heavy alcohol use (Squeglia et al., 2015). That study observed a similar pattern of accelerated GMV-c in heavy alcohol initiators along with an attenuated growth of several white matter structures. The current study expands on these findings, demonstrating that continued heavy drinking in emerging adulthood leads to excessive gray matter loss in brain structures relevant to everyday functioning. Also, compared to the above study, we employed a voxel-wise whole brain analysis that should enable us to visualize GMV-c with greater spatial specificity.

Previous studies have shown that disruptions to adolescent brain maturation might adversely impact developmental cognitive and motor performance (Burgaleta et al., 2014). In the current study we noted both baseline decreases and accelerated GMV decline of the parahippocampal gyrus (a region primarily responsible for memory function) in the heavy drinking group, which is consistent with and expands results from cross-sectional reports showing reduced GMV in this medial temporal region for both individuals with alcohol dependence and those with family history of alcohol dependence (Suzuki et al., 2010; Sjoerds et al., 2013), The significant interaction of alcohol use on gray matter volume development as shown here might therefore help explain previous longitudinal studies showing worse attention, working memory, and visuospatial performance in adolescents after initiating alcohol use (Tapert et al., 2002; Hanson et al., 2011).

Interestingly, many of the significantly affected regions overlap with brain systems involved in reward, decision making, emotion and stress, that have been directly linked to addictive behavior (Schoenbaum and Shaham, 2008; Sinha, 2011; Droutman et al., 2015; O'Connor and Kenny, 2015; Silveri et al., 2016). Previous functional studies have shown increased activation to alcohol cues in medial frontal/ACC that underlie attention and motivation (Myrick et al., 2004; Dager et al., 2013). Altered interactions between ACC and parts of the striatum (also implicated in our current study) have shown to be related to motivational shift toward drug-induced cues, thus suggesting potential biological markers of addictive pathology (Myrick et al., 2004; Dager et al., 2013). Another key region identified in our study was inferior frontal gyrus (IFG), which functionally signals drug availability and triggers anticipation of use (Schoenbaum and Shaham, 2008). IFG over-reactivity has also been prospectively linked to escalating drinking in a previous study that used a subset of the current dataset (Worhunsky et al., 2016). It is interesting to note that our supplementary analyses show that some of these frontal differences existed at baseline and seemingly became worse over time. Insula, another region that showed exacerbated GMV loss in our heavy alcohol users, has been shown to play an important role in drug addiction (Droutman et al., 2015). Meta analyses of structural abnormalities in addicted individuals have described significantly reduced insular volume (Ersche et al., 2013). Functional studies have repeatedly observed blunted insular activity in substance-dependent individuals when engaged in decision-making tasks, and have also been shown to predict relapse (Sinha, 2011). The substantial overlap of excess gray matter loss with critical brain systems implicated in addiction might suggest that some of these differences may have been pre-existing. Compulsive drug taking due to poorly modulated decision making as a consequence of inability to learn from negative consequences is a hallmark of addiction. Baseline differences noted in our study were primarily limited to the pre-frontal cortex (PFC) which plays a key role in such decision making processes among other critical executive functions (George and Koob, 2010). Indeed, frontal lobe volumetric differences may be both a pre-existing risk factor as well as consequence of heavy alcohol use in adolescence (Silveri et al., 2016). It is also possible that such volumetric changes might contribute to differential neurochemical transmission sensitivity to alcohol that might in-turn enhance vulnerability to addictive-like behaviors into young adulthood. Given the longitudinal design here, our findings support the view that exacerbated gray matter loss is a consequence of continued heavy use. Although sustained heavy use might have an adverse impact on neurodevelopment, many studies in adolescent and adult alcoholics have demonstrated that certain brain structures and pathways show potential for recovery with alcohol abstinence or curtailment (Gazdzinski et al., 2005; Durazzo et al., 2011, 2016; Dresler et al., 2012; Segobin et al., 2014). Future longitudinal studies should determine the degree of volumetric recovery if drinking is reduced during earlier phases of brain development.

A number of additional factors in college including illicit substance use, stress levels, academic performance, peer pressure

TABLE 2 | Significant regions of GMV decreases for both **(A)** within- and **(B)** between-group analyses.

(Hemisphere) Region	Brodmann area	x	y	z	Max (−log p)	Cluster size (mm^3)
(A) WITHIN-GROUP RESULTS						
Sustained light users						
LH Fusiform Gyrus	20	−45	−30	−24	1.71	170
LH Inferior Temporal Gyrus	20	−60	−27	−30	1.33	10
RH Fusiform Gyrus	20	51	−27	−24	1.76	61
RH Inferior Temporal Gyrus	20	57	−30	−15	1.79	165
RH Middle Temporal Gyrus	21	54	−21	−6	2.13	827
Sustained heavy users						
LH Anterior Cingulate	32	0	39	6	3.70	76.41
LH Caudate	Caudate body	−12	15	9	3.10	45.36
LH Claustrum		−27	24	9	3.70	148.23
LH Fusiform Gyrus	20	−54	−21	−21	3.70	152.82
LH Fusiform Gyrus	37	−39	−45	−15	3.22	118.26
LH Inferior Frontal Gyrus	11	−18	36	−18	3.70	153.09
LH Insula	13	−36	0	15	3.70	99.36
LH Medial Frontal Gyrus	10	−3	54	0	3.70	116.91
LH Middle Frontal Gyrus	46	−36	27	21	1.84	14.58
LH Middle Frontal Gyrus	9	−33	12	30	1.57	11.88
LH Middle Occipital Gyrus	19	−45	−60	−6	2.18	63.45
LH Middle Temporal Gyrus	21	−45	−33	0	3.70	93.96
LH Middle Temporal Gyrus	37	−42	−63	6	1.71	14.85
LH Pyramis	–	−15	−63	−27	1.31	13.5
LH Superior Temporal Gyrus	38	−48	12	−9	3.70	68.04
LH Superior Temporal Gyrus	22	−48	−15	−9	3.70	69.39
LH Superior Temporal Gyrus	39	−42	−51	21	3.22	79.11
LH Superior Temporal Gyrus	41	−54	−30	9	2.49	44.82
LH Thalamus	–	−12	−33	3	1.79	12.69
LH Thalamus	Medial dorsal nucleus	0	−15	9	1.76	13.23
RH Anterior Cingulate	32	12	48	−9	3.70	118.8
RH Anterior Cingulate	25	3	18	−9	3.70	120.69
RH Cingulate Gyrus	24	12	−15	42	3.70	118.8
RH Cingulate Gyrus	31	6	−45	27	3.70	109.89
RH Cingulate Gyrus	32	3	21	36	3.70	57.78
RH Fusiform Gyrus	37	36	−39	−12	2.49	66.96
RH Inferior Frontal Gyrus	47	48	24	−3	3.70	199.8
RH Inferior Frontal Gyrus	45	42	18	9	3.70	88.56
RH Inferior Frontal Gyrus	44	51	12	18	3.10	27
RH Insula	13	42	−18	3	3.70	44.01
RH Medial Frontal Gyrus	25	9	6	−15	3.40	26.19
RH Medial Frontal Gyrus	9	3	33	30	3.40	44.01
RH Middle Frontal Gyrus	10	42	57	−9	3.70	129.87
RH Middle Frontal Gyrus	47	51	42	−6	3.40	44.01
RH Middle Frontal Gyrus	6	39	6	57	2.27	27.81
RH Middle Frontal Gyrus	8	30	24	48	2.22	29.7
RH Middle Frontal Gyrus	46	45	30	18	1.57	11.34
RH Middle Temporal Gyrus	22	69	−30	3	3.70	133.65
RH Middle Temporal Gyrus	21	66	−15	−3	3.70	150.39
RH Parahippocampal Gyrus	30	24	−51	6	3.10	20.52
RH Posterior Cingulate	31	9	−54	24	3.70	150.66
RH Posterior Cingulate	30	18	−54	18	3.22	26.19

(Continued)

TABLE 2 | Continued

(Hemisphere) Region	Brodmann area	x	y	z	Max (−log p)	Cluster size (mm^3)
RH Precentral Gyrus	6	48	−3	9	3.70	67.23
RH Precentral Gyrus	9	39	9	36	2.38	34.02
RH Superior Temporal Gyrus	22	60	3	−6	3.70	156.06
RH Superior Temporal Gyrus	13	51	−45	21	3.70	79.92
(B) BETWEEN-GROUP RESULTS						
LH Anterior Cingulate	24	0	36	6	1.47	8.37
LH Anterior Cingulate	32	−12	39	9	1.45	1.35
LH Caudate	Caudate head	−12	18	−9	3.70	109.35
LH Caudate	Caudate body	−15	12	18	3.70	28.62
LH Cingulate Gyrus	31	−6	−36	33	3.22	48.87
LH Claustrum	–	−27	24	9	3.70	74.52
LH Inferior Frontal Gyrus	11	−18	36	−18	3.70	60.21
LH Inferior Frontal Gyrus	46	−39	39	6	3.70	98.55
LH Inferior Frontal Gyrus	9	−42	9	21	3.70	66.15
LH Insula	13	−39	0	−6	3.70	262.44
LH Lentiform Nucleus	Putamen	−27	−15	3	3.70	18.63
LH Medial Frontal Gyrus	11	0	36	−12	3.70	76.95
LH Medial Frontal Gyrus	10	−3	57	6	3.70	29.16
LH Medial Frontal Gyrus	6	−3	−21	63	2.27	18.63
LH Middle Frontal Gyrus	9	−33	12	30	2.09	1.35
LH Paracentral Lobule	5	−3	−33	57	1.67	6.48
LH Parahippocampal Gyrus	30	−12	−36	6	3.70	26.19
LH Parahippocampal Gyrus	34	−15	−12	−15	3.10	7.56
LH Posterior Cingulate	29	−6	−45	18	3.10	7.83
LH Precuneus	31	−12	−51	27	1.54	1.35
LH Superior Frontal Gyrus	10	−12	69	−6	3.70	33.75
LH Superior Frontal Gyrus	11	−18	48	−15	3.70	38.34
LH Superior Temporal Gyrus	38	−48	12	−9	3.70	43.74
LH Transverse Temporal Gyrus	41	−33	−27	9	3.70	14.31
RH Anterior Cingulate	25	6	18	−3	3.70	39.96
RH Anterior Cingulate	24	3	24	18	1.33	1.08
RH Caudate	Caudate head	18	24	0	3.70	50.22
RH Inferior Frontal Gyrus	47	48	24	−3	3.70	71.01
RH Inferior Frontal Gyrus	13	45	21	6	3.70	26.19
RH Inferior Frontal Gyrus	46	51	45	0	2.09	2.97
RH Inferior Frontal Gyrus	9	51	12	24	1.52	3.51
RH Insula	13	45	6	0	3.70	76.14
RH Medial Frontal Gyrus	6	9	−18	51	3.70	233.28
RH Medial Frontal Gyrus	11	3	57	−18	2.09	2.43
RH Middle Frontal Gyrus	8	39	21	45	3.70	52.65
RH Middle Frontal Gyrus	11	30	39	−9	3.70	75.87
RH Precentral Gyrus	6	36	−9	63	3.22	34.29
RH Precentral Gyrus	4	36	−15	51	2.10	33.21
RH Superior Temporal Gyrus	22	45	−6	−3	3.70	27
RH Thalamus	–	3	−6	6	3.70	39.69

and psychiatric status could have an interactive effect with alcohol consumption (Meda et al., 2017). Although the concurrent use of other commonly abused substances such as marijuana were not analyzed here (due to excessive missing rate ~40%), prior studies that performed similar analyses to ours noted no significant interactions between alcohol and drug use with gray matter loss patterns (Squeglia et al., 2014). We measured personality and psychiatric metrics such as the STAI, BDI, MDD, and ADHD and found them to be balanced across our diagnostic groups. Also, cigarette

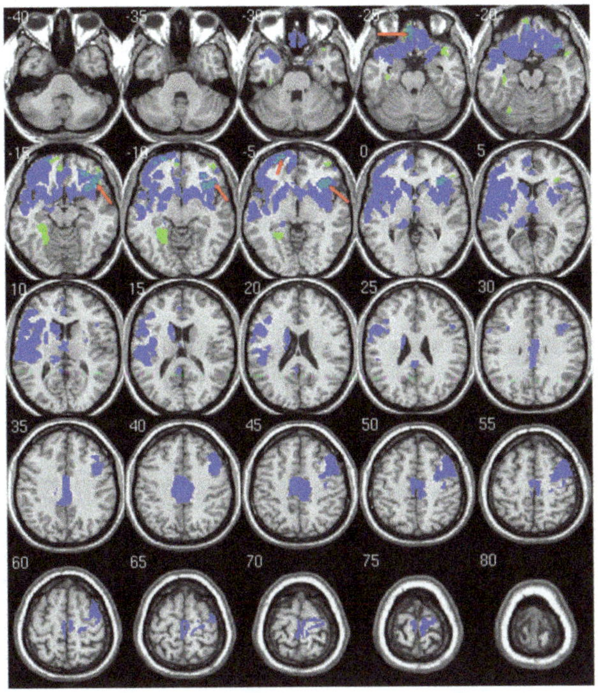

FIGURE 3 | Overlap of significant between-group differences at baseline and longitudinal follow up. Regions marked in green show lower GMV in heavy drinking group compared to abstainers/light at baseline. Regions in blue are the same longitudinal results as shown in **Figure 2**. Overlap between baseline and longitudinal differences are shown in light blue (red arrows). Results are displayed at $p < 0.05$ FWE corrected across the whole brain. Images are on a negative log P scale.

smoking, which is often co-morbid with alcohol use and has been associated with gray matter changes (Franklin et al., 2014) was not significantly different between our groups. The proportions of smokers/non-smokers in our sample can be seen in **Table 1**. Given that previous cross-sectional studies have suggested differential alcohol effects exerted across sexes (Squeglia et al., 2014, 2015), we looked at potential group by sex and group by sex by time interactions in our dataset, but found none.

Despite its current strengths, our study had several limitations to consider. We did not have sufficient numbers of individuals who transitioned from heavy to light or light to heavy alcohol use, and were therefore unable to examine gray matter changes associated with other trajectories of alcohol use that are of great interest. We also did not capture longitudinal behavioral data that might help better understand relationships between GMV-c and cognitive functioning, which might be a good avenue for future studies. There may be other important interacting variables, such as stress levels, personality factors, or other substance use, which were not examined here but would be critical areas for future inquiries. We did not scan participants before the onset of drinking, making it difficult to determine whether gray matter volume differences were pre-existing; future studies such as the ongoing ABCD project will help delineate patterns of gray matter development in relation to varying patterns of substance use initiation and escalation.

CONCLUSION

In summary, our study provides important longitudinal evidence regarding excessive gray matter loss in regions related to cognitive control, emotional regulation, and memory that might have both short and long-term implications on student life success. Importantly, regions of abnormal gray matter decline overlapped with those implicated previously in substance abuse, thus providing more evidence toward the theory that initiation and continued alcohol use during young adulthood might confer vulnerability for future, ongoing substance dependence.

AUTHOR CONTRIBUTIONS

SM and AD contributed to design, analysis, and drafting of the manuscript. KH, HT, SR, RW, CA, CF, and GP contributed to the study funding, design, and drafting of the manuscript.

ACKNOWLEDGMENTS

This research was made possible by grant support from the National Institute on Alcohol Abuse and Alcoholism (AA016599 and AA19036, Pearlson).

REFERENCES

Ahmadi, A., Pearlson, G. D., Meda, S. A., Dager, A., Potenza, M. N., Rosen, R., et al. (2013). Influence of alcohol use on neural response to Go/No-Go task in college drinkers. *Neuropsychopharmacology* 38, 2197–2208. doi: 10.1038/npp.2013.119

Alfonso-Loeches, S., Pascual, M., Gomez-Pinedo, U., Pascual-Lucas, M., Renau-Piqueras, J., and Guerri, C. (2012). Toll-like receptor 4 participates in the myelin disruptions associated with chronic alcohol abuse. *Glia* 60, 948–964. doi: 10.1002/glia.22327

Arnett, J. J. (2000). Emerging adulthood. A theory of development from the late teens through the twenties. *Am. Psychol.* 55, 469–480. doi: 10.1037/0003-066X.55.5.469

Ashburner, J., and Ridgway, G. R. (2012). Symmetric diffeomorphic modeling of longitudinal structural MRI. *Front. Neurosci.* 6:197. doi: 10.3389/fnins.2012.00197

Barkley, R. A., Knouse, L. E., and Murphy, K. R. (2011). Correspondence and disparity in the self- and other ratings of current and childhood ADHD symptoms and impairment in adults with ADHD. *Psychol. Assess.* 23, 437–446. doi: 10.1037/a0022172

Beck, A. T., Ward, C. H., Mendelson, M., Mock, J., and Erbaugh, J. (1961). An inventory for measuring depression. *Arch. Gen. Psychiatry* 4, 561–571. doi: 10.1001/archpsyc.1961.01710120031004

Bennett, C. M., and Baird, A. A. (2006). Anatomical changes in the emerging adult brain: a voxel-based morphometry study. *Hum. Brain Mapp.* 27, 766–777. doi: 10.1002/hbm.20218

Best, J. R., Miller, P. H., and Naglieri, J. A. (2011). Relations between executive function and academic achievement from ages 5 to 17 in a large, representative national sample. *Learn. Individ. Differ.* 21, 327–336. doi: 10.1016/j.lindif.2011.01.007

Bucholz, K. K., Cadoret, R., Cloninger, C. R., Dinwiddie, S. H., Hesselbrock, V. M., Nurnberger, J. I. Jr., et al. (1994). A new, semi-structured psychiatric interview for use in genetic linkage studies: a report on the reliability of the SSAGA. *J. Stud. Alcohol* 55, 149–158. doi: 10.15288/jsa.1994.55.149

Burgaleta, M., Johnson, W., Waber, D. P., Colom, R., and Karama, S. (2014). Cognitive ability changes and dynamics of cortical thickness development in healthy children and adolescents. *Neuroimage* 84, 810–819. doi: 10.1016/j.neuroimage.2013.09.038

Casey, B. J., Giedd, J. N., and Thomas, K. M. (2000). Structural and functional brain development and its relation to cognitive development. *Biol. Psychol.* 54, 241–257. doi: 10.1016/S0301-0511(00)00058-2

Crews, F. T., and Nixon, K. (2009). Mechanisms of neurodegeneration and regeneration in alcoholism. *Alcohol Alcohol.* 44, 115–127. doi: 10.1093/alcalc/agn079

Crews, F. T., Mdzinarishvili, A., Kim, D., He, J., and Nixon, K. (2006). Neurogenesis in adolescent brain is potently inhibited by ethanol. *Neuroscience* 137, 437–445. doi: 10.1016/j.neuroscience.2005.08.090

Dager, A. D., Anderson, B. M., Rosen, R., Khadka, S., Sawyer, B., Jiantonio-Kelly, R. E., et al. (2014). Functional magnetic resonance imaging (fMRI) response to alcohol pictures predicts subsequent transition to heavy drinking in college students. *Addiction* 109, 585–595. doi: 10.1111/add.12437

Dager, A. D., Anderson, B. M., Stevens, M. C., Pulido, C., Rosen, R., Jiantonio-Kelly, R. E., et al. (2013). Influence of alcohol use and family history of alcoholism on neural response to alcohol cues in college drinkers. *Alcohol. Clin. Exp. Res.* 37(Suppl. 1), E161–E171. doi: 10.1111/j.1530-0277.2012.01879.x

De Bellis, M. D., Narasimhan, A., Thatcher, D. L., Keshavan, M. S., Soloff, P., and Clark, D. B. (2005). Prefrontal cortex, thalamus, and cerebellar volumes in adolescents and young adults with adolescent-onset alcohol use disorders and comorbid mental disorders. *Alcohol. Clin. Exp. Res.* 29, 1590–1600. doi: 10.1097/01.alc.0000179368.87886.76

Dresler, T., Schecklmann, M., Ernst, L. H., Pohla, C., Warrings, B., Fischer, M., et al. (2012). Recovery of cortical functioning in abstinent alcohol-dependent patients: prefrontal brain oxygenation during verbal fluency at different phases during withdrawal. *World J. Biol. Psychiatry* 13, 135–145. doi: 10.3109/15622975.2011.564654

Droutman, V., Read, S. J., and Bechara, A. (2015). Revisiting the role of the insula in addiction. *Trends Cogn. Sci.* 19, 414–420. doi: 10.1016/j.tics.2015.05.005

Durazzo, T. C., Mon, A., Gazdzinski, S., and Meyerhoff, D. J., (2016). Regional brain volume changes in alcohol-dependent individuals during early abstinence: associations with relapse following treatment. *Addict Biol.* 22, 1416–1425. doi: 10.1111/adb.12420

Durazzo, T. C., Tosun, D., Buckley, S., Gazdzinski, S., Mon, A., Fryer, S. L., et al. (2011). Cortical thickness, surface area, and volume of the brain reward system in alcohol dependence: relationships to relapse and extended abstinence. *Alcohol. Clin. Exp. Res.* 35, 1187–1200. doi: 10.1111/j.1530-0277.2011.01452.x

Ersche, K. D., Williams, G. B., Robbins, T. W., and Bullmore, E. T. (2013). Meta-analysis of structural brain abnormalities associated with stimulant drug dependence and neuroimaging of addiction vulnerability and resilience. *Curr. Opin. Neurobiol.* 23, 615–624. doi: 10.1016/j.conb.2013.02.017

Fein, G., Greenstein, D., Cardenas, V. A., Cuzen, N. L., Fouche, J. P., Ferrett, H., et al. (2013). Cortical and subcortical volumes in adolescents with alcohol dependence but without substance or psychiatric comorbidities. *Psychiatry Res.* 214, 1–8. doi: 10.1016/j.pscychresns.2013.06.001

First, M. B., Frances, A. J., Pincus, H. A., Vettorello, N., and Davis, W. W. (1994). DSM-IV in progress. Changes in substance-related, schizophrenic, and other primarily adult disorders. *Hosp. Community Psychiatry* 45, 18–20.

Franklin, T. R., Wetherill, R. R., Jagannathan, K., Johnson, B., Mumma, J., Hager, N., et al. (2014). The effects of chronic cigarette smoking on gray matter volume: influence of sex. *PLoS ONE* 9:e104102. doi: 10.1371/journal.pone.0104102

Gazdzinski, S., Durazzo, T. C., and Meyerhoff, D. J., (2005). Temporal dynamics and determinants of whole brain tissue volume changes during recovery from alcohol dependence. *Drug Alcohol Depend.* 78, 263–273. doi: 10.1016/j.drugalcdep.2004.11.004

George, O., and Koob, G. F. (2010). Individual differences in prefrontal cortex function and the transition from drug use to drug dependence. *Neurosci. Biobehav. Rev.* 35, 232–247. doi: 10.1016/j.neubiorev.2010.05.002

Gogtay, N., Giedd, J. N., Lusk, L., Hayashi, K. M., Greenstein, D., Vaituzis, A. C., et al. (2004). Dynamic mapping of human cortical development during childhood through early adulthood. *Proc. Natl. Acad. Sci. U.S.A.* 101, 8174–8179. doi: 10.1073/pnas.0402680101

Hanson, K. L., Medina, K. L., Padula, C. B., Tapert, S. F., and Brown, S. A. (2011). Impact of adolescent alcohol and drug use on neuropsychological functioning in young adulthood: 10-year outcomes. *J. Child Adolesc. Subst. Abuse* 20, 135–154. doi: 10.1080/1067828X.2011.555272

Hansson, A. C., Nixon, K., Rimondini, R., Damadzic, R., Sommer, W. H., Eskay, R., et al. (2010). Long-term suppression of forebrain neurogenesis and loss of neuronal progenitor cells following prolonged alcohol dependence in rats. *Int. J. Neuropsychopharmacol.* 13, 583–593. doi: 10.1017/S1461145710000246

Heikkinen, N., Niskanen, E., Kononen, M., Tolmunen, T., Kekkonen, V., Kivimaki, P., et al. (2017). Alcohol consumption during adolescence is associated with reduced grey matter volumes. *Addiction* 112, 604–613. doi: 10.1111/add.13697

Jacobus, J., McQueeny, T., Bava, S., Schweinsburg, B. C., Frank, L. R., Yang, T. T., et al. (2009). White matter integrity in adolescents with histories of marijuana use and binge drinking. *Neurotoxicol. Teratol.* 31, 349–355. doi: 10.1016/j.ntt.2009.07.006

Jacobus, J., Squeglia, L. M., Bava, S., and Tapert, S. F. (2013). White matter characterization of adolescent binge drinking with and without co-occurring marijuana use: a 3-year investigation. *Psychiatry Res.* 214, 374–381. doi: 10.1016/j.pscychresns.2013.07.014

Koss, W. A., Sadowski, R. N., Sherrill, L. K., Gulley, J. M., and Juraska, J. M. (2012). Effects of ethanol during adolescence on the number of neurons and glia in the medial prefrontal cortex and basolateral amygdala of adult male and female rats. *Brain Res.* 1466, 24–32. doi: 10.1016/j.brainres.2012.05.023

Luciana, M., Collins, P. F., Muetzel, R. L., and Lim, K. O. (2013). Effects of alcohol use initiation on brain structure in typically developing adolescents. *Am. J. Drug Alcohol Abuse* 39, 345–355. doi: 10.3109/00952990.2013.837057

McQueeny, T., Schweinsburg, B. C., Schweinsburg, A. D., Jacobus, J., Bava, S., Frank, L. R., et al. (2009). Altered white matter integrity in adolescent binge drinkers. *Alcohol. Clin. Exp. Res.* 33, 1278–1285. doi: 10.1111/j.1530-0277.2009.00953.x

Meda, S. A., Gueorguieva, R. V., Pittman, B., Rosen, R. R., Aslanzadeh, F., Tennen, H., et al. (2017). Longitudinal influence of alcohol and marijuana use on academic performance in college students. *PLoS ONE* 12:e0172213. doi: 10.1371/journal.pone.0172213

Medina, K. L., McQueeny, T., Nagel, B. J., Hanson, K. L., Schweinsburg, A. D., and Tapert, S. F. (2008). Prefrontal cortex volumes in adolescents with alcohol use disorders: unique gender effects. *Alcohol. Clin. Exp. Res.* 32, 386–394. doi: 10.1111/j.1530-0277.2007.00602.x

Morris, S. A., Eaves, D. W., Smith, A. R., and Nixon, K. (2010). Alcohol inhibition of neurogenesis: a mechanism of hippocampal neurodegeneration in an adolescent alcohol abuse model. *Hippocampus* 20, 596–607. doi: 10.1002/hipo.20665

Myrick, H., Anton, R. F., Li, X., Henderson, S., Drobes, D., Voronin, K., et al. (2004). Differential brain activity in alcoholics and social drinkers to alcohol cues: relationship to craving. *Neuropsychopharmacology* 29, 393–402. doi: 10.1038/sj.npp.1300295

O'Connor, R. M., and Kenny, P. J. (2015). Neuroscience: binge drinking and brain stress systems. *Nature* 520, 168–169. doi: 10.1038/520168a

Rice, J. P., Reich, T., Bucholz, K. K., Neuman, R. J., Fishman, R., Rochberg, N., et al. (1995). Comparison of direct interview and family history diagnoses of alcohol dependence. *Alcohol. Clin. Exp. Res.* 19, 1018–1023. doi: 10.1111/j.1530-0277.1995.tb00983.x

SAMHSA (2016). *Key Substance Use and Mental Health Indicators in the United States: Results from the 2015 National Survey on Drug Use and Health (No. HHS*

Publication No. SMA 16-4984). Rockville, MD: Center for Behavioral Health Statistics and Quality.

Schoenbaum, G., and Shaham, Y. (2008). The role of orbitofrontal cortex in drug addiction: a review of preclinical studies. *Biol. Psychiatry* 63, 256–262. doi: 10.1016/j.biopsych.2007.06.003

Segobin, S. H., Chetelat, G., Le Berre, A. P., Lannuzel, C., Boudehent, C., Vabret, F., et al. (2014). Relationship between brain volumetric changes and interim drinking at six months in alcohol-dependent patients. *Alcohol. Clin. Exp. Res.* 38, 739–748. doi: 10.1111/acer.12300

Sheehan, D. V., Lecrubier, Y., Sheehan, K. H., Amorim, P., Janavs, J., Weiller, E., et al. (1998). The Mini-International Neuropsychiatric Interview (M.I.N.I.): the development and validation of a structured diagnostic psychiatric interview for DSM-IV and ICD-10. *J. Clin. Psychiatry* 59(Suppl. 20), 22–33.

Silveri, M. M., Dager, A. D., Cohen-Gilbert, J. E., and Sneider, J. T. (2016). Neurobiological signatures associated with alcohol and drug use in the human adolescent brain. *Neurosci. Biobehav. Rev.* 70, 244–259. doi: 10.1016/j.neubiorev.2016.06.042

Sinha, R. (2011). New findings on biological factors predicting addiction relapse vulnerability. *Curr. Psychiatry Rep.* 13, 398–405. doi: 10.1007/s11920-011-0224-0

Sjoerds, Z., Van Tol, M. J., Van den Brink, W., Van der Wee, N. J., Van Buchem, M. A., Aleman, A., et al. (2013). Family history of alcohol dependence and gray matter abnormalities in non-alcoholic adults. *World J. Biol. Psychiatry* 14, 565–573. doi: 10.3109/15622975.2011.640942

Spielberger, C. D., Gorssuch, R. L., Lushene, P. R., Vagg, P. R., and Jacobs, G. A. (1983). *Manual for the State-Trait Anxiety Inventory*. Palo Alto, CA: Consulting Psychologists Press, Inc.

Squeglia, L. M., Rinker, D. A., Bartsch, H., Castro, N., Chung, Y., Dale, A. M., et al. (2014). Brain volume reductions in adolescent heavy drinkers. *Dev. Cogn. Neurosci.* 9, 117–125. doi: 10.1016/j.dcn.2014.02.005

Squeglia, L. M., Tapert, S. F., Sullivan, E. V., Jacobus, J., Meloy, M. J., Rohlfing, T., et al. (2015). Brain development in heavy-drinking adolescents. *Am. J. Psychiatry* 172, 531–542. doi: 10.1176/appi.ajp.2015.14101249

Suzuki, Y., Oishi, M., Ogawa, K., and Mizutani, T. (2010). Atrophy of the parahippocampal gyrus and regional cerebral blood flow in the limbic system in chronic alcoholic patients. *Alcohol* 44, 439–445. doi: 10.1016/j.alcohol.2010.05.003

Tapert, S. F., Granholm, E., Leedy, N. G., and Brown, S. A. (2002). Substance use and withdrawal: neuropsychological functioning over 8 years in youth. *J. Int. Neuropsychol. Soc.* 8, 873–883. doi: 10.1017/S1355617702870011

Whelan, R., Watts, R., Orr, C. A., Althoff, R. R., Artiges, E., Banaschewski, T., et al. (2014). Neuropsychosocial profiles of current and future adolescent alcohol misusers. *Nature* 512, 185–189. doi: 10.1038/nature13402

Worhunsky, P. D., Dager, A. D., Meda, S. A., Khadka, S., Stevens, M. C., Austad, C. S., et al. (2016). A preliminary prospective study of an escalation in 'maximum daily drinks', fronto-parietal circuitry and impulsivity-related domains in young adult drinkers. *Neuropsychopharmacology* 41, 1637–1647. doi: 10.1038/npp.2015.332

3

Psychiatric Diagnoses Differ Considerably in their Associations with Alcohol/Drug-Related Problems Among Adolescents

Ove Heradstveit[1,2], Jens Christoffer Skogen[1,3], Jørn Hetland[4], Robert Stewart[5,6] and Mari Hysing[2,4]*

[1] Center for Alcohol and Drug Research, Stavanger University Hospital, Stavanger, Norway, [2] Regional Centre for Child and Youth Mental Health and Child Welfare, Norwegian Research Centre, Bergen, Norway, [3] Department of Health Promotion, Norwegian Institute of Public Health, Bergen, Norway, [4] Department of Psychosocial Science, Faculty of Psychology, University of Bergen, Bergen, Norway, [5] Institute of Psychiatry, Psychology and Neuroscience, King's College London, London, United Kingdom, [6] South London and Maudsley NHS Foundation Trust, London, United Kingdom

Edited by:
Danny Horesh,
Bar-Ilan University, Israel

Reviewed by:
Sherry Stewart,
Dalhousie University, Canada
Ahmad Hatim Sulaiman,
University of Malaya, Malaysia

***Correspondence:**
Ove Heradstveit
ovhe@norceresarch.no

The aim of this study was to examine alcohol/drug use and problems across psychiatric diagnoses and to what extent associations between each psychiatric diagnosis and alcohol/drug use and problems were independent from the potential confounding effects of psychiatric comorbidity, socioeconomic status, sex and age. We used a dataset comprising a linkage between a large population-based and cross-sectional study among Norwegian adolescents (the youth@hordaland conducted in 2012) and national registry-based data on specialist mental health care use during the 4 years prior to the survey (2008 to 2011). The study sample included 16 to 19 year olds who participated in the youth@hordaland survey and consented to the linkage with patient registry data (n = 9,408). Among these, 853 (9%) had received specialist mental health care and comprised the clinical group, while the rest (n = 8,555) comprised the comparison group. The main outcome variables were several self-reported indicators for alcohol/drug use, including any alcohol use, frequent alcohol intoxication, high-level alcohol consumption, and lifetime illicit drug use, as well as one indicator for potential alcohol/drug-related problems: a positive CRAFFT-score. Adolescents receiving specialist mental health care (n = 853) reported more frequently alcohol/drug use and problems compared to adolescents not receiving these services (Cohens d's ranging from 0.09 to 0.29, all $p \leq 0.01$). Anxiety, depression, conduct disorders, eating disorders, ADHD, and trauma-related disorders were all associated with single measures of alcohol/drug use and problems, with odds ratios (ORs) ranging from 1.58 to 4.63, all $p < 0.05$) in unadjusted models. Trauma-related disorders, depression and conduct disorders were also positively associated with higher scores on a combined indicator of alcohol/drug use and problems (ORs ranging from 1.89 to 3.15, all $p < 0.01$), even after the full adjustment from psychiatric comorbidity and sociodemographic variables (adjusted odds ratios ranging from 1.61 to 2.79, $p < 0.05$). These results suggest that alcohol/drug use and problems were slightly more common among adolescents who received specialist mental health care during the past 4 years compared with the general adolescent population, and adolescents with trauma-related disorders, depression and conduct disorders were high-risk groups for alcohol/drug use and problems.

Keywords: alcohol use, illicit drug use, alcohol/drug-related problems, mental health problems, psychiatric diagnoses, adolescence, registry-based data, population-based sample

INTRODUCTION

Mental health problems are prevalent among children and adolescents, with one in five fulfilling criteria for a psychiatric diagnosis (Canino et al., 2004; Belfer, 2008; Merikangas et al., 2010; Barkmann and Schulte-Markwort, 2012). Approximately, 25% of adolescents with a psychiatric diagnosis have at least one additional psychiatric diagnosis (Costello et al., 2003), indicating that psychiatric comorbidity is common. Psychiatric diagnoses are particularly frequent among adolescents with alcohol/drug-related problems, and it is estimated that 37–80% of adolescents with alcohol/drug-related problems have at least one psychiatric diagnosis (e.g., Regier et al., 1990; Rohde et al., 1996; Armstrong and Costello, 2002). Similarly, among adolescents within a psychiatric inpatient setting, one third of the adolescents fulfilled criteria for a substance use disorder (SUD) (Deas-Nesmith et al., 1998).

Previous studies have demonstrated positive associations between a range of psychiatric diagnoses and adolescent alcohol/drug-related problems. Specifically, these findings include anxiety (Kedzior and Laeber, 2014; Stapinski et al., 2016), attention-deficit/hyperactivity disorder (ADHD) (Groenman et al., 2013; Zulauf et al., 2014), eating disorders (Castro-Fornieles et al., 2009; Bisetto et al., 2011), post-traumatic stress disorder (PTSD) (Wolitzky-Taylor et al., 2012; Haller and Chassin, 2014), conduct disorders (Khoddam et al., 2016), depression (Wolitzky-Taylor et al., 2012; Heron et al., 2013; Edlund et al., 2015), and psychotic disorders (Ferdinand et al., 2005; Addington and Addington, 2007). The majority of previous literature has focused on selected associations between single psychiatric diagnoses and symptoms and alcohol/drug-related problems, and few studies have investigated the full range of common psychiatric diagnoses in a single model.

A notable exception is a recent Norwegian study which reported that illicit drug use was four times higher among adolescents receiving psychiatric services compared to the general population (Mangerud et al., 2014). They also reported that depression was the diagnosis associated with the highest frequencies of alcohol and drug use and autism with the lowest; however, participation in the clinical group was low and psychiatric comorbidity was not investigated. Similarly, a study by Wu et al. (2011) investigated associations between a range of psychiatric diagnoses and SUDs. They reported positive associations with SUDs for mood disorders, ADHD, and conduct disorders, while the role of psychiatric comorbidity was not investigated. A study by Boys et al. (2003) on a broad range of psychiatric diagnoses in relation to alcohol/drug-related problems, reported that there was an increased risk of substance use among those with a psychiatric disorder. However, small numbers did not allow differentiation between separate disorders. In sum, there is still limited knowledge on which psychiatric diagnoses are associated with the highest risk for alcohol/drug use and problems among adolescents.

It is also important to consider psychiatric comorbidity in order to clarify whether specificity of risk is indicative of potentially unique psychological mechanisms, or whether "general mental distress" is primarily driving an increased vulnerability for alcohol/drug-related problems. Although some studies have adjusted for psychiatric comorbidity in associations between single psychiatric diagnoses and selected comorbid psychiatric diagnoses (August et al., 2006; Maslowsky and Schulenberg, 2013), the inclusion of psychiatric comorbidity is overall rare. To our knowledge, no previous studies have analyzed associations between a broad range of psychiatric diagnoses and alcohol/drug use and problems among adolescents, while also attempting to adjust these associations from the potential confounding effects of comorbid psychiatric diagnoses. In addition, socioeconomic status (SES), age and gender have been shown to be associated with both mental health and substance use during adolescence (e.g., Van Oers et al., 1999; Schulte et al., 2009), and are as such important co-variates to be considered.

In the present study, we aimed to examine the frequencies of alcohol/drug use and problems among adolescents receiving specialist mental health care compared with a general population of adolescents. In addition, we investigated associations between a broad range of psychiatric diagnoses and alcohol/drug use and problems, while also accounting for the potential confounding effects of other comorbid psychiatric diagnoses, as well as sex, age, and SES. We hypothesized that all psychiatric diagnostic categories – except autism – would be associated with some measure of alcohol/drug use and problems. The lack of similar studies did not allow for specific hypotheses on which diagnoses would have the strongest associations with substance use after the adjustment for psychiatric comorbidity and demographics.

MATERIALS AND METHODS

Study Population

We employed data from the youth@hordaland-survey, which includes information on child and adolescent mental health, lifestyle, school performance and use of health services. Of all 19,430 adolescents born between 1993 and 1995 living in Hordaland County in Western Norway, 10,253 (53%) agreed to participate. The youth@hordaland-survey is a cross-sectional population-based study carried out during early 2012, when the adolescents ranged from 16 to 19 years of age. Participants received information by email and one school hour was used to complete the questionnaires. In addition, adolescents not going to school received the questionnaires by mail at their home address, and mental health services and other institutions were contacted to allow participation for adolescents in these settings. The questionnaires used in the youth@hordaland-survey were web-based.

We linked data from the youth@hordaland-survey to data from the National Patient Registry (NPR) through the participants' personal identification number. The NPR is the official national registry in Norway on specialist mental health care services, and includes information on specialist mental health care use and Axis 1 psychiatric diagnoses from January 2008 to December 2011, at a time when the adolescents ranged from 12 to 18 years of age, and before youth@hordaland participation. 845 (8.2%) of the adolescents did not provide consent for merging the data from the youth@hordaland-survey with other registries, and were excluded from the analyses. The final sample therefore included 9,408 participants, of whom 853 (9.1%) had at least one registration in NPR.

The Regional Committee for Medical and Health Research Ethics (REC) in Western Norway approved the study. In accordance with the regulations from the REC and Norwegian health authorities, adolescents aged 16 years and older can make decisions regarding their own health (including participation in research). All participants of the study gave written informed consent themselves to participate in the current study. Parents/guardians have the right to be informed, and in the current study, all parents/guardians received written information about the study in advance.

Measures and Instruments

Explanatory Variables: Psychiatric Disorders

The adolescents who had received specialist mental health care (n = 853), were assigned to the following diagnostic categories: anxiety (n = 132), depression (n = 172), conduct disorders (n = 32), attention-deficit/hyperactivity disorder (ADHD, n = 154), autism spectrum disorders (n = 46), eating disorders (n = 40), trauma-related disorders (n = 66), psychotic disorders (n = 10), other diagnoses (n = 84), and no Axis 1 psychiatric diagnosis (n = 329). 133 adolescents had psychiatric diagnoses from more than one of the specified diagnostic categories, and were assigned to multiple diagnostic categories. **Appendix I** details the operationalization of the diagnostic categories. Of note, none of the participants who were registered with mental health care use were given a substance-related disorder diagnosis.

Self-reported mental health problems were measured in order to examine differences between individuals that consented (n = 9,408) to the linkage between the youth@hordaland-survey and the NPR, and those that did not consent to this linkage (n = 845). Specifically, the short version of the Mood and Feelings Questionnaire (SMFQ) (Thapar and McGuffin, 1998) was used to measure symptoms of depression; the SCARED inventory (Birmaher et al., 1999) was used for anxiety symptoms; the Adult ADHD Self-report Scale (ASRS) (Kessler et al., 2007) for symptoms of hyperactivity/inattention; and the Youth Conduct Disorder (YCD) instrument (Lucas et al., 2001) for symptoms of conduct disorders.

Outcome Variables: Alcohol/Drug Use and Problems

We constructed a variable for *lifetime alcohol use* based on a single item: 'Have you ever tried alcohol?' (Yes/No). Similarly, we constructed a variable for *lifetime illicit drug use* based on a single item: 'Have you ever tried hash, marijuana or other narcotic substances?' (Yes/No). We measured *frequent alcohol intoxication* with the question: 'Have you ever consumed so much alcohol that you were clearly intoxicated (drunk)?' The original item had five categories ranging from 'No, never' to 'Yes, more than 10 times.' Frequent alcohol intoxication was defined as drinking so much that one was clearly intoxicated more than 10 times, and on this basis, a dichotomous variable was created. We added up five items that measured how many glasses of (i) beer, (ii) cider, (iii) wine, (iv) spirits, and (v) illegally distilled spirits the adolescents usually consumed during a time period of 14 days. 5,058 adolescents reported any usual alcohol consumption. The *high-level alcohol consumption* variable was defined as the above 90th sex-specific percentile alcohol consumption among the adolescents with any usual alcohol consumption, and a dichotomous variable was created for high-level alcohol consumption (Heradstveit et al., 2017). We also used the six-item, validated CRAFFT scale, in order to indicate adolescents that had a *positive CRAFFT score*. CRAFFT stands for the key words of the six items included in the scale – Car, Relax, Alone, Forget, Friends, Trouble. This scale has been designed to identify potential alcohol-and drug related problems among adolescents and has been demonstrated to have acceptable sensitivity and specificity at a cut-off of ≥ 2 relative to classifications of problem substance use, substance abuse or substance dependence as identified in structured clinical interviews (Knight et al., 2002; Dhalla et al., 2011). A previous publication based on the youth@hordaland-sample investigated the factor structure and concurrent validity of CRAFFT in relation to self-reported excessive alcohol consumption, frequent binge drinking, and any illicit drug use – and demonstrated a good fit with a single latent construct of alcohol/drug-related problems (Skogen et al., 2013). A dichotomous variable separating those above the cut-off of ≥ 2 on CRAFFT from those below the cut-off were calculated. In our sample the omega internal consistency coefficient (McDonald, 2013) of the CRAFFT scale was 0.88.

Finally, an ordinal variable for level of *risky substance use* was constructed (ranging from 0 to 4), in which we summed up the number of positive scores on lifetime illicit drug use, frequent alcohol intoxication, high-level alcohol consumption, and CRAFFT-scores ≥ 2.

Included Co-variates

Age and sex were retrieved from the Norwegian Population Registry, and were available for all participants in the youth@hordaland-sample. In addition, self-reported family financial circumstances was collected as either (1) 'about the same as others,' (2) 'better than others,' or (3) 'worse than others.' Self-reported information on maternal and paternal educational attainment was divided into primary school, high school, or more than 4 years of university or higher education. The variables of self-reported family financial circumstances, paternal educational attainment, and maternal educational attainment were used as a compound measure for SES (Skogen et al., 2014).

Statistical Analyses

All analyses were performed using STATA V.14.0 (StataCorp, 2015), with the exception that the omega internal consistency coefficient for the CRAFFT questionnaire was calculated in R Core Team (2018). First, frequencies of alcohol/drug use and problems, self-reported symptoms of mental health problems, and sociodemographic variables were examined across individuals who gave their consent to the linkage between the youth@hordaland-survey and the NPR, and those who refused to consent to this linkage (**Table 1**). Second, the sample was described according to age, sex, SES, and alcohol/drug use and problems among adolescents that had received specialist mental health care services compared to the adolescents that had not receiving these services during the past 4 years (**Table 2**). Third, psychiatric comorbidity rates within each diagnostic category were described, and all investigated psychiatric diagnoses were analyzed in terms of Spearman's Rank correlations with other psychiatric diagnoses (**Table 3**). Fourth, logistic regression models were employed to calculate associations between psychiatric diagnoses received within specialist mental health care and single measures of alcohol/drug use and problems. We then adjusted for the potential confounding effects of comorbid psychiatric diagnoses, in order to determine the independence of associations between each psychiatric diagnosis and substance use. For each psychiatric diagnosis that was investigated, all other psychiatric diagnostic categories were separately entered as potential confounding variables. Finally, we adjusted the analyses for the confounding effects of comorbid psychiatric diagnoses, as well as age, sex and SES (**Table 4**). Finally, ordered logistic regression models were employed to calculate unadjusted and adjusted odds ratios for the associations between psychiatric diagnoses and the total degree of risky substance use (**Table 5**). Due to the small size of the psychotic disorders group (n = 10), and due to considerable conceptual heterogeneity within the "other diagnoses" group and the "no Axis 1 diagnosis" group, we did not perform analyses of associations between these categories and substance use.

RESULTS

For the most part, adolescents who consented to the linkage between the youth@hordaland-survey and the NPR and which therefore constituted the final study sample (n = 9,408), were similar to those that did not consent (n = 845) (**Table 1**). However, the individuals that refused consent had somewhat higher frequencies of high-level alcohol consumption (8.5 versus 5.9%, d = 0.11, $p < 0.01$), higher mean symptom levels of self-reported conduct problems (0.68 versus 0.54, d = 0.11, $p < 0.01$), and were somewhat older (17.6 versus 17.4, $p < 0.001$).

In the study sample (n = 9,408), 9.1% (n = 853) of the adolescents had received services from Norwegian specialist health care during the past 4 years (2008 to 2011). As outlined in **Table 2**, adolescents who had received specialist mental health care services were more often female (58.5 versus 52.3%, p = 0.001) and of low SES (d = 0.17, $p < 0.001$). In addition, adolescents who had received specialist mental health care services had higher frequencies of most alcohol/drug use and problems (d's ranging from 0.09 to 0.29, all $p < 0.05$) compared with adolescents that had not received specialist mental health care services. The only exception was on the measure for having ever used alcohol, which was non-significant (p = 0.571).

Frequencies of comorbidity with other psychiatric diagnoses were examined for each of the included psychiatric diagnoses. Among adolescents who had received a psychiatric diagnosis from a specialist mental health care clinic (n = 524), a total of 133 (25.4%) had at least one comorbid psychiatric diagnosis from another diagnostic category (data not shown). Specifically, the prevalence of psychiatric comorbidity were 59.1% (n = 78) for anxiety, 62.2% (n = 107) for depression, 62.5% (n = 20) for conduct disorders, 42.9% (n = 66) for ADHD, 60.1% (n = 28) for autism, 52.5% (n = 21) for eating disorders, 28.8% (n = 19) for trauma-related disorders, 70.0% (n = 7) for psychotic disorders, and 11.8% (n = 39) for "other psychiatric diagnoses." **Table 3** presents the correlation coefficients between the psychiatric diagnoses. Anxiety and depression had the strongest correlation (r_s = 0.246, $p < 0.001$), while all other correlations were either non-significant or had a very small magnitude, spanning from r_s = 0.069 to r_s = 0.108.

In unadjusted models (**Table 4**), anxiety was associated with illicit drug use (odds ratio [OR] = 1.97, $p < 0.01$); depression was associated with frequent alcohol intoxication (OR = 1.58, $p < 0.001$), a positive CRAFFT score (OR = 2.04, $p < 0.001$) and illicit drug use (OR = 2.54, $p < 0.01$); conduct disorders were associated with a positive CRAFFT score (OR = 2.48, $p < 0.05$) and illicit drug use (OR = 4.63, $p < 0.001$); ADHD was associated with illicit drug use (OR = 1.81, $p < 0.01$); eating disorders were associated with frequent alcohol intoxication (OR = 2.08, $p < 0.05$) and a positive CRAFFT score (OR = 2.00, $p < 0.05$); trauma-related disorders were associated with all alcohol/drug measures (ORs ranging from 1.88 to 4.60, all $p < 0.05$). Additionally, autism was negatively associated with frequent alcohol intoxication (OR = 0.30, $p < 0.05$).

After adjustment for psychiatric comorbidity, anxiety was only negatively associated with frequent alcohol intoxication (adjusted odds ratio [AOR] = 0.48, $p < 0.01$). Depression was still significantly associated with frequent alcohol intoxication, a positive CRAFFT score and illicit drug use (AORs ranging from

TABLE 1 | Frequencies of alcohol/drug use and problems, mental health problems, and sociodemographic characteristics in adolescents excluded from the study sample (n = 845), compared with adolescents in the study sample (n = 9,408).

	Youth@hordaland-sample (n = 10,253)			
	Study sample: **Consented to linkage with NPR (n = 9,408)**	***Excluded individuals:*** **Refused consent to linkage with NPR (n = 845)**	**Cohens d**	***p*-Value**
Alcohol/drug use and problems				
Ever tried alcohol, *n* (%)	6, 948 (77.2)	573 (77.6)	0.01	0.803
Ever tried drugs, *n* (%)	917 (10.2)	82 (11.1)	0.03	0.436
Frequent alcohol intoxication, *n* (%)	1, 766 (18.8)	168 (19.9)	0.03	0.429
High-level alcohol consumption, *n* (%)[1]	495 (5.9)	56 (8.5)	0.11	0.008
CRAFFT ≥ 2, *n* (%)	1, 901 (21.2)	161 (21.9)	0.02	0.636
Mental health problems				
Anxiety (SCARED), mean (95% CI)	1.51 (1.47, 1.55)	1.55 (1.42, 1.69)	0.02	0.522
Depression (SMFQ), mean (95% CI)	5.88 (5.76, 6.00)	6.30 (5.85, 6.76)	0.07	0.058
Hyperactivity/inattention (ASRS), mean (95% CI)	26.90 (26.68, 27.12)	27.25 (26.39, 28.11)	0.03	0.396
Conduct problems (YCD), mean (95% CI)	0.54 (0.52, 0.57)	0.68 (0.57, 0.79)	0.11	0.004
Sociodemographic variables				
Girls, *n* (%)	4, 974 (52.9)	425 (50.3)	0.05	0.151
Age, mean (95% CI)	17.4 (17.4, 17.4)	17.6 (17.6, 17.7)	0.26	<0.001
Poor family economy, *n* (%)[2]	650 (7.1)	57 (7.2)	0.00	0.953
Low maternal education, *n* (%)[3]	718 (10.1)	71 (12.8)	0.09	0.050
Low paternal education, *n* (%)[4]	743 (10.7)	55 (10.1)	0.02	0.649

[1] *Includes individuals above 90th percentile sex-specific alcohol consumption levels in the full youth@hordaland sample (n = 10,253).*
[2] *Includes individuals reporting family economy as "worse than others."*
[3] *Includes individuals reporting maternal education as restrictred to only primary school.*
[4] *Includes individuals reporting paternal education as restrictred to only primary school.*

1.74 to 2.14, all $p < 0.05$). Conduct disorders were positively associated with a positive CRAFFT score (AOR = 2.19, $p < 0.05$) and illicit drug use (AOR = 3.54, $p < 0.01$). ADHD and eating disorders were no longer associated with any substance use or problems. Autism was still negatively associated with frequent alcohol intoxication (AOR = 0.25, $p < 0.05$). Trauma-related disorders were positively associated with all measures of substance use/problems (AORs ranging from 1.76 to 4.35, all $p < 0.05$).

In fully adjusted models, adjusting for the potential confounding effects of psychiatric comorbidity, SES, sex and age, neither anxiety nor ADHD were significantly associated with any measures of alcohol/drug use and problems. Depression was associated only with a positive CRAFFT score (AOR = 2.10, $p < 0.01$); conduct disorders were associated only with illicit drug use (AOR = 6.90, $p < 0.01$); eating disorders were associated only with frequent alcohol intoxication (AOR = 2.29, $p < 0.05$); and trauma-related disorders were associated with high-level alcohol consumption, frequent alcohol intoxication and a positive CRAFFT-score (AORs ranging from 2.15 to 4.77, all $p < 0.05$). In addition, autism was negatively associated with frequent alcohol intoxication (AOR = 0.28, $p < 0.05$).

Using likelihood-ratio tests of proportionality of odds across response categories, we found only non-significant differences between all the psychiatric diagnoses listed in **Table 5** and each ordinal level of indicators for risky substance use in the crude models (p-values ranging from 0.27 to 0.93), indicating that the proportional odds assumption underlying the ordered logistic regression models were met (Liao, 1994, p. 41). Autism diagnoses were excluded from this analysis as the proportional odds assumption was not met for this diagnosis.

In unadjusted models employing ordered logistic regression analyses, we found positive associations with the total degree of risky substance use and depression (OR = 1.89, $p < 0.001$), conduct disorders (OR = 3.15, $p < 0.01$), and trauma-related disorders (OR = 2.78, $p < 0.001$). Depression, conduct disorders and trauma-related disorders remained positively associated with the total degree of risky substance use after adjustment for psychiatric comorbidity (AORs ranging from 1.93 to 2.86, $p < 0.01$). Even in fully adjusted models, accounting for the confounding effects of psychiatric comorbidity, SES, sex and age, we found positive associations with the total degree of risky substance use for trauma-related disorders (AOR = 2.53, $p < 0.01$), depression (AOR = 1.61, $p < 0.05$), and conduct disorders (AOR = 2.79, $p < 0.05$).

DISCUSSION

The present study is to our knowledge the first to compare a broad range of psychiatric diagnoses and their associations with alcohol/drug use and problems during adolescence, while also addressing the role of psychiatric comorbidity. Frequencies of alcohol/drug use and problems were higher among adolescents who had received specialist mental health care services compared

TABLE 2 | Alcohol/drug use and sociodemographic characteristics of the study sample (n = 9,408).

Demographics	Study sample (n = 9,408)		Cohens d	p-value
	Received specialist mental health care services[1] (n = 853)	Did not receive specialist mental health care services (n = 8,555)		
Girls, n (%)	499 (58.5)	4, 475 (52.3)	0.124	0.001
Age, mean (SD)[2]	17.4 (0.8)	17.4 (0.8)	0.047	0.189
Family financial circumstances, n (%)			0.173	<0.001
Below average	115 (13.9)	535 (6.4)		–
Average	531 (64.4)	5, 623 (67.6)		–
Above average	179 (21.7)	2, 165 (26.0)		–
Mothers education, %[3]			0.159	<0.001
University/college	258 (43.8)	3, 174 (48.9)		–
High school	242 (41.1)	2, 687 (41.4)		–
Primary school	89 (15.1)	629 (9.7)		–
Fathers education, %[4]			0.174	<0.001
University/college	190 (35.9)	2, 770 (43.4)		–
High school	264 (49.8)	2, 953 (46.2)		–
Primary school	76 (14.3)	667 (10.4)		–
Alcohol/drug use and problems				
Ever used alcohol, n (%)	636 (78.0)	6, 312 (77.2)	−0.021	0.571
Tried illicit drugs, n (%)	148 (18.2)	769 (9.4)	−0.292	<0.001
Frequent drinking to intoxication[5], n (%)	188 (22.0)	1, 578 (18.5)	−0.092	0.010
High-level alcohol consumption, n (%)	65 (8.7)	442 (5.8)	−0.122	0.001
CRAFFT-score $\geq$ 2, n (%)	233 (28.7)	1, 668 (20.4)	−0.202	<0.001
Total degree of risky substance use			−0.269	<0.001
No indicators of alcohol/drug use and problems, n (%)	419 (56.3)	5, 002 (65.4)		–
1 indicator of alcohol/drug use and problem, n (%)	136 (18.3)	1, 454 (19.0)		–
2 indicators of alcohol/drug use and problems, n (%)	103 (13.8)	738 (9.6)		–
3 indicators of alcohol/drug use and problems, n (%)	70 (9.4)	375 (4.9)		–
4 indicators of alcohol/drug use and problems, n (%)	16 (2.2)	83 (1.1)		–

CRAFFT: screening scale for identification of potential problematic alcohol and drug use among adolescents.
[1]Received specialist mental health care services during the 4 years (2008–2011) prior to the youth@hordaland-survey (2012).
[2]Age at the time that the youth@hordaland-survey was collected.
[3]Only includes those who with valid response on mother's education (n = 7,079), excluding those having answered that they don't know (n = 2,187).
[4]Only includes those who with valid response on father's education (n = 6,920), excluding those having answered that they don't know (n = 2,325).
[5]Above 90th percentile alcohol consumption among those adolescents with a present alcohol consumption (n = 5,058).

TABLE 3 | Correlation matrix of psychiatric diagnoses (n = 853).

	ANX	DEP	COND	ADHD	AUT	EAT	TRA	PSY
ANX (n = 132)	–							
DEP (n = 172)	**0.246*****	–						
COND (n = 32)	0.001	−0.038	–					
ADHD (n = 154)	**−0.091****	−0.038	**0.100***	–				
AUT (n = 46)	−0.059	**−0.**004	0.008	**0.090****	–			
EAT (n = 40)	−0.049	**0.096****	−0.044	**−0.090****	−0.028	–		
TRA (n = 66)	−0.051	−0.047	0.012	**−0.102****	**−0.069***	−0.043	–	
PSY (n = 10)	**0.074***	**0.108****	−0.022	−0.023	−0.026	−0.024	−0.032	–

ANX, anxiety disorders; DEP, depression/mood disorders; COND, conduct disorders; ADHD, attention deficit/hyperactivity disorder; AUT, autism spectrum disorders; EAT, eating disorders; TRA, trauma-related disorders; PSY, psychotic disorders.
*Bold fonts signify statistically significant associations. *p < 0.05; **p < 0.01; ***p < 0.001.*

to adolescents who had not received such services during the past 4 years; however, the magnitude of these differences was small overall. Importantly, adolescents receiving treatment for a psychiatric disorder differed from controls on all measures of substance use and problems except any alcohol use. This finding may suggest that experimenting with alcohol is normative

TABLE 4 | Logistic regression analyses of associations between psychiatric diagnoses and alcohol/drug use and problems (*n* = 9,408)[1].

	High-level alcohol consumption OR (95%CI)	Frequent alcohol intoxication OR (95%CI)	CRAFFT-score ≥2 OR (95%CI)	Illicit drug use OR (95%CI)
Anxiety (*n* = 132)				
Crude model	1.12 (0.55, 2.32)	0.68 (0.41, 1.11)	1.21 (0.81, 1.83)	**1.97 (1.25, 3.12)****
Adj for comorbidity[2]	0.74 (0.33, 1.64)	**0.48 (0.28, 0.82)****	0.81 (0.51, 1.28)	1.10 (0.65, 1.87)
+Adj for SES+sex+age	1.40 (0.55, 3.57)	0.75 (0.38, 1.49)	0.88 (0.48, 1.60)	1.50 (0.74, 3.01)
Depression (*n* = 172)				
Crude model	1.45 (0.83, 2.53)	**1.58 (1.13, 2.23)****	**2.04 (1.48, 2.81)*****	**2.54 (1.76, 3.69)*****
Adj for comorbidity[2]	1.42 (0.76, 2.67)	**1.74 (1.18, 2.58)****	**2.14 (1.48, 3.09)*****	**2.12 (1.36, 3.29)****
+Adj for SES+sex+age	1.02 (0.44, 2.39)	1.31 (0.77, 2.23)	**2.10 (1.30, 3.38)****	1.68 (0.92, 3.08)
Conduct disorders (*n* = 32)				
Crude model	1.82 (0.55, 6.05)	1.96 (0.93, 4.14)	**2.48 (1.19, 5.16)***	**4.63 (2.15, 10.00)*****
Adj for comorbidity[2]	1.44 (0.41, 5.11)	1.88 (0.86, 4.11)	**2.19 (1.02, 4.71)***	**3.54 (1.58, 7.92)****
+Adj for SES+sex+age	0.73 (0.08, 6.29)	1.68 (0.51, 5.47)	2.12 (0.69, 6.55)	**6.90 (2.25, 21.17)****
ADHD (*n* = 154)				
Crude model	0.85 (0.40, 1.84)	1.32 (0.90, 1.92)	1.09 (0.73, 1.62)	**1.81 (1.16, 2.83)****
Adj for comorbidity[2]	0.74 (0.33, 1.64)	1.30 (0.87, 1.94)	0.92 (0.61, 1.40)	1.37 (0.85, 2.22)
+Adj for SES+sex+age	0.81 (0.28, 2.37)	1.25 (0.71, 2.20)	0.98 (0.56, 1.71)	1.72 (0.93, 3.19)
Autism disorders (*n* = 46)				
Crude model	0.82 (0.20, 3.40)	**0.30 (0.09, 0.96)***	0.49 (0.19, 1.24)	0.43 (0.10, 1.76)
Adj for comorbidity[2]	0.79 (0.18, 3.39)	**0.25 (0.08, 0.81)***	0.39 (0.15, 1.02)	0.28 (0.07, 1.19)
+Adj for SES+sex+age	0.85 (0.11, 6.73)	**0.28 (0.06, 1.24)***	0.35 (0.10, 1.25)	0.18 (0.02, 1.41)
Eating disorders (*n* = 40)				
Crude model	1.34 (0.41, 4.37)	**2.08 (1.07, 4.03)***	**2.00 (1.04, 3.84)***	1.25 (0.49, 3.20)
Adj for comorbidity[2]	1.04 (0.30, 3.63)	1.78 (0.89, 3.56)	1.48 (0.74, 2.93)	0.85 (0.32, 2.26)
+Adj for SES+sex+age	0.96 (0.21, 4.43)	**2.29 (1.01, 5.18)***	1.20 (0.54, 2.69)	1.06 (0.34, 3.29)
Trauma-related disorders (*n* = 66)				
Crude model	**4.60 (2.52, 8.41)*****	**1.88 (1.11, 3.18)***	**2.43 (1.25, 4.71)*****	**2.47 (1.36, 4.48)****
Adj for comorbidity[2]	**4.35 (2.35, 8.04)*****	**1.76 (1.03, 3.00)***	**2.43 (1.46, 4.05)****	**2.01 (1.09, 3.72)***
+Adj for SES+sex+age	**4.77 (2.17, 10.49)*****	**2.15 (1.06, 4.35)***	**2.31 (1.20, 4.43)****	2.05 (0.92, 4.54)

CRAFFT: screening scale for identification of potential problematic alcohol and drug use among adolescents.
[1]Analyses for psychotic disorders (n = 11) and other psychiatric diagnoses (n = 84) are not shown in the table.
[2]For each diagnostic category, psychiatric diagnoses from any other category are included as confounding comorbid diagnoses.
*Bold fonts signify statistically significant associations. *p < 0.05; **p < 0.01; ***p < 0.001.*

in adolescence but that excessive use of alcohol, use of other substances, and substance-related negative consequences are occurring at higher rates in those receiving services for psychiatric disorders. Furthermore, the investigated psychiatric diagnoses varied widely in the extent to which they were associated with alcohol/drug use and problems, particularly when the influence of other comorbid psychiatric diagnoses and demographic variables was accounted for.

Depression and Alcohol/Drug Use and Problems

In unadjusted models, depression was among the psychiatric diagnoses with the most consistent positive associations with alcohol/drug use and problems. Specifically, we found positive associations between depression and all single measures of alcohol/drug use and problems except high-level alcohol consumption. These associations remained significant after adjustment for psychiatric comorbidity. However, the only independent association between depression and alcohol/drug use and problems, after the additional adjustment for sociodemographic factors, was in relation to a positive CRAFFT-score. These findings lend some support to previous studies that have reported positive associations between depression and self-reported adolescent alcohol-related problems (Harrell et al., 2009) and general alcohol/drug use (Crum et al., 2008; Maslowsky and Schulenberg, 2013). Our study adds to previous findings that report positive associations between depression and alcohol intoxication (Crum et al., 2008; Pedersen, 2013), as our findings suggest that the association between depression and frequent alcohol intoxication was significant in the unadjusted model and after the adjustment of psychiatric comorbidity. However, this association was non-significant after the additional adjustment of sociodemographic factors. Moreover, depression was associated with the total degree of risky substance use, and this association was independent from psychiatric comorbidity and sociodemographic factors. In sum, these findings suggest that depression is a robust indicator for the total degree of risky substance use among adolescents.

TABLE 5 | Ordered logistic regression analyses of associations between psychiatric diagnoses and the total degree of risky substance use (*n* = 9,408)[1].

	Unadjusted model OR (95%CI)	Adjusted for psychiatric comorbidity[2] AOR (95%CI)	Adjusted for psychiatric comorbidity[2] + SES, sex and age AOR (95%CI)
Anxiety (*n* = 132)	1.08 (0.74, 1.56)	0.71 (0.48, 1.07)	0.92 (0.54, 1.58)
Depression (*n* = 172)	**1.89 (1.40, 2.55)*****	**1.93 (1.37, 2.71)*****	**1.61 (1.03, 2.54)***
Conduct disorders (*n* = 32)	**3.15 (1.62, 6.12)****	**2.86 (1.43, 5.73)****	**2.79 (1.02, 7.66)***
ADHD (*n* = 154)	1.34 (0.95, 1.88)	1.20 (0.84, 1.72)	1.44 (0.90, 2.31)
Eating disorders (*n* = 40)	1.81 (0.98, 3.34)	1.33 (0.70, 2.52)	1.34 (0.64, 2.80)
Trauma disorders (*n* = 66)	**2.78 (1.72, 4.48)*****	**2.48 (1.52, 4.03)*****	**2.62 (1.37, 5.02)****

[1]Analyses for psychotic disorders (n = 11) and other psychiatric diagnoses (n = 84) are not conducted. Autism diagnoses (n = 46) were also excluded as the proportional odds assumption was not met.
[2]For each diagnostic category, psychiatric diagnoses from any other category are included as confounding comorbid diagnoses.
*Bold fonts signify statistically significant associations. *p < 0.05; **p < 0.01; ***p < 0.001.*

Anxiety and Alcohol/Drug Use and Problems

We found that anxiety was positively associated with illicit drug use in unadjusted models. However, this association were non-significant after adjustment for psychiatric comorbidity. This finding suggests that no unique association between anxiety and illicit drug use was present in our data. Interestingly, anxiety was negative associated with frequent alcohol intoxication after adjustment for psychiatric comorbidity, but this association was no longer significant after the additional adjustment for sociodemographic variables. In sum, the present study lends little support to an independent association between anxiety and alcohol/drug use or problems among adolescents, and adjustment of psychiatric comorbidity tended to reduce the positive direction of the associations between anxiety and alcohol/drug use and problems, while the additional adjustment of sociodemographic variables did not affect the estimates in a consistent direction. Importantly, the previous literature is characterized by highly inconsistent findings, pointing to both negative (Schmits et al., 2015, 2016; Nelemans et al., 2016; Savage et al., 2016) and positive associations between anxiety and adolescent alcohol/drug use (Pardee et al., 2014; Birrell et al., 2015; Stapinski et al., 2016). Some studies have suggested that different anxiety disorders (Wu et al., 2010; Ohannessian, 2014) and different anxiety typologies within a given disorder (Tomlinson et al., 2013) yield different prediction of alcohol/drug use and problems, and anxiety may also have a role on adolescent alcohol/drug use and problems through interactions with other diagnoses (Lansford et al., 2008). Future studies should expand the scope to also distinguish between subtypes of anxiety disorders (e.g., social anxiety and generalized anxiety) and their independent associations with alcohol/drug use and problems during adolescence. Also of note, future studies could expand with measures of substance use/problems related to drugs with anxiolytic effects (e.g., alcohol and benzodiazepines), as our study did not include measures of alcohol-problems in particular (as CRAFFT is related to potential alcohol and/or drug-related problems) or benzodiazepine use/problems.

Autism and Alcohol/Drug Use and Problems

In the present study, autism was negatively associated with frequent alcohol intoxication after the adjustment of both psychiatric comorbidity and sociodemographic variables. In addition, all other single measures of alcohol/drug use and problems tended to go in a negative direction; however, these associations were non-significant. A limited number of previous studies have to our knowledge explored associations between autism and alcohol/drug use and problems among adolescents (Ramos et al., 2013; Mangerud et al., 2014), suggesting a low alcohol/drug use in this group. The present study support these findings by indicating that adolescents with autism had significantly lower odds for frequent alcohol intoxication compared with the general adolescent population. A possible explanation for this finding is that the social skills deficits of autistic adolescents may keep them out of the social situations and/or peer relations typically associated with alcohol consumption in adolescence (Santosh and Mijovic, 2006). However, autism may be associated with alcohol/drug use and problems beyond the adolescent years (Butwicka et al., 2017).

Eating Disorders and Alcohol/Drug Use and Problems

Our findings suggest that eating disorders were positively associated with frequent alcohol intoxication and a positive CRAFFT-score in unadjusted analyses. However, eating disorders were no longer significantly associated with any alcohol/drug use and problems measures after the adjustment for psychiatric comorbidity, while eating disorders were positively associated with frequent alcohol intoxication after the additional adjustment for demographic variables. This finding supports previous studies linking eating disorders with specific patterns of alcohol use characterized by a loss of control, such as frequent intoxication (Mustelin et al., 2016) and binge drinking (Khaylis et al., 2009). Previous studies indicate that elevated alcohol/drug use and problems are more likely amongst those with bulimia nervosa and binge eating disorders relative to those with anorexia nervosa (e.g., Gadalla and Piran, 2007). The present study did not, however, distinguish between different subtypes of eating disorders, something that should be considered in future research.

ADHD and Alcohol/Drug Use and Problems

Previous studies have linked both childhood ADHD symptoms (Lee et al., 2011; Heradstveit et al., 2018) and ADHD symptoms during adolescence (August et al., 2006) with adolescent alcohol/drug use and problems. However, several researchers have highlighted that most studies have not controlled for associated psychopathology (August et al., 2006; Lee et al., 2011; Bidwell et al., 2014), therefore leaving doubt on the independence of this association. Our findings were that ADHD was associated with illicit drug use alone; however, this association was non-significant after the adjustment of psychiatric comorbidity as well as after the additional adjustment of sociodemographic variables. These findings suggest that no unique association between ADHD and alcohol/drug use and problems were present in our data, lending support to a study by August et al. (2006). They demonstrated that adolescent ADHD was positively associated with illicit drug use only for individuals with a comorbid externalizing disorder, primarily oppositional defiant disorder. A recent literature review similarly indicated that ADHD does not increase the risk of illicit drug use beyond the effect of conduct-related disorders (Serra-Pinheiro et al., 2013). In sum, our results suggest that ADHD was not independently associated with alcohol/drug use and problems among adolescents, and that comorbid psychiatric disorders may be important confounders in association between ADHD and illicit drug use. However, future studies are encouraged to test whether certain features of ADHD (e.g., impulsivity) might show more unique relations to alcohol/drug use and problems.

Conduct Disorders and Alcohol/Drug Use and Problems

A range of previous studies have pointed to positive associations between externalizing problems and alcohol/drug use and problems (e.g., Heron et al., 2013; Hopfer et al., 2013; Cerda et al., 2016; Heradstveit et al., 2018; Pedersen et al., 2018), while studies exploring the independence of these associations with respect to comorbidity are more limited. In the present study, we found that conduct disorders were associated with illicit drug use, a positive CRAFFT score, and the total degree of risky substance use in unadjusted models, while we also found independent associations between conduct problems and illicit drug use and the total degree of risky substance use. Hence, conduct disorders appeared to be an important indicator for alcohol/drug use and problems in this study. Also of note, conduct disorders were the only specific psychiatric diagnosis that had an independent association with illicit drug use, highlighting the importance of this diagnosis in relation to illicit drug use among adolescents. This finding lends support to the deviancy proneness model that highlights deviant behaviors as an important risk factor for illicit drug use among adolescents (Tarter et al., 2006).

Trauma-Related Disorders and Alcohol/Drug Use and Problems

In unadjusted models, trauma-related disorders were positively associated with all single measures of alcohol/drug use and problems, while they were positively associated with all single measures except illicit drug use after the combined adjustment for psychiatric comorbidity and sociodemographic variables. This latter finding suggest that psychiatric comorbidity and sociodemographic variables should be taken into account as potential confounders in the associations between trauma-related disorders and illicit drug use. Additionally, trauma-related disorders were independently associated with the total degree of risky substance use. This finding supports previous studies that report positive associations between trauma-related disorders and alcohol/drug use and problems among adolescents (Giaconia et al., 2000; Haller and Chassin, 2014). The mechanisms behind associations between trauma-related problems and alcohol/drug-related problems are complex. A longitudinal, community-based study by Haller and Chassin (2014) found that PTSD symptoms increased the risk for later alcohol/drug-related problems among adolescents, and the authors argued that these results supported a self-medication hypothesis. However, other mechanisms may potentially be at work. For example, early alcohol/drug-related problems often involves chaotic and violent lifestyles, which could possibly increase the risk for trauma exposure (Deykin and Buka, 1997).

Strengths and Limitations

The study described here has several strengths. First, the sample consists of a well-defined population-based sample of adolescents aged 16 to 19 years, and was sufficiently large to enable a detailed investigation of the associations of interest. Second, a unique linkage with official registry data on specialist mental health care services was utilized, facilitating an investigation of formal psychiatric diagnoses independently determined according to the ICD-10 by professional mental health practitioners. However, the diagnoses are based on clinical judgment and no inter-rater reliability between the raters exists. Third, we investigated alcohol/drug use and problems across a broad range of diagnostic groups, which is rare in previous research (Mangerud et al., 2014), and enabled us to evaluate the independence of associations with alcohol/drug use and problems across several psychiatric diagnoses. Finally, due to the relatively large sample and comprehensive information about psychiatric diagnoses, we were able to adjust our analyses for psychiatric comorbidity, SES, sex, and age.

Some limitations require consideration when drawing inferences from this study. First, although the measures of psychiatric diagnoses preceded those of alcohol/drug use and problems, the study does not have a stringent longitudinal design, and it is not possible to draw conclusions on the causality between psychiatric diagnoses and alcohol/drug use and problems in this study, since some substance use may have predated the mental health care contacts. Second, the response rate in the population-based sample was 53% and included a relatively low proportion of adolescents with self-reported low SES, who in previous studies are found to have higher levels of mental health problems (e.g., Bøe et al., 2012). Official Norwegian statistics indicate that in 2012, 92% of all adolescents in Norway aged 16 to 18 years of age attended high school, compared with 98% in the youth@hordaland-sample (Hysing et al., 2015). The sample may therefore not have been fully representative of adolescents with psychiatric diagnoses due to selective participation. However, a previous publication from the Bergen Child Study indicated that although non-participation in the survey affected the estimated frequency of mental health problems, it did not affect patterns of associations between sociodemographic characteristics and mental health problems (Heiervang and Goodman, 2011). Nevertheless, our findings on associations between the broad range of psychiatric diagnoses and alcohol/drug use and problems require replication within more comprehensively ascertained clinical samples. Third, we did not differentiate between subtypes of psychiatric diagnoses. Fourth, psychiatric comorbidity was significantly higher within some of the diagnostic categories, particularly anxiety, depression, and conduct disorders. We may therefore have underestimated the independent associations between these psychiatric diagnoses and alcohol/drug use and problems. Fifth, alcohol/drug use and problems were measured by self-report, and does not imply the presence of diagnosable SUDs. In addition, the summed variable of the total degree of risky substance use included both substance use (illicit drug use, high-level alcohol consumption, frequent alcohol intoxication) and substance problems (a positive CRAFFT score). The use of a compound measure can be considered as a limitation, as it is difficult to differentiate between substance use and substance problems. Moreover, this summed variable did not specifically include prescription drug misuse as well as tobacco use. The results may therefore not be generalized to all types of drug use. Sixth, although adolescents that did not consent to the linkage between the youth@hordaland-survey and the NPR were overall similar to those that consented to this linkage, they reported somewhat higher frequency of high-level alcohol consumption, self-reported conduct problems, and higher age. Hence, this limitation may affect the generalizability of our findings. Seventh, the present study included many sets of analyses of associations. Multiple testing might therefore be an issue to consider when interpreting the results. Finally, an important limitation related to the generalizability of the findings from the present study is that individuals with untreated mental health problems in the general youth@hordaland-population were not identified. Psychiatric diagnoses in the present study was restricted to individuals that had received specialist mental health care services during the past 4 years. However, some adolescents in the general population may be suffering from undetected and/or untreated psychiatric disorders, or may have received treatment for psychiatric disorders elsewhere other than through specialist mental health care services (e.g., in private practice or through community-based psychologist services). A range of factors may potentially affect specialist mental health care use, such as functional impairment levels (Hintzpeter et al., 2015) and sociodemographic characteristics (Zwaanswijk et al., 2003). Also, a former wave of the Bergen Child Study concluded that specialist mental health care use differed considerably across psychiatric diagnoses, in which children with emotional disorders were underrepresented in mental health care services (Heiervang et al., 2007). Therefore, our findings on associations between psychiatric diagnoses and alcohol/drug use and problems should be interpreted with caution, particularly in relation to anxiety and depression disorders.

CONCLUSION

Alcohol/drug use and problems were slightly more common among adolescents who received specialist mental health care during the past 4 years compared with the general adolescent population. All investigated psychiatric diagnoses - except autism - were associated with some measure of hazardous alcohol/drug use and problems, and adolescents with trauma-related disorders, depression, and conduct disorders had particularly high odds for alcohol/drug use and problems.

ETHICS STATEMENT

The Regional Committee for Medical and Health Research Ethics (REC) in Western Norway approved the study. In accordance with the regulations from the REC and Norwegian health authorities, adolescents aged 16 years and older can make decisions regarding their own health (including participation in research), and thus gave consent themselves to participate in the current study. Parents/guardians have the right to be informed, and in the current study, all parents/guardians received written information about the study in advance.

AUTHOR CONTRIBUTIONS

OH has carried out the literature review for the introduction and the discussion section, conducted the statistical analyses, and has written the manuscript. OH, MH, and JS have been involved in the preparation and conduct of the statistical analyses, while all authors (OH, MH, JS, JH, and RS) have reviewed the project and participated in manuscript writing.

FUNDING

This work was supported by the Health Ministry of Western Norway, Fund for Strategic Research on Alcohol and Drug Use (Grant No. 912002). RS was partly funded by the National Institute for Health Research (NIHR) Biomedical Research Centre at South London and Maudsley NHS Foundation Trust and King's College London.

REFERENCES

Addington, J., and Addington, D. (2007). Patterns, predictors and impact of substance use in early psychosis: a longitudinal study. *Acta Psychiatr. Scand.* 115, 304–309. doi: 10.1111/j.1600-0447.2006.00900.x

Armstrong, T. D., and Costello, E. J. (2002). Community studies on adolescent substance use, abuse, or dependence and psychiatric comorbidity. *J. Consult. Clin. Psychol.* 70, 1224–1239. doi: 10.1037//0022-006x.70.6.1224

August, G. J., Winters, K. C., Realmuto, G. M., Fahnhorst, T., Botzet, A., and Lee, S. (2006). Prospective study of adolescent drug use among community samples of ADHD and non-ADHD participants. *J. Am. Acad. Child Adolesc. Psychiatry* 45, 824–832. doi: 10.1097/01.chi.0000219831.16226.f8

Barkmann, C., and Schulte-Markwort, M. (2012). Prevalence of emotional and behavioural disorders in German children and adolescents: a meta-analysis. *J. Epidemiol. Commun. Health* 66, 194–203. doi: 10.1136/jech.2009.102467

Belfer, M. L. (2008). Child and adolescent mental disorders: the magnitude of the problem across the globe. *J. Child Psychol. Psychiatry* 49, 226–236. doi: 10.1111/j.1469-7610.2007.01855.x

Bidwell, L. C., Henry, E. A., Willcutt, E. G., Kinnear, M. K., and Ito, T. A. (2014). Childhood and current ADHD symptom dimensions are associated with more severe cannabis outcomes in college students. *Drug Alcohol Depend.* 135, 88–94. doi: 10.1016/j.drugalcdep.2013.11.013

Birmaher, B., Brent, D. A., Chiappetta, L., Bridge, J., Monga, S., and Baugher, M. (1999). Psychometric properties of the screen for child anxiety related emotional disorders (SCARED): a replication study. *J. Am. Acad. Child Adolesc. Psychiatry* 38, 1230–1236. doi: 10.1097/00004583-199910000-00011

Birrell, L., Newton, N. C., Teesson, M., Tonks, Z., and Slade, T. (2015). Anxiety disorders and first alcohol use in the general population. Findings from a nationally representative sample. *J. Anxiety Disord.* 31, 108–113. doi: 10.1016/j.janxdis.2015.02.008

Bisetto, P. D., Botella, G. Á., and Sancho, M. A. (2011). Eating disorders and drug use in adolescents. *Adicciones* 24, 9–16.

Bøe, T., Øverland, S., Lundervold, A. J., and Hysing, M. (2012). Socioeconomic status and children's mental health: results from the bergen child study. *Soc. Psychiatry Psychiatr. Epidemiol.* 47, 1557–1566. doi: 10.1007/s00127-011-0462-9

Boys, A., Farrell, M., Taylor, C., Marsden, J., Goodman, R., Brugha, T., et al. (2003). Psychiatric morbidity and substance use in young people aged 13–15 years: results from the child and adolescent survey of mental health. *Br. J. Psychiatry* 182, 509–517. doi: 10.1192/bjp.182.6.509

Butwicka, A., Långström, N., Larsson, H., Lundström, S., Serlachius, E., Almqvist, C., et al. (2017). Increased risk for substance use-related problems in autism spectrum disorders: a population-based cohort study. *J. Autism Dev. Disord.* 47, 80–89. doi: 10.1007/s10803-016-2914-2

Canino, G., Shrout, P. E., Rubio-Stipec, M., Bird, H. R., Bravo, M., Ramirez, R., et al. (2004). The DSM-IV rates of child and adolescent disordersin puerto rico: prevalence, correlates, service use, and the effects of impairment. *Arch. Gen. Psychiatry* 61, 85–93.

Castro-Fornieles, J., Díaz, R., Goti, J., Calvo, R., Gonzalez, L., Serrano, L., et al. (2009). Prevalence and factors related to substance use among adolescents with eating disorders. *Eur. Addic. Res.* 16, 61–68. doi: 10.1159/000268106

Cerda, M., Prins, S. J., Galea, S., Howe, C. J., and Pardini, D. (2016). When psychopathology matters most: identifying sensitive periods when within-person changes in conduct, affective and anxiety problems are associated with male adolescent substance use. *Addiction* 111, 924–935. doi: 10.1111/add.13304

Costello, E. J., Mustillo, S., Erkanli, A., Keeler, G., and Angold, A. (2003). Prevalence and development of psychiatric disorders in childhood and adolescence. *Arch. Gen. Psychiatry* 60, 837–844.

Crum, R. M., Green, K. M., Storr, C. L., Chan, Y.-F., Ialongo, N., Stuart, E. A., et al. (2008). Depressed mood in childhood and subsequent alcohol use through adolescence and young adulthood. *Arch. Gen. Psychiatry* 65, 702–712. doi: 10.1001/archpsyc.65.6.702

Deas-Nesmith, D., Campbell, S., and Brady, K. T. (1998). Substance use disorders in an adolescent inpatient psychiatric population. *J. Natl. Med. Assoc.* 90, 233–238.

Deykin, E. Y., and Buka, S. L. (1997). Prevalence and risk factors for posttraumatic stress disorder among chemically dependent adolescents. *Am. J. Psychiatry* 154, 752–757. doi: 10.1176/ajp.154.6.752

Dhalla, S., Zumbo, B., and Poole, G. (2011). A review of the psychometric properties of the CRAFFT instrument: 1999-2010. *Curr. Drug Abuse Rev.* 4, 57–64. doi: 10.2174/1874473711104010057

Edlund, M. J., Forman-Hoffman, V. L., Winder, C. R., Heller, D. C., Kroutil, L. A., Lipari, R. N., et al. (2015). Opioid abuse and depression in adolescents: results from the national survey on drug use and health. *Drug Alcohol Depend.* 152, 131–138. doi: 10.1016/j.drugalcdep.2015.04.010

Ferdinand, R. F., Sondeijker, F., Van Der Ende, J., Selten, J. P., Huizink, A., and Verhulst, F. C. (2005). Cannabis use predicts future psychotic symptoms, and vice versa. *Addiction* 100, 612–618. doi: 10.1111/j.1360-0443.2005.01070.x

Gadalla, T., and Piran, N. (2007). Co-occurrence of eating disorders and alcohol use disorders in women: a meta analysis. *Arch. Womens Ment. Health* 10, 133–140. doi: 10.1007/s00737-007-0184-x

Giaconia, R. M., Reinherz, H. Z., Hauf, A. C., Paradis, A. D., Wasserman, M. S., and Langhammer, D. M. (2000). Comorbidity of substance use and post-traumatic stress disorders in a community sample of adolescents. *Am. J. Orthopsychiatry* 70, 253–262. doi: 10.1037/h0087634

Groenman, A. P., Oosterlaan, J., Rommelse, N., Franke, B., Roeyers, H., Oades, R. D., et al. (2013). Substance use disorders in adolescents with attention deficit hyperactivity disorder: a 4-year follow-up study. *Addiction* 108, 1503–1511. doi: 10.1111/add.12188

Haller, M., and Chassin, L. (2014). Risk pathways among traumatic stress, posttraumatic stress disorder symptoms, and alcohol and drug problems: a test of four hypotheses. *Psychol. Addic. Behav.* 28, 841–851. doi: 10.1037/a0035878

Harrell, Z. A., Slane, J. D., and Klump, K. L. (2009). Predictors of alcohol problems in college women: the role of depressive symptoms, disordered eating, and family history of alcoholism. *Addic. Behav.* 34, 252–257. doi: 10.1016/j.addbeh.2008.10.019

Heiervang, E., and Goodman, R. (2011). Advantages and limitations of web-based surveys: evidence from a child mental health survey. *Soc. Psychiatry Psychiatr. Epidemiol.* 46, 69–76. doi: 10.1007/s00127-009-0171-9

Heiervang, E., Stormark, K. M., Lundervold, A. J., Heimann, M., Goodman, R., Posserud, M.-B., et al. (2007). Psychiatric disorders in Norwegian 8-to 10-year-olds: an epidemiological survey of prevalence, risk factors, and service use. *J. Am. Acad. Child Adolesc. Psychiatry* 46, 438–447.

Heradstveit, O., Skogen, J. C., Bøe, T., Hetland, J., Pedersen, M. U., and Hysing, M. (2018). Prospective associations between childhood externalising and internalising problems and adolescent alcohol and drug use: the bergen child study. *Nord. Stud. Alcohol Drugs* 35, 357–371. doi: 10.1177/1455072518789852

Heradstveit, O., Skogen, J. C., Hetland, J., and Hysing, M. (2017). Alcohol and illicit drug use are important factors for school-related problems among adolescents. *Front. Psychol.* 8:1023. doi: 10.3389/fpsyg.2017.01023

Heron, J., Barker, E. D., Joinson, C., Lewis, G., Hickman, M., Munafò, M., et al. (2013). Childhood conduct disorder trajectories, prior risk factors and cannabis use at age 16: birth cohort study. *Addiction* 108, 2129–2138. doi: 10.1111/add.12268

Hintzpeter, B., Klasen, F., Schön, G., Voss, C., Hölling, H., Ravens-Sieberer, U., et al. (2015). Mental health care use among children and adolescents in Germany: results of the longitudinal BELLA study. *Eur. Child Adolesc. Psychiatry* 24, 705–713. doi: 10.1007/s00787-015-0676-6

Hopfer, C., Salomonsen-Sautel, S., Mikulich-Gilbertson, S., Min, S. J., McQueen, M., Crowley, T., et al. (2013). Conduct disorder and initiation of substance use: a prospective longitudinal study. *J. Am. Acad. Child Adolesc. Psychiatry* 52, 511–518.

Hysing, M., Pallesen, S., Stormark, K. M., Jakobsen, R., Lundervold, A. J., and Sivertsen, B. (2015). Sleep and use of electronic devices in adolescence: results from a large population-based study. *BMJ Open* 5:e006748. doi: 10.1136/bmjopen-2014-006748

Kedzior, K. K., and Laeber, L. T. (2014). A positive association between anxiety disorders and cannabis use or cannabis use disorders in the general population: a meta-analysis of 31 studies. *BMC Psychiatry* 14:136. doi: 10.1186/1471-244X-14-136

Kessler, R. C., Adler, L. A., Gruber, M. J., Sarawate, C. A., Spencer, T., and Van Brunt, D. L. (2007). Validity of the world health organization adult ADHD self-report scale (ASRS) screener in a representative sample of health plan members. *Int. J. Methods Psychiatr. Res.* 16, 52–65. doi: 10.1002/mpr.208

Khaylis, A., Trockel, M., and Taylor, C. B. (2009). Binge drinking in women at risk for developing eating disorders. *Int. J. Eat. Disord.* 42, 409–414. doi: 10.1002/eat.20644

Khoddam, R., Jackson, N. J., and Leventhal, A. M. (2016). Internalizing symptoms and conduct problems: redundant, incremental, or interactive risk factors for adolescent substance use during the first year of high school? *Drug Alcohol Depend.* 169, 48–55. doi: 10.1016/j.drugalcdep.2016.10.007

Knight, J. R., Sherritt, L., Shrier, L. A., Harris, S. K., and Chang, G. (2002). Validity of the CRAFFT substance abuse screening test among adolescent clinic patients. *Arch. Pediatr. Adolesc. Med.* 156, 607–614.

Lansford, J. E., Erath, S., Yu, T., Pettit, G. S., Dodge, K. A., and Bates, J. E. (2008). The developmental course of illicit substance use from age 12 to 22: links with depressive, anxiety, and behavior disorders at age 18. *J. Child Psychol. Psychiatry* 49, 877–885. doi: 10.1111/j.1469-7610.2008.01915.x

Lee, S. S., Humphreys, K. L., Flory, K., Liu, R., and Glass, K. (2011). Prospective association of childhood attention-deficit/hyperactivity disorder (ADHD) and substance use and abuse/dependence: a meta-analytic review. *Clin. Psychol. Rev.* 31, 328–341. doi: 10.1016/j.cpr.2011.01.006

Liao, T. F. (1994). *Interpreting Probability Models: Logit, Probit, and Other Generalized Linear Models.* Thousand Oaks, CA: Sage.

Lucas, C. P., Zhang, H., Fisher, P. W., Shaffer, D., Regier, D. A., Narrow, W. E., et al. (2001). The DISC predictive scales (DPS): efficiently screening for diagnoses. *J. Am. Acad. Child Adolesc. Psychiatry* 40, 443–449. doi: 10.1097/00004583-200104000-00013

Mangerud, W. L., Bjerkeset, O., Holmen, T. L., Lydersen, S., and Indredavik, M. S. (2014). Smoking, alcohol consumption, and drug use among adolescents with psychiatric disorders compared with a population based sample. *J. Adolesc.* 37, 1189–1199. doi: 10.1016/j.adolescence.2014.08.007

Maslowsky, J., and Schulenberg, J. E. (2013). Interaction matters: quantifying conduct problem x depressive symptoms interaction and its association with adolescent alcohol, cigarette, and marijuana use in a national sample. *Dev. Psychopathol.* 25, 1029–1043. doi: 10.1017/S0954579413000357

McDonald, R. P. (2013). *Test Theory: A Unified Treatment: Psychology Press.* New York, NY: Routledge.

Merikangas, K. R., He, J. P., Burstein, M., Swanson, S. A., Avenevoli, S., Cui, L., et al. (2010). Lifetime prevalence of mental disorders in US adolescents: results from the national comorbidity survey replication–adolescent supplement (NCS-A). *J. Am. Acad. Child Adolesc. Psychiatry* 49, 980–989. doi: 10.1016/j.jaac.2010.05.017

Mustelin, L., Latvala, A., Raevuori, A., Rose, R. J., Kaprio, J., and Keski-Rahkonen, A. (2016). Risky drinking behaviors among women with eating disorders: a longitudinal community-based study. *Int. J. Eat. Disord.* 49, 563–571. doi: 10.1002/eat.22526

Nelemans, S. A., Hale, W. W. III, Raaijmakers, Q. A. W., Branje, S. J. T., van Lier, P. A. C., and Meeus, W. H. J. (2016). Longitudinal associations between social anxiety symptoms and cannabis use throughout adolescence: the role of peer involvement. *Eur. Child Adolesc. Psychiatry* 25, 483–492. doi: 10.1007/s00787-015-0747-8

Ohannessian, C. M. (2014). Anxiety and substance use during adolescence. *Subs. Abuse* 35, 418–425. doi: 10.1080/08897077.2014.953663

Pardee, C. S., Colder, C. R., and Bowker, J. C. (2014). Dynamic associations among alcohol use and anxiety symptoms in early adolescence. *Psychol. Addic. Behav.* 28, 1246–1252. doi: 10.1037/a0038372

Pedersen, D. E. (2013). Gender differences in college binge drinking: examining the role of depression and school stress. *Soc. Sci. J.* 50, 521–529. doi: 10.1016/j.soscij.2013.03.003

Pedersen, M. U., Thomsen, K. R., Heradstveit, O., Skogen, J. C., Hesse, M., and Jones, S. (2018). Externalizing behavior problems are related to substance use in adolescents across six samples from Nordic countries. *Eur. Child Adolesc. Psychiatry* 27, 1551–1561. doi: 10.1007/s00787-018-1148-6

R Core Team (2018). *R: A Language and Environment for Statistical Computing.* Vienna: R Foundation for Statistical Computing.

Ramos, M., Boada, L., Moreno, C., Llorente, C., Romo, J., and Parellada, M. (2013). Attitude and risk of substance use in adolescents diagnosed with asperger syndrome. *Drug Alcohol Depend.* 133, 535–540. doi: 10.1016/j.drugalcdep.2013.07.022

Regier, D. A., Farmer, M. E., Rae, D. S., Locke, B. Z., Keith, S. J., Judd, L. L., et al. (1990). Comorbidity of mental disorders with alcohol and other drug abuse: results from the epidemiologic catchment area (ECA) study. *JAMA* 264, 2511–2518. doi: 10.1001/jama.264.19.2511

Rohde, P., Lewinsohn, P. M., and Seeley, J. R. (1996). Psychiatric comorbidity with problematic alcohol use in high school students. *J. Am. Acad. Child Adolesc. Psychiatry* 35, 101–109. doi: 10.1097/00004583-199601000-00018

Santosh, P. J., and Mijovic, A. (2006). Does pervasive developmental disorder protect children and adolescents against drug and alcohol use? *Eur. Child Adolesc. Psychiatry* 15, 183–188. doi: 10.1007/s00787-005-0517-0

Savage, J. E., Kaprio, J., Korhonen, T., Pulkkinen, L., Rose, R. J., Verhulst, B., et al. (2016). The effects of social anxiety on alcohol and cigarette use across adolescence: results from a longitudinal twin study in Finland. *Psychol. Addic. Behav.* 30, 462–474. doi: 10.1037/adb0000183

Schmits, E., Mathys, C., and Quertemont, E. (2015). A longitudinal study of cannabis use initiation among high school students: effects of social anxiety, expectancies, peers and alcohol. *J. Adolesc.* 41, 43–52. doi: 10.1016/j.adolescence.2015.02.009

Schmits, E., Mathys, C., and Quertemont, E. (2016). Is social anxiety associated with cannabis use? The role of cannabis use effect expectancies in middle adolescence. *J. Child Adolesc. Subs. Abuse* 25, 348–359. doi: 10.1080/1067828x.2015.1039683

Schulte, M. T., Ramo, D., and Brown, S. A. (2009). Gender differences in factors influencing alcohol use and drinking progression among adolescents. *Clin. Psychol. Rev.* 29, 535–547. doi: 10.1016/j.cpr.2009.06.003

Serra-Pinheiro, M. A., Coutinho, E. S., Souza, I. S., Pinna, C., Fortes, D., Araújo, C., et al. (2013). Is ADHD a risk factor independent of conduct disorder for illicit substance use? A meta-analysis and metaregression investigation. *J. Attent. Disord.* 17, 459–469. doi: 10.1177/1087054711435362

Skogen, J. C., Bøe, T., Knudsen, A. K., and Hysing, M. (2013). Psychometric properties and concurrent validity of the CRAFFT among Norwegian adolescents. Ung@hordaland, a population-based study. *Addict. Behav.* 38, 2500–2505. doi: 10.1016/j.addbeh.2013.05.002

Skogen, J. C., Sivertsen, B., Lundervold, A. J., Stormark, K. M., Jakobsen, R., and Hysing, M. (2014). Alcohol and drug use among adolescents: and the co-occurrence of mental health problems. Ung@hordaland, a population-based study. *BMJ Open* 4:e005357. doi: 10.1136/bmjopen-2014-005357

Stapinski, L. A., Montgomery, A. A., and Araya, R. (2016). Anxiety, depression and risk of cannabis use: examining the internalising pathway to use among chilean adolescents. *Drug Alcohol Depend.* 166, 109–115. doi: 10.1016/j.drugalcdep.2016.06.032

StataCorp (2015). *Stata Statistical Software: Release 14.* College Station, TX: StataCorp LP.

Tarter, R. E., Vanyukov, M., Kirisci, L., Reynolds, M., and Clark, D. B. (2006). Predictors of marijuana use in adolescents before and after licit drug use: examination of the gateway hypothesis. *Am. J. Psychiatry* 163, 2134–2140. doi: 10.1176/ajp.2006.163.12.2134

Thapar, A., and McGuffin, P. (1998). Validity of the shortened mood and feelings questionnaire in a community sample of children and adolescents: a preliminary research note. *Psychiatry Res.* 81, 259–268. doi: 10.1016/s0165-1781(98)00073-0

Tomlinson, K. L., Cummins, K. M., and Brown, S. A. (2013). Social anxiety and onset of drinking in early adolescence. *J. Child Adolesc. Subs. Abuse* 22, 163–177. doi: 10.1080/1067828x.2012.747994

Van Oers, J., Bongers, I., Van de Goor, L., and Garretsen, H. (1999). Alcohol consumption, alcohol-related problems, problem drinking, and socioeconomic status. *Alcohol Alcohol.* 34, 78–88. doi: 10.1093/alcalc/34.1.78

Wolitzky-Taylor, K., Bobova, L., Zinbarg, R. E., Mineka, S., and Craske, M. G. (2012). Longitudinal investigation of the impact of anxiety and mood disorders in adolescence on subsequent substance use disorder onset and vice versa. *Addict. Behav.* 37, 982–985. doi: 10.1016/j.addbeh.2012.03.026

Wu, L.-T., Gersing, K., Burchett, B., Woody, G. E., and Blazer, D. G. (2011). Substance use disorders and comorbid Axis I and II psychiatric disorders among young psychiatric patients: findings from a large electronic health records database. *J. Psychiatr. Res.* 45, 1453–1462. doi: 10.1016/j.jpsychires.2011.06.012

Wu, P., Goodwin, R. D., Fuller, C., Liu, X., Comer, J. S., Cohen, P., et al. (2010). The relationship between anxiety disorders and substance use among adolescents in the community: specificity and gender differences. *J. Youth Adolesc.* 39, 177–188. doi: 10.1007/s10964-008-9385-5

Zulauf, C. A., Sprich, S. E., Safren, S. A., and Wilens, T. E. (2014). The complicated relationship between attention deficit/hyperactivity disorder and substance use disorders. *Curr. Psychiatry Rep.* 16, 1–11.

Zwaanswijk, M., Van Der Ende, J., Verhaak, P. F., Bensing, J. M., and Verhulst, F. C. (2003). Factors associated with adolescent mental health service need and utilization. *J. Am. Acad. Child Adolesc. Psychiatry* 42, 692–700. doi: 10.1097/01.chi.0000046862.56865.b7

APPENDIX I

TABLE A1 | Full range of ICD-10 psychiatric diagnoses (F and R codes) in the clinical sample, and the psychiatric diagnostic categories employed in the study.

Diagnostic category	ICD-10 code	ICD-10 diagnosis
ADHD	F900	Hyperkinetic disorders
	F901	Disturbance of activity and attention
	F908	Other hyperkinetic disorders
	F909	Attention-deficit hyperactivity disorder, unspecified type
Conduct disorders	F910	Conduct disorder confined to family context
	F911	Unsocialized conduct disorder
	F913	Oppositional defiant disorder
	F918	Other conduct disorders
	F919	Conduct disorder, unspecified
	F920	Depressive conduct disorder
	F928	Other mixed disorders of conduct and emotions
	F929	Mixed disorder of conduct and emotions, unspecified
Anxiety disorders	F401	Social phobias
	F402	Specific (isolated) phobias
	F408	Other phobic anxiety disorders
	F410	Panic disorder (episodic paroxysmal anxiety)
	F411	Generalized anxiety disorder
	F412	Mixed anxiety and depressive disorder
	F413	Other mixed anxiety disorders
	F418	Other specified anxiety disorders
	F419	Anxiety disorder, unspecified
	F420	Predominantly obsessional thoughts or ruminations
	F421	Predominantly compulsive acts (obsessional rituals)
	F422	Mixed obsessional thoughts and acts
	F429	Obsessive-compulsive disorder, unspecified
	F452	Hypochondriacal disorders
	F930	Separation anxiety disorder of childhood
	F931	Phobic anxiety disorder of childhood
	F932	Social anxiety disorder of childhood
	F940	Elective mutism
	F932	Social anxiety disorder of childhood
	F940	Elective mutism
Depression/mood disorders	F310	Bipolar affective disorder, current episode hypomanic
	F311	Bipolar affective disorder, current episode manic without psychotic symptoms
	F313	Bipolar affective disorder, current episode mild or moderate depression
	F316	Bipolar affective disorder, current episode mixed
	F317	Bipolar affective disorder, currently in remission
	F319	Bipolar affective disorder, unspecified
	F320	Mild depressive episode
	F3200	Mild depressive episode
	F321	Moderate depressive episode
	F322	Severe depressive episode without psychotic symptoms
	F328	Other depressive episodes
	F329	Depressive episode, unspecified
	F331	Recurrent depressive disorder, current episode moderate

(Continued)

TABLE A1 | Continued

Diagnostic category	ICD-10 code	ICD-10 diagnosis
	F332	Recurrent depressive disorder, current episode severe without psychotic symptoms
	F333	Recurrent depressive disorder, current episode severe with psychotic symptoms
	F338	Other recurrent depressive disorders
	F349	Persistent mood (affective) disorder, unspecified
	F381	Other recurrent mood (affective) disorders
	F412	Mixed anxiety and depressive disorder
Trauma-related disorders	F430	Acute stress reaction
	F431	Post-traumatic stress disorder
	F4320	Adjustment disorder, unspecified
	F4321	Adjustment disorder with depressed mood
	F4322	Adjustment disorder with anxiety
	F4323	Adjustment disorder with mixed anxiety and depressed mood
	F4325	Adjustment disorder with mixed disturbance of emotions and conduct
	F438	Other reactions to severe stress
	F439	Reaction to severe stress, unspecified
Psychotic disorders	F2090	Schizophrenia, unspecified
	F21	Schizotypal disorder
	F231	Acute polymorphic psychotic disorder with symptoms of schizophrenia
	F239	Acute and transient psychotic disorder, unspecified
	F2390	Acute and transient psychotic disorder, unspecified
	F29	Unspecified non-organic psychosis
	F333	Recurrent depressive disorder, current episode severe with psychotic symptoms
Autistic disorders	F840	Childhood autism
	F841	Atypical autism
	F845	Asperger syndrome
	F849	Pervasive developmental disorder, unspecified
Eating disorders	F500	Anorexia nervosa
	F501	Atypical anorexia nervosa
	F502	Bulimia nervosa
	F503	Atypical bulimia nervosa
	F509	Eating disorder, unspecified
Other psychiatric diagnoses	F449	Dissociative (conversion) disorder, unspecified
	F454	Persistent somatoform pain disorder
	F489	Neurotic disorder, unspecified
	F510	Non-organic insomnia
	F512	Non-organic disorder of the sleep-wake schedule
	F54	Psychological and behavioral factors associated with disorders or diseases classified elsewhere
	F601	Schizoid personality disorder
	F633	Trichotillomania
	F640	Transsexualism
	F659	Disorder of sexual preference, unspecified
	F933	Sibling rivalry disorder
	F938	Other childhood emotional disorders
	F939	Childhood emotional disorder, unspecified
	F941	Reactive attachment disorder of childhood
	F942	Disinhibited attachment disorder of childhood
	F951	Chronic motor or vocal tic disorder
	F952	Combined vocal and multiple motor tic disorder (de la Tourette)
	F980	Non-organic enuresis

(Continued)

TABLE A1 | Continued

Diagnostic category	ICD-10 code	ICD-10 diagnosis
	F981	Non-organic encopresis
	F988	Other specified behavioral and emotional disorders with onset usually occurring in childhood and adolescence
	F989	Unspecified behavioral and emotional disorders with onset usually occurring in childhood and adolescence
	R418	Other symptoms and signs involving cognitive functions and awareness
	R452	Unhappiness
	R454	Irritability and anger
	R457	State of emotional shock and stress, unspecified
	R458	Other symptoms and signs involving emotional state
	R466	Undue concern and preoccupation with stressful events
Non-diagnosis	1000	No proven diagnosis on Axis I
	1999	Not sufficient information to code on Axis I
	–	No F- or R-codes on Axis I

4

The Relationship Between Childhood Physical and Sexual Abuse and Adolescent Cannabis Use

Víctor De la Peña-Arteaga [1,2], Sarah O. Nogueira [1,2], Michael Lynskey [3] and Lindsey A. Hines [4]**

[1] Bellvitge Biomedical Research Institute, Barcelona, Spain, [2] Faculty of Medicine and Health Sciences, University of Barcelona, Barcelona, Spain, [3] Addictions Department, Institute of Psychiatry, Psychology & Neuroscience (IoPPN), King's College London, London, United Kingdom, [4] Centre for Academic Mental Health, Population Health Sciences, University of Bristol, Bristol, United Kingdom

Edited by:
Daniel Feingold,
Ariel University, Israel

Reviewed by:
Daria Piacentino,
National Institutes of Health (NIH),
United States
Bruno Kluwe Schiavon,
University of Minho, Portugal

***Correspondence:**
Víctor De la Peña-Arteaga
vdelapena@idibell.cat
Lindsey A. Hines
Lindsey.hines@bristol.ac.uk

Background: Among adolescents, cannabis use is a health concern due to associations with drug addiction and mental health disorders across the life course. It has been shown that childhood maltreatment is associated with drug addiction in adulthood. However, a better understanding of the relationship between maltreatment and drug use may improve targeted prevention and interventions. The aim of this systematic review is to describe the association between exposure to childhood maltreatment, specifically physical and sexual abuse, with adolescent cannabis use.

Methods: A systematic search strategy was applied to Embase, PsycINFO, and Ovid MEDLINE(R) databases. Methods followed Preferred Reporting Items for Systematic Reviews and Meta-Analyses (PRISMA) guidelines. Abstract and title screening was performed to identify papers which reported an estimate of the association between childhood physical or sexual abuse and adolescent cannabis use. Full text screening of each paper was performed, and data were extracted and study quality assessed. Weighted means meta-analysis was performed on studies reporting odds ratios as effect estimates.

Results: Of 8,780 screened articles, 13 were identified for inclusion. Eight papers received a quality rating score indicating lower risk of bias. Eleven papers reported the relationship between childhood sexual abuse and adolescent cannabis use; effect estimates ranged from AOR 0.53–AOR 2.18 (weighted mean OR 1.29, 95% CI 1.08–1.49). The relationship between childhood physical abuse and adolescent cannabis use was reported in 7 papers; effect estimates ranged from AOR 1.25–AOR 1.87 (weighted mean OR 1.39, 95% CI 1.12–1.66). Differences in the strength of the evidence were observed by the method of exposure ascertainment, and there was some evidence of differences in association by gender, age of cannabis initiation, and the severity of the abuse.

Conclusions: This systematic review indicates childhood physical or sexual abuse may increase risk of adolescent-onset cannabis use. Few studies considered variation in timing of onset, or by gender. Adolescent cannabis use precedes is strongly associated with increased risk of negative mental health outcomes; further exploration of adolescent cannabis use's place on the causal pathway between childhood abuse and adult mental health problems is warranted to improve intervention.

Keywords: childhood maltreatment, physical abuse, sexual abuse, adolescence, cannabis, drug use, systematic review

INTRODUCTION

Globally, cannabis is the most commonly used internationally regulated drug (1). Adolescence is a key period for initiation of cannabis use (2). Cannabis use in adolescence is considered an area of public health concern as adolescence is recognised as a key period for development (3, 4) and there is research associating drug abuse with neurobiological changes in the developing brain of adolescents (5). There are notable recent changes regarding cannabis; policy on its use is becoming more liberal worldwide (6), and cannabis use is increasing amongst young Europeans, with prevalence of past-month use amongst those aged 15–34 years estimated at 5.4% in 2017 (7).

Adolescent cannabis use is a key target for early intervention strategies (8). Recent reviews have identified that adolescent cannabis use raises likelihood of depression and suicide attempts in later life (9), and cannabis use is consistently associated with increased likelihood of psychosis (10). Additionally, adolescent cannabis use is associated with poorer education and employment outcomes (11–13), and with acute risks from use such as car accidents (14). In a stage-sequential model of drug use and addiction, initiation of drug use is a necessary stage before individuals can escalate in frequency of use and problematic use (15). Exploring the early stages of drug use can have implications for better understanding of the pathways that lead to adult addiction and mental health disorders. Consequently, there is value in identifying risk factors for adolescent cannabis use in order to target prevention and intervention efforts.

A known risk factor for addiction is childhood adversity. Meta-analyses have shown that experiencing Adverse Childhood Experiences (ACEs) can raise the likelihood of experiencing negative physical and mental health outcomes (16, 17). Recent systematic reviews and meta-analysis (18–20) have found evidence for an association between childhood maltreatment or past traumatic events and drug problems later in life. However, these reviews have focussed mainly on dependence across the life course. The authors are unaware of a review which has focussed exclusively on non-problematic cannabis use during adolescence.

Previous reviews have focussed on broad conceptualisations of childhood adversity and trauma, but it is not clear that all childhood ACEs (classically conceptualised as sexual, physical or emotional abuse, emotional neglect, substance abuse by the parents, parental mental illness or suicide attempt, violence between parents, parental separation, bullying and parental criminal conviction) have the same relationship to outcomes. In the present review, we explore childhood physical abuse (CPA) and childhood sexual abuse (CSA) as risk factors. It is estimated that, globally, half of all children will experience or witness some form of violence in childhood (21). Although global meta-analyses estimate the prevalence of physical and sexual abuse to be minimal to moderate severity (22), childhood physical and sexual abuse in childhood are both public health concerns given their association with negative outcomes across the life course (23). In relation to cannabis use and dependence, a study breaking down risk factors by stages of drug use found a relationship between CSA and exposure to cannabis, but not progression to dependence (24). Studies of these risk factors for illicit drug use have contradictory findings, with physical abuse more strongly associated than sexual abuse in some studies (25, 26), while others show the opposite relationship (27).

This systematic review focusses on general population studies to describe the association between exposure to the adverse childhood experiences of physical and sexual abuse and adolescent cannabis use. We explore the quality of the literature on the relationship between childhood physical and sexual abuse and discuss the consistency of findings and the implications for cannabis use.

METHODS

Research Design

The present study consists of a systematic review of the literature based on the Preferred Reporting Items for Systematic Reviews and Meta-Analyses (PRISMA) guidelines.

Information Sources

The electronic databases used for this systematic review were Embase, PsycINFO and Ovid MEDLINE(R). The search was performed at two different points in time: June 2017 and September 2020.

Search

The following search terms were used to perform the search in the electronic databases [selected using a Participants, Interventions, Comparators, Outcomes, and Study design approach (28)]:

[(Teenage or Adolescent or Adolescence or Youth or Child) and (Maltreatment or "Child abuse" or "Sexual abuse" or "Physical abuse" or "Adverse experience" or Trauma or Stress) and ("Misuse" or "First use" or Initiation or "Illicit use" or "Use" or "Abuse" or Experimentation) and (Drug or "Illicit drug" or

Cannabis or Marijuana or Hash* or Skunk or Opiate or Heroin or Stimulant or Alcohol or Chemsex or "Novel Psychoactive Substance" or "Legal high" or Ecstasy or Cocaine or Meth or Tobacco or Nicotine or Cigarette)].tw.

The search was limited by title and abstract content (.tw.). No further limits were used. Alcohol, tobacco and other illegal drugs search terms were included to ensure capture of papers where cannabis use was a secondary focus.

Eligibility Criteria

Inclusion/Exclusion Criteria

Studies were included if they met the following inclusion criteria:

1. Reported as part of a peer reviewed journal and as part of the databases used to the search or their references.
2. Individuals were up to 26 years old. This age range encompasses contemporary patterns of adolescent growth and their social role transitions (29), as well as capturing a period in which neuronal connexions are continuing to develop (30).
3. Papers published in English.
4. General population samples.
5. Included a measure of association between childhood physical or sexual abuse and cannabis use.

Studies were excluded if:

1. Reviews, meta-analysis, conference abstracts, dissertations, lectures, book chapters or incomplete articles.
2. Regarding sample: excluding
    a. Individuals diagnosed with addiction or substance use disorder.
    b. Animal studies, due to the aim of researching human adolescence.
    c. Groups of drug using participants only or inpatients of an addiction clinic.

Study Selection

Once the search was run, by two researchers (VDA and SON), results were exported into a reference manager software. Duplicates were removed using the same software and afterwards an abstract and title screening was performed to obtain the relevant full text studies. During this stage, papers were excluded using the criteria stated above.

Subsequently full text screening was performed by researcher review (VDA and SON) of each paper. Inclusion and exclusion criteria were applied as above to determine suitability for inclusion in review. Papers excluded at this stage mainly represented the ones outside of the age range or focused exclusively on cannabis use disorders rather than cannabis use.

As mentioned, the full search and screenings were performed by two researchers independently. Afterwards, each inconsistency was examined by another researcher (LH) to obtain a final list of included papers. To finalise, references of key papers were manually screened to ensure review completeness.

Quality Assessment

An adapted version of the Newcastle-Ottawa Scale (NOS) for assessing the quality of non-randomised studies in meta-analyses [by Wells et al. (31)] was used for this review. With this tool, each study was judged on three broad perspectives: the selection of the study groups; the comparability of the groups; and the ascertainment of either the exposure or outcome of interest for case-control or cohort studies, respectively. Once again, papers were rated for quality by two researchers independently (VDA and SON) and inconsistencies were reviewed by a third researcher (LH).

Weighted Mean Meta-Analysis

The studies reporting Odds Ratios (OR) and Confidence Intervals (CI) were entered into a weighted mean meta-analysis. Weights were assigned to each study taking into account each sample size and OR. This was obtained to summarise the global magnitude of effect sizes with the available data.

RESULTS

Study Selection

The final study selection of 13 papers is fully shown in **Figure 1**. Characteristics of each of the included studies can be seen in both quality assessment table (**Table 1**) and data extraction table (**Table 2**) (32–44).

Quality Assessment and Risk of Bias

According to the quality rating scale, one paper achieved the maximum rating of eight (42), and three got a very high grade of seven (38–40). A further eight papers received five or more of the available quality rating points and only one paper obtained a very low score of two (43).

Studies did not consistently differ by the representativeness of the cohort or the selection method of participants. Contrastingly, other rated categories, as control for confounders, ascertainment of childhood abuse, or data collection's start point were very different among studies. These differences created most of the variations seen in the final ratings. The interrater reliability between researchers was 0.42 (Kappa value).

Definition of Physical and Sexual Abuse

Nine out of 13 papers used non-structured and structured self-reported scales (**Table 2**). Only one of these papers (39) included interviews as part of the assessment. The remaining four papers (33, 40, 41, 44) used data from child protective services records.

Three studies (34, 35, 44) differentiated outcomes based on the number or type of traumatic events. One study (34) made a differentiation between being sexually abused once or twice, three or more times and raped. When comparing frequency of events in adjusted models; occasional cannabis use Adjusted Odds Ratios (AOR) was 1.4 (95% CI 1.0–2.0) when sexual abuse was once or twice, compared to an AOR of 2.1 (95% CI 1.4–3.3) when sexual abuse was experienced three or more times. In contrast, frequent cannabis use AOR was 2.8 (95% CI 1.7–4.4) when sexual abuse was once or twice compared to an AOR of

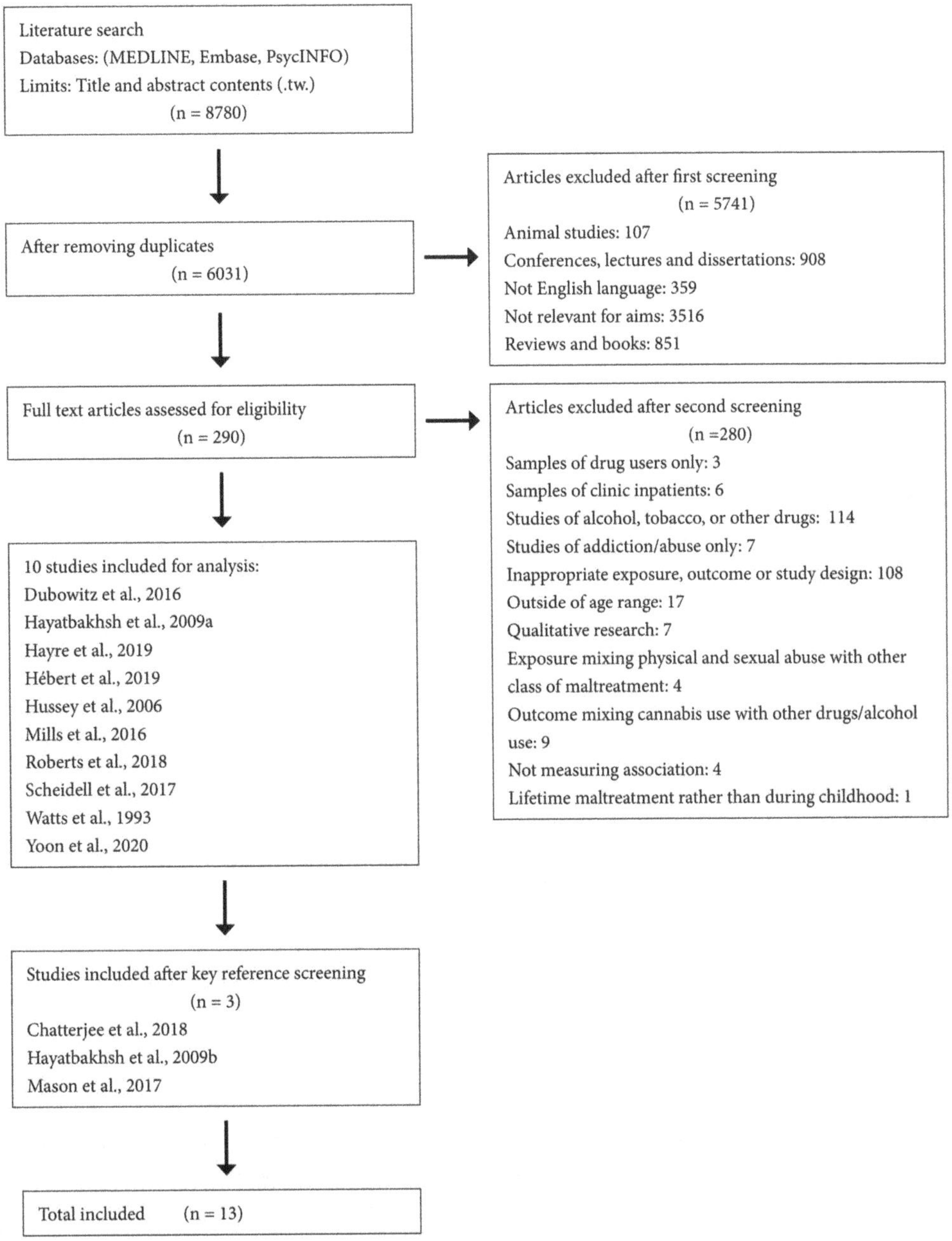

FIGURE 1 | Flowchart of search results.

3.6 (95% CI 2.0–6.4) when sexual abuse was experienced three or more times.

Additionally, one study (35) explored differences between the type of sexual abuse, comparing non-penetrative or penetrative. It did not identify differences for type of sexual abuse (35), finding an effect of AOR 1.7 (95% CI 1.3–2.2) for non-penetrative sexual abuse on any cannabis use, compared to AOR 1.8 (95% CI 1.3–2.7) for penetrative sexual abuse on any cannabis use.

One study (44) differentiated between timing of abuse for the association with cannabis use. Odds of recent cannabis use aged 12–18 were increased amongst those reporting adolescent physical abuse (AOR 1.87, 95% CI 1.06–3.32), but were not significantly different among those reporting early childhood physical abuse (AOR 1.72, 95% CI 0.95–3.10), early childhood sexual abuse (AOR 0.55, 95% CI 0.25–1.21) and middle childhood sexual abuse (AOR 0.53, 95% CI 0.22–1.26).

Association Between Childhood Maltreatment and Adolescent Cannabis Use

For sexual abuse, a significant association between the exposure and adolescent cannabis use was observed in 5 of the 11 studies which focussed on this form of abuse (34, 35, 38, 39, 43), and

TABLE 1 | Quality rating.

References	Representativeness of the cohort	Selection of participants who did not experience childhood abuse	Ascertainment of childhood abuse	Did data collection start before participants started using cannabis?	Did the study control for confounders that will make samples comparable?	Was follow-up long enough for outcomes to occur	Adequacy of sample retention	Total
Chatterjee et al. (32)	1	1	0	0	2	0	0	4
Dubowitz et al. (33)	1	1	1	1	0	0	1	5
Hayatbakhsh et al. (34)	1	1	0	1	2	0	1	6
Hayatbakhsh et al. (35)	1	1	0	1	1	0	0	4
Hayre et al. (36)	1	1	0	0	1	0	1	4
Hébert et al. (37)	1	1	0	0	1	0	1	4
Hussey et al. (38)	1	1	1	1	2	0	1	7
Mason et al. (39)	1	1	1	1	1	1	1	7
Mills et al. (40)	1	1	1	1	2	0	1	7
Roberts et al. (41)	1	0	1	1	1	1	1	6
Scheidell et al. (42)	1	1	1	1	2	1	1	8
Watts et al. (43)	1	1	0	0	0	0	0	2
Yoon et al. (44)	1	1	1	1	0	0	1	5

Selection	***Max 4****
Representativeness of the cohort.	**truly/somewhat representative cohort sample; 0 selected group e.g., volunteers/no sampling description.*
Selection of the participants who did not experience childhood abuse.	**from the same community as the exposed cohort; 0 different source/no description.*
Ascertainment of childhood abuse.	**secure record (government record)/structured interview; 0 written self-report/no description.*
Did data collection start before participants started using cannabis?	**yes; 0 no.*
Comparability	***Max 2****
Did the study control for confounders that will make samples comparable?	**study controls for sex/gender; * study controls for SES.*
Outcome	***Max 3****
Was follow-up long enough for outcomes to occur.	**yes - followed up past age 25; 0 no.* **complete follow up - all subjects accounted for.*
Adequacy of sample retention.	**subjects lost to follow up unlikely to introduce bias – > 60 % follow up, or description provided of those lost;* *0 follow up rate <60% and no description of those lost/no description of retention or sample loss.*
Total maximum: 8*	

5 of the 11 studies reported weaker, non-significant evidence (33, 40–42, 44). One study (37) stratified by gender and found a significant association in females (OR 2.18, 95% CI 1.84–2.59), but a non-significant association for males (OR 1.28, 95% CI 0.88–1.84). Adjusted odds ratios ranged from AOR 1.4 (95% CI 1.0–2.0) (34) to AOR 2.00 ($P \leq 0.001$) (38) in longitudinal studies, and as high as AOR 2.18 (95% CI 1.84–2.59) in a cross-sectional study (analysis restricted to females only) (37). Significant correlations of 0.19–0.2 between sexual abuse and lifetime adolescent cannabis use by age 18 were also reported (39, 43). In longitudinal studies the non-significant effect estimates ranged from AOR 0.53 (95% CI 0.22–1.26) (44) to AOR 1.52 (0.98–2.36) (33). Notably, all the studies reporting a significant association relied on self-report of sexual abuse from participants and the majority of the studies that identified weaker evidence used child protection records of childhood sexual abuse to determine the exposure (33, 40, 41, 44). Six studies reporting AOR and 95% CI (33–35, 40, 42, 44) were entered into a meta-analysis, producing a weighted mean effect of OR 1.29 (95% CI 1.08–1.49) for the relationship between childhood sexual abuse and adolescent cannabis use.

For physical abuse, a significant association between the exposure and adolescent cannabis use was observed in 4 of the 7 studies which focussed on this form of abuse (36, 38, 41, 42), and weaker evidence was reported in 2 of the 7 studies (33, 40). One study (44) differentiated timing of abuse, and consequently reported both significant and non-significant findings dependent on the timing of exposure (see discussion in section Definition of Physical and Sexual Abuse). Significant effect estimates ranged from AOR 1.38 (95% CI 1.09–1.76) (42) to AOR 1.87 (95% CI 1.06–3.32) when exposure to abuse was in early adolescence (44) in longitudinal studies. A Beta of 0.62 (95% CI 0.25–0.99) was reported in a cross-sectional study (36). This stronger evidence for an association between physical abuse and adolescent cannabis use came from studies with both self-reported abuse and child protection records as outcomes. All of the studies providing weaker, non-significant evidence were longitudinal, and used child protection records as their exposure.

TABLE 2 | Data extraction.

References	Country	Study design	Measure of childhood abuse	% female	Mean age of sample (range)	Sample size	Cannabis use measure (lifetime, past year, frequency)	Statistical method	Univariable effect estimate (CI): composite measure of physical/ sexual abuse	Univariable effect estimate (CI): physical abuse	Univariable effect estimate (CI): sexual abuse	Covariate adjustment	Adjusted effect estimate (CI): composite measure of physical/ sexual abuse	Adjusted effect estimate (CI): physical abuse	Adjusted effect estimate (CI): sexual abuse	Notes
Chatterjee et al. (32)	USA	Cross-sectional	Self-reported, semi-structured scale	49.7	9th, and 11th grade	79,339	First use age 14 and under	Multivariable logistic regression analysis	na	na	na	Race/ethnicity, poverty status, grade, family composition, school location, and connexions to parents	Female 1.24 (1.04–1.43) Male 1.21 (1.03–1.42)	na	na	
Dubowitz et al. (33)	USA	Prospective cohort study	Child protective services records	Not specified	18 and under	702	Some use	Multinomial logistic regression analysis	na	na	na	Peer use, neglect, emotional maltreatment, extent of childhood maltreatment, sex, site, ethnicity/race	na	1.25 (0.80–1.95)	1.52 (0.98–2.36)	
	As above	As above	As above	As above	As above	As above	Heavy Use	Multinomial logistic regression analysis	na	na	na	Peer use, neglect, emotional maltreatment, extent of childhood maltreatment, sex, site, ethnicity/race	na	1.23 (0.72–2.08)	0.80 (0.47–1.37)	
Hayatbakhsh et al. (34)	Australia	Prospective cohort study	Self-reported	52.1	21	3,285	Occasional use	Multinomial logistic regression	—	—	SA Once or twice 1.7 (1.2–2.3) SA 3+ times 2.5 (1.7–3.9) Raped 2.2 (1.4–3.3)	Gender, mother's age, mother's education measured at the child's birth, family income, marital status and quality mother-child communication measured at 14 years, maternal anxiety, depression, smoking, alcohol consumption measured at 14 years, child internalising and externalising measured at 14 years	—	—	SA Once or twice 1.4 (1.0–2.0) SA 3+ times 2.1 (1.4–3.3) Raped 1.6 (1.0–2.6)	
	As above	As above	As above	As above	As above	As above	Frequent use	As above	na	na	SA Once or twice 2.2 (1.5–3.5) SA 3+ times 3.3 (1.9–5.7) Raped 2.7 (1.6–4.7)	Gender, mother's age, mother's education measured at the child's birth, family income, marital status and quality mother-child communication measured at 14 years, maternal anxiety, depression, smoking, alcohol consumption measured at 14 years, child internalising and externalising measured at 14 years	na	na	SA Once or twice 2.8 (1.7–4.4) SA 3+ times 3.6 (2.0–6.4) Raped 3.1 (1.7–5.8)	

(Continued)

TABLE 2 | Continued

References	Country	Study design	Measure of childhood abuse	% female	Mean age of sample (range)	Sample size	Cannabis use measure (lifetime, past year, frequency)	Statistical method	Univariable effect estimate (CI): composite measure of physical/ sexual abuse	Univariable effect estimate (CI): physical abuse	Univariable effect estimate (CI): sexual abuse	Covariate adjustment	Adjusted effect estimate (CI): composite measure of physical/ sexual abuse	Adjusted effect estimate (CI): physical abuse	Adjusted effect estimate (CI): sexual abuse	Notes
Hayatbakhsh et al. (35)	Australia	Longitudinal (MUSP), general population	Self-reported	34.3	21	3,754	Lifetime use	Multinomial logistic regression	na	na	Non-penetrative: 1.9 (1.4–2.5) Penetrative: 2.5 (1.8–3.5)	Gender, mother's age, changes in marital status, family income, problems in residential area, anxiety/depression, aggression/delinquency, nonverbal reasoning ability, school performance, puberty activity, child smoking, child alcohol use, TV watching, rule breaking at school, maternal smoking, maternal alcohol use, paternal history of crime, openness family communication	na	na	Non-penetrative: 1.7 (1.3–2.2) Penetrative: 1.8 (1.3–2.7)	
Hayre et al. (36)	Canada	Cross-sectional	Self-reported, semi-structured scale	59.3	12–18	528	Use in past month	Mediation sequential regression analysis	na	0.619 (0.245–0.993)	na	na	na	na	na	
Hébert et al. (37)	Canada	Cross-sectional school population	Self-reported, semi-structured scale	57.8	15.35 (grades 10–12)	8,194	Past year	Multivariable logistic regression analysis	na	na	na	Grade level, family structure, ethnicity. physical and emotional abuse, exposure to violence, exposure to interparental violence	na	na	Girls 2.18 (1.84–2.59) Boys 1.28 (0.88–1.84)	
Hussey et al. (38)		Prospective cohort study	Self-reported, structured, computerised	na	Grades 7–11	10,828	Last month	Binary logistic regression	—	1.65 $p \leq 0.001$	1.76 $p \leq 0.001$	Gender, age, race/ethnicity, parent's education, family income, immigrant generation, and US region	—	1.57 $p \leq 0.001$	2.00 $p \leq 0.001$	
Mason et al. (39)	US	Prospective cohort study	Interview, self-reported, childhood and adolescence	46	18	457	Life time	Path analysis	—	—	—	Mother's educational level, family after-tax income, mother's occupational level	—	—	r0.203 $p < 0.01$	
Mills et al. (40)	Australia	Prospective cohort study	State child protection agency records	52.6	21	3,778	Lifetime use	Logistic regression analysis	na	na	na	Age, gender, race, family income, maternal age, education, marital status, alcohol use, smoking, anxiety, depression	na	1.74 (0.91–3.34)	1.45 (0.77–2.72)	

(Continued)

TABLE 2 | Continued

References	Country	Study design	Measure of childhood abuse	% female	Mean age of sample (range)	Sample size	Cannabis use measure (lifetime, past year, frequency)	Statistical method	Univariable effect estimate (CI): composite measure of physical/ sexual abuse	Univariable effect estimate (CI): physical abuse	Univariable effect estimate (CI): sexual abuse	Covariate adjustment	Adjusted effect estimate (CI): composite measure of physical/ sexual abuse	Adjusted effect estimate (CI): physical abuse	Adjusted effect estimate (CI): sexual abuse	Notes
	As above	As above	As above	As above	As above	As above	Early initiation	Logistic regression analysis	na	na	na	Age, gender, race, family income, maternal age, education, marital status, alcohol use, smoking, anxiety, depression	na	2.59 (1.37–4.89)	2.11 (1.13–3.94)	
	As above	As above	As above	As above	As above	As above	Daily use	Logistic regression analysis	na	na	na	Age, gender, race, family income, maternal age, education, marital status, alcohol use, smoking, anxiety, depression	na	2.94 (1.24–6.99)	3.08 (1.14–8.29)	
Roberts et al. (41)	US	Prospective cohort study	Child protective services records	55.6	18	847	Last month	Multilevel linear models	na	na	na	Gender, race, exposure to maltreatment	na	Beta: 0.06, SE: 0.14	Beta: −0.23, SE: 0.16	
Scheidell et al. (42)	USA	Prospective cohort study	Self-reported, structured, computerised	54.3	Age 11–21	12,288	Lifetime use	Logistic regression analysis	na	1.89 (1.60–2.24)	1.69 (1.39–2.05)	Each other type of trauma, age, gender, race, and poverty	na	1.38 (1.09–1.76)	1.29 (0.97–1.71)	Only took adolescent wave results, as the other ages fell outside of the review age range
Watts et al. (43)	US	Cross-sectional	Self-reported, non-structured	100	Grades 7–12	670	Lifetime use	Analysis of variance	na	na	r0.185	na	na	na	na	Results only presented for females, consequently analysis sample N 670
Yoon et al. (44)	USA	Prospective cohort study	Child protective services records	52.9	ages 12–18	903	Past year cannabis use	Binary logistic regression	na	na	na	Gender, race, household income	na	Early childhood abuse: 1.72 (0.95–3.10) Adolescent abuse: 1.87 (1.06–3.32)	Early childhood abuse: 0.55 (0.25–1.21) Middle childhood abuse: 0.53 (0.22–1.26)	

The non-significant effect estimates ranged from AOR 1.25 (95% CI 0.80–1.95) (33) to AOR 1.74 (95% CI 0.91–3.34) (40). Four studies reporting adjusted odds ratios and confidence intervals (33, 40, 42, 44) were entered into a meta-analysis, producing a weighted mean effect of OR 1.39 (95% CI 1.12–1.66) for the relationship between childhood physical abuse and adolescent cannabis use.

Association Between Physical/Sexual Abuse and Age of Cannabis Initiation

Although not the primary focus of the review, some studies allowed an examination of the association between exposure to childhood maltreatment and age of onset of cannabis use. In a prospective cohort study, early onset of cannabis use (defined as prior to 17 years of age) was more than twice as likely amongst those who had experienced either physical abuse or sexual abuse (respectively, AOR 2.59, 95% CI 1.37–4.89 and AOR 2.11, 95% CI 1.13–3.94) (40). These effect estimates were significant, and stronger than for the association between either physical or sexual abuse and lifetime cannabis use (respectively, AOR 1.45, 95% CI 0.77–2.72 and AOR 1.45, 95% CI 0.77–2.72) (40). There was no clear linear pattern between sexual molestation and age of cannabis use in a cross-sectional study in U.S. school populations, with correlations reported by grade (7th—8th grade r0.19, 9th grade r0.03, 10th grade r0.15, 11th grade r0.09, 12th grade r0.35) (43), but it is notable that this study was rated low on quality.

Gender Differences in the Relationship Between Childhood Abuse and Adolescent Cannabis Use

Two cross-sectional studies provided separate estimates of the relationship between childhood physical/sexual abuse and adolescent cannabis use for males and females. Experiencing physical or sexual childhood abuse was associated with a significantly increased likelihood of cannabis use at age 14 or under for both males and females (32). Effect estimates were similar across genders, with an AOR of 1.24 (95% CI 1.04–1.43) for females and AOR 1.21(95% CI 1.03–1.42) for males. Experiencing sexual abuse was significantly associated with over twice the likelihood of past-year cannabis use in Canadian school grades 10–12 for females (AOR 2.18, 95% CI 1.84–2.59), but with only a slight and non-significant increase in likelihood for males (AOR 1.28, 95% CI 0.88–1.84) (37).

DISCUSSION

This review identified 13 papers reporting an association between childhood physical or sexual abuse and adolescent cannabis use (defined in the search as use up to age 26) (29). There was good evidence for a relationship between both physical and sexual abuse in childhood and increased likelihood of adolescent cannabis use in studies where abuse was self-reported. The reported range of effect sizes was similar for both physical and sexual abuse, indicating that those who experience these forms of childhood abuse may be around twice as likely to report adolescent cannabis use. However, evidence was weaker in studies where abuse was determined using child protection records. There were more papers reporting associations for sexual abuse than for physical abuse, and most of the thirteen selected papers for this systematic review had a quality rating that indicated lower risks of bias.

The range of effect sizes was similar for the association between both physical and sexual abuse and adolescent cannabis use. However, of the papers that did report both measurements, those with better quality ratings for lifetime use (40, 42), showed a stronger effect size for the association with physical abuse in comparison with sexual abuse. Physical abuse has been identified as a risk factor for adolescent drug use (20) and subsequent transition to use disorders (45), but the present results demonstrate that it has received less focus in the literature than sexual abuse (reported in 7 studies, compared to 11 for sexual abuse).

The review identified differences in the strength of the evidence for the relationship between childhood physical/sexual abuse and adolescent cannabis use were related to the method of ascertainment of abuse. In this sense, studies with data from child protective services should be interpreted carefully. Although the reliability of this source is high, detection of exposed individuals may be lower due to unreported cases to authorities. As some researchers (40) have previously observed, "rates of retrospective self-report of child maltreatment are generally much higher than rates of agency confirmation, which raises the possibility of maltreated youth being misclassified." Previous research has indicated that substantiated childhood maltreatment is no better at predicting outcomes than alleged (46). A recent review has identified that individuals who report abuse prospectively and retrospectively may represent different populations (47); consequently, it is important to compare differences between cross-sectional and prospective studies. In the present review cross-sectional and longitudinal designs were mostly in agreement, indicating that timing of reporting did not influence results.

Variations in exposure, such as the form and timing of the abuse, and the individual's gender may affect the relationship to adolescent cannabis use, but this is not widely explored in the literature. In the present review, one study (44) made a differentiation between early and middle childhood abuse, as well as adolescent abuse; only finding significant associations with past year cannabis use and physical adolescent abuse. Differences in the association with cannabis use were observed by frequency of the abuse and severity of the sexual abuse (34, 35). There were conflicting findings on whether effects may differ by gender (32, 40). Another recent review of this topic, focusing on cannabis abuse, also highlights the need for additional research on potential gender differences (19).

Adverse childhood experiences such as physical and sexual abuse are known to raise risks for life course negative mental health and addiction outcomes, and the present results indicate that adolescent cannabis use may be a plausible intervention target to mitigate these risks. A recent meta-analysis of the relationship between childhood physical/sexual abuse and adolescent cannabis abuse and dependence indicated that cannabis abuse/dependence is more likely amongst those experiencing physical abuse (OR: 1.58, 95% CI 1.01–2.46), and more than twice as likely amongst those experiencing sexual abuse (OR: 2.35, 95% CI 1.64–3.35) (19). Similarly, a comprehensive meta-analysis indicated likelihood of experiencing depression or anxiety was more than twice as high amongst those reporting childhood physical abuse (OR 2.00, 95% CI 1.25–3.19) or sexual abuse (OR 2.66, 95% CI 1.88–3.75) (48), and similar results have been found in relation to the likelihood of reporting psychotic experiences in a longitudinal cohort (physical abuse AOR, 2.24 95% CI, 1.75–2.87, sexual abuse AOR, 2.04 95% CI, 1.42–2.91) (49).

Adolescent cannabis use is a necessary step in the progression to the development of cannabis abuse/dependence (24), and is a commonly identified risk factor for anxiety, depression and psychosis (9, 50). The results of the present review add to the evidence that preventing adolescent cannabis use may be a viable intervention target for reducing risks of these negative outcomes amongst those experiencing early adversities such as physical and sexual abuse.

LIMITATIONS

This review aimed to improve on previous studies by focussing the exposure to specific forms of adversity. However, a result of this approach was that we excluded studies which included composite measures of childhood abuse including non-physical abuses (e.g., emotional abuse and neglect). Future reviews may benefit from exploring the clustering of adversities. Our conclusions regarding sex differences and age of onset are weak considering the final number of studies that provided this information. To focus on cannabis use, distinct from abuse or dependence, studies of problematic use were excluded. However, this may have precluded us from identifying variation in frequency of use, which is an important consideration in the development of addiction and mental health. Studies did not commonly report unadjusted odds ratios, with the result that odds ratios included in the meta-analysis of weighted average have different adjustment patterns. A further limitation of the meta-analyses was the exclusion of studies that did not report odds ratios. Finally, we limited the search to studies published in the English language which may have excluded some relevant literature.

CONCLUSIONS

There is some evidence both physical and sexual abuse may represent important risk factors for adolescent cannabis use. Adolescent cannabis use precedes the development of dependence, and is strongly associated with increased risk of negative mental health outcomes; further exploration of adolescent cannabis use's place on the causal pathway between childhood abuse and adult addiction and mental health problems is warranted to improve intervention.

AUTHOR CONTRIBUTIONS

VD, LH, and ML developed the concept and scope of the paper. VD and LH produced the search strategy. VD and SN ran searches, screened papers, and completed quality rating and data extraction. LH oversaw these processes and resolved any conflicting decisions. VD drafted the manuscript, and LH performed meta-analyses. All authors made substantial contributions to the interpretation of the data and contributed to revising the manuscript critically. All authors approved the final version of the study to be published and are accountable for all aspects of the work.

FUNDING

The project that gave rise to these results received the support of a fellowship from la Caixa Foundation (ID 100010434). The fellowship code for VD is LCF/BQ/DI17/11620071 and for SN LCF/BQ/DI17/11620022. LH was supported by a Wellcome Trust Sir Henry Wellcome Postdoctoral Fellowship (209158/Z/17/Z).

REFERENCES

1. United Nations Office on Drugs and Crime. *World Drug Report 2020.* (2020). United Nations Publication. Available online at: https://wdr.unodc.org/wdr2020/ (accessed November 10, 2020).
2. Behrendt S, Wittchen H, Höfler M, Lieb R, Beesdo K. Transitions from first substance use to substance use disorders in adolescence: is early onset associated with a rapid escalation? *Drug Alcohol Depend.* (2009) 99:68–78. doi: 10.1016/j.drugalcdep.2008.06.014
3. Patton G, Sawyer S, Santelli J, Ross D, Afifi R, Allen N, et al. Our future: a Lancet commission on adolescent health and wellbeing. *Lancet.* (2016) 387:2423–78. doi: 10.1016/S0140-6736(16)00579-1
4. Romeo R. The teenage brain. *Curr Dir Psychol Sci.* (2013) 22:140–5. doi: 10.1177/0963721413475445
5. Puetz V, McCrory E. Exploring the relationship between childhood maltreatment and addiction: a review of the neurocognitive evidence. *Curr Addict Rep.* (2015) 2:318–25. doi: 10.1007/s40429-015-0073-8
6. Hall W, Lynskey M. Why it is probably too soon to assess the public health effects of legalisation of recreational cannabis use in the USA. *Lancet Psychiatry.* (2016) 3:900–6. doi: 10.1016/S2215-0366(16)30071-2
7. United Nations Office on Drugs and Crime. *World Drug Report 2019.* (2019). United Nations Publication. Available online at: https://wdr.unodc.org/wdr2019/ (accessed November 10, 2020).
8. Golick J. Shifting the paradigm: adolescent cannabis abuse and the need for early intervention. *J Psychoactive Drugs.* (2016) 48:24–7. doi: 10.1080/02791072.2015.1119916

9. Gobbi G, Atkin T, Zytynski T, Wang S, Askari S, Boruff J, et al. Association of cannabis use in adolescence and risk of depression, anxiety, and suicidality in young adulthood. *JAMA Psychiatry.* (2019) 76:426–34. doi: 10.1001/jamapsychiatry.2018.4500
10. Moore T, Zammit S, Lingford-Hughes A, Barnes T, Jones P, Burke M, et al. Cannabis use and risk of psychotic or affective mental health outcomes: a systematic review. *Lancet.* (2007) 370:319–28. doi: 10.1016/S0140-6736(07)61162-3
11. Fergusson D, Horwood L. Early onset cannabis use and psychosocial adjustment in young adults. *Addiction.* (1997) 92:279–96. doi: 10.1111/j.1360-0443.1997.tb03198.x
12. Lynskey M, Hall W. The effects of adolescent cannabis use on educational attainment: a review. *Addiction.* (2000) 95:1621–30. doi: 10.1046/j.1360-0443.2000.951116213.x
13. Rodwell L, Romaniuk H, Nilsen W, Carlin J, Lee K, Patton G. Adolescent mental health and behavioural predictors of being NEET: a prospective study of young adults not in employment, education, or training. *Psychol Med.* (2017) 48:861–71. doi: 10.1017/S0033291717002434
14. Li M, Brady J, DiMaggio C, Lusardi A, Tzong K, Li G. Marijuana use and motor vehicle crashes. *Epidemiol Rev.* (2011) 34:65–72. doi: 10.1093/epirev/mxr017
15. Hines L, Morley K, Mackie C, Lynskey M. Genetic and environmental interplay in adolescent substance use disorders. *Curr Addict Rep.* (2015) 2:122–9. doi: 10.1007/s40429-015-0049-8
16. Hughes K, Bellis M, Hardcastle K, Sethi D, Butchart A, Mikton C, et al. The effect of multiple adverse childhood experiences on health: a systematic review and meta-analysis. *Lancet Public Health.* (2017) 2:e356–e66. doi: 10.1016/S2468-2667(17)30118-4
17. Petruccelli K, Davis J, Berman T. Adverse childhood experiences and associated health outcomes: a systematic review and meta-analysis. *Child Abuse Negl.* (2019) 97:104127. doi: 10.1016/j.chiabu.2019.104127
18. Konkolÿ Thege B, Horwood L, Slater L, Tan M, Hodgins D, Wild T. Relationship between interpersonal trauma exposure and addictive behaviors: a systematic review. *BMC Psychiatry.* (2017) 17:164. doi: 10.1186/s12888-017-1323-1
19. Martínez-Mota L, Jiménez-Rubio G, Hernández Hernández O, Páez-Martínez N. Influence of the type of childhood violence on cannabis abuse and dependence among adolescents: a systematic review and meta-analysis. *Adicciones.* (2020) 32:63–76. doi: 10.20882/adicciones.1050
20. Norman R, Byambaa M, De R, Butchart A, Scott J, Vos T. The long-term health consequences of child physical abuse, emotional abuse, and neglect: a systematic review and meta-analysis. *PLoS Med.* (2012) 9:e1001349. doi: 10.1371/journal.pmed.1001349
21. Hillis S, Mercy J, Amobi A, Kress H. Global prevalence of past-year violence against children: a systematic review and minimum estimates. *Pediatrics.* (2016) 137:e20154079. doi: 10.1542/peds.2015-4079
22. Viola T, Salum G, Kluwe-Schiavon B, Sanvicente-Vieira B, Levandowski M, Grassi-Oliveira R. The influence of geographical and economic factors in estimates of childhood abuse and neglect using the childhood trauma questionnaire: a worldwide meta-regression analysis. *Child Abuse Negl.* (2016) 51:1–1. doi: 10.1016/j.chiabu.2015.11.019
23. Springer K, Sheridan J, Kuo D, Carnes M. The long-term health outcomes of childhood abuse. *J Gen Intern Med.* (2003) 18:864–70. doi: 10.1046/j.1525-1497.2003.20918.x
24. Hines L, Morley K, Strang J, Agrawal A, Nelson E, Statham D, et al. Onset of opportunity to use cannabis and progression from opportunity to dependence: are influences consistent across transitions? *Drug Alcohol Depend.* (2016) 160:57–64. doi: 10.1016/j.drugalcdep.2015.12.032
25. Benjet C, Borges G, Medina-Mora M, Méndez E. Chronic childhood adversity and stages of substance use involvement in adolescents. *Drug Alcohol Depend.* (2013) 131:85–91. doi: 10.1016/j.drugalcdep.2012.12.002
26. Huang S, Trapido E, Fleming L, Arheart K, Crandall L, French M, et al. The long-term effects of childhood maltreatment experiences on subsequent illicit drug use and drug-related problems in young adulthood. *Addict. Behav.* (2011) 36:95–102. doi: 10.1016/j.addbeh.2010.09.001
27. Moran P, Vuchinich S, Hall N. Associations between types of maltreatment and substance use during adolescence. *Child Abuse Negl.* (2004) 28:565–74. doi: 10.1016/j.chiabu.2003.12.002
28. Liberati A, Altman D, Tetzlaff J, Mulrow C, Gøtzsche P, Ioannidis J, et al. The PRISMA statement for reporting systematic reviews and meta-analyses of studies that evaluate health care interventions: explanation and elaboration. *J Clin Epidemiol.* (2009) 62:e1–e34. doi: 10.1016/j.jclinepi.2009.06.006
29. Sawyer S, Azzopardi P, Wickremarathne D, Patton G. The age of adolescence. *Lancet Child Adolesc Health.* (2018) 2:223–8. doi: 10.1016/S2352-4642(18)30022-1
30. Pfefferbaum A, Mathalon D, Sullivan E, Rawles J, Zipursky R, Lim K. A quantitative magnetic resonance imaging study of changes in brain morphology from infancy to late adulthood. *Arch Neurol.* (1994) 51:874–87. doi: 10.1001/archneur.1994.00540210046012
31. Wells G, Shea B, O'Connell D, Peterson J, Welch V, Losos M, et al. *The Newcastle-Ottawa Scale (NOS) for Assessing The Quality of Nonrandomised Studies in Meta-Analyses [Internet].* Available online at: http://www.ohri.ca/programs/clinical_epidemiology/oxford.asp
32. Chatterjee D, McMorris B, Gower A, Forster M, Borowsky I, Eisenberg M. Adverse childhood experiences and early initiation of marijuana and alcohol use: the potential moderating effects of internal assets. *Subst Use Misuse.* (2018) 53:1624–32. doi: 10.1080/10826084.2017.1421224
33. Dubowitz H, Thompson R, Arria A, English D, Metzger R, Kotch J. Characteristics of child maltreatment and adolescent marijuana use. *Child Maltreat.* (2016) 21:16–25. doi: 10.1177/1077559515620853
34. Hayatbakhsh M, Najman J, Jamrozik K, Mamun A, O'Callaghan M, Williams G. Childhood sexual abuse and cannabis use in early adulthood: findings from an australian birth cohort study. *Arch Sex Behav.* (2009) 38:135–42. doi: 10.1007/s10508-007-9172-5
35. Hayatbakhsh M, Najman J, Bor W, O'Callaghan M, Williams G. Multiple risk factor model predicting cannabis use and use disorders: a longitudinal study. *Am J Drug Alcohol Abuse.* (2009) 35:399–407. doi: 10.3109/00952990903353415
36. Hayre R, Goulter N, Moretti M. Maltreatment, attachment, and substance use in adolescence: direct and indirect pathways. *Addict Behav.* (2019) 90:196–203. doi: 10.1016/j.addbeh.2018.10.049
37. Hébert M, Amédée L, Blais M, Gauthier-Duchesne A. Child sexual abuse among a representative sample of Quebec high school students: prevalence and association with mental health problems and health-risk behaviors. *Can J Psychiatry.* (2019) 64:846–54. doi: 10.1177/0706743719861387
38. Hussey J, Chang J, Kotch J. Child maltreatment in the United States: prevalence, risk factors, and adolescent health consequences. *Pediatrics.* (2006) 118:933–42. doi: 10.1542/peds.2005-2452
39. Mason W, Russo M, Chmelka M, Herrenkohl R, Herrenkohl T. Parent and peer pathways linking childhood experiences of abuse with marijuana use in adolescence and adulthood. *Addict Behav.* (2017) 66:70–5. doi: 10.1016/j.addbeh.2016.11.013
40. Mills R, Kisely S, Alati R, Strathearn L, Najman J. Child maltreatment and cannabis use in young adulthood: a birth cohort study. *Addiction.* (2016) 112:494–501. doi: 10.1111/add.13634
41. Roberts Y, English D, Thompson R, White C. The impact of childhood stressful life events on health and behavior in at-risk youth. *Child Youth Serv Rev.* (2018) 85:117–26. doi: 10.1016/j.childyouth.2017.11.029
42. Scheidell J, Quinn K, McGorray S, Frueh B, Beharie N, Cottler L, et al. Childhood traumatic experiences and the association with marijuana and cocaine use in adolescence through adulthood. *Addiction.* (2017) 113:44–56. doi: 10.1111/add.13921
43. Watts W, Ellis A. Sexual abuse and drinking and drug use: implications for prevention. *J Drug Educ.* (1993) 23:183–200. doi: 10.2190/00GX-84JY-3N4M-48EG
44. Yoon S, Shi Y, Yoon D, Pei F, Schoppe-Sullivan S, Snyder S. Child maltreatment, fathers, and adolescent alcohol and marijuana use trajectories. *Subst Use Misuse.* (2020) 55:721–33. doi: 10.1080/10826084.2019.1701033
45. Werner K, McCutcheon V, Agrawal A, Sartor C, Nelson E, Heath A, et al. The association of specific traumatic experiences with cannabis initiation and transition to problem use: differences between African-American

and European-American women. *Drug Alcohol Depend.* (2016) 162:162–9. doi: 10.1016/j.drugalcdep.2016.03.003

46. Dubowitz H, Roesch S, Lewis T. Child maltreatment, early adult substance use, and mediation by adolescent behavior problems. *Child Maltreat.* (2020) 26:238–48. doi: 10.1177/1077559520941919
47. Baldwin J, Reuben A, Newbury J, Danese A. Agreement between prospective and retrospective measures of childhood maltreatment. *JAMA Psychiatry.* (2019) 76:584. doi: 10.1001/jamapsychiatry.2019.0097
48. Li M, D'Arcy C, Meng X. Maltreatment in childhood substantially increases the risk of adult depression and anxiety in prospective cohort studies: systematic review, meta-analysis, and proportional attributable fractions. *Psychol Med.* (2016) 46:717. doi: 10.1017/S0033291715002743
49. Croft J, Heron J, Teufel C, Cannon M, Wolke D, Thompson A, et al. Association of trauma type, age of exposure, and frequency in childhood and adolescence with psychotic experiences in early adulthood. *JAMA Psychiatry.* (2019) 76:79. doi: 10.1001/jamapsychiatry.2018.3155
50. Radhakrishnan R, Wilkinson S, D'Souza D. Gone to pot - a review of the association between cannabis and psychosis. *Front Psychiatry.* (2014) 5:54. doi: 10.3389/fpsyt.2014.00054

5

Age-Related Differences in Alcohol Intake and Control Over Alcohol Seeking in Rats

Maaike Labots[1], *Janna Cousijn*[2,3], *Linda A. Jolink*[1], *J. Leon Kenemans*[4], *Louk J. M. J. Vanderschuren*[1] *and Heidi M. B. Lesscher*[1*]

[1] Department of Animals in Science and Society, Division of Behavioural Neuroscience, Faculty of Veterinary Medicine, Utrecht University, Utrecht, Netherlands, [2] ADAPT-Lab, Department of Psychology, University of Amsterdam, Amsterdam, Netherlands, [3] Amsterdam Brain and Cognition (ABC), University of Amsterdam, Amsterdam, Netherlands, [4] Department of Experimental Psychology, Helmholtz Research Institute, Utrecht University, Utrecht, Netherlands

Edited by:
Cristina Cadoni,
Consiglio Nazionale Delle Ricerche (CNR), Italy

Reviewed by:
Erika Roman,
Uppsala University, Sweden
Valentina Vengeliene,
Zentralinstitut für Seelische Gesundheit (ZI), Germany

***Correspondence:**
Heidi M. B. Lesscher
h.m.b.lesscher@uu.nl

Alcohol use disorder (AUD) is characterized by excessive and persistent alcohol use, despite adverse consequences. AUD often originates during adolescence, as do other substance use disorders. However, despite periods of excessive alcohol intake, many adolescents reduce their alcohol use by early adulthood. Brain development, social context, personality traits, and genetic makeup are thought to play an important role in these age-dependent fluctuations in alcohol use. However, studies that directly investigate age-related differences in the effects of alcohol exposure on brain and behavior are sparse. Therefore, to better understand the relationship between adolescent alcohol consumption and AUD-like behavior, this study compared the degree of control over alcohol seeking in rats that differed in terms of age of onset of alcohol drinking and in their level of alcohol consumption. We hypothesized that control over alcohol seeking is more prominent in adolescent-onset rats than in adult-onset rats, and that control over alcohol seeking is related to the consumed amount of alcohol. To test this hypothesis, alcohol seeking in the presence of a conditioned aversive stimulus was assessed after 2 months of intermittent alcohol access (IAA) in rats that consumed alcohol from postnatal day 42 (adolescence) or day 77 (adulthood). The rats were subdivided into low (LD), medium (MD), or high (HD) alcohol drinking rats, in order to assess the impact of the extent of alcohol intake on control over alcohol seeking. The adolescent-onset animals consumed slightly, but significantly less alcohol compared to the adult-onset rats. In adult-onset rats, we found that conditioned suppression of alcohol seeking, i.e., reduction of alcohol seeking by presentation of a conditioned aversive stimulus, was most pronounced in LD. By contrast, in the adolescent-onset rats, MD and HD showed increased alcohol seeking compared to LD, which was suppressed by conditioned aversive stimuli. Taken together, these findings reveal a complex relationship between the age of onset and level of alcohol intake with control over alcohol seeking, whereby adolescent rats consume less alcohol than adults. In adult rats, control over alcohol seeking is negatively related to preceding levels of alcohol intake. By contrast, adolescent rats appear to retain control over alcohol seeking, even after a history of high levels of alcohol intake.

Keywords: alcohol, loss of control, adolescence, addiction-like behavior, conditioned suppression, individual differences, rats

INTRODUCTION

Alcohol is among the most widely used substances of abuse and alcohol use disorder (AUD) remains an enormous public health problem, affecting over 76 million people worldwide (1–3). AUD is characterized by excessive alcohol use and loss of control over alcohol intake, signified by persistent alcohol use despite adverse consequences (4). Considering that only a minority of the individuals that use alcohol develop an AUD, it is important to understand the factors that determine the transition from recreational and controlled, to compulsive and uncontrolled alcohol use. AUD often originates during adolescence and young adulthood, as do other substance use disorders. Adolescent alcohol use has been shown to be detrimental for brain development [for review see (5)]. At the same time, risk taking behavior during adolescence, which is expressed, amongst others, through substance use, is increasingly considered to be important for adolescents to mature and develop a degree of behavioral flexibility, that is necessary to thrive as adults [e.g., (6)]. Importantly, even after periods of excessive alcohol use, many adolescents show a reduction in their alcohol use by early adulthood (7). Brain development, social context, personality traits and genetic makeup are thought to play an important role in these age-dependent fluctuations in alcohol use (8).

Human literature suggests that the age of onset of alcohol use is associated with the risk to develop an AUD later in life. Population based studies have suggested that the earlier the onset of alcohol consumption, the greater the likelihood to develop heavy alcohol use, alcohol-related problems and an AUD (9–16). However, age of first alcohol use is not specifically associated with AUD but also with the development of other mental disorders (17). Moreover, recent systematic reviews suggest that the evidence for the association between age of first drink and AUD is less consistent and may be driven by confounding factors, such as socioeconomic status, a history of alcohol problems in the family or preceding mental health problems that may have contributed to the early onset of drinking and the risk for AUD (18, 19). The impact of adolescent alcohol exposure on alcohol consumption and other reward-related behaviors in adulthood has also been addressed in animal studies that have yielded a picture that is far from straightforward. For example, it has been shown that adolescent alcohol exposure enhances alcohol consumption and operant self-administration of alcohol in adulthood in rats and mice (20–24). However, other studies have found that adolescent alcohol exposure does not affect alcohol intake in adulthood (25), or only upon vapor-induced dependence (26) or alcohol deprivation (27). Moreover, direct comparison of adolescent vs. adult onset of alcohol intake suggests that alcohol intake is not different in animals with an adolescent onset of alcohol consumption, compared to rats that started to consume alcohol in adulthood (28, 29). With regard to the associative structure of alcohol use, Serlin and Torregrossa (30) have shown that rats that started to self-administer alcohol in adolescence were more goal-directed in their alcohol seeking (i.e., alcohol seeking was sensitive to the subjective value of alcohol) compared to adult-onset animals, that more readily developed habitual alcohol seeking. On the other hand, alcohol exposure during adolescence has been shown to enhance risky behavior in adulthood [(31–33); but see (34)], as well as the responsiveness to reward-predictive cues (35, 36). Importantly, the studies described above used different, often overlapping age ranges, making it unlikely that discrepancies in the findings can simply be explained by age differences, such as between early or late adolescence (37, 38).

Taken together, there is evidence that adolescent onset of alcohol use alters behavioral traits related to AUD, although the differential impact of adolescent- vs. adult-onset alcohol use on the development of AUD-like behavior remains largely unexplored. The aim of this study was therefore to compare the influence of age of onset of alcohol consumption on control over alcohol seeking in rats. To address this, alcohol consumption and control over alcohol seeking was determined in rats that initiated alcohol consumption during adolescence or adulthood. In order to also take individual variation in alcohol consumption into account, we used outbred Lister Hooded rats and an intermittent alcohol consumption paradigm, similar to previous studies in which we demonstrated individual differences in alcohol consumption that are associated with loss of control over alcohol seeking (39, 40). We hypothesized that control over alcohol seeking in rats would be related to the level of alcohol intake (39, 40), that control over alcohol seeking would be more prominent in adolescent-onset rats than in adult-onset rats and that the age related difference in control over alcohol seeking would be especially pronounced in high alcohol consuming animals.

MATERIALS AND METHODS

Animals

Male Lister Hooded rats (Charles River, Sulzfeld, Germany) arrived either at postnatal day (PND) 35 (adolescent, $N = 84$) or 70 (adult, $N = 84$) in the facility and were housed in type III Makrolon cages with matching type III-S lids under controlled conditions, with a reversed 12 h light/dark cycle (lights off 7.00 a.m.) and *ad libitum* access to water and chow. The cages were enriched with a homemade square PVC shelter and paper tissues. The rats were acclimatized to the facility for 1 week upon arrival. Thereafter, the rats were housed individually and they were weighed and handled at least once per week. All experiments were approved by the Animal Ethics Committee of Utrecht University and conducted in agreement with Dutch laws (Wet op de dierproeven, 2014) and European regulations (Guideline 86/609/EEC).

Voluntary Home-Cage Alcohol Consumption

The rats were allowed to consume alcohol according to an intermittent alcohol access (IAA) schedule. The rats were given access to 20% (v/v) alcohol (Klinipath, The Netherlands) and water in a two-bottle choice setup in the home-cage with IAA for 3 days a week (Monday–Wednesday–Friday). For voluntary alcohol consumption, transparent 250 ml bottles (Techniplast, Germany) were used and the position of the alcohol and water bottle was switched between sessions. On alcohol-free days the rats had only one 500 ml bottle, filled with water. The adolescent rats started to consume alcohol from PND 42, while the adult animals started with voluntary alcohol consumption from PND 77. We chose to start adolescent voluntary alcohol consumption at PND 42 because we wanted to capture the developmental period starting at puberty, which in male rats is around PND 40 (41). Moreover, we wanted to avoid social isolation during the period in life when rats show most social play behavior (i.e., PND 21-42), since we and others have previously shown that animals deprived from social play show increased sensitivity to the rewarding properties of substances of abuse (42–44). We therefore started the drinking study, which requires the rats to be housed individually, from PND 42. During the first month of IAA, alcohol was presented for 7 h/day (9.00 a.m. until 16.00 p.m.) and access to alcohol was extended to 24 h/day in the second month of the experiment [see (39)]. Alcohol intake (g/kg) and preference (% volume of alcohol over water) were calculated per rat per session and subsequently averaged per week. After 2 months of voluntary home-cage alcohol consumption, the rats were classified into low (LD), medium (MD), or high (HD) alcohol drinking groups based on their average home cage alcohol intake per week across the 2 months using a tertile split of the population.

Operant Alcohol Self-Administration

After 2 months of voluntary home-cage alcohol consumption, operant responding for alcohol in the presence of an aversive conditioned stimulus, i.e., conditioned suppression of alcohol seeking, was assessed in order to investigate the influence of adolescent-onset vs. adult-onset alcohol exposure on control over alcohol use.

Operant Training

The rats were trained to lever press for alcohol in operant conditioning chambers (Med-Associates, USA) 3 days/week (Monday–Wednesday–Friday) as previously described (40). The position of the active and inactive levers was counterbalanced between rats. Upon meeting the response requirement, the dipper cup containing alcohol (0.1 ml, 20% v/v) was raised, the cue light above the active lever was illuminated and the house light was switched off. Ten seconds after a head entry into the magazine, access to alcohol was terminated, the cue light was turned off and 5 s later a new trial started. Pressing the inactive lever was recorded, but had no programmed consequences. The rats were initially trained to respond for alcohol under a Fixed Ratio 1 (FR1) schedule of reinforcement for three sessions. Thereafter, the rats were trained under a random interval (RI) schedule of reinforcement, whereby the first active lever press initiated a RI during which lever pressing was recorded but was without consequences. After the RI had elapsed, the first active lever press resulted in the delivery of alcohol. The rats were trained in 30 min RI sessions with increasing RI durations (3 sessions with a 5 s RI, followed by 3 sessions with a 15 s RI, 2–3 sessions with a 30 s RI and then 2–3 sessions with a 60 s RI). Finally, the rats were trained in five 60 min RI 120 s sessions. Thereafter, the data were analyzed to verify stable responding under the RI120 schedule of reinforcement, i.e., <25% variation in active responses during the last three RI 120 s sessions. To determine the stability of alcohol seeking, only the first 15 min of the last three RI 120 s sessions were considered to match the duration of the conditioned suppression tests (see below). Experimental events and data recording were controlled using MED-PC software.

Conditioned Suppression of Alcohol Seeking

After the RI training was completed, conditioned suppression was performed according to previously described procedures (40, 45–47). Thus, the LD, MD, or HD rats were assigned to subgroups that either underwent fear conditioning, with conditioned stimulus - footshock pairings (CS+), or underwent control conditioning (CS–). A CS-shock conditioning session started with a 5 min period in which only the house light was illuminated, followed by two periods of 10 min during which a 85 dB, 2,900 Hz tone (separated by a 10 min inter-trial-interval) was constantly presented. During the 10 min tone presentations, 10 unpredictable footshocks (1 s duration) were delivered, resulting in a total of 20 shocks for each CS+ rat. The conditioning session was completed after a final 5 min period without tone presentation. Rats in the CS– control group underwent the same procedure, but without footshocks. To ensure equal mean seeking rates for CS+ and CS– groups prior to conditioning, the rats' mean seeking responses per minute during the first 15 min of the last three RI 120 s sessions, chosen to align with the duration of the conditioned suppression tests, were used to assign the rats to the respective CS- and CS+ groups. From the adolescent-onset rats, a total of 14 LD, 14 MD, and 14 HD underwent control conditioning (CS–) and 14 LD, 14 MD, and 14 HD were fear-conditioned with 0.4 mA footshocks. In the adult group, 3 animals were lost due health problems prior to conditioned suppression, leaving a total of 14 LD, 13 MD, and 14 HD in the CS– groups and a total of 14 LD, 13 MD, and 13 HD in the CS+ groups, respectively. To prevent association of fear conditioning with the self-administration environment, acquisition of the CS-shock association was established in conditioning chambers that were physically different from operant self-administration (SA) chambers, in that the conditioning chamber had a curved wall with 5 nose poke holes and no levers and stimulus lights. To facilitate CS-shock associations, rather than context-shock associations, the rats were habituated to the conditioning chambers in three 30 min sessions on separate days prior to conditioning.

After conditioning, the rats received two additional RI 120 s training sessions. Subsequently, conditioned suppression of alcohol-seeking behavior was assessed in the SA chambers. The house light was illuminated and 2 min after the start of the session, the levers were extended for the remaining 12 min of the test. Alcohol seeking during the conditioned suppression test was examined in extinction, i.e., responding on the levers was recorded, but had no programmed consequences. To avoid altered responding due to the lack of (smell of) alcohol in the SA chamber, the cup containing 20% alcohol (v/v) was present underneath the liquid dipper but the rats did not have access to the solution. Three 2-min intervals in which the tone CS was presented (CS-ON interval) were alternated with 2-min intervals where the tone CS was absent (CS-OFF interval). Active lever presses and latency to the first lever press were recorded and compared for CS– and CS+ subgroups as a measure of control over alcohol seeking.

Conditioned Freezing

One week after completion of the conditioned suppression test, the rats underwent fear conditioning (CS+) or control conditioning (CS–); the rats were assigned to the same group as for conditioned suppression of alcohol seeking. Fear conditioning procedures were similar to those described in the previous section. After 24 h, the rats were placed in the conditioning chamber: 2 min without the CS+ tone and subsequently 2 min with the CS+ tone. The frequency and duration of freezing behavior, defined as the absence of any movement other than breathing (40, 48–50), was scored from DVD-taped behavior using Observer software (Noldus, Wageningen, NL) by an observer blind to age, alcohol drinking group and conditioning history.

Statistics

To compare the level of alcohol consumption in the two age groups and the subgroups of low, medium and high alcohol drinking rats, the alcohol intake (g/kg), preference (% choice for alcohol vs. water), and total volume of fluid intake (ml/kg) data were analyzed by three-way repeated measures ANOVA with month (1st- 7 h and 2nd- 24 h) as the within-subjects factor and age group (adolescent and adult onset) and group (LD, MD, HD) as the between-subjects factors. Moreover, to test our hypotheses that control over alcohol seeking in rats would be more prominent in adolescent-onset than in adult-onset rats and that the age related differences in control over alcohol seeking would be more pronounced in the high alcohol consuming animals, the conditioned suppression data were analyzed by four-way repeated measures ANOVA with tone (ON/OFF) and interval (3 repetitions for ON/OFF) as the within-subjects factors and age group (adolescent and adult onset), CS (CS+/CS–) and group (LD, MD, HD) as the between-subjects factors. Mauchly's test of sphericity was used to test if variances of the differences between treatment levels were equal. If the assumption of sphericity was violated, degrees of freedom were corrected using Huynh-Feldt estimates of sphericity to more conservative values; corrected degrees of freedom are presented rounded to the nearest integer. When appropriate, *post-hoc* analyses were conducted using multiple LSD pairwise comparisons. Each parameter was tested for normality with a Kolmogorov-Smirnov test. In case the behavioral parameters were not normally distributed (i.e., the latency data from the conditioned suppression test), data was log transformed prior to statistical analyses, which resulted in normal distribution of the data. Statistical analyses were conducted using IBM SPSS Statistics for Windows, version 22.0 (IBM Corp., Armonk, N.Y. USA). The threshold for statistical significance was set at $p < 0.05$. All data are presented as mean + SEM.

RESULTS

Alcohol Consumption

Analysis of the alcohol intake data (**Figure 1A**) revealed that, in line with previous studies (36, 39, 40, 44), alcohol intake was higher in the second month of the experiment [$F_{(1, 161)\text{month}} = 471$, $P < 0.001$], when access to alcohol was extended from 7 to 24 h. This escalation of alcohol intake during the second month of access was dependent on the age of onset, as is evident from a significant month × age group interaction [$F_{(1, 161)} = 20.1$, $P < 0.001$]; escalation of alcohol intake was more pronounced in adult-onset rats. Overall, the group that started to consume alcohol as adults consumed more alcohol compared to the rats that started to consume alcohol during adolescence [$F_{(1, 161)\text{ age group}} = 5.4$, $P < 0.05$]. *Post-hoc* pairwise comparisons showed that the difference in alcohol intake between the age groups was only significant for the second month, when the rats had 24 h access to alcohol. The increase in alcohol intake in the second month was also dependent on the level of alcohol consumption of the individual animals [$F_{(2, 161)\text{ month} \times \text{group}} = 65.7$, $P < 0.001$], in that HD showed a greater increment compared to LD and MD. Further, the selected HD overall consumed more alcohol than the LD and MD [$F_{(2, 161)\text{ group}} = 195.1$, $P < 0.001$], independent of the age of onset [$F_{(2, 161)\text{ age group} \times \text{group}} = 0.07$, N.S.]. Similar effects were observed for the preference for alcohol over water (**Figure 1B**) and overall, adolescent rats consumed more fluids when compared to their adult counterparts (**Figure 1C**).

Importantly, the groups remained different during operant alcohol self-administration. Analysis of the number of active responses confirmed overall effects of drinking group during the initial FR1 training sessions [**Figure 2A**; $F_{(2, 166)\text{ group}} = 21.0$, $P < 0.001$] and during the final RI 120 s sessions [**Figure 2B**; $F_{(2, 166)\text{ group}} = 11.7$, $P < 0.001$], with a trend for an age group effect on the number of active responses during RI120 training sessions [$F_{(1,166)\text{ age group}} = 3.3$, $P = 0.07$]. *Post-hoc* pairwise comparisons revealed that MD made more responses for alcohol than LD and HD made more responses for alcohol than LD and MD.

Conditioned Suppression of Alcohol Seeking

For the analysis of conditioned suppression of alcohol seeking (**Figures 3**, **4**), the LD, MD, and HD groups for both the adolescent- and adult-onset groups were further subdivided into CS– and CS+ animals ($N = 13$–14). Analysis of the number of active responses for the CS– control groups by age revealed that the adolescent-onset groups tend to differ in their responding during the conditioned suppression test [$F_{(2, 39)\text{ group}} = 3.21$, $P = 0.051$]. *Post-hoc* pairwise comparisons revealed that adolescent-onset LD made fewer responses compared to HD rats, but LD were not different from MD that in turn did not significantly differ from the HD. The differences in active responses between the groups were not dependent on tone presentation [$F_{(2, 39)\text{ tone} \times \text{group}} = 0.17$, N.S.; $F_{(4, 78)\text{tone} \times \text{interval} \times \text{group}} = 0.21$, N.S.]. By contrast, the adult CS– LD, MD, and HD did not differ in their number of

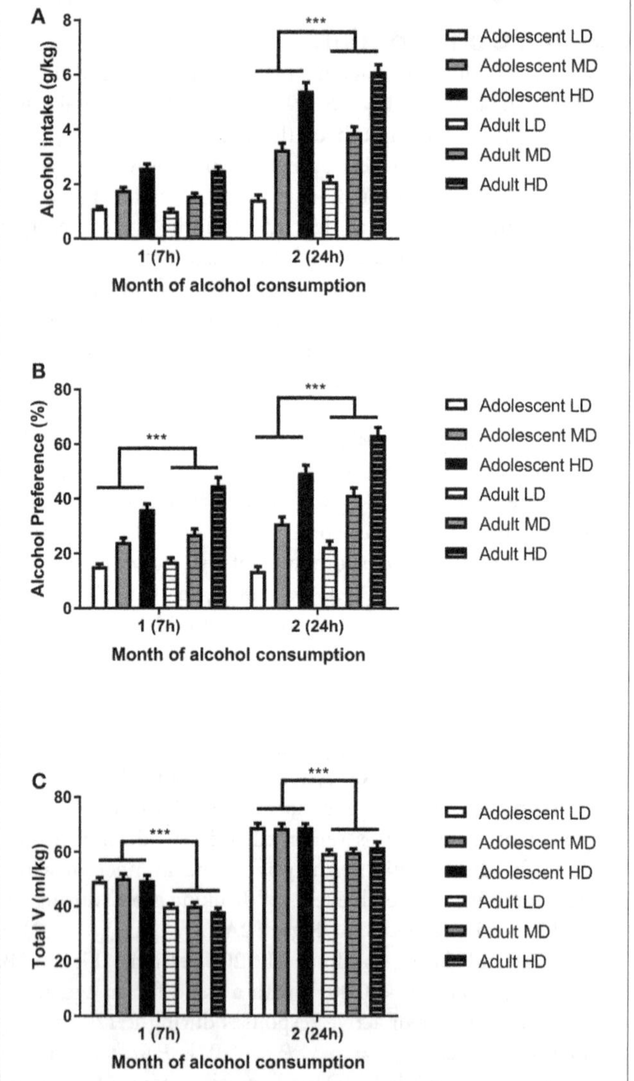

FIGURE 1 | Alcohol intake in adolescent onset and adulthood onset rats. Depicted are alcohol intake **(A)**, alcohol preference **(B),** and total volume (V) of fluid consumed **(C)** for selected low drinkers (LD), medium drinkers (MD), and high drinkers (HD) from both age groups. The data are shown as mean + SEM. ***Significant overall difference between adolescent-onset and adult-onset rats, independent of drinking group by *post-hoc* pairwise comparison, ($P < 0.001$).

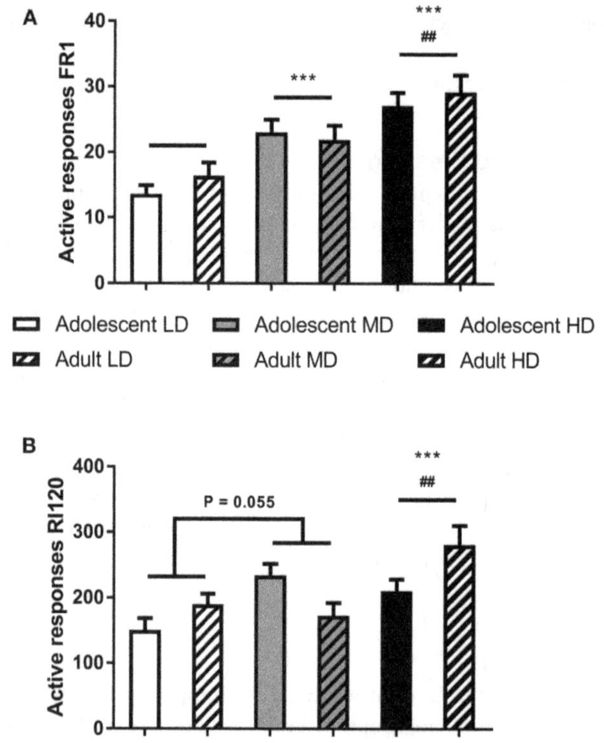

FIGURE 2 | Responding for alcohol under FR1 **(A)** and RI120 **(B)** schedules of reinforcement. Shown are the average number of active responses during the (last) three sessions of training on the respective schedules for adolescent-onset and adult-onset low (LD), medium (MD), and high alcohol drinking (HD) rats after 8 weeks of intermittent alcohol consumption. Data are presented as mean + SEM active responses. ***MD and HD made more active responses compared to LD, independent of age group (*post-hoc* pairwise comparisons, $P < 0.001$) and ##HD made more active responses than MD, independent of age group (*post-hoc* pairwise comparisons, $P < 0.01$).

active responses for alcohol [$F_{(2, 38)\text{tone} \times \text{group}} = 0.44$, N.S.; $F_{(4, 76)\text{ tone} \times \text{interval} \times \text{group}} = 1.9$, N.S.; $F_{(2, 38)\text{ group}} = 1.14$, N.S.].

Analysis of the active responses during the conditioned suppression test (**Figure 3**) revealed a significant effect of CS [$F_{(1, 153)\text{ CS}} = 15.7$, $P < 0.001$], which was dependent on the tone presentation [$F_{(1,153)\text{ tone} \times \text{CS}} = 28.9$, $P < 0.001$] and the interval [$F_{(2, 281)\text{ tone} \times \text{ interval} \times \text{CS}} = 6.4$, $P < 0.01$]. Moreover, conditioned suppression of alcohol seeking was dependent on the age of onset, as evident from a significant interval × age group × group × CS interaction [$F_{(3.4, 258)} = 3.1$, $P < 0.05$] and a significant age group × group × CS interaction [$F_{(2, 153)} = 3.4$, $P < 0.05$]. A similar pattern emerged after analysis of the data for the latency to the first response. There was an overall effect of CS [$F_{(1, 153)\text{ CS}} = 14$, $P < 0.001$], which was dependent on presentation of the tone [$F_{(1, 153)\text{ tone} \times \text{CS}} = 7.5$, $P < 0.01$] and the interval [$F_{(2, 306)\text{ interval} \times \text{CS}} = 8.1$, $P < 0.001$]. Moreover, conditioned suppression was dependent on age of onset and group, in an interval and CS dependent manner [$F_{(4, 306)\text{ interval} \times \text{age} \times \text{group} \times \text{CS}} = 2.8$, $P < 0.05$] and there was a significant tone x interval x age group x group interaction [$F_{(2, 306)} = 3.1$, $P < 0.05$]. To further explore the differences between the groups, we analyzed the data separately for the LD, MD, and HD in the two age groups.

Adolescent Onset

For the adolescent-onset LD (**Figure 3A**), there was no overall difference in responding between the CS– and CS+ groups [$F_{(1, 26)\text{ CS}} = 0.089$, N.S], but the number of active lever presses in the CS+ and CS– rats was different when tone presentation was taken into account [$F_{(1, 26)\text{ tone} \times \text{CS}} = 5.2$, $P < 0.05$]. *Post-hoc* pairwise comparisons revealed no significant differences between the CS– and CS+ animals for any of the intervals. For the MD (see **Figure 3B**), the CS+ group showed a near-significant

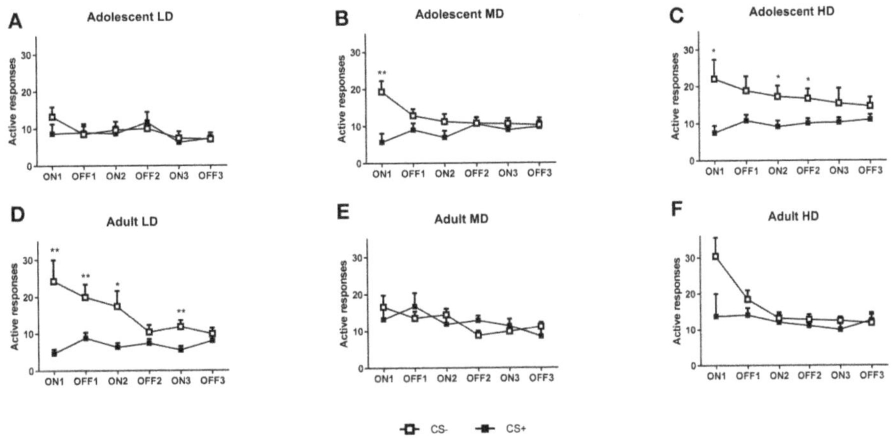

FIGURE 3 | Conditioned suppression of alcohol seeking in CS– and CS+ groups of adolescent-onset and adult-onset low (LD), medium (MD), and high alcohol drinking (HD) rats after 8 weeks of intermittent alcohol consumption. In **(A–C)**, the number of active responses during consecutive CS ON and CS OFF intervals are shown for adolescent-onset LD, MD, and HD, respectively. In **(D–F)**, the number of active responses during CS ON and CS OFF intervals are shown for adult-onset LD, MD, and HD, respectively. Data are presented as mean + SEM active responses, binned in 2 min intervals. Significant differences between CS– and CS+ groups are indicated by * and ** (*post-hoc* pairwise comparisons, $P < 0.05$ and $P < 0.01$, respectively).

reduction in the number of active lever presses compared to CS– controls [$F_{(1, 26)\ CS} = 3.6$, $P = 0.067$], which was dependent on the tone presentation [$F_{(1, 26)\ tone \times CS} = 10.8$, $P < 0.01$]. *Post-hoc* pairwise comparisons showed reduced responding in the CS+ group during the first tone ON interval. The HD group (**Figure 3C**) showed significant conditioned suppression, in that overall active responding during the conditioned suppression test was lower in the CS+ compared to the CS– animals [$F_{(1, 26)CS} = 5.6$, $P < 0.05$], independent of tone presentation [$F_{(1,26)\ tone \times CS} = 2.2$, N.S.]. *Post-hoc* pairwise comparisons showed decreased responding in the CS+ HD group during the first two tone ON intervals and the second tone OFF interval.

In agreement with the active response data, separate analyses of the latency data confirmed that adolescent-onset LD did not show suppression of alcohol seeking behavior, as evident from a lack of an overall difference between CS– and CS+ rats [**Figure 4A**; $F_{(1, 26)\ CS} = 0.98$, N.S.; $F_{(1, 26)tone \times CS} = 0.4$, N.S.]. The MD and HD CS– and CS+ animals also did not differ in their latency to respond during the conditioned suppression test [MD: **Figure 4B,** $F_{(1, 26)\ CS} = 3.4$, N.S.; $F_{(1, 26)\ tone \times CS} = 3.4$, N.S.; HD: **Figure 4C,** $F_{(1, 26)\ CS} = 0.5$, N.S.; $F_{(1, 26)\ tone \times CS} = 0.01$, N.S.].

Adult Onset

When comparing CS– and CS+ groups, only the LD animals showed conditioned suppression of alcohol seeking behavior. This was evident from an reduction in the number of active responses by the CS+ LD animals compared to the CS– controls [$F_{(1, 26)\ CS} = 9.3$, $P < 0.01$], which was dependent on tone presentation [$F_{(1, 26)\ tone \times CS} = 17.0$, $P < 0.001$]. *Post-hoc* pairwise comparisons for the LD (**Figure 3D**) showed reduced alcohol seeking during all tone ON intervals and during the first tone OFF interval. By contrast, the MD did not show significant conditioned suppression of alcohol seeking [**Figure 3E**; $F_{(1, 24)\ CS} = 0.0$, N.S.; $F_{(1, 24)\ tone \times CS} = 2.2$, N.S.]. Analysis of the active seeking responses for the HD (**Figure 3F**) showed no significant CS effect [$F_{(1, 25)\ CS} = 2.7$, $P < 0.05$; $F_{(1, 25)\ tone \times CS} = 2.9$, N.S.].

Separate analyses of the latency data revealed that the adult-onset LD rats displayed a suppression of alcohol seeking when confronted with the shock-paired tone (**Figure 4D**) in that the latency to respond was greater for the CS+ compared to the CS– rats [$F_{(1, 26)\ CS} = 7.7$, $P < 0.01$; $F_{(2, 52)\ tone \times CS} = 2.4$, N.S.]. By contrast, the adult-onset MD and HD rats did not show an altered latency to respond [MD: **Figure 4E,** $F_{(1, 24)\ CS} = 2.1$, N.S.; $F_{(1, 24)\ tone \times CS} = 0.8$, N.S.; HD: **Figure 4F,** $F_{(1, 25)\ CS} = 2.6$, N.S.; $F_{(1, 25)\ tone \times CS} = 3.7$, N.S.].

Conditioned Freezing Behavior

After the conditioned suppression test, the rats were re-conditioned and conditioned freezing was determined. Analysis of freezing behavior of the rats during 2 min before (no-tone) and during CS (tone) presentation revealed that the time spent freezing was higher in CS+ rats compared to the CS– control animals [$F_{(1, 152)\ CS} = 272$, $P < 0.001$] (**Figure 5**). Moreover, conditioned freezing behavior was increased upon presentation of the footshock CS+ [$F_{(1, 152)\ tone \times CS} = 192$, $P < 0.001$]. The degree of freezing behavior was comparable across age and groups [$F_{(2, 152)\ tone \times age\ group \times group \times CS} = 0.44$, N.S.; $F_{(1, 152)\ tone \times age\ group \times CS} = 0.33$, N.S.; $F_{(2, 152)\ tone \times group \times CS} = 1.5$, N.S.; $F_{(2, 152)\ age\ group \times group \times CS} = 0.57$, N.S.].

DISCUSSION

The consumption of alcohol and the development of AUD often starts during adolescence. However, the relative impact of alcohol exposure during adolescence, as compared to adulthood, on the emergence of AUD later in life is poorly understood. Therefore, in the present study, we compared alcohol intake and control over alcohol seeking in animals that started to consume alcohol

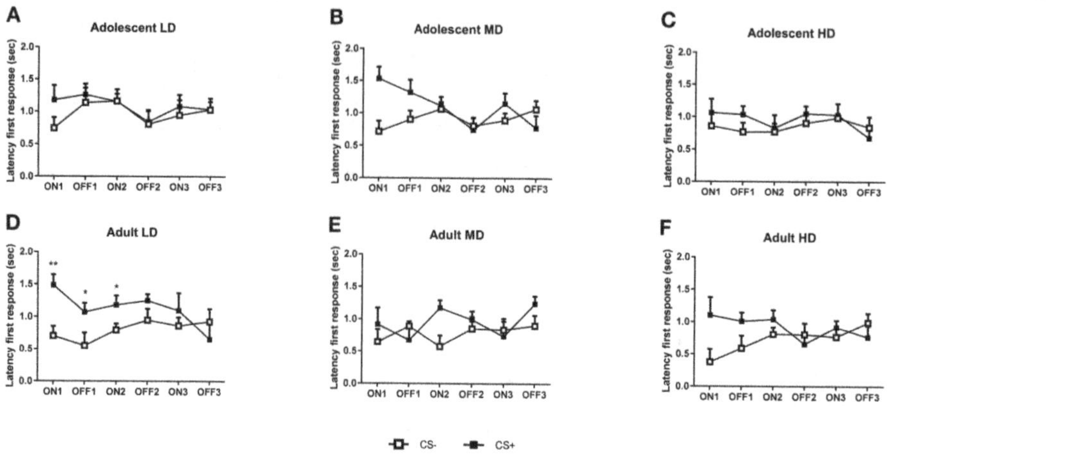

FIGURE 4 | Conditioned suppression of alcohol seeking in CS– and CS+ groups of adult-onset and adolescent-onset low (LD), medium (MD), and high alcohol drinking (HD) rats after 8 weeks of intermittent alcohol consumption. In **(A–C)**, the latency to the first active response during consecutive CS ON and CS OFF intervals are shown for adolescent-onset LD, MD, and HD, respectively. In **(D–F)**, the latencies to respond during CS ON and CS OFF intervals are shown for adult-onset LD, MD, and HD, respectively. Data are presented as mean + SEM active responses, binned in 2 min intervals. Significant differences between CS– and CS+ groups are indicated by * and** (*post-hoc* pairwise comparisons, $P < 0.05$ and $P < 0.01$, respectively).

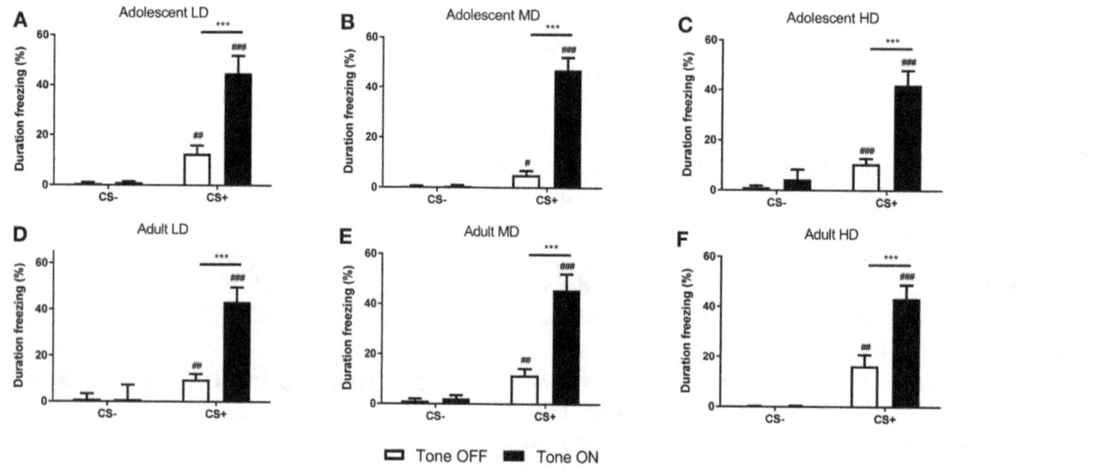

FIGURE 5 | Freezing behavior in adolescent-onset low (LD; **A**), medium (MD; **B**), and high (HD; **C**) alcohol drinking rats and adult-onset LD **(D)**, MD **(E)**, and HD **(F)**. Shown is the duration of freezing in the conditioning chamber, expressed as a percentage of the 2 min prior to (Tone OFF) and during presentation of the footshock-associated CS+ (Tone ON) period. The conditioned rats (CS+) showed significant context- and CS-induced freezing, while the respective CS– control groups did not. This was comparable for all age and alcohol drinking groups. Data are presented as mean + SEM. #, ##, ###Significant difference between CS– and CS+ groups (*post-hoc* pairwise comparisons, $P < 0.05$, $P < 0.01$, and $P < 0.001$, respectively). ***Significant difference between tone ON and tone OFF periods (*post-hoc* pairwise comparisons, $P < 0.001$).

in either adolescence or adulthood. Rats with an adolescent onset of alcohol drinking consumed less alcohol than rats that started to drink alcohol in adulthood. In addition, we found that control over alcohol seeking was differentially related to the level of alcohol intake in the two age groups. In adult-onset rats, conditioned suppression of alcohol seeking was observed in the LD, but not the MD or HD, i.e., being negatively related to levels of alcohol intake. In the adolescent-onset group the MD and HD, that showed higher levels of alcohol seeking compared to the LD, showed significantly reduced alcohol seeking upon presentation of conditioned aversive stimuli. These findings indicate a complex relationship between age of alcohol drinking onset, level of alcohol intake, and control over alcohol seeking.

Alcohol Intake in Adolescent and Adult Rats

We observed a modest but significant difference in alcohol intake when comparing the two age groups. The adolescent-onset rats consumed less alcohol when compared to adult rats. This was most pronounced during the second month of alcohol intake, when rats had 24 h access to alcohol. Perhaps the age differences were more prominent during this phase of the experiment because alcohol consumption levels are higher when access time to alcohol is extended, as we have shown previously (39). Other studies that directly compared alcohol intake in age groups that were tested in parallel, comparable to our approach, showed that adolescent rats consumed equal or lower amounts of alcohol than rats with an adult onset of alcohol intake (24, 28, 51), although adolescent rats have been shown to respond more for alcohol in an operant task (30). The adolescent rats also showed a lower preference for alcohol and the adolescents overall consumed more water compared to the adult rats, which is in line with previous reports (28, 51). Taken together, our findings show that adolescent rats do not drink more alcohol than their adult counterparts. These findings are in apparent contrast to the human literature, which shows that alcohol use peaks during adolescence (7). Although speculative, it is likely that this discrepancy is related to the housing conditions. While adolescent alcohol use in humans is thought to be driven in part by the social environment, for example by social attunement (8), the rats in this study were individually housed, precluding a potential impact of social factors.

In apparent contrast to our present, and other observations (24, 28, 51), it has previously been suggested that alcohol intake in adolescence promotes the development of AUD-like behavior. This was based on studies that reported augmented alcohol intake or operant responding for alcohol in adult rats that were exposed to alcohol during adolescence (20–24). However, it should be borne in mind that in these experiments, alcohol intake after adolescent pre-exposure was compared to adolescent non-exposure to alcohol. Moreover, alcohol intake or operant responding was determined after an abstinence period of 3–6 weeks. It is therefore possible that the increase in alcohol intake after adolescent alcohol exposure reflects an alcohol deprivation effect, i.e., an increase in alcohol intake after an abstinence phase [e.g., (52–60)], rather than an age-dependent risk for AUD. In fact, Siegmund et al. (28) have shown that the alcohol deprivation effect is comparable in adolescent- and adult-onset drinking rats. Therefore, reports of adolescent alcohol exposure-induced changes in alcohol intake may reflect the impact of adolescent exposure to alcohol, but may also mirror the effect of an alcohol deprivation phase.

Age of Drinking Onset Influences Control Over Alcohol Seeking

To determine the impact of adolescent vs. adult onset of alcohol exposure on the individuals' risk to develop AUD-like behavior, we directly compared two age groups, i.e., commencing alcohol intake at PND 42 vs. PND 77, in a parallel design. We assessed the degree of control over alcohol seeking in these age groups using a conditioned suppression test. In this test, animals are exposed to a conflict situation where they can seek alcohol but at the same time are confronted with a warning sign that has previously been associated with unpredictable mild electric footshocks. Continued substance seeking under these conditions is interpreted as loss of control over alcohol seeking (40, 45, 47). The adult rats displayed a similar pattern to what we have previously reported (40), in that adult LD showed a clear suppression of alcohol seeking, while MD and HD did not. This was apparent both from the active response data and from the latency data, where LD CS+ rats show reduced lever pressing and a longer latency to press upon presentation of the aversive stimulus. These differences between the groups were not due to differences in baseline responding, which were comparable for the LD, MD, and HD CS− groups. By contrast, the adolescent MD and HD, but not the LD rats showed significant conditioned suppression of alcohol seeking. Importantly, the differences in alcohol intake between adolescents and adults were only modest. Moreover, adolescent-onset rats consumed less alcohol compared to adult-onset rats, but adolescent HD rats consumed more alcohol than adult MD, that did not display suppression of alcohol seeking. Therefore, the suppression of alcohol seeking in adolescent MD and HD cannot be explained by low levels of preceding alcohol consumption. The remarkable absence of conditioned suppression in the adolescent-onset LD could indicate reduced control over alcohol use in rats that consume low amounts of alcohol. However, this is not likely, given that our previous studies demonstrate more control over alcohol use in low alcohol drinking animals, in comparison to their high alcohol drinking counterparts (39, 40). Rather, we think that the absence of conditioned suppression in the adolescent-onset LD reflects a floor-effect, due to the low baseline levels of responding in this group.

Taken together, these results indicate that whereas in adult-onset rats, control over alcohol seeking is inversely related to the level of preceding alcohol intake, adolescent-onset alcohol exposure less readily leads to loss of control over alcohol seeking. The neural and behavioral mechanisms underlying this age difference remain to be elucidated, but comparable findings have previously been reported. For example, Jeanblanc et al. (61) characterized rats, with or without a neonatal ventral hippocampus lesion (NVHL), that were exposed to low levels of alcohol during adolescence for the expression of AUD-like behavioral characteristics (61). The sham rats in this study did not develop AUD-like behavior, i.e., did not show greater motivation for alcohol, resistance to extinction or an increase in reinstatement of alcohol seeking. Moreover, Serlin and Torregrossa (30) have shown reduced habit formation in rats that were exposed to alcohol during adolescence. This latter observation may reflect a relative resilience to AUD, considering that habit formation is thought to contribute to the development of substance use disorders [e.g., (62)].

Our findings suggest that rats that are exposed to alcohol during adolescence are more flexible in the conditioned suppression task, as they adjust their alcohol seeking behavior in this conflict situation. It is tempting to speculate about the implications of adolescent alcohol exposure for the development of behavioral flexibility in general. Intermittent exposure to intoxicating levels of alcohol during adolescence has been shown to result in impaired performance in a reversal learning task in rats (63), but similar findings have been reported for adult rats (64). Therefore, high levels of alcohol may be detrimental for behavioral flexibility, independent of age. There is some evidence from human studies, which suggests that binge drinking during adolescence (13–18 years) does not impair the performance in executive tasks, while binge drinking during young adulthood (19–22 years) does (65), suggesting that the adolescent brain may compensate for alcohol intoxication to maintain behavioral flexibility. However, this age range only partly overlaps with early adolescent onset of alcohol use, i.e., before the age of 15, which has been shown to increase the likelihood for developing an AUD (9–16). Therefore, it remains unclear whether and how adolescent alcohol exposure alters behavioral flexibility, as a potential mechanism underlying the apparent adolescent resilience to loss of control over alcohol use. Future studies are necessary to fully understand the consequences of adolescent vs. adult alcohol exposure on control over behavior and the underlying neural mechanisms.

A limitation of the present study is the use of males only. Considering the gender differences in alcohol use and AUD, follow-up studies should be extended to determine the impact of age in females. A further limitation is that loss of control was determined when the rats reached adulthood and we have no data on adolescent behavior. This is inherent to the paradigms that we have used. Previously, we have shown that HD develop loss of control after 8 weeks of alcohol consumption (40), which is the exposure time to alcohol that was used here. In the present study, the adolescent-onset animals started to consume alcohol (for 8 consecutive weeks) when they were 6 weeks of age (PND 42) and were subsequently trained to respond for alcohol under fixed and random interval schedules of reinforcement for at least 7 consecutive weeks. Rats are considered adult from 8 to 10 weeks of age. Therefore, our adolescent-onset rats were adults when we assessed loss of control over alcohol seeking. To overcome this limitation, future studies should determine the duration of alcohol consumption after which rats develop resistance to conditioned suppression.

In conclusion, the present findings reveal a complex age-dependence of alcohol drinking and control over alcohol seeking, whereby adolescent rats consume less alcohol than adults. Moreover, while control over alcohol seeking in adult-onset rats is negatively related to preceding levels of alcohol intake, adolescent-onset rats appear to retain control over alcohol seeking, even after consuming high levels of alcohol. These findings support our hypothesis that rats are less susceptible to lose control over alcohol seeking when alcohol intake is initiated during adolescence as compared to adulthood. Future studies should be directed at understanding the underlying mechanisms of a possible, relative resilience to AUD in adolescents. This may inform prevention and treatment strategies for AUD, aimed at both the young and the adult.

AUTHOR CONTRIBUTIONS

HL, JC, JK, and LV designed the study. ML and LJ performed the experiments. ML and HL analyzed the data. HL, JC, JK, and LV wrote the paper with input from all authors.

FUNDING

This work was supported by a seed grant from the Utrecht University strategic research theme Dynamics of Youth to HL and an Amsterdam Brain and Cognition project grant to JC.

REFERENCES

1. Anderson P. Global use of alcohol, drugs and tobacco. *Drug Alcohol Rev.* (2006) 25:489–502. doi: 10.1080/09595230600944446
2. Rehm J, Mathers C, Popova S, Thavorncharoensap M, Teerawattananon Y, Patra J. Global burden of disease and injury and economic cost attributable to alcohol use and alcohol-use disorders. *Lancet* (2009) 373:2223–33. doi: 10.1016/S0140-6736(09)60746-7
3. WHO. *RE: Global Status Report on Alcohol and Health.* World Health Organization (2011).
4. American Psychiatric Association. *Diagnostic and Statistical Manual of Mental Disorders.* 5th ed. Washington, DC: American Psychiatric Association (2013).
5. Squeglia LM, Jacobus J, Tapert SF. The effect of alcohol use on human adolescent brain structures and systems. *Handb Clin Neurol.* (2014) 125:501–10. doi: 10.1016/B978-0-444-62619-6.00028-8
6. Crone EA, Dahl RE. Understanding adolescence as a period of social-affective engagement and goal flexibility. *Nat rev Neurosci.* (2012) 13:636–50. doi: 10.1038/nrn3313
7. Dennis M, Scott CK. Managing addiction as a chronic condition. *Addict Sci Clin Pract.* (2007) 4:45–55. doi: 10.1151/ascp074145
8. Cousijn J, Luijten M, Feldstein Ewing SW. Adolescent resilience to addiction: a social plasticity hypothesis. *Lancet Child Adolesc Health* (2018) 2:69–78. doi: 10.1016/S2352-4642(17)30148-7
9. Grant BF, Dawson DA. Age at onset of alcohol use and its association with DSM-IV alcohol abuse and dependence: results from the National Longitudinal alcohol epidemiologic survey. *J Subst Abuse* (1997) 9:103–10. doi: 10.1016/S0899-3289(97)90009-2
10. Pedersen W, Skrondal A. Alcohol consumption debut: predictors and consequences. *J Stud Alcohol* (1998) 59:32–42. doi: 10.15288/jsa.1998.59.32
11. DeWit DJ, Adlaf EM, Offord DR, Ogborne AC. Age at first alcohol use: a risk factor for the development of alcohol disorders. *Am J Psychiatry* (2000) 157:745–50. doi: 10.1176/appi.ajp.157.5.745
12. Pitkanen T, Lyyra AL, Pulkkinen L. Age of onset of drinking and the use of alcohol in adulthood: a follow-up study from age 8-42 for females and males. *Addiction* (2005) 100:652–61. doi: 10.1111/j.1360-0443.2005.01053.x
13. Dawson DA, Goldstein RB, Chou SP, Ruan WJ, Grant BF. Age at first drink and the first incidence of adult-onset DSM-IV alcohol use disorders. *Alcohol Clin Exp Res.* (2008) 32:2149–60. doi: 10.1111/j.1530-0277.2008.00806.x
14. Sartor CE, Lynskey MT, Bucholz KK, Madden PA, Martin NG, Heath AC. Timing of first alcohol use and alcohol dependence: evidence of common genetic influences. *Addiction* (2009) 104:1512–8. doi: 10.1111/j.1360-0443.2009.02648.x
15. Liang W, Chikritzhs T. Age at first use of alcohol and risk of heavy alcohol use: a population-based study. *Biomed Res Int.* (2013) 2013:721761. doi: 10.1155/2013/721761
16. Asbridge M, Cartwright J, Wilson K, Langille D. Age at first drink, experiences of drunkenness, and alcohol-related problems in Canadian youth: Is early onset bad if you are a moderate drinker? *J Stud Alcohol Drugs* (2016) 77:974–9. doi: 10.15288/jsad.2016.77.974
17. McGue M, Iacono WG, Legrand LN, Malone S, Elkins I. Origins and consequences of age at first drink. I. Associations with substance-use disorders, disinhibitory behavior and psychopathology, and P3 amplitude. *Alcohol Clin Exp Res.* (2001) 25:1156–65. doi: 10.1111/j.1530-0277.2001.tb02330.x
18. Maimaris W, McCambridge J. Age of first drinking and adult alcohol problems: systematic review of prospective cohort studies. *J Epidemiol Commun Health* (2014) 68:268–74. doi: 10.1136/jech-2013-203402

19. Kuntsche E, Rossow I, Engels R, Kuntsche S. Is 'age at first drink' a useful concept in alcohol research and prevention? We doubt that. *Addiction* (2016) 111:957–65. doi: 10.1111/add.12980
20. Alaux-Cantin S, Warnault V, Legastelois R, Botia B, Pierrefiche O, Vilpoux C, et al. Alcohol intoxications during adolescence increase motivation for alcohol in adult rats and induce neuroadaptations in the nucleus accumbens. *Neuropharmacology* (2013) 67:521–31. doi: 10.1016/j.neuropharm.2012.12.007
21. Milivojevic V, Covault J. Alcohol exposure during late adolescence increases drinking in adult Wistar rats, an effect that is not reduced by finasteride. *Alcohol Alcohol.* (2013) 48:28–38. doi: 10.1093/alcalc/ags105
22. O'Tousa DS, Matson LM, Grahame NJ. Effects of intoxicating free-choice alcohol consumption during adolescence on drinking and impulsivity during adulthood in selectively bred high-alcohol preferring mice. *Alcohol Clini Exp Res.* (2013) 37:141–9. doi: 10.1111/j.1530-0277.2012.01857.x
23. Pandey SC, Sakharkar AJ, Tang L, Zhang H. Potential role of adolescent alcohol exposure-induced amygdaloid histone modifications in anxiety and alcohol intake during adulthood. *Neurobiol Dis.* (2015) 82:607–19. doi: 10.1016/j.nbd.2015.03.019
24. Amodeo LR, Kneiber D, Wills DN, Ehlers CL. Alcohol drinking during adolescence increases consumptive responses to alcohol in adulthood in wistar rats. *Alcohol* (2017) 59:43–51. doi: 10.1016/j.alcohol.2016.12.002
25. Varlinskaya EI, Kim EU, Spear LP. Chronic intermittent ethanol exposure during adolescence: effects on stress-induced social alterations and social drinking in adulthood. *Brain Res.* (2017) 1654:145–56. doi: 10.1016/j.brainres.2016.03.050
26. Gilpin NW, Karanikas CA, Richardson HN. Adolescent binge drinking leads to changes in alcohol drinking, anxiety, and amygdalar corticotropin releasing factor cells in adulthood in male rats. *PLoS ONE* (2012) 7:e31466. doi: 10.1371/journal.pone.0031466
27. Schramm-Sapyta NL, DiFeliceantonio AG, Foscue E, Glowacz S, Haseeb N, Wang N, et al. Aversive effects of ethanol in adolescent versus adult rats: potential causes and implication for future drinking. *Alcohol. Clin. Exp Res.* (2010) 34:2061–9. doi: 10.1111/j.1530-0277.2010.01302.x
28. Siegmund S, Vengeliene V, Singer MV, Spanagel R. Influence of age at drinking onset on long-term ethanol self-administration with deprivation and stress phases. *Alcohol. Clin. Exp Res.* (2005) 29:1139–45. doi: 10.1097/01.ALC.0000171928.40418.46
29. Vetter CS, Doremus-Fitzwater TL, Spear LP. Time course of elevated ethanol intake in adolescent relative to adult rats under continuous, voluntary-access conditions. *Alcohol Clin Exp Res.* (2007) 31:1159–68. doi: 10.1111/j.1530-0277.2007.00417.x
30. Serlin H, Torregrossa MM. Adolescent rats are resistant to forming ethanol seeking habits. *Dev Cogn Neurosci.* (2015) 16:183–90. doi: 10.1016/j.dcn.2014.12.002
31. Nasrallah NA, Yang TW, Bernstein IL. Long-term risk preference and suboptimal decision making following adolescent alcohol use. *Proc Nat Acad Sci USA.* (2009) 106:17600–4. doi: 10.1073/pnas.0906629106
32. Nasrallah NA, Clark JJ, Collins AL, Akers CA, Phillips PE, Bernstein IL. Risk preference following adolescent alcohol use is associated with corrupted encoding of costs but not rewards by mesolimbic dopamine. *Proc Nat Acad Sci USA.* (2011) 108:5466–71. doi: 10.1073/pnas.1017732108
33. Schindler AG, Tsutsui KT, Clark JJ. Chronic alcohol intake during adolescence, but not adulthood, promotes persistent deficits in risk-based decision making. *Alcohol Clin Exp Res.* (2014) 38:1622–9. doi: 10.1111/acer.12404
34. Miller KM, Risher ML, Acheson SK, Darlow M, Sexton HG, Schramm-Sapyta N, et al. Behavioral inefficiency on a risky decision-making task in adulthood after adolescent intermittent ethanol exposure in rats. *Sci Rep.* (2017) 7:4680. doi: 10.1038/s41598-017-04704-7
35. McClory AJ, Spear LP. effects of ethanol exposure during adolescence or in adulthood on pavlovian conditioned approach in sprague-dawley rats. *Alcohol* (2014) 48:755–63. doi: 10.1016/j.alcohol.2014.05.006
36. Spoelder M, Tsutsui KT, Lesscher HMB, Vanderschuren LJMJ, Clark JJ. Adolescent alcohol exposure amplifies the incentive value of reward-predictive cues through potentiation of phasic dopamine signaling. *Neuropsychopharmacology* (2015) 40:2873–85. doi: 10.1038/npp.2015.139
37. Spear LP. Adolescent alcohol exposure: are there separable vulnerable periods within adolescence? *Physiol Behav.* (2015) 148:122–30. doi: 10.1016/j.physbeh.2015.01.027
38. Crews FT, Vetreno RP, Broadwater MA, Robinson DL. Adolescent alcohol exposure persistently impacts adult neurobiology and behavior. *Pharmacol Rev.* (2016) 68:1074–109. doi: 10.1124/pr.115.012138
39. Spoelder M, Vanderschuren LJMJ, Lesscher HMB. Individual variation in alcohol intake predicts reinforcement, motivation, and compulsive alcohol use in rats. *Alcohol Clin Exp Res.* (2015b) 39:2427–37. doi: 10.1111/acer.12891
40. Spoelder M, Pol S, Janssen BSG, Baars AM, Vanderschuren LJMJ, Lesscher HMB. Loss of control over alcohol seeking in rats depends on individual vulnerability and duration of alcohol consumption experience. *Behav Pharmacol.* (2017) 28:334–44. doi: 10.1097/FBP.0000000000000304
41. Vetter-O'Hagen CS, Spear LP. The effects of gonadectomy on sex- and age-typical responses to novelty and ethanol-induced social inhibition in adult male and female Sprague-Dawley rats. *Behav Brain Res.* (2012) 227:224–32. doi: 10.1016/j.bbr.2011.10.023
42. Whitaker LR, Degoulet M, Morikawa H. Social deprivation enhances VTA synaptic plasticity and drug-induced contextual learning. *Neuron* (2013) 77:335–45. doi: 10.1016/j.neuron.2012.11.022
43. Baarendse PJ, Limpens JH, Vanderschuren LJMJ. Disrupted social development enhances the motivation for cocaine in rats. *Psychopharmacology* (2014) 231:1695–704. doi: 10.1007/s00213-013-3362-8
44. Lesscher HMB, Spoelder M, Rotte MD, Janssen MJ, Hesseling P, Lozeman-van 't Klooster, JG, et al. Early social isolation augments alcohol consumption in rats. *Behav Pharmacol.* (2015) 26:673–80. doi: 10.1097/FBP.0000000000000165
45. Vanderschuren LJMJ, Everitt BJ. Drug seeking becomes compulsive after prolonged cocaine self-administration. *Science* (2004) 305:1017–9. doi: 10.1126/science.1098975
46. Limpens JHW, Damsteegt R, Broekhoven MH, Vanderschuren LJMJ. Pharmacological inactivation of the prelimbic cortex emulates compulsive cocaine seeking in rats. *Brain Res.* (2014) 1628:210–8. doi: 10.1016/j.brainres.2014.10.045
47. Limpens JHW, Schut EHS, Vanderschuren LJMJ. Using conditioned suppression to investigate compulsive drug seeking in rats. *Drug Alcohol Depend.* (2014) 142:314–24. doi: 10.1016/j.drugalcdep.2014.06.037
48. Blanchard RJ, Blanchard DC. Passive and active reactions to fear-eliciting stimuli. *J. Comp Physiol Psychol.* (1969) 68:129–35. doi: 10.1037/h0027676
49. Bouton ME, Bolles RC. Conditioned fear assessed by freezing and by the suppression of three different baselines. *Anim Learn Behav.* (1980) 8:429–34. doi: 10.3758/BF03199629
50. LeDoux JE, Sakaguchi A, Reis DJ. Subcortical efferent projections of the medial geniculate nucleus mediate emotional responses conditioned to acoustic stimuli. *J Neurosci.* (1984) 4:683–98. doi: 10.1523/JNEUROSCI.04-03-00683.1984
51. Bell RL, Rodd ZA, Sable HJ, Schultz JA, Hsu CC, Lumeng L, et al. Daily patterns of ethanol drinking in peri-adolescent and adult alcohol-preferring (P) rats. *Pharmacol Biochem Behav.* (2006) 83:35–46. doi: 10.1016/j.pbb.2005.12.004
52. Spanagel R, Hölter SM. Long-term alcohol self-administration with repeated alcohol deprivation phases: an animal model of alcoholism? *Alcohol Alcohol.* (1999) 34:231–43.
53. Rodd-Henricks ZA, McKinzie DL, Murphy JM, McBride WJ, Lumeng L, Li TK. The expression of an alcohol deprivation effect in the high-alcohol-drinking replicate rat lines is dependent on repeated deprivations. *Alcohol Clin Exp Res.* (2000) 24:747–53. doi: 10.1111/j.1530-0277.2000.tb02051
54. Rodd-Henricks ZA, McKinzie DL, Shaikh SR, Murphy JM, McBride WJ, Lumeng L, et al. Alcohol deprivation effect is prolonged in the alcohol preferring (P) rat after repeated deprivations. *Alcohol Clin Exp Res.* (2000) 24:8–16. doi: 10.1111/j.1530-0277.2000.tb04546.x
55. Spanagel R, Hölter SM. Pharmacological validation of a new animal model of alcoholism. *J Neural Transm.* (2000) 107:669–80. doi: 10.1007/s007020070068
56. Serra S, Brunetti G, Pani M, Vacca G, Carai MA, Gessa GL, et al. Blockade by the cannabinoid CB(1) receptor antagonist, SR 141716, of alcohol deprivation effect in alcohol-preferring rats. *Eur J Pharmacol.* (2002) 443:95–7. doi: 10.1016/S0014-2999(02)01594-7

57. Colombo G, Serra S, Brunetti G, Vacca G, Carai MA, Gessa GL. Suppression by baclofen of alcohol deprivation effect in Sardinian alcohol-preferring (sP) rats. *Drug Alcohol Depend.* (2003) 70:105–8. doi: 10.1016/S0376-8716(02)00333-2
58. McBride WJ, Rodd ZA, Bell RL, Lumeng L, Li TK. The alcohol-preferring (P) and high-alcohol-drinking (HAD) rats–animal models of alcoholism. *Alcohol* (2014) 48:209–15. doi: 10.1016/j.alcohol.2013.09.044
59. Momeni S, Roman E. Subgroup-dependent effects of voluntary alcohol intake on behavioral profiles in outbred Wistar rats. *Behav Brain Res.* (2014) 275:288–96. doi: 10.1016/j.bbr.2014.08.058
60. Vengeliene V, Bilbao A, Spanagel R. The alcohol deprivation effect model for studying relapse behavior: a comparison between rats and mice. *Alcohol* (2014) 48:313–20. doi: 10.1016/j.alcohol.2014.03.002
61. Jeanblanc J, Balguerie K, Coune F, Legastelois R, Jeanblanc V, Naassila M. Light alcohol intake during adolescence induces alcohol addiction in a neurodevelopmental model of schizophrenia. *Addict Biol.* (2015) 20:490–9. doi: 10.1111/adb.12146
62. O'Tousa D, Grahame N. Habit formation: implications for alcoholism research. *Alcohol* (2014) 48:327–35. doi: 10.1016/j.alcohol.2014.02.004
63. Fernandez GM, Lew BJ, Vedder LC, Savage LM. Chronic intermittent ethanol exposure leads to alterations in brain-derived neurotrophic factor within the frontal cortex and impaired behavioral flexibility in both adolescent and adult rats. *Neuroscience* (2017) 348:324–34. doi: 10.1016/j.neuroscience.2017.02.045
64. Fernandez GM, Stewart WN, Savage LM. Chronic drinking during adolescence predisposes the adult rat for continued heavy drinking: neurotrophin and behavioral adaptation after long-term, continuous ethanol exposure. *PLoS ONE* (2016) 11:e0149987. doi: 10.1371/journal.pone.0149987
65. Gil-Hernandez S, Mateos P, Porras C, Garcia-Gomez R, Navarro E, Garcia-Moreno LM. Alcohol Binge Drinking and Executive Functioning during Adolescent Brain Development. *Front Psychol.* (2017) 8:1638. doi: 10.3389/fpsyg.2017.01638

6

Neural Correlates of Rewarded Response Inhibition in Youth at Risk for Problematic Alcohol Use

Brenden Tervo-Clemmens[1,2], Alina Quach[1], Beatriz Luna[1,2,3], William Foran[3], Tammy Chung[3], Michael D. De Bellis[4] and Duncan B. Clark[3]*

[1] Department of Psychology, University of Pittsburgh, Pittsburgh, PA, United States, [2] Center for the Neural Basis of Cognition, University of Pittsburgh, Pittsburgh, PA, United States, [3] Department of Psychiatry, University of Pittsburgh, Pittsburgh, PA, United States, [4] Department of Psychiatry and Behavioral Sciences, Duke University Medical Center, Durham, NC, United States

Edited by:
Shannon Leigh Gourley,
Emory University School of Medicine,
United States

Reviewed by:
Seth Davin Norrholm,
Emory University School of Medicine,
United States
Manuela Sellitto,
Heinrich Heine Universität Düsseldorf,
Germany

***Correspondence:**
Brenden Tervo-Clemmens
bct16@pitt.edu

Risk for substance use disorder (SUD) is associated with poor response inhibition and heightened reward sensitivity. During adolescence, incentives improve performance on response inhibition tasks and increase recruitment of cortical control areas (Geier et al., 2010) associated with SUD (Chung et al., 2011). However, it is unknown whether incentives moderate the relationship between response inhibition and trait-level psychopathology and personality features of substance use risk. We examined these associations in the current project using a rewarded antisaccade (AS) task (Geier et al., 2010) in youth at risk for substance use. Participants were 116 adolescents and young adults (ages 12–21) from the University of Pittsburgh site of the National Consortium on Adolescent Neurodevelopment and Alcohol [NCANDA] study, with neuroimaging data collected at baseline and 1 year follow up visits. Building upon previous work using this task in normative developmental samples (Geier et al., 2010) and adolescents with SUD (Chung et al., 2011), we examined both trial-wise BOLD responses and those associated with individual task-epochs (cue presentation, response preparation, and response) and associated them with multiple substance use risk factors (externalizing and internalizing psychopathology, family history of substance use, and trait impulsivity). Results showed that externalizing psychopathology and high levels of trait impulsivity (positive urgency, SUPPS-P) were associated with general decreases in antisaccade performance. Accompanying this main effect of poor performance, positive urgency was associated with reduced recruitment of the frontal eye fields (FEF) and inferior frontal gyrus (IFG) in both a priori regions of interest and at the voxelwise level. Consistent with previous work, monetary incentive improved antisaccade behavioral performance and was associated with increased activation in the striatum and cortical control areas. However, incentives did not moderate the association between response inhibition behavioral performance and any trait-level psychopathology and personality factor of substance use risk. Reward interactions were observed for BOLD responses at the task-epoch level, however, they were inconsistent across substance use risk types. The results from this study may suggest poor response inhibition and heightened reward sensitivity are not overlapping neurocognitive features of substance use risk. Alternatively, more subtle, common longitudinal processes might jointly explain reward sensitivity and response inhibition deficits in substance use risk.

Keywords: adolescence, response inhibition, reward, substance use, risk factors, functional magnetic resonance imaging (fMRI)

INTRODUCTION

Poor response inhibition and heightened reward sensitivity have been suggested as neurobiological risk factors for problematic substance use (Heitzeg et al., 2015). During adolescence, functional brain development supports the integration of these processes, which may influence risk for substance use initiation (Heitzeg et al., 2015; Luna and Wright, 2016). However, it is unclear how brain processes supporting cognitive-reward integration may incur risk for substance use disorders and whether these are associated with trait-level psychopathology and personality features of substance use risk.

Neuroimaging research in adolescents suggests substance use risk is associated with reduced BOLD activation in cortical brain regions supporting cognitive control. During response inhibition tasks, reduced prefrontal BOLD activation has been observed in youth who would later transition to heavy alcohol use (Norman et al., 2011) (Mahmood et al., 2013) and adolescents with a family history of alcoholism (Schweinsburg et al., 2004; see Heitzeg et al., 2015 for review). Response inhibition continues to improve through adolescence across a range of tasks (e.g., antisaccade; see Luna et al., 2010 for review), accompanied by functional changes in cortical control regions (Ordaz et al., 2013). Accordingly, poor response inhibition (c.f., Nigg et al., 2006) and reduced prefrontal BOLD activation (Norman et al., 2011) during adolescence may serve as risk factors for escalation to problematic substance use later in development.

Reduced engagement of cognitive control circuitry in youth at risk for substance use may underlie common behavioral associations between laboratory measures of response inhibition and trait-level psychopathology features of substance use risk (c.f., Young et al., 2009). To this end, neurobehavioral disinhibition (ND), a latent construct designed to asses an individual's general level of inhibition across affective, personality, and cognitive domains (c.f., Tarter et al., 2003), predicts substance use initiation (Tarter et al., 2003) and has been associated with reductions in BOLD activation in frontal cortex (McNamee et al., 2008).

Although poorer response inhibition and reduced prefrontal function have received support as neurocognitive indicators of adolescent substance use risk, previous work has typically investigated these associations in the absence of incentives on performance. However, a number of studies have demonstrated that adolescents' performance on response inhibition tasks improves when working toward an incentive (Jazbec et al., 2006; Hardin et al., 2007; Geier and Luna, 2012). Furthermore, rewarded response inhibition tasks increase BOLD activation in cortical control regions in adolescents with substance use disorder (SUD; Chung et al., 2011). This enhanced BOLD activation in youth with SUD in the context of reward may occur through enhanced reward signals from the ventral striatum, a brain region involved in the salience of reward cues (Berridge, 2007). Previous work suggests compulsive drug use is associated with a sensitization of ventral-striatal reward pathways (Robinson and Berridge, 1993). Alternatively, reward sensitivity may precede substance use initiation, as trait-level psychopathology features of substance use risk (externalizing symptoms: Bjork et al., 2010a; impulsivity: see Plichta and Scheres, 2014 review) are associated with increased BOLD activation in the ventral striatum.

In the current project, we utilized a rewarded antisaccade (AS) task to examine whether incentives enhanced response inhibition in youth at risk for substance use in a large adolescent neuroimaging sample with two time points. Building on previous work using this rewarded AS task in a normative developmental sample (Geier et al., 2010) and adolescents with SUD (Chung et al., 2011, 2015), we hypothesized that incentives would improve performance and reduce the association between substance use risk and poorer response inhibition. We first examined the relative prediction of multiple substance use risk factors on AS performance and BOLD activation. Based on the neurobehavioral disinhibition model, we predicted substance use risk factors representing poor impulse control (e.g., trait impulsivity and externalizing symptoms) would be associated with poorer AS performance and lower BOLD activation in cortical control areas. We further hypothesized these differences would be moderated by incentives, with at-risk youth showing greater reward-related improvement in response inhibition and smaller differences in inhibition-related BOLD activation during reward, relative to neutral conditions.

METHODS

Participants

Participants were recruited at the University of Pittsburgh site of the National Consortium on Adolescent Neurodevelopment and Alcohol (NCANDA) study, using procedures detailed in Brown et al. (2015). In brief, targeted catchment area calling was used to initially identify eligible youth (e.g., ages 12–21). In order to study prospective prediction for substance use risk, NCANDA recruited youth with limited substance use. However, sampling also prioritized adolescents at increased risk for alcohol use disorder (AUD) (e.g., family history of SUD), such that youth with increased risk represented 47% of the total NCANDA sample. Exclusion criteria included MRI contraindications (e.g., claustrophobia, pregnancy, non-removable metal in the body), medical history that may influence MRI (e.g., head injury with loss of consciousness), current or persistent psychiatric disorder that may influence study completion (e.g., psychosis), and psychiatric medication (see Brown et al., 2015). The University of Pittsburgh's Institutional Review Board approved the study. Adult participants provided informed consent. For minors, parents provided informed consent and youth provided assent. Participants were compensated for completing research assessments.

Based on study-specific exclusion criteria (see below), the current analyses included 116 participants who provided useable data at baseline and/or 1-year follow up. This final analysis sample spanned adolescence into young adulthood (baseline age: 12.27–21.96, mean = 17.10, $SD = 2.60$); 56.90% ($n = 66$) female; and represented 80.17% White ($n = 93$), 18.10% ($n = 21$) Black, and 1.72 % ($n = 2$) multi-racial or other race/ethnicity (see **Table 1** for sample description). A majority (58%) of participants contributed data at both baseline and follow up (total sessions: $N = 183$; total subjects: $N = 116$; subjects at baseline: $n = 101$; subjects at follow up: $n = 82$; subjects with data at both visits: $n = 67$). As detailed below, we utilize methods robust to missing data (linear and generalized mixed effects models) and therefore include all available data (subject at visit).

Measures

Exceeds Threshold Drinking

At baseline, based on self-report from the Customary Drinking and Drug Use Record (CCDR) (Brown et al., 1998), 31 participants in the analysis sample reported alcohol use that exceeded age-adjusted National Institute on Alcohol Abuse and Alcoholism (NIAAA) guidelines for risky drinking (see Brown et al., 2015), and are considered "exceeds threshold drinkers" (ETD).

Risk Factors for Substance Use

As with other sites, the NCANDA Pittsburgh sample was recruited such that approximately half of the participants were at increased risk for problematic alcohol use. The current sample utilizes participants with increased substance use risk based on one or more of the following: early substance use onset (EOS; $n = 9$), family history of substance use disorder (FH; $n = 21$), externalizing symptoms (EXT, $n = 31$), or internalizing symptoms (INT, $n = 26$). In the current analyses, EOS, FH, EXT, and INT were categorical variables (Risk vs. No Risk) and were defined at the baseline visit as in Brown et al. (2015).

EOS was defined as consuming the first full drink of alcohol prior to age 15, based on the child's report on the CDDR (Brown et al., 1998). FH was defined as having at least one biological parent with a history suggesting a substance use disorder (SUD), based on parent report using the Family History Assessment Module (Rice et al., 1995). EXT was defined as having endorsed at least one symptom of conduct disorder or antisocial personality disorder on the Computerized Semi-Structured Assessment for the Genetics of Alcoholism (SSAGA, Bucholz et al., 1994; Hesselbrock et al., 1999) or having an Achenbach System of Empirically Based Assessment (ASEBA; Achenbach, 2009) externalizing age- and gender-adjusted t-score

TABLE 1 | Subject characteristics in risk categories.

	EXT		INT		FH		ETD		Any Risk (Non-ETD)	
	Risk	**No risk**	**Risk**	**No risk**	**Risk**	**No risk**	**ETD**	**Non-ETD**	**Any risk**	**No risk**
Number of Participants	31	85	26	90	21	95	31	35	40	45
Gender n female	19	47	18	48	9	57	19	47	21	26
Age (years)	17.35 (2.55)	16.98 (2.64)	17.72 (2.25)	16.89 (2.69)	17.38 (2.85)	17.01 (2.57)	19.20 (1.47)	16.30 (2.51)	16.30 (2.34)	16.30 (2.67)
Socioeconomic status (standard score)	81.13 (15.97)	92.73 (12.31)	88.31 (15.83)	89.82 (13.95)	84.80 (15.50)	90.50 (13.97)	89.28 (15.75)	89.53 (13.93)	84.88 (14.74)	94.07 (11.55)
Generalized ability (z-score)	−0.389 (0.967)	0.085 (0.796)	0.191 (0.795)	−0.105 (0.880)	0.038 (0.820)	−0.055 (0.880)	0.199 (0.839)	−0.172 (0.865)	−0.205 (0.938)	−0.049 (0.800)
Positive urgency	1.96 (0.612)	1.77 (0.608)	1.85 (0.629)	1.82 (0.611)	1.89 (0.671)	1.81 (0.602)	1.85 (0.756)	1.82 (0.557)	1.96 (0.562)	1.69 (0.526)
Negative urgency	2.10 (0.621)	1.85 (0.641)	2.03 (0.609)	1.88 (0.652)	1.82 (0.520)	1.93 (0.667)	1.98 (0.699)	1.89 (0.628)	2.06 (0.559)	1.74 (0.657)

*All scores from baseline visit. In addition to EXT, INT, and FH, Any Risk (Non-ETD) additionally excludes EOS ($n = 9$). See **Table 2** for associations between variables.*

above 60. Similarly, INT was defined as having endorsed two or more symptoms or having an ASEBA internalizing t-score above 60. In the current analysis, we did not examine EOS because of the few participants meeting criteria in the Pittsburgh sample ($n = 9$).

Trait Impulsivity

In addition to risk factors described by Brown et al. (2015), we also examined associations between AS performance and BOLD activation and trait impulsivity as measured by the short version of the UPPS-P (SUPPS-P, Cyders et al., 2014). Trait impulsivity is associated with increased vulnerability to SUD (c.f., Verdejo-García et al., 2008) and has been conceptualized as having shared underlying features with antisocial behavior and substance use (Krueger et al., 2007). Although trait impulsivity and response inhibition have both been considered measures of inhibitory control, it has been suggested trait personality measures of impulsivity likely represent more global differences in impulsive choice whereas behavioral measures of response inhibition reflect specific cognitive processes (Reynolds et al., 2006). We focused on the SUPPS-P scales of negative and positive *urgency* as the urgency domain has been associated with substance use (Zapolski et al., 2009) and BOLD activation in a rewarded stop signal task (Wilbertz et al., 2014). Participants completed the SUPPS-P at both baseline and follow up visits.

Generalized Cognitive Ability

As part of the NCANDA test protocol, participants completed the Penn Computerized Neurocognitive Battery (WebCNP: Gur et al., 2010) and traditional "pencil and paper" neuropsychological tests (Sullivan et al., 2016). We utilized a composite score, generalized ability accuracy (GA; see Sullivan et al., 2016), as an outcome variable and covariate when examining substance use risk factors in our analyses. The GA measure was derived from several domains of neuropsychological function, allowing us to examine whether associations among substance use risk factors, AS performance, and BOLD activation were specific to response inhibition or instead, reflected reduced generalized cognitive ability.

Socioeconomic Status

The socioeconomic status (SES) variable was determined by both parental education and income (see Brown et al., 2015). SES was expressed as a standard score (mean = 100, $SD = 15$) and included as a covariate in secondary analyses.

Baseline and Follow up Coding of Primary Variables of Interest

In order to harmonize our analytic approach with previous work with NCDANDA baseline data (c.f., Brown et al., 2015; Müller-Oehring et al., 2017), at both baseline and follow up we utilized scores from study initiation for the primary substance use risk categories (FH, EXT, INT) and exceeds threshold drinking (ETD) as outlined in Brown et al. (2015). This approach allows our results to be interpreted more readily with other projects describing cognitive differences with baseline risk group definitions (c.f., Sullivan et al., 2016). Continuous primary measures (participant age and trait-impulsivity) were treated as time-varying covariates, with the unique scores entered at baseline and follow up.

Missing Data from Primary Variables of Interest

Based on the random effects structure of our modeling framework (see below), we were able to utilize participants that only had data at one visit (baseline or follow up). However, some participants were missing primary variables of interest. In the final behavioral sample (see below), SUPPS-P data was missing for two participants at baseline and eight participants at follow up. In the final neuroimaging sample two participants were missing SUPPS-P at baseline. As SUPPS-P was collected at both baseline and follow up, missing sessions (subject at visit) were excluded from analyses of SUPPS-P variables. One subject included in both behavioral and neuroimaging analysis was missing GA data. Six participants were missing SES data. As GA and SES were defined at baseline these participants were excluded from all analyses using these variables. No participants were missing FH, EXT, INT, or ETD data.

Rewarded Antisaccade Task

Participants completed the same rewarded antisaccade task as used in Geier et al. (2010) and Chung et al. (2011) (See **Figure 1**). The full protocol included 56 full reward trials and 56 full neutral trials, completed across four neuroimaging runs (14 reward and 14 neutral trials per run), which included three epochs (cue, preparation, and response). Full trials began with a cue epoch (1.5 s), where participants viewed a white central fixation cross, surrounded by a circle of green "$" symbols (reward trials) or blue "#" symbols (neutral trials). Next, a red fixation cross appeared, indicating the preparation epoch (1.5 s), where subjects prepared to stop an impending eye movement to an unknown location. Finally, in the response epoch (1.5 s), a peripheral cue (yellow circle) was presented along the horizontal meridian at 1 of 6 eccentricities (±3, 6, and 9 degrees visual angle, relative to fixation) and participants were instructed to perform a saccade away from the circle toward the mirror location. An additional 24 (12 rewarded; 12 neutral) partial trials that presented either

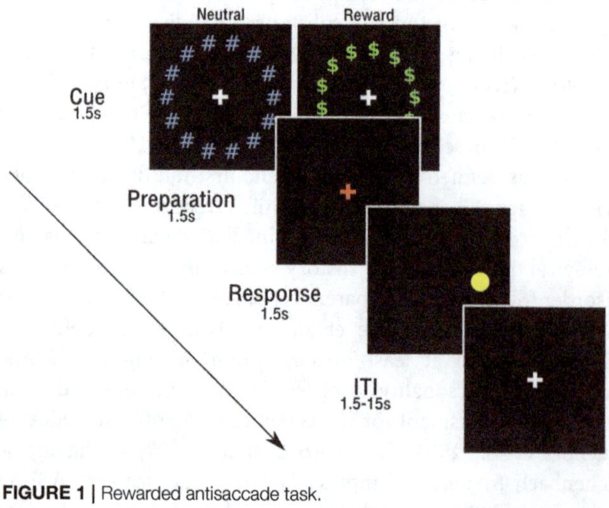

FIGURE 1 | Rewarded antisaccade task.

the cue alone (6 of each reward type) or the cue and prep epoch (6 of each reward type) but not the response epoch were included in order to estimate the hemodynamic response for each trial epoch (c.f., Ollinger et al., 2001).

Prior to the session, participants were informed they could earn a small monetary reward during trials with the "$." As in Chung et al. (2011), participants were told they could win up to $10 for correct antisaccade performance in the session and that there would be no monetary loss for incorrect responses. However, participants were not told the value of a specific response in reward trials and feedback was not provided. This prevented participants from attempting to keep track of an ongoing reward tally. At the end of the session, all participants received the full $10 reward.

Eye Movement Measurement and Scoring

Stimuli from the AS task were presented on a flat screen behind the MRI scanner with E-Prime software (Schneider et al., 2002) and made visible to the subject with a mirror mounted on the head coil. Eye-tracking was performed using a long-range optics eye-tracking system (Applied Science Laboratories, Bedford, MA) and eye-position was measured through corneal reflection. Video monitoring was performed to ensure task compliance. Prior to the test session, a 9-point calibration was performed for each subject.

Eye movements in the response epoch were a scored as a correct AS if the first eye movement during the response epoch had a velocity greater than or equal to 30°/s (Gitelman, 2002) and was made in the mirror location of the peripheral cue and extended at least 2.5° visual angle from central fixation. In contrast, eye movements were marked as an incorrect AS if the first saccade in the response epochs was made toward the peripheral cue and extended at least 2.5° visual angle from central fixation, but then later directed toward the correct location, suggesting task compliance. Trials in which no saccade occurred or if the eye-tracker lost fixation were excluded from all analyses. Scan sessions were excluded from all behavioral and fMRI analysis if the proportion of excluded trials was greater than 33%.

Within the final analysis sample ($N = 116$), the overall proportion of excluded trials was 11.4% at baseline and 12.1% at follow up. Utilizing linear mixed effects models (see below for methods), the proportion of excluded trials was positively associated with the trait impulsivity measure of negative urgency [$t = 2.01$, $\chi^2_{(1)} = 4.02$, $p = 0.045$], suggesting that those with higher levels of negative urgency had more excluded trials. Those with a family history of substance use had a significantly lower proportion of excluded trials [$t = -1.97$, $\chi^2_{(1)} = 3.87$, $p = 0.049$]. Age at visit, EXT, INT, ETD, and positive urgency were not associated with the proportion of excluded eye tracking trials (see Supplemental Table 1).

fMRI Data Acquisition

Imaging data were collected using a 3.0-T Siemens Magnetom TIM Trio at the Magnetic Resonance Research Center at the University of Pittsburgh. Structural images used for functional registration and conversion to a standardized template were collected using a magnetization prepared rapid acquisition gradient-echo (MP-RAGE) pulse sequence with a 160 slices (1.2 × 0.938 × 0.938 mm). Functional data were collected using an echo-planar imaging (EPI) sequence with the following parameters: TR = 1.5 s, TE = 28 ms, Flip Angle = 73°, and 64 × 64 acquisition matrix with a field of view of 200 mm. Twenty-nine slices were collected in the axial plane with 3.125 × 3.125 by 3.200 mm anisotropic voxels.

fMRI Data Preprocessing

Preprocessing of functional data followed standard procedures. This included slice timing correction, despiking (AFNI 3dDespike), motion correction (mcflirt; Jenkinson et al., 2002), brain extraction, non-linear registration of functional data to a standardized anatomical brain (3 mm MNI-152 template: 2009c), spatial smoothing with FWHM of 5 mm (SUSAN; Smith and Brady, 1997), high pass filtering at 80 volumes (0.00625 Hz), and scaling by 10,000 of the global median.

Data Analysis

Associations among Participant Characteristics

Associations among participant characteristics were analyzed for sample description and covariate selection (**Table 2**). In order to provide standardized associations across all

TABLE 2 | Correlations among participant characteristics.

	EXT	INT	FH	ETD	PUG	NUG	Gender	Age	SES	GA
EXT		Polychoric	Polychoric	Polychoric	Polyserial	Polyserial	Polychoric	Polyserial	Polyserial	Polyserial
INT	**0.467****		Polychoric	Polychoric	Polyserial	Polyserial	Polychoric	Polyserial	Polyserial	Polyserial
FH	0.133	0.032		Polychoric	Polyserial	Polyserial	Polychoric	Polyserial	Polyserial	Polyserial
ETD	0.056	−0.085	0.223		Polyserial	Polyserial	Polychoric	Polyserial	Polyserial	Polyserial
PUG	0.176	0.031	0.068	0.032		Pearson	Polyserial	Pearson	Pearson	Pearson
NUG	0.231	0.135	−0.103	0.075	**0.686****		Polyserial	Pearson	Pearson	Pearson
Gender	0.091	0.238	−0.241	0.091	**−0.282***	−0.095		Polyserial	Polyserial	Polyserial
Age	0.086	0.194	0.080	**0.705****	**−0.244***	−0.095	0.136		Pearson	Pearson
SES	**−0.432***	−0.060	−0.210	−0.010	−0.162	−0.109	−0.014	−0.005		Pearson
GA	**−0.306***	0.209	0.062	0.226	**−0.296***	**−0.272***	0.033	**0.433***	**0.411***	

*$p < 0.05$, **$p < 0.01$. Lower triangle displays correlations. Upper triangle displays correlation type. EXT, INT, FH, and ETD were coded with meeting criteria/risk as 1. Gender was coded with women as 1. See (Data Analysis for further discussion). Significant relationships are bolded.*

variable types, Pearson (continuous-continuous), polyserial (continuous-categorical), and polychoric (categorical-categorical) correlation values (Fox, 2010) are reported (see **Table 2**). Significance testing utilized Pearson correlation for continuous-continuous associations, Welch's *t*-test for continuous-categorical associations and chi-square testing for categorical-categorical associations.

Antisaccade Behavioral Performance

Behavioral analysis was performed using R 3.1.2 (R Core Team, 2014). Mixed effects models (lme4 package; Bates et al., 2013) were used to examine associations between antisaccade (AS) correct response rates (accuracy) and latency and exceeds threshold drinking (ETD), substance use risk factors (FH, INT, EXT), and trait impulsivity (positive and negative urgency) and whether these associations were moderated by reward.

AS correct response rates were analyzed with generalized mixed-effects models with a logit link function as trial level data was binomially distributed (correct vs. incorrect). AS latencies were analyzed with linear mixed effects models and only included correct trials. Both linear and generalized-linear mixed-effects models used maximum likelihood estimation. Random intercepts were estimated for each subject. Reward condition (reward/neutral), visit (baseline/follow up), age at visit, exceeds threshold drinking (ETD), substance use risk factors (FH, EXT, INT), trait impulsivity measures (positive and negative urgency), generalized ability (GA), and socioeconomic status (SES) were included as fixed effects in three types of models. In the first type (Type A), ETD, FH, EXT, INT, and impulsivity measures were examined as predictors of AS performance in separate models. Second (Type B), ETD, FH, EXT, INT, and impulsivity measures were examined as joint predictors of AS performance in the same model. Third (Type C), GA and SES were included as additional covariates to the joint model. Reward, visit, and age at visit were included in all three model types. Secondary analysis included gender as a covariate in analysis of positive urgency (see below). Significance values for fixed effects were obtained through the car package in R (Fox et al., 2016; Wald chi-square test). Given the correlation between our variables of interest and our goal of defining sensitive and specific associations between substance use risk factors and AS performance, we highlight predictors that are significant across all three model types (A-C).

fMRI

Twelve sessions were excluded from all fMRI analyses due to poor EPI coverage across imaging runs ($n = 4$) or technical errors ($n = 8$). Accordingly, the final neuroimaging sample consisted of 171 scan sessions distributed across 111 participants (participants at baseline, $n = 95$; participants at follow up, $n = 76$; participants with data at both visits, $n = 60$). Subject-level fMRI analyses were performed with Analysis and Visualization of Functional Neuroimages (AFNI, Bethesda, MD) software. In order to estimate the BOLD response at the trial- and individual AS epoch-level (cue, preparation, response), two level 1 GLM analyses were run for each subject at each visit using AFNI's 3dDeconvolve tool.

GLM-1

Reward and neutral trial-level BOLD responses were estimated with a 4,500 ms boxcar convolved with a gamma function (AFNI's block 4) and scaled to have an amplitude of 1. Separate regressors were included for correct, incorrect, and dropped/poor eye-tracking AS trials. Partial trials were modeled in the same manner but with 1,500 ms (cue partial trial) or 3,000 ms (cue and preparation partial trial) boxcars. Six rigid-body head motion parameters and their derivatives and run-wise 0 through 3rd order polynomials were used as nuisance regressors. The current and preceding TR were censored if the Euclidean norm head motion distance surpassed 0.9 mm, based on suggestions for task-based neuroimaging outlined in Siegel et al. (2014). Parameter estimates were examined both as main effects (Task > Fixation) and in comparisons with reward type (Reward > Neutral).

GLM-2

As reward-related changes in BOLD activation have been shown to vary according to demand characteristics (c.f., Geier et al., 2010), we also estimated BOLD activation in individual task-epochs (cue, preparation, and response). Epoch-level BOLD responses were estimated in a second model with individual regressors for cue, preparation, and response epochs. Relevant partial trials were included as examples of the epoch in question to aid in epoch-specific HRF estimation. All three epochs (cue, preparation, and response) were modeled with a 1,500 ms boxcar convolved with a gamma function (AFNI's block 4). The same nuisance regressors and motion censoring were used as in GLM-1.

Regions of Interest

We first examined associations of BOLD activation with ETD and substance use risk (FH, EXT, INT, impulsivity) in a priori regions of interest (ROIs) (**Table 3**). Regions were selected based on their association with the AS task in previous voxelwise analyses (Velanova et al., 2009; Geier et al., 2010), including the frontal and supplementary eye fields (FEF and SEF), pre supplementary motor area (pre-SMA), and executive function more generally (c.f., Wesley and Bickel, 2014), including posterior parietal cortices (PPC), dorsolateral prefrontal cortex (DLPFC), ventrolateral prefrontal cortex (VLPFC), inferior frontal gyrus (IFG) and dorsal anterior cingulate cortex (dACC). Additionally, given the focus on interactions with reward, we also selected regions of interest from the striatum, including the caudate, putamen, and nucleus accumbens (NAcc), which have previously been associated with reward effects and externalizing symptoms (Bjork et al., 2010b) and rewarded response inhibition tasks (Wilbertz et al., 2014).

Cortical ROIs were taken from a previous longitudinal neuroimaging study utilizing an AS task in adolescents (Ordaz et al., 2013), where the full methods are provided. Briefly, central coordinates were identified using topic and term searches in Neurosynth (http://neurosynth.org/), a meta-analysis tool for functional neuroimaging. Minor corrections to coordinates were made to ensure final ROIs overlapped with canonical eye movement regions (c.f., Munoz and Everling, 2004). From

TABLE 3 | Regions of interest and BOLD characteristics.

	MNI X, Y, Z	Radius (mm)	Voxels (*n*)	Sessions excluded (*n*)	Neutral (*t*)	Reward (*t*)	Reward > Neutral (*t*)	Reward by hemisphere (*t*)
SUBCORTICAL								
Caudate		–		0	3.22**	5.56**	3.15**	−0.02
Left	−13.7, 13.5, 9.5		137					
Right	12.0, 13.1, 11.0		154					
Putamen		–		1	18.63**	20.02**	2.01*	<0.01
Left	−25.1, 6.8, 0.5		136					
Right	24.3, 7.0, 0.4	–	150					
NAcc		–		3	−2.28*	1.17	3.86**	0.75
Left	−9.2, 12.4, −6.9		14					
Right	8.5, 13.4, −6.5		14					
CORTICAL								
PPC				0	14.65**	16.23**	2.23*	−0.01
Left	−32, −48, 50	10	85					
Right	32, −54, 48	10	97					
FEF				0	20.18**	21.76**	2.45*	0.08
Left	−25.5, −1.5, 46	10	122					
Right	26.5, −1.5, 58	10	89					
SEF	0.0, −4.6, 62.0	7	46	0	9.37**	10.74**	2.02*	–
pre-SMA	0.0, 5.0, 52.1	7	38	0	10.48**	11.38**	1.24	–
dACC	0.0, 19.5, 40.5	10	156	0	11.43**	13.80**	2.38*	–
DLPFC				0	−0.53	2.04*	2.78**	−0.49
Left	−41.0, 19.0, 41.0	12	103					
Right	42.0, 18.0, 42.0	12	169					
VLPFC				0	6.71**	7.83**	1.36	0.03
Left	−46.5, 10.5, 24.0	10	80					
Right	49.5, 12.0 22.0	10	95					
IFG				1	7.99**	8.11**	0.13	0.17
Left	−40.0, 6.0, 0.0	12	220					
Right	40.0, 10, 2.0	12	230					

*$p < 0.05$, **$p < 0.01$.

each central coordinate, spheres were grown, with the radius determined based on anatomical size and to avoid overlap (see **Table 3**). Striatum ROIs were taken from the Harvard-Oxford Atlas distributed through FSL software (Jenkinson et al., 2012). All ROIs were eroded such that they only included voxels with a 50% or greater probability of being gray matter in the MNI-152 template.

Our final list of ROIs included several pairs of bilateral regions (**Table 3**). In order to reduce the number of comparisons and because our hypotheses were not hemisphere specific, our primary analyses utilized left and right ROI pairs in one model with hemisphere as a within-subject factor. No ROI pair had a significant reward by hemisphere interaction (**Table 3**).

Region of Interest Testing

Nonzero mean BOLD activation (parameter estimates from GLM-1 & 2; see above) from correct trials were extracted from ROIs for each subject at each visit. As in the AS behavioral analysis, linear mixed effects models were utilized to examine the association of BOLD activation with ETD and substance use risk factors (FH, EXT, INT, impulsivity) and whether these associations were moderated by reward. Random intercepts were estimated for each subject and fixed effects were included in three phases (Type A, B, C). Additionally, session-wise motion estimates (proportion of censored volumes due to head motion) were used as a covariate in all models. Secondary analysis of positive urgency included gender as a covariate, as positive urgency was higher in males than females (see below). Scan sessions (subject at a particular visit) were excluded from analysis of an ROI if it did not have at least 90% epi coverage of the ROI or ROI pair. This exclusion never resulted in more than three scan sessions being omitted. In order to maximize the precision of individual subject estimates, we first examined main effects of ETD and risk factors (FH, EXT, INT, impulsivity) and their interactions with reward on trial-wise BOLD responses (GLM-1). Subsequently, we examined whether reward effects varied by AS epoch (reward by epoch interaction) using individual BOLD estimates of cue, preparation, and response from GLM-2. In order to assist in the interpretation of the direction of effects with BOLD activation, we additionally examined the association between BOLD activation and antisaccade correct response rate (accuracy). In all cases, significance values across ROIs were corrected for multiple comparisons using the false-discovery rate (FDR; $q < 0.05$).

Voxelwise Testing

To ensure the selection of ROIs did not bias our results we also performed voxelwise linear mixed effects analysis (3dLME; Chen et al., 2013) with age at visit and session-wise motion as covariates (model Type A). As in ROI analysis, voxelwise analysis only used data from correct trials. Voxelwise testing was limited to voxels that met each of the following criteria: 50% or greater probability of being gray matter in the MNI-152 template, full EPI coverage in all participants across all runs, and a significant simple effect of the task in reward or neutral trials (task vs. fixation), suggesting activation to the AS task significantly differed (positively or negatively). When examining ETD and risk factors (FH, INT, EXT, impulsivity), multiple comparison correction within this voxelwise space was performed using the intersection of voxelwise FDR correction ($q < 0.05$) and cluster size. AFNI's 3dClustsim program was used to determine cluster size threshold through a Monte Carlo simulation with parameters derived from mean spatial autocorrelation parameters from GLM-1 residuals.

RESULTS

Associations among Participant Characteristics

Based on the significant association of GA with EXT, PUG, and NUG and SES with EXT (**Table 2**), these variables were used as covariates in the step-wise modeling procedure (Type A-C). Additionally given that female participants had lower levels of positive urgency (mean female positive urgency baseline: 1.70; mean male positive urgency baseline: 1.98; polyserial correlation: −0.282, welch's *t*: −2.49, $p = 0.014$), secondary analysis of positive urgency included gender as a covariate.

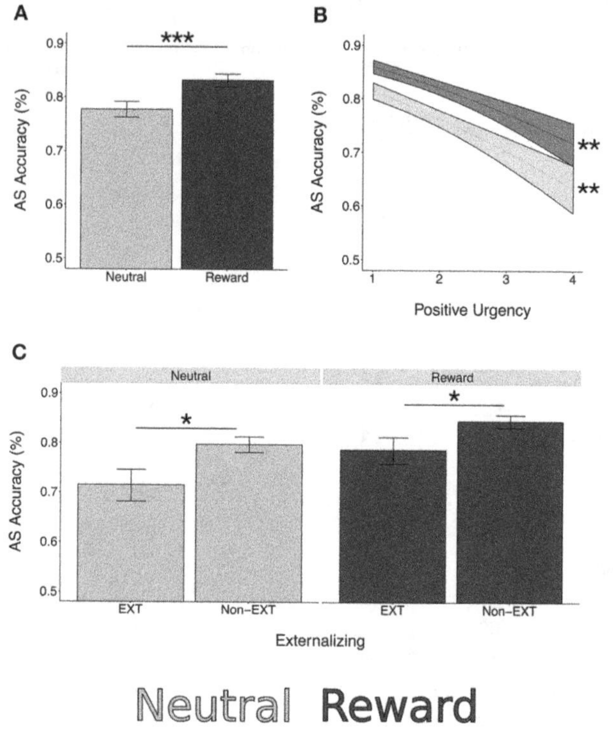

FIGURE 2 | Rewarded antisaccade behavioral performance. $^{*}p < 0.05$, $^{**}p < 0.01$, $^{***}p < 0.0001$. **(A)** Antisaccade correct response rate (accuracy) is significantly higher in reward trials compared to neutral [$z = 9.01$, $\chi^2_{(1)} = 81.16$, $p < 0.0001$]. **(B)** Positive urgency is a significant negative predictor of AS accuracy [$z = -4.19$, $\chi^2_{(1)} = 17.53$, $p < 0.001$]. This association is not moderated by reward [$z = 0.32$, $\chi^2_{(1)} = 0.12$, $p = 0.750$]. **(C)** Those with externalizing risk have lower AS accuracy [$z = -2.34$, $\chi^2_{(1)} = 5.50$, $p = 0.019$]. This does not differ by reward type [$z = 0.66$, $\chi^2_{(1)} = 0.43$, $p = 0.510$]. Simple effects testing confirmed significant effects of externalizing risk and positive urgency in both reward and neutral trials (externalizing neutral: $z = -2.43$, $p = 0.015$; externalizing reward: $z = -2.10$, $p = 0.036$; positive urgency neutral: $z = -4.06$, $p = 0.001$; positive urgency reward: $z = -3.73$, $p = 0.002$).

Antisaccade Behavioral Performance

Accuracy

Overall, antisaccade (AS) correct response rate (accuracy) (mean = 75.31%, *SD* = 16.67%) was comparable with previous work (Geier et al., 2010). Consistent with previous work (Geier et al., 2010), participant age was a significant positive predictor of AS accuracy [$z = 5.36$, $\chi^2_{(1)} = 28.70$, $p < 0.001$], with increased performance in older participants. Furthermore, as in Geier et al. (2010), AS accuracy was significantly higher in reward trials compared to neutral [$z = 9.01$, $\chi^2_{(1)} = 81.16$, $p < 0.001$; **Figure 2**].

Substance Use and Risk Factors

Externalizing risk [$z = -2.34$, $\chi^2_{(1)} = 5.50$, $p = 0.019$] and higher levels of the trait impulsivity measure of positive urgency [$z = -4.19$, $\chi^2_{(1)} = 17.53$, $p < 0.001$] were associated with lower AS accuracy while controlling for age and reward condition (model type A; **Figure 2**). Externalizing risk and positive urgency remained significant predictors when ETD and the other substance use risk factors were entered into a multivariate model (model type B; **Table 4**), suggesting that EXT and positive urgency were each independently associated with AS correct response rate controlling for other variables. INT, FH, ETD, and negative urgency were not significantly associated with AS accuracy (see **Table 4**).

Neither externalizing risk nor positive urgency had significant interaction terms with the AS reward condition [externalizing risk by reward: $z = 0.66$, $\chi^2_{(1)} = 0.43$, $p = 0.510$; positive urgency by reward: $z = 0.32$, $\chi^2_{(1)} = 0.12$, $p = 0.750$], suggesting equivalent performance effects in reward and neutral trials (**Table 4**, **Figure 2**). Supporting this, simple effects testing revealed externalizing risk and positive urgency were significant predictors of AS accuracy in both neutral and reward trials [externalizing neutral: $z = -2.43$, $p = 0.015$; externalizing reward: $z = -2.10$, $p = 0.036$; positive urgency neutral: -4.06, $p < 0.001$; positive urgency reward: $z = -3.73$, $p < 0.001$]. Reward interactions were also not significant for INT, FH, ETD, or negative urgency (**Table 4**).

TABLE 4 | Main effects and reward interactions from models of antisaccade performance.

	EXT	INT	FH	ETD	PUG	NUG	Age	SES	GA
ACCURACY (z)									
Main effect	**−2.34***[B]	1.12	−0.62	1.33	**−4.19****[B,C,G]	−1.39	**5.36****[B,C]	0.82	**2.93****
Reward interaction	0.66	0.58	−0.63	−0.24	0.32	0.66	−1.56	0.42	−0.09
LATENCY (t)									
Main effect	0.04	0.32	−1.14	0.07	**−2.80****[B,C,G]	−0.26	**−3.32****[B,C]	0.55	0.25
Reward interaction	0.81	0.56	−1.30	0.45	0.42	0.69	−0.89	1.01	0.11

*$p < 0.05$, **$p < 0.01$. Displayed estimates are test statistics from models with the specific factor, subject age, visit, and reward condition (Type A). [B]$p < 0.05$ (Type B) model with all risk factors, subject age, visit, and reward condition; [C]$p < 0.05$ (Type C) model with all risk factors, subject age, visit, reward condition, and socioeconomic status (SES) and GA (generalized ability). Significant estimates are bolded. [G]Positive Urgency $p < 0.05$ while covarying gender.

Covariate Relationships

SES was not associated with AS accuracy [$z = 0.82$, $\chi^2_{(1)} = 0.68$, $p = 0.410$]. Generalized cognitive ability (GA) was positively associated with AS accuracy [$z = 2.93$, $\chi^2_{(1)} = 8.57$, $p = 0.003$]. When covarying GA (i.e., model type A + GA), the association between externalizing risk and AS accuracy was reduced to a trend [$z = -1.69$, $\chi^2_{(1)} = 2.84$, $p = 0.092$], but positive urgency remained a significant negative predictor of AS accuracy [$z = -3.88$, $\chi^2_{(1)} = 15.09$, $p < 0.001$].These results were unchanged in the full model with all other predictors (model Type C; see **Table 4**). Secondary analysis further showed positive urgency remained a significant negative predictor of AS accuracy while covarying gender [type A + gender: $z = -4.30$, $\chi^2_{(1)} = 18.52$, $p < 0.001$]. Gender was not a significant predictor in this model [$z = 1.17$, $\chi^2_{(1)} = 1.17$, $p = 0.279$].

Latency

AS latency on correct trials (mean = 440.86, SD = 59.62) had a negative relationship with participant age [$t = -3.32$, $\chi^2_{(1)} = 11.01$, $p = 0.001$]. AS latency was significantly shorter in rewarded trials compared to neutral trials [$t = -6.99$, $\chi^2_{(1)} = 48.89$, $p < 0.001$].

Substance Use and Risk Factors

Of the substance use and risk measures, only positive urgency was significantly associated with AS latency, where higher positive urgency scores were associated with shorter latencies [$t = -2.80$, $\chi^2_{(1)} = 7.84$, $p = 0.005$] (see **Table 4**). The relationship between positive urgency and AS latency did not vary by reward condition [$t = 0.42$, $\chi^2_{(1)} = 0.18$, $p = 0.676$].

Covariate Relationships

Neither SES [$t = 0.55$, $\chi^2_{(1)} = 0.30$, $p = 0.583$] nor GA [$t = 0.24$, $\chi^2_{(1)} = 0.06$, $p = 0.809$] was associated with AS latency. Gender was associated with AS latency, where males (least-squares mean: 421.74 ms) were faster than females (least-squares mean: 457.55 ms) on correct trials [Type A: $t = -3.55$, $\chi^2_{(1)} = 12.57$, $p = 0.0003$]. When entered as joint predictors (Type A + positive urgency and gender), positive urgency [$t = -2.47$, $\chi^2_{(1)} = 6.13$, $p = 0.013$] and gender [$t = -3.22$, $\chi^2_{(1)} = 10.35$, $p = 0.001$] remained significant predictors of AS latency.

fMRI

Head Motion

The proportion of censored volumes due to head motion was negatively associated with age [$t = -2.07$, $\chi^2_{(1)} = 4.287$, $p = 0.038$] and positively associated with both trait impulsivity measures [positive urgency: $t = 2.86$, $\chi^2_{(1)} = 8.18$, $p = 0.004$; negative urgency: $t = 2.80$ $\chi^2_{(1)} = 7.86$, $p = 0.005$]. There was also trend for those in the externalizing risk group to have more motion [$t = 1.94$ $\chi^2_{(1)} = 3.77$, $p = 0.052$]. In contrast, the proportion of censored volumes due to motion was not associated with exceeding threshold drinking [$t = 0.35$, $\chi^2_{(1)} = 0.12$, $p = 0.728$], internalizing risk [$t = -1.16$, $\chi^2_{(1)} = 1.35$, $p = 0.244$], or family history of SUD [$t = 0.50$, $\chi^2_{(1)} = 0.25$ $p = 0.617$]. As detailed in the method section, the proportion of censored volumes due to head motion was used as a covariate in all fMRI analyses.

Task Effects

Robust activation in response to the task (task > fixation) was observed in canonical AS and cognitive control regions, including bilateral frontal eye fields (FEF), posterior parietal cortices (PPC), as well as in the anterior cingulate cortex (ACC) and striatum (see **Figure 3**). All selected ROIs had significant positive BOLD activation (task > fixation) in either the neutral or reward condition (**Table 3**). Increased activation to reward was observed at the voxelwise level in the striatum, bilateral PPC, and the right middle frontal gyrus/dorsolateral prefrontal cortex (DLPFC; **Figure 3**). The majority of ROIs had greater activation in reward trials, compared to neutral (**Table 3**).

Main Effects of ETD and Substance Use Risk Factors

Within a priori ROIs, positive urgency was associated with reduced BOLD activation in the putamen [$t = -4.68$, $\chi^2_{(1)} = 21.86$, $p < 0.001$, corrected], FEF [$t = -2.64$, $\chi^2_{(1)} = 6.96$, $p = 0.031$, corrected], and inferior frontal gyrus [IFG; $t = -3.00$, $\chi^2_{(1)} = 8.99$, $p = 0.015$, corrected] (**Table 5**). Family history of SUD was associated with reduced activation in the posterior parietal cortex, although this was only a trend after multiple comparison correction [$t = -2.74$, $\chi^2_{(1)} = 7.49$, $p = 0.006$ uncorrected, $p = 0.068$ corrected]. These effects were unchanged with ETD and all substance use risk measures entered in a multivariate model (Type B) or when including SES and GA

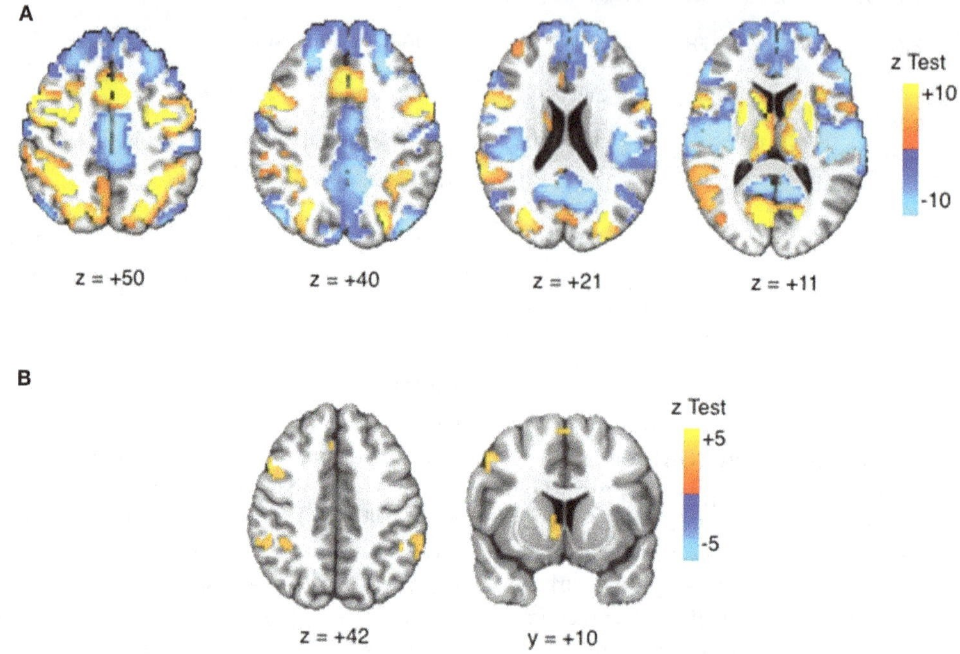

FIGURE 3 | Task BOLD effects. Activation maps displayed at voxelwise threshold $p < 0.005$, number of contiguous voxels (faces touching) > 24, cluster-level alpha <0.05. **(A)** Task > Fixation: Robust BOLD activation is observed in canonical eye movement and executive function areas. **(B)** Reward > Neutral: Increased BOLD activation is observed in striatal reward areas and attentions areas.

TABLE 5 | BOLD main effects in regions of interest (*t*-values): trial-wise (GLM-1).

	EXT	INT	FH	ETD	PUG	NUG	Age	SES	GA	AS Acc
SUBCORTICAL										
Caudate$^{L.R.}$	−1.36	−0.41	−1.03	0.04	−1.00	1.55	−1.65	−0.47	0.41	**2.48***
Putamen$^{L.R.}$	**−2.29**	−1.24	−1.33	−0.19	**−4.68***^{B,C,G}	−1.35	0.87	−0.30	0.44	**3.08***
NAcc$^{L.R.}$	−1.38	−0.21	0.06	0.45	1.39	1.68	−0.86	0.70	0.81	−0.14
CORTICAL										
PPC$^{L.R.}$	−0.91	−0.33	**−2.74**+^{B,C}	**−2.42**	−0.51	−0.20	0.10	−0.58	0.64	1.72
FEF$^{L.R.}$	**−2.05**	−0.79	−0.78	0.20	**−2.64***^{B,C,G}	−0.87	1.03	0.23	**2.09**	**2.34+**
SEF	−1.45	−0.63	−0.23	0.89	−1.06	−0.75	−0.34	−0.77	−0.55	**2.04+**
Pre-SMA	−1.79	0.25	−0.26	−1.22	−1.70	−1.88	0.34	0.06	0.84	**2.14+**
dACC	−1.53	−0.54	−0.88	−0.55	−1.59	−0.93	−0.94	−0.30	1.11	**2.57***
DLPFC$^{L.R.}$	−0.36	−0.10	−1.51	−1.25	−1.65	−0.12	−1.34	−0.62	−1.46	0.49
VLPFC$^{L.R.}$	−0.90	−1.31	−1.04	0.07	−1.34	−0.64	1.35	−1.28	0.47	−1.21
IFG$^{L.R.}$	0.43	−0.48	−1.47	−0.80	**−3.00***^{B,C,G}	−0.26	−0.05	−1.03	−1.31	1.16

*$^{+}p < 0.10$ (corrected), *$p < 0.05$ (corrected). Displayed estimates are test statistics from models with the specific factor, subject age, visit, and reward condition (Type A). $^{B}p < 0.05$ (Type B) model with all risk factors, subject age, visit, and reward condition; $^{C}p < 0.05$ (Type C) model with all risk factors, subject age, visit, reward condition, and SES and GA. ^{G}Positive Urgency $p < 0.05$ while covarying gender. $^{L.R.}$, Left/Right ROIs are included within one model. Estimates with uncorrected p's < 0.05 are bolded.*

as covariates (Type C). Furthermore, the association between positive urgency and BOLD activation in the putamen, FEF, and IFG, remained significant while covarying gender. No other measures had significant or trending, corrected main effects.

At the voxelwise level, positive urgency had a negative relationship with BOLD activation in the left inferior frontal gyrus (IFG) and right frontal eye field [FEF; voxelwise threshold (p) = 0.0012, $q < 0.05$, number of contiguous voxels (faces touching) > 24] (**Figure 4**), confirming results from a priori ROIs. Negative urgency had two voxels that reached FDR corrected significance ($q < 0.05$). EXT, INT, FH, ETD, and negative urgency did not have significant voxelwise BOLD main effects (minimum q's > 0.072).

Reward Interactions of Substance Use and Risk Factors

Trial-Wise Reward Interactions

With trial-wise BOLD responses (GLM-1), ETD and substance use risk measures did not have a significant, corrected interaction with reward in a priori ROIs (**Table 6**) or at the voxelwise level (minimum q's > 0.876).

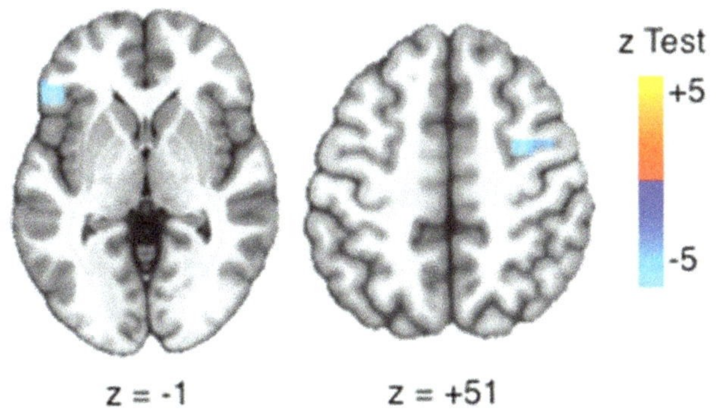

FIGURE 4 | Voxelwise main effects of positive urgency. Positive urgency had a significant, voxelwise main effect with BOLD activation in the left inferior frontal gyrus (IFG: $x = 49.5$, $y = 28.5$, $z = -1.5$; 32 voxels; peak test statistic = −5.93) and right frontal eye field (FEF; $x = -31.5$, $y = 1.5$, $z = 49.5$, 25 voxels, peak test statistic = −5.52). Significance based on intersection of FDR-correction and cluster size [voxelwise threshold (p) = 0.0012, $q < 0.05$, number of contiguous voxels (faces touching) > 24].

Epoch Reward Interactions

Significant BOLD reward interactions for AS task epochs in ROIs are presented in **Table 7**. See Supplemental Tables 2–4 for full list. No reward interactions were observed in the cue epoch. In the preparation epoch, there was a significant interaction between subject age and reward condition in the NAcc ROI [$t = 2.85$, $\chi^2_{(1)} = 8.10$, $p = 0.048$, corrected]. *Post hoc* testing revealed a significant simple effect of age in reward trials [$t_{(204.03)} = 2.38$, $p = 0.018$] but a non-significant simple effect of age in neutral trials [$t_{(204.03)} = -0.45$, $p = 0.651$]. A significant reward interaction was also observed in the preparation epoch for exceeds threshold drinking in the FEF ROI [$t = -2.92$, $\chi^2_{(1)} = 8.54$, $p = 0.038$, corrected] with *post-hoc* testing demonstrating that those who exceeded threshold drinking had higher BOLD activation than those not meeting criteria in the neutral trials [$t_{(150.98)} = 3.47$, $p < 0.001$], but not reward trials [$t_{(150.98)} = 1.41$, $p = 0.158$] (**Figure 5**).

In the response epoch, there was a significant reward interaction for positive urgency in the SEF [$t = 3.06$, $\chi^2_{(1)} = 9.35$, $p = 0.024$, corrected], with *post-hoc* testing demonstrating a significant simple effect of positive urgency in reward trials [$t_{(323.86)} = 2.24$, $p = 0.026$] but a non-significant simple effect in neutral trials [$t_{(323.86)} = -1.10$, $p = 0.274$] (**Figure 5**). A reward interaction was also observed for externalizing risk in the IFG during the response epoch [$t = 2.96$, $\chi^2_{(1)} = 8.75$, $p = 0.034$, corrected], but *post-hoc* testing revealed non-significant simple effects in both reward and neutral trials (p's > 0.0998). However, no reward interactions were significant at the voxelwise level (minimum q's > 0.107).

DISCUSSION

In this study, we examined neural correlates of rewarded response inhibition in youth at risk for problematic substance use. Within a two time point adolescent neuroimaging dataset, we tested whether incentives moderated the association between response inhibition and trait-level psychopathology and personality features of substance use risk. In multivariate models, the trait impulsivity measure of positive urgency and externalizing risk were significant negative predictors of AS correct response rate. Positive urgency was associated with reduced trial-wise BOLD activation in a priori ROIs representing frontal eye fields and inferior frontal gyrus, which were confirmed at the voxelwise level. However, contrary to our hypothesis, limited evidence suggested differential associations between response inhibition and substance use risk factors in the context of reward. Significant interactions between reward and substance use risk factors were not observed with AS behavioral performance or trial-wise BOLD estimates. When examining reward effects in discrete stages of the AS task (e.g., cue, preparation, response), some reward interactions were observed in a priori ROIs, but no reward interaction effects were observed at the voxelwise level.

Substance Use Risk and Brain Systems Supporting Response Inhibition

Consistent with previous work (Young et al., 2009), externalizing risk was associated with poorer response inhibition. However, externalizing risk was also associated with lower general cognitive ability (GA) and when GA was included as a covariate, the association between externalizing risk and AS performance was reduced to a trend. This suggests the association between externalizing risk and AS performance may be driven in part, by aspects of cognition that are not specific to inhibition. In contrast, higher levels of the trait impulsivity measure of positive urgency were associated with poorer AS performance, while accounting for GA. Higher scores of positive urgency also predicted shorter latencies to correct AS responses. This pattern is consistent with the notion of high levels of trait impulsivity predicting a speed-accuracy tradeoff in cognitive tests (Dickman and Meyer, 1988). We further demonstrate positive urgency is associated with reduced BOLD activation in the inferior frontal gyrus (IFG), frontal eye fields (FEF), and putamen. The negative association between urgency and BOLD activation in the IFG is consistent with recent work examining UPPS-P urgency domain score in a rewarded go/no-go task (Wilbertz et al., 2014). We extend this result by demonstrating this association may be specific to positive urgency, rather than negative urgency.

Positive urgency is conceptualized as the tendency to act rashly/impulsively in response to high levels of positive affect (Cyders et al., 2007). Theoretical models implicate the ventromedial prefrontal cortex (VMPFC) in affective instability and impulsivity (see Cyders and Smith, 2008), highlighting evidence from patients with damage to this region (Bechara, 2004). However, in the absence of a significant interaction between positive urgency and reward in AS behavioral performance, our results suggest positive urgency is associated with a general response inhibition deficit. Accordingly, we observed negative associations between positive urgency and BOLD activation in multiple regions associated with response inhibition, including IFG (c.f., Aron et al., 2003) and FEF (c.f.,

TABLE 6 | BOLD reward interactions in regions of interest (*t*-values): trial-wise (GLM-1).

	EXT	INT	FH	ETD	PUG	NUG	Age	SES	GA	AS Acc
SUBCORTICAL										
Caudate[L,R.]	−1.12	1.01	0.85	−0.54	0.27	−1.36	0.31	−1.39	−0.28	−1.11
Putamen[L,R.]	0.47	1.75	−0.05	−0.40	−0.11	−0.88	0.28	−1.77	0.30	−0.44
NAcc[L,R.]	−0.21	0.48	0.91	−0.10	−0.27	−1.42	0.09	−1.39	−0.02	0.58
CORTICAL										
PPC[L,R.]	0.29	1.26	0.56	0.15	0.84	0.12	−0.11	−0.66	−0.53	−0.03
FEF[L,R.]	−0.21	0.79	0.97	−0.43	1.31	0.18	−0.35	−0.76	0.06	−0.28
SEF	−0.55	0.31	1.73	−0.32	**2.11**	0.16	−0.54	−1.02	−0.30	−0.53
Pre-SMA	−0.64	0.71	1.17	−0.62	0.76	−0.35	−0.15	−0.74	−0.21	−0.43
dACC	−0.71	0.84	0.20	−0.05	0.60	−0.77	0.04	−0.82	−0.26	−0.45
DLPFC[L,R.]	−0.68	1.08	0.97	−0.45	0.35	−1.33	−0.22	−0.82	−0.45	−1.37
VLPFC[L,R.]	−0.21	1.14	−0.10	−0.50	−0.74	−1.74	0.07	−0.58	−0.16	−0.70
IFG[L,R.]	−0.35	1.92	−0.56	0.01	−0.24	−1.13	0.30	−1.13	−0.64	−0.64

Displayed estimates are test statistics from models with the specific factor, subject age, visit, and reward condition (Type A). [L,R.]*, Left/Right ROIs are included within one model. Estimates with uncorrected p's < 0.05 are bolded.*

TABLE 7 | BOLD reward interactions of antisaccade epochs in regions of interest (GLM-2).

	Variable	Reward interaction (*t*)	Simple effect: neutral (*t*)	Simple effect: reward (*t*)
PREPARATION				
NAcc[L,R.]	Age	2.85*[B,C]	−0.45	2.38*
FEF[L,R.]	ETD	−2.92*[B,C]	3.47**	1.41
RESPONSE				
SEF	PUG	3.06*[B,C,G]	−1.10	2.24*
IFG[L,R.]	EXT	2.96*[B,C]	−1.65	0.93

Reward interaction estimates are test statistics from models with the specific variable, subject age, visit, and reward condition (Type A) that were significant after multiple comparison correction. See Supplemental Tables 2–4 for full epoch reward interactions. [B]*p < 0.05 (Type B) model with all risk factors, subject age, visit, and reward condition;* [C]*p < 0.05 (Type C) model with all risk factors, subject age, visit, reward condition, and SES and GA.* [G]*Positive Urgency p < 0.05 while covarying gender.* [L,R.]*, Left/Right ROIs are included within one model. Simple effect neutral and reward refer to test statistics from association between variable and BOLD activation in neutral and reward trials, respectively: *p < 0.05, **p < 0.01.*

Muggleton et al., 2010) and the putamen ROI (Zandbelt and Vink, 2010).

Both positive urgency and externalizing risk were significant negative predictors of AS correct response rate. This is consistent with an association between disinhibited psychopathology and poorer response inhibition (Young et al., 2009). Moreover, although not significant after correction for multiple comparisons, externalizing risk was associated with lower BOLD activation in a priori FEF and putamen ROIs. To this end, our data provide some support for a notion of common neurocognitive correlates to disinhibited psychopathology and substance use risk. Moreover, associations between positive urgency and externalizing risk and AS response inhibition appear functionally distinct from other forms of psychopathology, as no other risk factors had significant (corrected or uncorrected) associations with AS behavioral performance or BOLD activation in FEF or the putamen.

Reward Interactions and Substance Use Risk

Consistent with previous work utilizing this rewarded AS task (Geier et al., 2010) and other response inhibition tasks (Hardin et al., 2007), the availability of reward improved response inhibition performance (increased correct response rate and reduced latency). However, no substance use risk measures had significant interactions with reward in AS behavioral performance or trial-wise BOLD estimates. This result may suggest that response inhibition deficits and reward sensitivity may be non-overlapping features of substance use risk, which is consistent with factor analytic work suggesting substance use risk is a multidimensional construct (Woicik et al., 2009).

Previous work suggests BOLD activation associated with reward modulation may vary according to the cognitive processes engaged during different epochs of the AS task (c.f., Geier et al., 2010; Chung et al., 2011). To this end, we observed significant BOLD reward modulation when examining specific AS epochs in a priori ROIs, with exceeding threshold drinking associated with increased BOLD activation in FEF during response preparation in neutral trials, but not reward trials. This result is consistent with previous work using this task in adolescents with SUD (Chung et al., 2011) and provides some support for the notion that incentives may normalize response inhibition differences in SUD. Given the pattern of greater differences in neutral trials compared to reward trials was specific to SUD and not substance use risk factors, its possible this effect reflects a sensitization to rewards following substance use initiation. To this end, positive urgency was associated with increased BOLD activation during response preparation in the supplementary eye fields during reward trials, but not neutral trials. However, reward interactions were not observed at the voxelwise level, indicating the need for caution in interpreting possible effects of reward on regional BOLD activation.

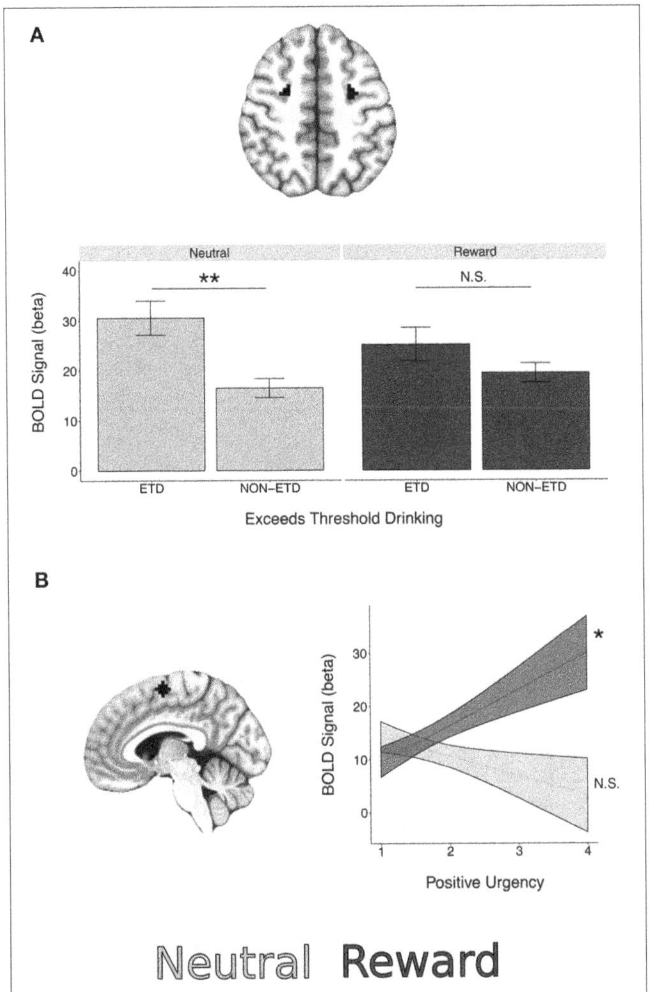

FIGURE 5 | BOLD epoch reward interactions in regions of interest. **(A)** A significant interaction between reward and exceeds threshold drinking was observed in the FEF ROIs during the preparation epoch. **(B)** A significant interaction between reward and positive urgency was observed in the SEF ROI during the response epoch. See **Table 7** for interaction statistics and simple effects testing. $^{*}p < 0.05$, $^{**}p < 0.01$.

A possible explanation for a lack of reward modulation of the association between response inhibition and substance use risk factors in this study may be from our focus on general associations across development. Previous work suggests developmental changes within reward circuitry during adolescence (Larsen and Luna, 2015). Supporting this we found age by reward interactions in the NAcc during the preparation epoch, with greater age-related changes in reward trials compared to neutral. This result is consistent with previous work (Bjork et al., 2010b) suggesting adults have greater NAcc activation during reward anticipation. Accordingly, reward interactions with substance use risk may emerge later in development (Müller et al., 2015). The degree of the moderating effect of reward on the association between substance use risk factors and response inhibition may also depend on the magnitude of the incentive offered. Given the ongoing data-collection within the NCANDA sample, future work may explore within-subject, longitudinal changes during development in relation to reward interactions with substance use risk.

Limitations

This project was characterized by a number of strengths, including a relatively large sample size, multiple time points (baseline and follow up visits), and extensive characterization of psychopathology and personality variables associated with substance use risk. However, it is worth noting a few limitations. First, we coded participants risk scores at both baseline and follow-up visits based on baseline risk factors established by NCANDA. Combined with the use of mixed effects models, this procedure allowed us to increase the precision of between-subject estimates of risk factors groups as defined in previous NCANDA projects (c.f., Brown et al., 2015) and utilize all data from baseline and follow up visits. Nevertheless, subtle variation in meeting criteria for certain risk factors (e.g., externalizing and internalizing risk and exceeding threshold drinking) may have occurred between baseline and follow up visits and we did not examine within-subject change (difference scores between baseline and 1-year follow-up). Accordingly, future work may utilize more complex modeling frameworks with random growth terms to better characterize within-subject changes and joint maturation of substance use risk and brain activation.

Another potential limitation of the analyses is the focus on bivariate relationships between substance use risk factors and AS performance and BOLD activation. Although we examined interactions between substance use risk and reward processes, these were completed iteratively across risk factors. This procedure, combined with multivariate regression, allowed us to examine the specificity of associations between particular substance use risk factors and AS performance and BOLD activation. However, several of our risk factors were significantly correlated with one another. To this end, previous work suggests substance use risk may be characterized by higher-order, latent dimensions that may explain risk factor covariation (c.f., Tarter et al., 2003; Woicik et al., 2009). Future work could utilize latent variable analysis to examine whether higher-order factors of substance use risk display significant interactions with reward on response inhibition tasks.

CONCLUSION

Utilizing a rewarded antisaccade task during fMRI acquisition, the results from this project confirm previous work suggesting substance use risk, and specifically externalizing psychopathology and trait impulsivity, are associated with poorer response inhibition. Furthermore, we found that higher levels of positive urgency are associated with reduced BOLD activation in FEF and IFG. However, we found little evidence that monetary incentive moderated the association between substance use risk factors and AS behavioral performance or BOLD activation. Further work is needed to determine the parameters (e.g., type, magnitude of reward) under which incentives increase response inhibition, examine overlap between substance use risk factors, and investigate within-subject longitudinal change in the interplay between sensitivity to reward and response inhibition.

AUTHOR CONTRIBUTIONS

BT, BL, and DC designed analysis. BT and AQ completed analysis. BT and WF performed preprocessing and quality assurance on imaging data. BT constructed manuscript with input and feedback from BL, TC, MD, and DC.

REFERENCES

Achenbach, T. M. (2009). *The Achenbach System of Empirically Based Assessemnt (ASEBA): Development, Findings, Theory, and Applications*. Burlington, VT: University of Vermont Research Center for Children, Youth, and Families.

Aron, A. R., Fletcher, P. C., Bullmore, E. T., Sahakian, B. J., and Robbins, T. W. (2003). Stop-signal inhibition disrupted by damage to right inferior frontal gyrus in humans. *Nat. Neurosci.* 6, 115–116. doi: 10.1038/nn1003

Bates, D., Maechler, M., and Bolker, B. (2013). *lme4: Linear Mixed-Effects Models Using S4 Classes*. Available online at: http://CRAN.R-project.org/package=lme4

Bechara, A. (2004). The role of emotion in decision-making: evidence from neurological patients with orbitofrontal damage. *Brain Cogn.* 55, 30–40. doi: 10.1016/j.bandc.2003.04.001

Berridge, K. C. (2007). The debate over dopamine's role in reward: the case for incentive salience. *Psychopharmacology* 191, 391–431. doi: 10.1007/s00213-006-0578-x

Bjork, J. M., Chen, G., Smith, A. R., and Hommer, D. W. (2010a). Incentive-elicited mesolimbic activation and externalizing symptomatology in adolescents. *J. Child Psychol. Psychiatry* 51, 827–837. doi: 10.1111/j.1469-7610.2009.02201.x

Bjork, J. M., Smith, A. R., Chen, G., and Hommer, D. W. (2010b). Adolescents, adults and rewards: comparing motivational neurocircuitry recruitment using fMRI. *PLoS ONE* 5:e11440. doi: 10.1371/journal.pone.0011440

Brown, S. A., Brumback, T., Tomlinson, K., Cummins, K., Thompson, W. K., and Nagel, B. J., et al. (2015). The National Consortium on Alcohol and NeuroDevelopment in Adolescence (NCANDA): a multisite study of adolescent development and substance use. *J. Stud. Alcohol Drugs* 76, 895–908. doi: 10.15288/jsad.2015.76.895

Brown, S. A., Myers, M. G., Lippke, L., Tapert, S. F., Stewart, D. G., and Vik, P. W. (1998). Psychometric evaluation of the Customary Drinking and Drug Use Record (CDDR): a measure of adolescent alcohol and drug involvement. *J. Stud. Alcohol* 59, 427–438. doi: 10.15288/jsa.1998.59.427

Bucholz, K. K., Cadoret, R., Cloninger, C. R., Dinwiddie, S. H., Hesselbrock, V. M., Nurnberger, J. I., et al. (1994). A new, semi-structured psychiatric interview for use in genetic linkage studies: a report on the reliability of the SSAGA. *J. Stud. Alcohol* 55, 149–158. doi: 10.15288/jsa.1994.55.149

Chen, G., Saad, Z. S., Britton, J. C., Pine, D. S., and Cox, R. W. (2013). Linear mixed-effects modeling approach to FMRI group analysis. *Neuroimage* 73, 176–190. doi: 10.1016/j.neuroimage.2013.01.047

Chung, T., Geier, C., Luna, B., Pajtek, S., Terwilliger, R., Thatcher, D., et al. (2011). Enhancing response inhibition by incentive: comparison of adolescents with and without substance use disorder. *Drug Alcohol Depend.* 115, 43–50. doi: 10.1016/j.drugalcdep.2010.10.017

Chung, T., Paulsen, D. J., Geier, C. F., Luna, B., and Clark, D. B. (2015). Regional brain activation supporting cognitive control in the context of reward is associated with treated adolescents' marijuana problem severity at follow-up: a preliminary study. *Dev. Cogn. Neurosci.* 16, 93–100. doi: 10.1016/j.dcn.2015.05.004

Cyders, M. A., Littlefield, A. K., Coffey, S., and Karyadi, K. A. (2014). Examination of a short English version of the UPPS-P Impulsive Behavior Scale. *Addict. Behav.* 39, 1372–1376. doi: 10.1016/j.addbeh.2014.02.013

Cyders, M. A., and Smith, G. T. (2008). Emotion-based dispositions to rash action: positive and negative urgency. *Psychol. Bull.* 134:807. doi: 10.1037/a0013341

Cyders, M. A., Smith, G. T., Spillane, N. S., Fischer, S., Annus, A. M., and Peterson, C. (2007). Integration of impulsivity and positive mood to predict risky behavior: Development and validation of a measure of positive urgency. *Psychol. Assess.* 19:107. doi: 10.1037/1040-3590.19.1.107

Dickman, S. J., and Meyer, D. E. (1988). Impulsivity and speed-accuracy tradeoffs in information processing. *J. Pers. Soc. Psychol.* 54:274. doi: 10.1037/0022-3514.54.2.274

Fox, J. (2010). *Polycor: Polychoric and Polyserial Correlations. R Package Version 0.7-8.* [*Online*]. Available online at: https://cran.r-project.org/web/packages/polycor/index.html (Accessed August 31, 2010).

Fox, J., Weisberg, S., Adler, D., Bates, D., Baud-Bovy, G., and Ellison, S., et al. (2016). *Package "car." Companion to Applied Regression*. R Package Version, 2–1.

Geier, C. F., and Luna, B. (2012). Developmental effects of incentives on response inhibition. *Child Dev.* 83, 1262–1274. doi: 10.1111/j.1467-8624.2012.01771.x

Geier, C. F., Terwilliger, R., Teslovich, T., Velanova, K., and Luna, B. (2010). Immaturities in reward processing and its influence on inhibitory control in adolescence. *Cereb. Cortex* 20, 1613–1629. doi: 10.1093/cercor/bhp225

Gitelman, D. R. (2002). ILAB: a program for postexperimental eye movement analysis. *Behav. Res. Methods*, 34, 605–612. doi: 10.3758/BF03195488

Gur, R. C., Richard, J., Hughett, P., Calkins, M. E., Macy, L., Bilker, W. B., et al. (2010). A cognitive neuroscience-based computerized battery for efficient measurement of individual differences: standardization and initial construct validation. *J. Neurosci. Methods* 187, 254–262. doi: 10.1016/j.jneumeth.2009.11.017

Hardin, M. G., Schroth, E., Pine, D. S., and Ernst, M. (2007). Incentive-related modulation of cognitive control in healthy, anxious, and depressed adolescents: development and psychopathology related differences. *J. Child Psychol. Psychiatry Allied Discip.* 48, 446–454. doi: 10.1111/j.1469-7610.2006.01722.x

Heitzeg, M. M., Cope, L. M., Martz, M. E., and Hardee, J. E. (2015). Neuroimaging risk markers for substance abuse: recent findings on inhibitory control and reward system functioning. *Curr. Addict. Rep.* 2, 91–103. doi: 10.1007/s40429-015-0048-9

Hesselbrock, M., Easton, C., Bucholz, K. K., Schuckit, M., and Hesselbrock, V. (1999). A validity study of the SSAGA-a comparison with the SCAN. *Addiction* 94, 1361–1370. doi: 10.1046/j.1360-0443.1999.94913618.x

Jazbec, S., Hardin, M. G., Schroth, E., McClure, E., Pine, D. S., and Ernst, M. (2006). Age-related influence of contingencies on a saccade task. *Exp. Brain Res.* 174, 754–762. doi: 10.1007/s00221-006-0520-9

Jenkinson, M., Bannister, P., Brady, M., and Smith, S. (2002). Improved optimization for the robust and accurate linear registration and motion correction of brain images. *Neuroimage* 17, 825–841. doi: 10.1006/nimg.2002.1132

Jenkinson, M., Beckmann, C. F., Behrens, T. E., Woolrich, M. W., and Smith, S. M. (2012). FSL. *Neuroimage* 62, 782–790. doi: 10.1016/j.neuroimage.2011.09.015

Krueger, R. F., Markon, K. E., Patrick, C. J., Benning, S. D., and Kramer, M. D. (2007). Linking antisocial behavior, substance use, and personality: an integrative quantitative model of the adult externalizing spectrum. *J. Abnorm. Psychol.* 116:645. doi: 10.1037/0021-843X.116.4.645

Larsen, B., and Luna, B. (2015). *In vivo* evidence of neurophysiological maturation of the human adolescent striatum. *Dev. Cogn. Neurosci.* 12, 74–85. doi: 10.1016/j.dcn.2014.12.003

Luna, B., Padmanabhan, A., and O'Hearn, K. (2010). What has fMRI told us about the development of cognitive control through adolescence? *Brain Cogn.* 72, 101–113. doi: 10.1016/j.bandc.2009.08.005

Luna, B., and Wright, C. (2016). "Adolescent brain development: implications for the juvenile criminal justice system," in *APA Handbook of Psychology and Juvenile Justice*, eds K. Heilbrun, D. De-Matteo, and N. Goldstein (Washington, DC: American Psychological Association), 91–116.

Mahmood, O. M., Goldenberg, D., Thayer, R., Migliorini, R., Simmons, A. N., and Tapert, S. F. (2013). Adolescents' fMRI activation to a response inhibition task predicts future substance use. *Addict. Behav.* 38, 1435–1441. doi: 10.1016/j.addbeh.2012.07.012

McNamee, R. L., Dunfee, K. L., Luna, B., Clark, D. B., Eddy, W. F., and Tarter, R. E. (2008). Brain activation, response inhibition, and increased risk for substance use disorder. *Alcohol. Clin. Exp. Res.* 32, 405–413. doi: 10.1111/j.1530-0277.2007.00604.x

Muggleton, N. G., Chen, C. Y., Tzeng, O. J., Hung, D. L., and Juan, C.-H. (2010). Inhibitory control and the frontal eye fields. *J. Cogn. Neurosci.* 22, 2804–2812. doi: 10.1162/jocn.2010.21416

Müller, K. U., Gan, G., Banaschewski, T., Barker, G. J., Bokde, A. L., and Büchel, C., et al. (2015). No differences in ventral striatum responsivity between adolescents with a positive family history of alcoholism and controls. *Addict. Biol.* 20, 534–545. doi: 10.1111/adb.12136

Müller-Oehring, E. M., Kwon, D., Nagel, B. J., Sullivan, E. V., Chu, W., Rohlfing, T., et al. (2017). Influences of age, sex, and moderate alcohol drinking on the intrinsic functional architecture of adolescent brains. *Cereb. Cortex.* doi: 10.1093/cercor/bhx014. [Epub ahead of print].

Munoz, D. P., and Everling, S. (2004). Look away: the anti-saccade task and the voluntary control of eye movement. *Nat. Rev. Neurosci.* 5, 218–228. doi: 10.1038/nrn1345

Nigg, J. T., Wong, M. M., Martel, M. M., Jester, J. M., Puttler, L. I., Glass, J. M., et al. (2006). Poor response inhibition as a predictor of problem drinking and illicit drug use in adolescents at risk for alcoholism and other substance use disorders. *J. Am. Acad. Child Adolesc. Psychiatry* 45, 468–475. doi: 10.1097/01.chi.0000199028.76452.a9

Norman, A. L., Pulido, C., Squeglia, L. M., Spadoni, A. D., Paulus, M. P., and Tapert, S. F. (2011). Neural activation during inhibition predicts initiation of substance use in adolescence. *Drug Alcohol Depend.* 119, 216–223. doi: 10.1016/j.drugalcdep.2011.06.019

Ollinger, J. M., Shulman, G. L., and Corbetta, M. (2001). Separating processes within a trial in event-related functional MRI: I. The method. *Neuroimage* 13, 210–217. doi: 10.1006/nimg.2000.0710

Ordaz, S. J., Foran, W., Velanova, K., and Luna, B. (2013). Longitudinal growth curves of brain function underlying inhibitory control through adolescence. *J. Neurosci.* 33, 18109–18124. doi: 10.1523/JNEUROSCI.1741-13.2013

Plichta, M. M., and Scheres, A. (2014). Ventral–striatal responsiveness during reward anticipation in ADHD and its relation to trait impulsivity in the healthy population: a meta-analytic review of the fMRI literature. *Neurosci. Biobehav. Rev.* 38, 125–134. doi: 10.1016/j.neubiorev.2013.07.012

R Core Team (2014). *R: A Language and Environment for Statistical Computing.* Vienna: R Foundation for Statistical Computing.

Reynolds, B., Ortengren, A., Richards, J. B., and de Wit, H. (2006). Dimensions of impulsive behavior: Personality and behavioral measures. *Pers. Individ. Dif.* 40, 305–315. doi: 10.1016/j.paid.2005.03.024

Rice, J. P., Reich, T., Bucholz, K. K., Neuman, R. J., Fishman, R., Rochberg, N., et al. (1995). Comparison of direct interview and family history diagnoses of alcohol dependence. *Alcoholism* 19, 1018–1023. doi: 10.1111/j.1530-0277.1995.tb00983.x

Robinson, T. E., and Berridge, K. C. (1993). The neural basis of drug craving: an incentive-sensitization theory of addiction. *Brain Res. Rev.* 18, 247–291. doi: 10.1016/0165-0173(93)90013-P

Schneider, W., Eschman, A., and Zuccolotto, A. (2002). *E-Prime: User's Guide.* Pittsburgh, PA: Psychology Software Tools Inc.

Schweinsburg, A. D., Paulus, M. P., Barlett, V. C., Killeen, L. A., Caldwell, L. C., Pulido, C., et al. (2004). An FMRI study of response inhibition in youths with a family history of alcoholism. *Ann. N. Y. Acad. Sci.* 1021, 391–394. doi: 10.1196/annals.1308.050

Siegel, J. S., Power, J. D., Dubis, J. W., Vogel, A. C., Church, J. A., Schlaggar, B. L., et al. (2014). Statistical improvements in functional magnetic resonance imaging analyses produced by censoring high-motion data points. *Hum. Brain Mapp.* 35, 1981–1996. doi: 10.1002/hbm.22307

Smith, S., and Brady, J. (1997). SUSAN - a new approach to low level image processing. *Int. J. Comput. Vis.* 23, 45–78. doi: 10.1023/A:1007963824710

Sullivan, E. V., Brumback, T., Tapert, S. F., Fama, R., Prouty, D., and Brown, S. A., et al. (2016). Cognitive, emotion control, and motor performance of adolescents in the NCANDA study: contributions from alcohol consumption, age, sex, ethnicity, and family history of addiction. *Neuropsychology* 30:449. doi: 10.1037/neu0000259

Tarter, R. E., Kirisci, L., Mezzich, A., Cornelius, J. R., Pajer, K., Vanyukov, M., et al. (2003). Neurobehavioral disinhibition in childhood predicts early age at onset of substance use disorder. *Am. J. Psychiatry* 160, 1078–1085. doi: 10.1176/appi.ajp.160.6.1078

Velanova, K., Wheeler, M. E., and Luna, B. (2009). The maturation of task set-related activation supports late developmental improvements in inhibitory control. *J. Neurosci.* 29, 12558–12567. doi: 10.1523/JNEUROSCI.1579-09.2009

Verdejo-García, A., Lawrence, A. J., and Clark, L. (2008). Impulsivity as a vulnerability marker for substance-use disorders: review of findings from high-risk research, problem gamblers and genetic association studies. *Neurosci. Biobehav. Rev.* 32, 777–810. doi: 10.1016/j.neubiorev.2007.11.003

Wesley, M. J., and Bickel, W. K. (2014). Remember the future II: meta-analyses and functional overlap of working memory and delay discounting. *Biol. Psychiatry* 75, 435–448. doi: 10.1016/j.biopsych.2013.08.008

Wilbertz, T., Deserno, L., Horstmann, A., Neumann, J., Villringer, A., Heinze, H. J., et al. (2014). Response inhibition and its relation to multidimensional impulsivity. *Neuroimage*, 103, 241–248. doi: 10.1016/j.neuroimage.2014.09.021

Woicik, P. A., Stewart, S. H., Pihl, R. O., and Conrod, P. J. (2009). The substance use risk profile scale: a scale measuring traits linked to reinforcement-specific substance use profiles. *Addict. Behav.* 34, 1042–1055. doi: 10.1016/j.addbeh.2009.07.001

Young, S. E., Friedman, N. P., Miyake, A., Willcutt, E. G., Corley, R. P., Haberstick, B. C., et al. (2009). Behavioral disinhibition: liability for externalizing spectrum disorders and its genetic and environmental relation to response inhibition across adolescence. *J. Abnorm. Psychol.* 118, 117–130. doi: 10.1037/a0014657

Zandbelt, B. B., and Vink, M. (2010). On the role of the striatum in response inhibition. *PLoS ONE* 5:e13848. doi: 10.1371/journal.pone.0013848

Zapolski, T. C., Cyders, M. A., and Smith, G. T. (2009). Positive urgency predicts illegal drug use and risky sexual behavior. *Psychol. Addict. Behav.* 23:348. doi: 10.1037/a0014684

7

Consequences of Adolescent Exposure to the Cannabinoid Receptor Agonist WIN55,212-2 on Working Memory in Female Rats

Erin K. Kirschmann[1†], *Daniel M. McCalley*[1†], *Caitlyn M. Edwards*[1,2] *and Mary M. Torregrossa*[1,2*]

[1]*Department of Psychiatry, Translational Neuroscience Program, University of Pittsburgh, Pittsburgh, PA, United States,*
[2]*Center for Neuroscience, University of Pittsburgh, Pittsburgh, PA, United States*

Edited by:
Valérie Doyère, Centre National de la Recherche Scientifique (CNRS), France

Reviewed by:
James David Jentsch, Binghamton University, United States
Arnau Busquets-Garcia, Neurocentre Magendie, France

***Correspondence:**
Mary M. Torregrossa
torregrossam@upmc.edu

†*Co-first authors.*

Marijuana is a prevalent illicit substance used by adolescents, and several studies have indicated that adolescent use can lead to long-term cognitive deficits including problems with attention and memory. However, preclinical animal studies that observe cognitive deficits after cannabinoid exposure during adolescence utilize experimenter administration of doses of cannabinoids that may exceed what an organism would choose to take, suggesting that contingency and dose are critical factors that need to be addressed in translational models of consequences of cannabinoid exposure. Indeed, we recently developed an adolescent cannabinoid self-administration paradigm in male rats, and found that prior adolescent self-administration of the cannabinoid receptor agonist WIN55,212-2 (WIN) resulted in improved working memory performance in adulthood. In addition, the doses self-administered were not as high as those that are found to produce memory deficits. However, given known sex differences in both drug self-administration and learning and memory processes, it is possible that cannabinoid self-administration could have different cognitive consequences in females. Therefore, we aimed to explore the effects of self-administered vs. experimenter-administered WIN in adolescent female rats on adult cognitive function. Female rats were trained to self-administer WIN daily throughout adolescence (postnatal day 34–59). A control group self-administered vehicle solution. The acute effects of adolescent WIN self-administration on memory were determined using a short-term spatial memory test 24 h after final SA session; and the long-term effects on cognitive performance were assessed during protracted abstinence in adulthood using a delayed-match-to-sample working memory task. In a separate experiment, females were given daily intraperitoneal (IP) injections of a low or high dose of WIN, corresponding to self-administered and typical experimenter-administered doses, respectively, or its vehicle during adolescence and working memory was assessed under drug-free conditions in adulthood. While self-administration of WIN in adolescence had no significant effects on short-term spatial memory or adult working memory, experimenter administration of WIN resulted in improved adult working memory performance that was more pronounced in the low dose group. Thus, low-dose adolescent WIN exposure, whether self-administered or experimenter-administered, results in either improvements or no change in adult working memory performance in female rats, similar to previous results found in males.

Keywords: cannabis, WIN55,212-2, adolescence, female, working memory, self-administration

INTRODUCTION

Legal policy in the U.S. regarding both medicinal and recreational use of marijuana has become increasingly relaxed over the last decade. Considering that the prevalence of marijuana use among adolescents is between 35 and 40 percent (Moss et al., 2014; Salas-Wright et al., 2016), it is crucial to understand the long-term effects of marijuana exposure during adolescence in order to properly inform any potential policy changes. Adolescence is a period of substantial neuronal development. Of particular importance, the development of both the prefrontal cortex, a brain region required for higher-order cognitive processing, and the endocannabinoid system, responsible for modulating various physiological functions as well as the binding of exogenous cannabinoids, occur simultaneously (Spear, 2000; Schneider, 2008). The primary psychoactive components of marijuana are cannabinoids, particularly Δ^9-tetrahydrocannabinol (THC), that activate cannabinoid receptors CB1 and CB2. Therefore, considering the concurrent changes in neuronal and cannabinoid system development, there is potential for marijuana use to cause cannabinoid-induced interference in the carefully orchestrated development of the adolescent brain, possibly resulting in long-term effects on cognition.

Several studies have been conducted in order to assess the long-term effects of cannabinoid use during adolescence; however, the findings have been mixed. Some clinical work has linked adolescent THC use to reduced IQ, increased risk for psychosis, and impaired working memory (Meier et al., 2012; Becker et al., 2014; Gage et al., 2016; Marconi et al., 2016). In contrast, other clinical studies have failed to find differences in performance between cannabis users and controls on cognitive tasks (Jager et al., 2006; Buchy et al., 2015; Mokrysz et al., 2016). In preclinical animal studies, the most common application of cannabinoids has been via experimenter administration, which does not model the volitional control over intake and choice over dose of intake observed in human populations, bringing to question the translational value of these studies. Nevertheless, these studies have generally found a relationship between chronic cannabinoid exposure and cognitive deficits, especially in working memory, object recognition and short-term spatial memory capacity (Hampson and Deadwyler, 2000; O'Shea et al., 2004, 2006; Schneider and Koch, 2007; Abush and Akirav, 2012; Renard et al., 2016).

We recently developed a model of adolescent intravenous (IV) cannabinoid self-administration, which more closely models the voluntary nature of drug use in humans (Kirschmann et al., 2017). We trained rats to self-administer the synthetic cannabinoid receptor agonist WIN55,212-2 (WIN), a full agonist of CB1 and CB2 cannabinoid receptors that is more potent than THC, because previous studies have found that rats will readily self-administer this compound, whereas rats did not readily self-administer THC, which is a partial agonist (Takahashi and Singer, 1979; Fattore et al., 2001; Deiana et al., 2007; Pertwee, 2010; Lefever et al., 2014). Although WIN's effects may be more directly comparable to the frequently abused synthetic cannabinoids such as K2 and spice, it provides us with the opportunity to investigate the effects of self-directed cannabinoid receptor activation on behavior. Interestingly, adolescent self-administration of WIN did not lead to acute memory deficits or long-term effects on working memory performance using a delayed-match-to-sample task. In fact, we found that rats that self-administered WIN had better working memory performance in adulthood (after several weeks of abstinence) than control animals that responded for sucrose pellets. However, the doses of WIN that rats were willing to self-administer were much lower than doses used in previous studies identifying memory impairments after experimenter-administration. Thus, it is possible that cannabinoid-induced memory deficits are likely to only be found in very heavy users, and/or are not likely to be observed after long periods of abstinence. Another potential difference between findings in rodents and humans is that almost all previous preclinical work, including our own study, was conducted in male subjects. Given that there are known sex differences in both drug self-administration and learning and memory processes, it is possible that adolescent cannabinoid exposure could produce different results in males and females. Therefore, the current study aimed to explore the long-term cognitive effects of self-administered versus experimenter-administered cannabinoids in adolescent female rats.

MATERIALS AND METHODS

Animals

A total of 42 female, Sprague–Dawley (Harlan, Frederick, MD, USA) rats were delivered on postnatal day (PND) 22 and were housed in a climate-controlled room on a 12-h dark/light cycle (lights on at 4:30 am) throughout the duration of the experiment. All behavioral experiments were conducted during the light phase. Rats were pair-housed unless otherwise indicated, and were food restricted to about 85%–90% of normal, free-feeding weight for the duration of all behavioral experiments. Food portions were adjusted daily throughout adolescence with females receiving a range of 13–15 g/day. Food restriction was necessary to maintain responding in behavioral tasks. All procedures were performed in accordance with the recommendations of the National Institutes of Health *Guide for the Care and Use of Laboratory Animals*. The protocol was approved by the University of Pittsburgh's Institutional Animal Care and Use Committee.

Drugs

The synthetic cannabinoid receptor agonist WIN55,212-2 mesylate (WIN; NIMH Chemical Synthesis and Drug Supply Program; Cayman Chemical Company, Ann Arbor, MI, USA), was dissolved in sterile 0.9% saline with a drop of Tween 80. Fresh stock solutions were made every 2–3 days, and were diluted with saline daily to a working concentration for IV administration of 0.0125 mg/kg/infusion. A vehicle solution of 0.9% saline and a drop of Tween 80 was created daily and was diluted with saline for IV administration and intraperitoneal (IP) administration. Fresh working solutions of 1.2 mg/mL and 0.2 mg/mL were prepared daily for IP administration.

Surgical Procedures

In animals responding for IV WIN/vehicle, surgery was performed to implant indwelling jugular catheters on PND 27–28. Rats were anesthetized with ketamine (90 mg/kg) and xylazine (5 mg/kg) and given 5 mg/kg of the analgesic Rimadyl. Catheters were constructed with silastic tubing (11 cm; Braintree Scientific, Braintree, MA, USA) attached to a bent steel guide cannula (22 gauge; Plastics One Inc., Roanoke, VA, USA), surrounded by Loctite medical epoxy (Grainger, Pittsburgh, PA, USA) and attached to a 2 cm square piece of mesh (Bard Mesh; Davol Inc., Cranston, RI, USA). Catheters were implanted in the right jugular vein and fed subcutaneously to the back, where they exited through a small incision between the shoulder blades, and were flushed daily with 0.1 ml of Gentamicin in heparinized saline. A recovery period of 7 days was allowed before initiation of behavioral testing.

Self-Administration

Between PNDs 34–59, rats (n = 10) were trained to self-administer the synthetic cannabinoid receptor agonist WIN in standard operant conditioning chambers (Med Associates, St. Albans, VT, USA; see **Figure 1** for an experimental timeline). The chambers contained two retractable levers, a house light, two stimulus lights, a tone generator, a food magazine and a fan for background noise. A press on the active lever resulted in a 0.0125 mg/kg/infusion delivery of WIN at a rate of 0.03 ml/s paired with a 10 s tone and light stimulus in combination with a 10 s timeout, during which the house light was extinguished. Infusion times were adjusted daily based on individual rats' weights to maintain the 0.0125 mg/kg/infusion dose. A press on the inactive lever yielded no programmed consequences. Rats were trained on a 1-h fixed-ratio 1 (FR1) schedule of reinforcement during the first 4 days of self-administration, and were then switched to 2-h sessions (FR1) for the remaining 18 days of self-administration. Control rats (n = 8) responded for IV infusions of a vehicle solution using identical training procedures as for WIN.

Extinction and Reinstatement Testing

Following the last day of self-administration training, rats underwent instrumental extinction (1-h sessions), where lever presses produced no cue presentations or IV infusions. Rats underwent extinction for 8–9 days and until the rat had fewer than 20 lever presses. The day following the last day of extinction, and again 20 days later, rats were tested for cue-induced reinstatement of WIN seeking in 30 min sessions. During these sessions, lever presses resulted in a 10 s presentation of the audiovisual cue on an FR1 schedule. No infusions were given during reinstatement.

Experimenter-Administration

In a separate experiment, female rats (n = 24) received IP injections daily throughout adolescence (PND 34–53) between 2:00–3:00 pm during the light phase (**Figure 1**). Rats received either vehicle (n = 8), a low dose of WIN, 0.2 mg/kg, which corresponds to the average total daily dose that males received during self-administration (Kirschmann et al., 2017; n = 8), or

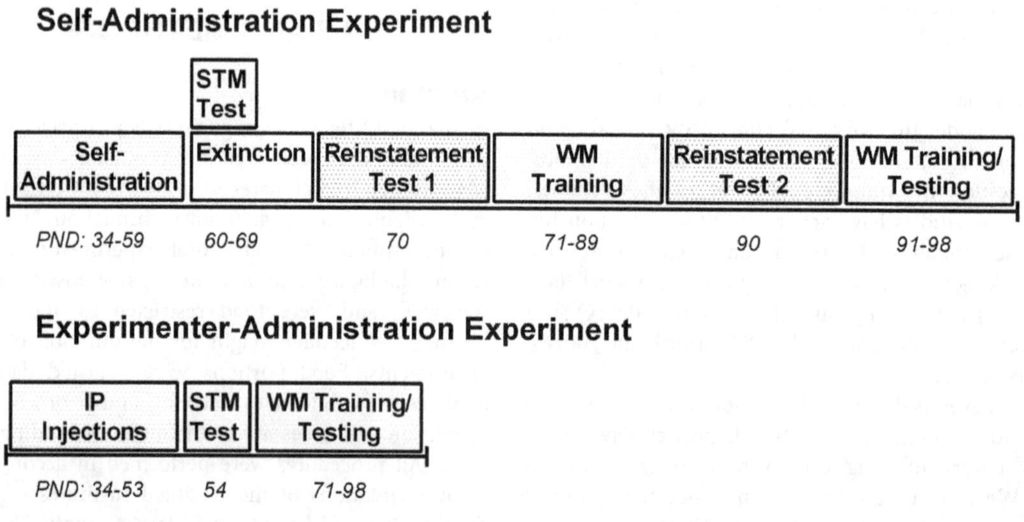

FIGURE 1 | Timeline of treatment and behavioral testing for both the self-administration and experimenter-administration experiments. PND, postnatal day; STM, short-term memory; WM, working memory; IP, intraperitoneal.

a high dose of WIN, 1.2 mg/kg, which corresponds to the dose commonly given in previous experiments that identified deficits in short-term memory (Schneider and Koch, 2003; O'Shea et al., 2006; $n = 8$). The total number of days of exposure to WIN was almost the same between the experimenter-administration and self-administration groups, though the age at which exposure ended varied by 6 days. The self-administration group did not have sessions on ~3 days during the study due to experimental conflicts, and rats that self-administered tended to get fewer infusions, and thus a lower dose of WIN, on the initial day of self-administration. Thus, the low dose IP group and the self-administration group are not perfectly equated, but received similar amounts of WIN overall.

Short-Term Spatial Memory Task

All rats were allowed to habituate to an empty, open field chamber (43 cm × 43 cm; Med Associates) under dim light for a period of 5 min on three occasions. Within 24 h of the last day of WIN exposure (PND 60 for self-administration (SA) rats, PND 54 for IP rats), all rats underwent short-term spatial memory testing in the same open field chamber. Two objects were placed evenly from opposing corners in the chamber, and rats were allowed to explore the objects for a period of 5 min. Objects were similar in material (glass/ceramic) and dimension (11 cm × 11 cm). Rats were returned to their home cages, and one of the objects was moved to a new spatial location. Following a 35-min delay, rats were again allowed to explore the objects in the chamber. Typically, rats prefer novelty; hence a rat with intact spatial memory will spend more time examining the object in the novel location, compared to the time spent examining the object in the familiar location. All rats performed this task and the chamber was cleaned with 70% ethanol between trials. Data were collected and analyzed offline using AnyMaze software (Stoelting, Wood Dale, IL, USA).

Delayed-Match-to-Sample Working Memory Task

Following 10–11 days of abstinence (which allowed the rats to age into adulthood), all rats began training in a delayed-match-to-sample working memory task. Training was performed during 1-h sessions in chambers (Med Associates) equipped with five nose poke apertures and a food dispenser. Initially, all five apertures were illuminated and rats received a sucrose pellet (45 mg, Bioserv, Flemington, NJ, USA) reward upon response on any of these five holes on an FR1 schedule. Next, a single aperture was illuminated and only a response in that hole resulted in reward. On the following days of training, a response on the single, illuminated "sample" aperture resulted in the immediate illumination of the "sample" and two additional "choice" apertures. The sample aperture for each trial was selected at random using Med Associates random number generator software code. The additional two apertures illuminated during the choice phase were always the two closest apertures to the sample, resulting in the two flanking apertures for the middle three apertures, and the next two innermost apertures for outer apertures. Following illumination of the choice aperture, a second response on the "sample" resulted in sucrose reward (FR1). Responses in any of the other apertures resulted in a 2 s timeout where all lights were extinguished. Once animals performed this task reliably with accuracy greater than 75% correct, delays were introduced between the "sample" phase and the "choice" phase. Rats performed blocks of trials in which seven delays (0.5–6 s) were presented in random order; each of the seven delays occurred before a new block of trials began. Once rats reached training criterion (≥80% correct 0.5 s delay), the range was increased (0.5–12 s; 0.5–24 s; See **Tables 1, 2** for summaries of SA and IP groups' training data). Working memory was assessed most critically on the first day in which the animals were presented with delays between 0.5 s and 24 s, ranging from age PND 93 to 98.

Estrous Cycle Monitoring

Vaginal lavage samples were taken by gently pipetting 150 μl of saline into the vagina to flush the vaginal canal. The saline

TABLE 1 | Training data for self-administration study.

		Days to meet criteria[a]	Reinforcers earned[b,c,d]	Accuracy across delays[e]
Phase 1	WIN	1.0 (±0)	60.1 (±4.3)	N/A
	VEH	1.0 (±0)	62.6 (±6.5)	
Phase 2	WIN	4.0 (±0.3)	59.1 (±6.0)	N/A
	VEH	4.1 (±0.1)	63.8 (±9.8)	
Phase 3	WIN	4.0 (±0.4)	58.2 (±2.3)	N/A
	VEH	3.9 (±0.3)	61.3 (±6.7)	
Phase 4	WIN	5.6 (±0.6)	49.9 (±2.3)	$F_{(1,16)} = 0.51, p = 0.49$
	VEH	5.6 (±0.5)	54.1 (±3.4)	
Phase 5	WIN	6.0 (±0.4)	47.2 (±2.4)	$F_{(1,16)} = 0.29, p = 0.60$
	VEH	6.0 (±0.2)	56.6 (±3.3)*	

*[a]Number of days WIN SA or VEH SA rats remained in current phase of training before advancing to next phase. Reinforcers earned: [b]Single day of phase 1; [c]Average over first 4 days in phases 2–3; [d]Average over first 6 days in phases 4–5. [e]Accuracy across delays on first day of training in phases 4–5. *$p < 0.05$, WIN vs. VEH.*

TABLE 2 | Training data for experimenter-administration study.

		Days to meet criteria[a]	Reinforcers earned[b,c,d]	Accuracy across delays[e]
Phase 1	Low	1.0 (±0)	23.9 (±2.8)	N/A
	High	1.0 (±0)	27.3 (±2.8)	
	Veh	1.0 (±0)	26.9 (±3.1)	
Phase 2	Low	7.0 (±0.6)	24.4 (±6.3)	N/A
	High	7.1 (±0.4)	18.4 (±4.4)*	
	Veh	6.0 (±0.5)	41.0 (±6.4)	
Phase 3	Low	3.9 (±0.7)	63.6 (±10.6)	N/A
	High	2.9 (±0.1)	84.0 (±7.6)	
	Veh	3.0 (±0.2)	95.3 (±23.7)	
Phase 4	Low	3.4 (±0.3)	57.5 (±5.3)	$F_{(2,21)} = 0.47, p = 0.63$
	High	4.0 (±0.3)	48.2 (±6.1)	
	Veh	4.0 (±0.3)	54.7 (±7.7)	
Phase 5	Low	5.6 (±0.3)	50.6 (±3.6)	$F_{(2,21)} = 0.78, p = 0.47$
	High	5.8 (±0.4)	45.8 (±5.8)	
	Veh	6.6 (±0.5)	52.0 (±6.0)	

*[a]Number of days Low WIN (0.2 mg/kg) IP, High WIN (1.2 mg/kg) IP or vehicle IP rats remained in current phase of training before advancing to next phase. Reinforcers earned: [b]Single day of phase 1; [c]Average over first 6 days in phases 2 and 5; [d]Average over first 3 days in phases 3–4. [e]Accuracy across delays on first day of training in phases 4–5. *$p < 0.05$, High WIN vs. VEH.*

was pipetted onto a clean microscope slide and covered with a coverslip. Cell morphology was examined under a compound microscope at a magnification of 100–200× to determine estrous cycle phase using standard procedures (Goldman et al., 2007). In order to allow for uninterrupted pubertal development, vaginal lavage sampling began on PND 46 (day 13 of the self-administration period) and was performed daily until the final day of self-administration. Samples were also taken on days of significant testing, specifically on the first day of each new delay range in working memory. Females were split into two groups of either high estradiol (proestrus or transitioning in or out of proestrus; PRO), or low estradiol (estrus, metestrus, or diestrus; EMD) and analyzed accordingly.

Statistical Analyses

Data were analyzed using Prism 6.0 Software (GraphPad Inc., LaJolla, CA, USA) and the SPSS software package version 21.0 (SPSS, Chicago, IL, USA). Self-administration and extinction data were analyzed using repeated measures (rm) ANOVA with a within-subjects factor of day of self-administration and between-subjects factor of group (WIN vs. VEH SA). Additionally, separate rmANOVA analyses of VEH and WIN SA groups were conducted with a within-subjects factor of day of self-administration and between-subjects factor of response type (active lever vs. infusions vs. inactive lever). Reinstatement data were analyzed by comparing within-subjects lever pressing on the last day of extinction to pressing across days of abstinence, comparing responses on the active and inactive levers by rmANOVA. Short-term spatial memory and working memory were also analyzed by rmANOVA, comparing test phase or delay length within-subjects and adolescent treatment type (WIN vs. VEH) between subjects. Fisher's least significant difference (LSD) test was used for *post hoc* analyses following identification of significant effects. Two-sided *t*-tests were used to determine if high or low estradiol phases of the estrous cycle [proestrus (PRO) vs. a combination of estrus, metestrus, and diestrus (EMD)] affected self-administration behaviors during the last 5 days of training.

RESULTS

Adolescent Self-Administration, Extinction and Cue-Induced Reinstatement

Analysis of infusions earned during self-administration by rmANOVA with group (WIN vs. VEH) as the between subjects factor showed that infusion number increased over the course of self-administration, regardless of whether responding was for WIN or for vehicle solution (VEH; main effect of SA day, $F_{(21,336)} = 5.41$, $p < 0.001$; no group × day interaction $F_{(21,336)} = 0.51$, $p = 0.97$). We also conducted separate rmANOVAs for WIN and VEH groups individually in order to compare the pattern of active vs. inactive lever pressing across days under each self-administration condition. Adolescent female rats that self-administered WIN reliably discriminated between the active and inactive levers (**Figure 2A**). Analysis by rmANOVA found a significant main effect of response type across days ($F_{(2,27)} = 14.83$, $p < 0.001$), and Fisher's LSD test indicated significant difference between inactive lever presses and both active lever presses ($p < 0.001$) and infusions earned ($p = 0.041$). Females responding for VEH did not significantly differ from WIN treated females in the number of active or inactive lever presses overall, and exhibited a significant main effect of response type ($F_{(2,21)} = 15.30$, $p < 0.001$). Further analysis indicated that only active and inactive lever presses significantly differed ($p < 0.001$), while there was no difference between infusions earned and inactive lever presses ($p = 0.65$; **Figure 2B**). Therefore, inactive pressing for VEH did not separate from infusions earned to the same degree as in the WIN group, though there were no overall between-drug differences. We hypothesize that the high degree of VEH responding was likely driven by presentation of the audiovisual cue. Importantly, the equatable levels of SA performance during adolescence in the VEH group serves as a better behavioral control for our later assessment of cognitive consequences, since both groups had similar experience with the cues. Females self-administered an average dose of 0.15–0.16 mg/kg WIN over the last 5 days of self-administration, similar to what we have previously observed in males, where the average daily dose was 0.22 mg/kg (Kirschmann et al., 2017).

Next, we examined extinction of the lever press response, where active lever presses produced neither the IV infusion, nor the audiovisual cue. Analysis of active lever responding by rmANOVA with day as within-subjects factor and group (WIN vs. VEH) as between subjects factor showed no effect of SA condition on extinction behavior (main effect of day ($F_{(7,112)} = 4.02$, $p = 0.001$), no group × day interaction ($F_{(7,112)} = 1.08$, $p = 0.384$)). We confirmed in separate rmANOVAs for WIN and VEH groups that both WIN and VEH self-administration groups exhibited a significant decrease in active lever responding over days (main effects of day ($F_{(7,126)} = 2.57$, $p = 0.017$) and ($F_{(7,98)} = 3.90$, $p < 0.001$), respectively), indicating acquisition of extinction (**Figures 2C,D**). However, the WIN group did not extinguish to as low of a degree of responding as the VEH group, exhibiting a significant difference between active and inactive lever presses across days of training ($F_{(1,18)} = 4.70$, $p = 0.044$), while the VEH group showed no significant differences between active and inactive lever responses over time ($F_{(1,14)} = 2.80$, $p = 0.12$).

Following extinction training, rats were tested for cue-induced reinstatement in two 30-min sessions where active lever presses resulted in presentation of the audiovisual cue. The first test occurred following the last day of extinction training, on day 9–10 of abstinence depending on when the rat met the extinction criterion. The second test occurred 20 days later, corresponding to day 29–30 of abstinence. Due to the difference in session length between extinction training and reinstatement tests, response rates were calculated (lever presses/minute) and compared between the last day of extinction (baseline) and the two reinstatement tests. Analysis by rmANOVA with group (WIN vs. VEH) as between-subjects factor identified a main effect of test phase ($F_{(2,32)} = 44.52$, $p < 0.001$), but no effect of group ($F_{(1,16)} = 0.616$, $p = 0.44$)

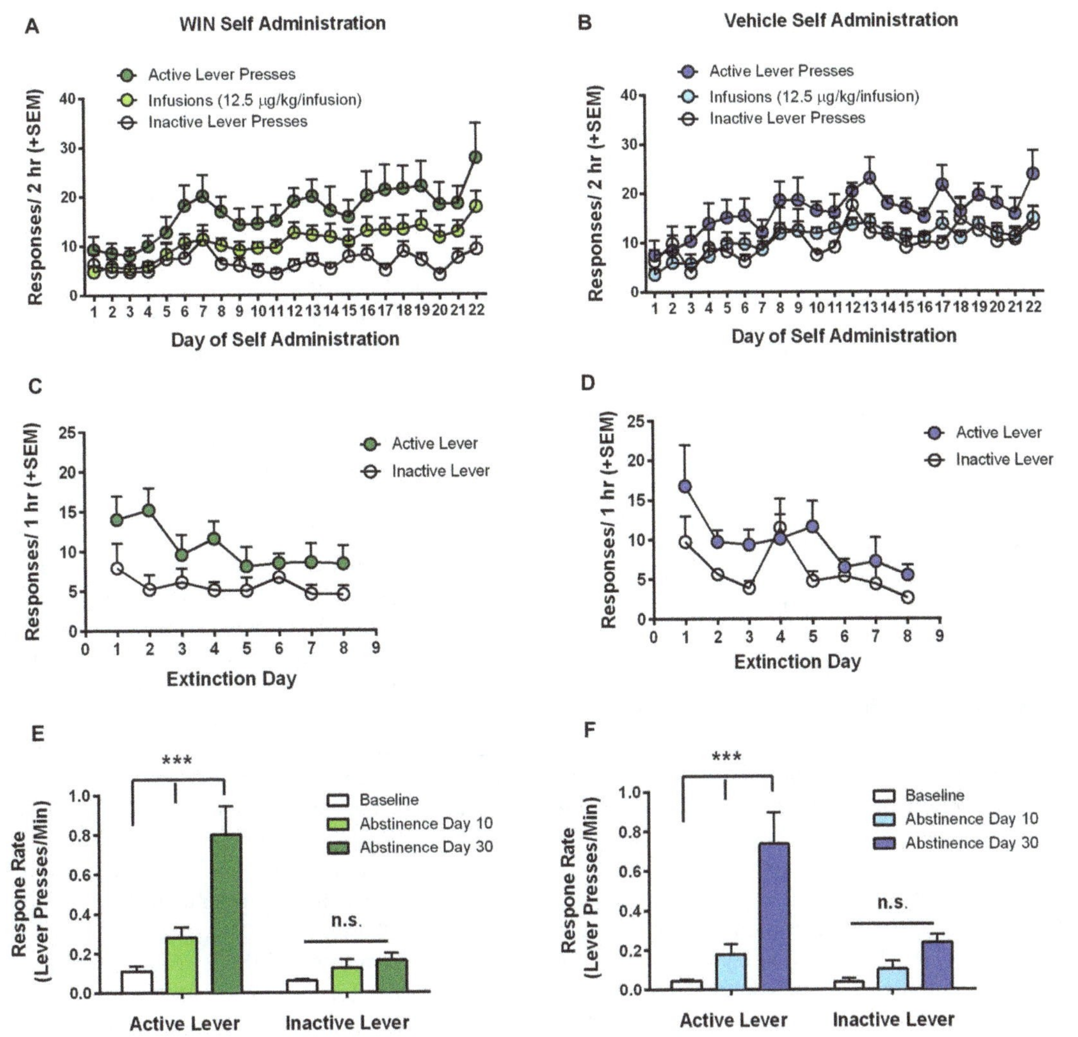

FIGURE 2 | Adolescent self-administration behaviors. **(A)** Rats self-administering WIN throughout adolescence showed clear discrimination between active and inactive lever responses over days, and rats earned significantly more infusions relative to inactive lever presses. **(B)** Rats self-administering vehicle showed a smaller, but significant differentiation between active and inactive lever responses, but no difference between inactive lever presses and infusions earned. **(C,D)** Significant extinction of the lever press response occurred in both the WIN **(C)** and VEH **(D)** groups. **(E)** Rats that self-administered WIN exhibited significant cue-induced reinstatement of lever pressing over response rates on the last day of extinction (i.e., baseline) on both 10 and 30 days of abstinence. Reinstatement on day 30 was also significantly greater than that observed on day 10. **(F)** Rats that self-administered VEH did not exhibit a significant cue-induced reinstatement of lever pressing on day 10, but responding on day 30 was significantly greater than baseline and day 10 response rates. ***$p < 0.001$.

or group × test phase interaction ($F_{(2,32)} = 0.04$, $p = 0.96$). Analysis of WIN and VEH SA groups separately by rmANOVA revealed that the WIN self-administration group exhibited significant differences based on test phase ($F_{(2,18)} = 26.09$, $p < 0.001$), and lever type ($F_{(1,9)} = 17.42$, $p = 0.002$), and a significant interaction between the two ($F_{(2,18)} = 23.60$, $p < 0.001$). *Post hoc* analysis indicated that there were no significant differences in inactive lever response rates across test days, but that there was a significant difference between baseline responding (i.e., on the last day of extinction) and response rates on day 10 ($p = 0.018$) and day 30 ($p < 0.001$) of abstinence, indicating significant cue-induced reinstatement of WIN seeking on both test days. Furthermore, there was also a significant increase in responding from day 10 to day 30 of abstinence ($p < 0.001$), indicating a significant incubation of craving effect (**Figure 2E**). Similar effects were observed in the VEH self-administration group, with significant effects of test day ($F_{(2,14)} = 28.02, p < 0.001$), lever type ($F_{(1,7)} = 9.48, p = 0.018$) and their interaction ($F_{(2,14)} = 7.28$, $p = 0.007$). However, on day 10 of "abstinence", there was no significant difference in response rate from the extinction baseline ($p = 0.20$). Nevertheless, on day 30 of "abstinence", response rates were significantly increased over both baseline ($p < 0.001$) and day 10 levels ($p < 0.001$). Therefore, while there was not a significant cue-induced reinstatement effect on day 10, there was still an increase in cue-motivated responding on day 30, despite the cue never being paired with a drug (**Figure 2F**). These data suggest that cues can be strong motivators of behavior (at least in adolescent females), independent of conditioning to a reinforcer.

Estrous Cycle Phase Does Not Impact Self-Administration

The present study was conducted in freely cycling females, thus making it difficult to explicitly assess the relationship between circulating hormones and motivation to self-administer WIN. However, we did monitor estrous cycle phase via observation of vaginal cytology during the last 9 days of self-administration and averaged the infusions earned, active and inactive lever presses of rats during the last 5 days of self-administration on days that they were in a high estradiol phase (PRO) and a low estradiol phase (EMD). Using two-sample *t*-tests (PRO vs. EMD), we found no significant differences based on estrous cycle in infusions ($t_{(16)} = 0.639$, $p = 0.53$) or active lever presses ($t_{(16)} = 0.445$, $p = 0.66$; **Figures 3A,B**). Inactive lever presses did appear to be reduced during proestrus, but this only reached a trend level of significance ($t_{(16)} = 1.783$, $p = 0.09$; **Figure 3C**).

Adolescent Cannabinoid Exposure Does Not Acutely Affect Short-Term Spatial Memory

We next tested whether or not females would exhibit acute deficits in short-term spatial memory 24 h following the last self-administration session. Since previous research has indicated that adolescent experimenter administration of WIN, at doses substantially higher than those obtained during self-administration, can produce short-term memory deficits in males (Kirschmann et al., 2017), a separate cohort of rats was exposed to chronic WIN in adolescence using an experimenter-administration procedure. We compared a dose of WIN comparable to that obtained during self-administration (0.2 mg/kg/day) to the commonly used "high" dose of WIN (1.2 mg/kg/day). Neither self-administration, nor experimenter-administration of WIN at either dose, produced any short-term memory deficits in females. Both WIN and VEH self-administration groups exhibited equivalent discrimination of novel from familiar spatial locations (main effect of location ($F_{(1,13)} = 68.09$, $p < 0.001$), but no effect of treatment ($F_{(1,13)} = 0.08$, $p = 0.78$; **Figure 4A**). Similar results were observed under experimenter-administration conditions, with a main effect of location ($F_{(1,20)} = 43.19$, $p < 0.001$), but no effect of treatment ($F_{(2,20)} = 0.29$, $p = 0.75$; **Figure 4B**).

Working Memory Performance

All rats began training on the delayed-match-to-sample working memory task 10–11 days after the last drug exposure day, which followed extinction and initial reinstatement testing in the self-administration group. All groups received between 22 days and 25 days of training prior to final working memory assessments. We observed no differences between the self-administration groups across different phases of training (**Table 1**). Analysis of working memory performance once rats reached the final test phase, where the delays between sample and choice phases are longest, revealed no significant effects of treatment ($F_{(1,17)} = 0.01$, $p = 0.91$). However, we did observe the expected effect of delay, with performance accuracy significantly decreasing as the delay length was increased ($F_{(6,102)} = 44.99$, $p < 0.001$; **Figure 5A**). Thus, female rats that self-administered WIN during adolescence showed neither an improvement nor a detriment in working memory performance in adulthood under drug-free conditions.

Conversely, analysis of working memory performance in rats that received experimenter-administered WIN in adolescence indicated that exposure to the low, but not the high dose, produced working memory improvements in adulthood (see **Table 2** for training data). Analysis by rmANOVA identified the expected decrease in performance with increasing delay length ($F_{(6,126)} = 40.29$, $p < 0.001$), and a strong trend toward a treatment effect when all three treatment groups were included in the analysis ($F_{(2,21)} = 3.19$, $p = 0.06$). Due to the fact that the potential treatment effect appeared to be driven by low dose WIN exposure and differences are not expected at very short and very long delays, a separate two-way rmANOVA comparing the vehicle and low dose groups across 4–16 s delays was conducted, which indicated a significant improvement in working memory performance after adolescent exposure to low dose WIN ($F_{(1,14)} = 10.57$, $p = 0.006$; **Figure 5B**). Similar analysis

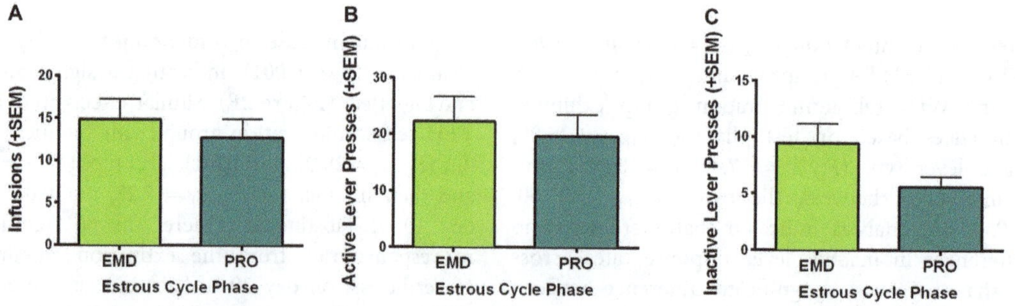

FIGURE 3 | Role of estrous cycle phase on WIN self-administration. Behaviors during the high estradiol phase of proestrus (PRO) were compared to behavior during the low estradiol phases of estrus, metestrus and diestrus (EMD). No significant differences were identified for **(A)** infusions earned, **(B)** active lever presses, or **(C)** inactive lever presses.

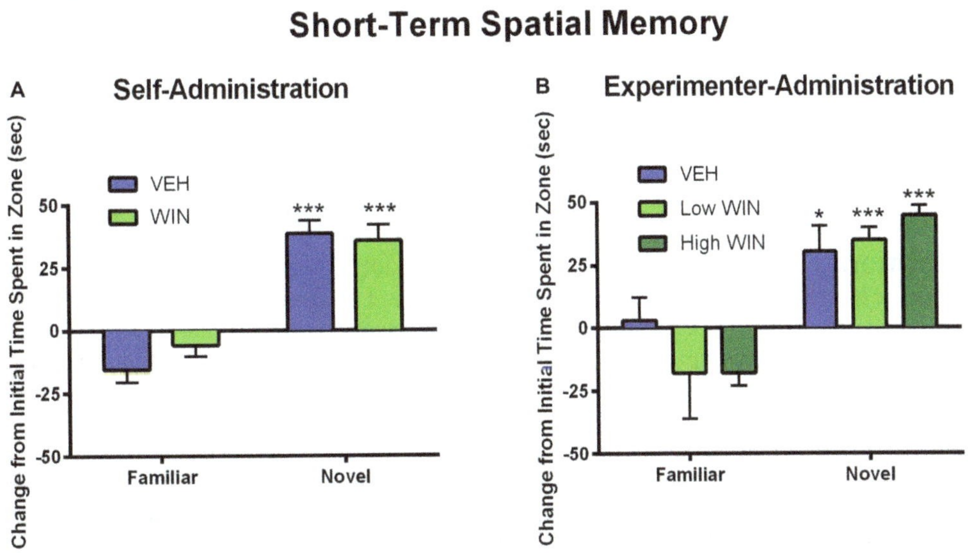

FIGURE 4 | Effect of adolescent WIN exposure on short-term spatial memory. **(A)** Self-administration of WIN did not result in any acute deficits in short-term spatial memory in an object location task in female rats tested 24 h after the last self-administration day. All rats showed a significant discrimination between the familiar and novel spatial locations, $^{***}p < 0.001$. **(B)** Experimenter-administration of either a low or high dose of WIN did not significantly alter short-term spatial memory 24 h after the last injection day. All groups exhibited significant discrimination between familiar and novel locations, indicating intact memory, $^{*}p \leq 0.05$, $^{***}p < 0.001$.

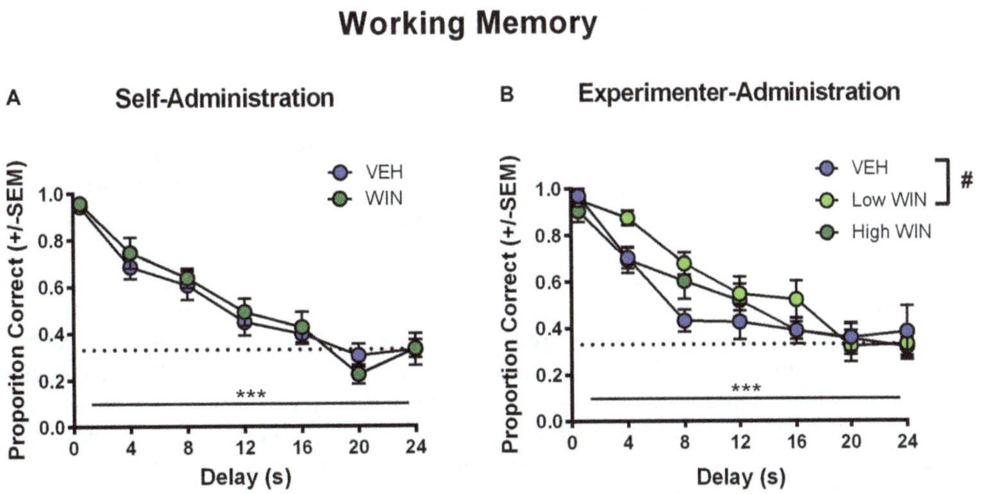

FIGURE 5 | Effect of adolescent WIN exposure on adult working memory. **(A)** Adult working memory performance in rats that self-administered WIN or VEH in adolescence. All working memory training and testing was conducted under drug-free conditions. As delay increased, performance decreased, $^{***}p < 0.001$. Adolescent WIN self-administration had no significant effect on working memory performance. **(B)** Adult working memory performance in rats that were exposed to WIN in adolescence via experimenter-administration (IP injection) of a low dose (0.2 mg/kg/day) or a high dose (1.2 mg/kg/day), or its vehicle. In all rats, as delay increased, performance decreased, $^{***}p < 0.001$. The low dose of WIN produced a strong trend toward improved working memory performance relative to vehicle, and separate analyses of delays from 4 s to 16 s, indicated a significant improvement in performance, $^{\#}p = 0.05$.

of the high WIN dose group did not reveal a significant treatment effect on performance ($F_{(1,14)} = 2.34, p = 0.15$).

DISCUSSION

The aims of the present study were to determine the long-term effects of self-administered cannabinoids in adolescence on adult cognitive function, and to explore the abuse liability of adolescent-onset cannabinoid use, in females. Additionally, we aimed to explore whether similar cognitive consequences arose from different routes of cannabinoid administration during adolescence. Similar to our previous findings in males, there were no detrimental effects of adolescent WIN self-administration on adult cognitive performance in females. Additionally, experimenter-administration of a low dose of WIN in adolescent females resulted in improved performance in a delayed-match-to-sample working memory task in adulthood. Together, our data provide further support towards the notion that cannabinoid exposure under self-administration conditions, or at behaviorally-relevant doses, is less detrimental than originally suspected.

Analysis of Female Cannabinoid Self-Administration

The National Institutes of Health now requires the consideration of sex as a relevant biological variable in all new applications for funding. To our knowledge, our current study in females, in conjunction with our previously published findings in males (Kirschmann et al., 2017), is one of the first analyses of males and females in adolescent cannabinoid self-administration (but see work in adults by Fattore et al., 2007, 2010). We show here that adolescent female rats will self-administer the synthetic cannabinoid receptor agonist WIN55,212-2, and will attain a daily dose similar to, though slightly less than, the daily dose that what male rats attained in our prior study (~0.15 mg/kg here in females vs. 0.22 mg/kg in males; Kirschmann et al., 2017). This is in contrast to rodent findings for other drugs of abuse such as cocaine, ethanol and opiates, where females take substantially higher amounts compared to males (e.g., Becker et al., 2007; Anker and Carroll, 2010; Becker and Koob, 2016; Bertholomey et al., 2016). However, our finding that females maintained a slightly lower daily dose of a cannabinoid receptor agonist than males is in line with human findings in which women report greater sensitivity to the subjective effects of inhaled or orally-administered cannabis (Cooper and Haney, 2014; Fogel et al., 2017). There were no significant differences in self-administration behaviors during the high estradiol phase (proestrus) compared to the low estradiol phases (estrus, metestrus and diestrus), indicating a lack of a role of estrous cycle in cannabinoid self-administration in adolescent females, at least to the degree to which we could assess estrous cycle in this study. In contrast, Fattore et al. (2007) found that ovariectomized adult females self-administered significantly less WIN compared to intact controls; however different strains and ages of rats were used in that study, and ovariectomy clamps estradiol at much lower levels than what occurs naturally during all phases of the estrous cycle, which could explain the difference in findings.

Female rats that self-administered WIN showed significant cue-induced lever pressing after a short abstinence period (10 days); and they exhibited even greater cue-induced lever pressing after an extended abstinence period (30 days), indicating an "incubation of craving" effect for a self-administered cannabinoid, similar to our previous findings in male rats (Kirschmann et al., 2017). However, female rats that self-administered the vehicle solution also exhibited increased cue-induced lever pressing after an extended period of "abstinence" (or lack of exposure to vehicle or cues). Few groups have ever examined incubation of craving in a vehicle group, particularly in females. The closest work may be that of Lee et al. (2013), and that of Werner et al. (2015), in which male rats trained to self-administer saline showed a lack of reinstatement for visual stimuli previously paired with infusion delivery; although in one case, if all reinstatement test days were collapsed, saline-trained animals did show a memory for the saline cue (Werner et al., 2015). Experiments with rodents responding for natural rewards (e.g., sucrose or food pellets) also have demonstrated reinstatement and incubation of craving for the cues previously paired with the natural rewards (e.g., Grimm et al., 2011; Darling et al., 2016; Dingess et al., 2017). Additionally, our paradigm utilized an audiovisual cue, and compound stimuli have themselves been shown to serve as conditioned reinforcers (Fuchs et al., 1998; See et al., 1999; Caggiula et al., 2002). Finally, adolescents have been shown to learn more about cues than adults (e.g., Meyer and Bucci, 2016). Thus, the increased cue-induced reinstatement after 30 days of abstinence in female rats that had previously self-administered the vehicle solution in adolescence is likely a reflection of compound cues serving as strong motivators of behavior in adolescent females, and makes it difficult to interpret if the incubation of craving observed in the WIN group is related specifically to the potential reinforcing property of WIN or to the compound cues. Future studies could examine if self-administration of other unit doses of WIN would produce greater self-administration and reinstatement in females, though the high level of responding in the vehicle group is still an important factor to consider when interpreting reinstatement and incubation of craving results across drug classes.

Cannabinoid Exposure in Adolescence Differentially Impacts Cognition

Similar to what we have shown in males, WIN self-administration did not cause acute deficits in short-term spatial memory in females. Contrary to findings in males (Abush and Akirav, 2012; Kirschmann et al., 2017), experimenter-administration of a high dose of WIN (1.2 mg/kg) in adolescence did not result in acute deficits in short-term spatial memory in females. This could reflect the differential sensitivity of females to cannabinoids; potentially, exposure to a higher or lower dose of WIN than was used in this study could have resulted in acute short-term memory deficits in females. We then examined the long-term effect of adolescent WIN exposure and we found a significant improvement in working memory in females that received the low dose (0.2 mg/kg) during adolescence. In contrast to what we previously reported in males, adolescent self-administration of WIN in females did not significantly impact adult working memory performance. It is not clear if this is due to sex differences in the impact of self-administered vs. experimenter-administered drugs, or if the lack of effect in the self-administration group is due to the fact that the females self-administered a lower dose of WIN (~0.15 mg/kg/day) than males. Thus, a very tight dose-effect relationship may exist between adolescent WIN exposure and improvements in adult working memory performance. Nevertheless, under no conditions by dose, sex, or route of administration have we observed long-lasting deficits in working memory after adolescent WIN exposure.

Limitations and Conclusions

The present set of experiments does have some caveats. First, it is clear that adolescent females will respond for cues, regardless of the solution they receive IV. This limits our interpretation of the self-administration data on the degree to which WIN is reinforcing in and of itself. However, because adolescent females responding for IV WIN tended to show better discrimination between the active and inactive levers, there is some indication that WIN carries at least somewhat greater reinforcing value than the vehicle solution. Future work that includes a full dose-response curve and examines differences in responding with and without cues for both male and female adolescents in the same experiment would be warranted. Additionally, because our main question was focused on the long-term cognitive consequences of cannabinoid self-administration during adolescence, the fact that the vehicle group exhibited similar levels of responding during SA provides for a more closely-matched control group. All rats received equivalent exposure to the cues, and therefore the differences we observed in later working memory performance can be attributed to the WIN exposure itself. Second, because we did not include males and females in a singular experiment, definitive conclusions about sex differences in cannabinoid self-administration and effects of adolescent cannabinoid exposure on later cognitive performance cannot be made. Overall, the response rates are similar in the females of the current experiment and the males we previously tested (Kirschmann et al., 2017); a larger study that includes both sexes run simultaneously would be necessary to confirm this. Third, all of our females were food restricted for the duration of behavioral experiments. Though this was necessary to maintain motivation to complete the tasks, this could interact with our behavioral findings. In line with this, we did not conduct a full panel of cognitive assessments in our rats. Future work could aim to complete additional investigations of cognitive ability using paradigms that do not require food restriction to ensure task performance. Fourth, all of our experiments utilized the synthetic cannabinoid receptor agonist WIN55,212-2, not the main psychoactive component of marijuana, Δ^9-THC. Although WIN does act on the same receptors as THC, its pharmacological properties may be distinct from THC, and its chemical structure may be more comparable to the frequently-abused synthetic cannabinoids K2 and spice (Pertwee, 2010). Nevertheless, there is evidence for similar effects of experimenter-administered THC or WIN on short-term memory that are blocked by nonselective cannabinoid receptor antagonists (Hampson and Deadwyler, 2000; O'Shea et al., 2004, 2006; Schneider and Koch, 2007; Abush and Akirav, 2012; Renard et al., 2016), suggesting that any effects of THC on cognition are likely to be recapitulated by WIN. Finally, we acknowledge that conclusions about self- vs. experimenter-administration are limited, in that these groups experience different daily conditions. The animals receiving daily IP injections were not exposed to any behavioral chambers prior to the start of working memory training, whereas the animals self-administering entered the behavioral chambers daily during the course of adolescence. Future work could include animals that receive IP injections but are then allowed daily exposure to the behavioral chambers, to ensure that experience is equated prior to working memory training. Despite the IP females taking a longer amount of time to reach training criteria than SA females in earlier phases of working memory training, by the time delays were introduced, all animals were performing at similar levels (see **Tables 1, 2**).

In conclusion, we report one of the first examinations of the effects of adolescent cannabinoid self-administration on cognitive function in females. We have found that adolescent cannabinoid exposure alone is not sufficient to produce long-lasting deficits in memory function. Our data are potentially consistent with human literature showing an increased sensitivity to cannabinoids in females, which may explain why females self-administered slightly less WIN, in contrast to other drugs of abuse. Finally, our data show some evidence for craving-like behavior after adolescent cannabinoid SA in females, suggesting the potential for abuse liability.

AUTHOR CONTRIBUTIONS

EKK and MMT contributed to the design of the experiments. DMM, EKK and CME were involved in data collection. EKK, DMM and MMT analyzed and interpreted the data with input from CME. EKK and DMM wrote the article with input from CME and MMT. All authors gave final approval for publication.

ACKNOWLEDGMENTS

The authors would like to acknowledge grant DA042029, and the NIMH Chemical Synthesis and Drug Supply Program for providing WIN55,212-2 for this study.

REFERENCES

Abush, H., and Akirav, I. (2012). Short- and long-term cognitive effects of chronic cannabinoids administration in late-adolescence rats. *PLoS One* 7:e31731. doi: 10.1371/journal.pone.0031731

Anker, J. J., and Carroll, M. E. (2010). Females are more vulnerable to drug abuse than males: evidence from preclinical studies and the role of ovarian hormones. *Curr. Top. Behav. Neurosci.* 8, 73–96. doi: 10.1007/7854_2010_93

Becker, M. P., Collins, P. F., and Luciana, M. (2014). Neurocognition in college-aged daily marijuana users. *J. Clin. Exp. Neuropsychol.* 36, 379–398. doi: 10.1080/13803395.2014.893996

Becker, J. B., and Koob, G. F. (2016). Sex differences in animal models: focus on addiction. *Pharmacol. Rev.* 68, 242–263. doi: 10.1124/pr.115.011163

Becker, J. B., Monteggia, L. M., Perrot-Sinal, T. S., Romeo, R. D., Taylor, J. R., Yehuda, R., et al. (2007). Stress and disease: is being female a predisposing factor? *J. Neurosci.* 27, 11851–11855. doi: 10.1523/JNEUROSCI.3565-07.2007

Bertholomey, M. L., Nagarajan, V., and Torregrossa, M. M. (2016). Sex differences in reinstatement of alcohol seeking in response to cues and yohimbine in rats with and without a history of adolescent corticosterone exposure. *Psychopharmacology* 233, 2277–2287. doi: 10.1007/s00213-016-4278-x

Buchy, L., Seidman, L. J., Cadenhead, K. S., Cannon, T. D., Cornblatt, B. A., McGlashan, T. H., et al. (2015). Evaluating the relationship between cannabis use and IQ in youth and young adults at clinical high risk of psychosis. *Psychiatry Res.* 230, 878–884. doi: 10.1016/j.psychres.2015.11.033

Caggiula, A., Donny, E., White, A., Chaudhri, N., Booth, S., Gharib, M., et al. (2002). Environmental stimuli promote the acquisition of nicotine self-administration in rats. *Psychopharmacology* 163, 230–237. doi: 10.1007/s00213-002-1156-5

Cooper, Z. D., and Haney, M. (2014). Investigation of sex-dependent effects of cannabis in daily cannabis smokers. *Drug Alcohol Depend.* 136, 85–91. doi: 10.1016/j.drugalcdep.2013.12.013

Darling, R. A., Dingess, P. M., Schlidt, K. C., Smith, E. M., and Brown, T. E. (2016). Incubation of food craving is independent of macronutrient composition. *Sci. Rep.* 6:30900. doi: 10.1038/srep30900

Deiana, S., Fattore, L., Spano, M. S., Cossu, G., Porcu, E., Fadda, P., et al. (2007). Strain and schedule-dependent differences in the acquisition, maintenance and extinction of intravenous cannabinoid self-administration in rats. *Neuropharmacology* 52, 646–654. doi: 10.1016/j.neuropharm.2006.09.007

Dingess, P. M., Darling, R. A., Derman, R. C., Wulff, S. S., Hunter, M. L., Ferrario, C. R., et al. (2017). Structural and functional plasticity within the nucleus accumbens and prefrontal cortex associated with time-dependent increases in food cue-seeking behavior. *Neuropsychopharmacology* doi: 10.1038/npp.2017.57 [Epub ahead of print].

Fattore, L., Cossu, G., Martellotta, C., and Fratta, W. (2001). Intravenous self-administration of the cannabinoid CB1 receptor agonist WIN 55,212-2 in rats. *Psychopharmacology* 156, 410–416. doi: 10.1007/s002130100734

Fattore, L., Spano, M. S., Altea, S., Angius, F., Fadda, P., and Fratta, W. (2007). Cannabinoid self-administration in rats: sex differences and the influence of ovarian function. *Br. J. Pharmacol.* 152, 795–804. doi: 10.1038/sj.bjp.0707465

Fattore, L., Spano, M. S., Altea, S., Fadda, P., and Fratta, W. (2010). Drug- and cue-induced reinstatement of cannabinoid-seeking behaviour in male and female rats: influence of ovarian hormones. *Br. J. Pharmacol.* 160, 724–735. doi: 10.1111/j.1476-5381.2010.00734.x

Fogel, J. S., Kelly, T. H., Westgate, P. M., and Lile, J. A. (2017). Sex differences in the subjective effects of oral Δ^9-THC in cannabis users. *Pharmacol. Biochem. Behav.* 152, 44–51. doi: 10.1016/j.pbb.2016.01.007

Fuchs, R. A., Tran-Nguyen, L. T. L., Specio, S. E., Groff, R. S., and Neisewander, J. L. (1998). Predictive validity of the extinction/reinstatement model of drug craving. *Psychopharmacology* 135, 151–160. doi: 10.1007/s002130050496

Gage, S. H., Hickman, M., and Zammit, S. (2016). Association between cannabis and psychosis: epidemiologic evidence. *Biol. Psychiatry* 79, 549–556. doi: 10.1016/j.biopsych.2015.08.001

Goldman, J. M., Murr, A. S., and Cooper, R. L. (2007). The rodent estrous cycle: characterization of vaginal cytology and its utility in toxicological studies. *Birth Defects Res. B Dev. Reprod. Toxicol.* 80, 84–97. doi: 10.1002/bdrb.20106

Grimm, J. W., Barnes, J., North, K., Collins, S., and Weber, R. (2011). A general method for evaluating incubation of sucrose craving in rats. *J. Vis. Exp.* 57:e3335. doi: 10.3791/3335

Hampson, R. E., and Deadwyler, S. A. (2000). Cannabinoids reveal the necessity of hippocampal neural encoding for short-term memory in rats. *J. Neurosci.* 20, 8932–8942.

Jager, G., Kahn, R. S., Van Den Brink, W., Van Ree, J. M., and Ramsey, N. F. (2006). Long-term effects of frequent cannabis use on working memory and attention: an fMRI study. *Psychopharmacology* 185, 358–368. doi: 10.1007/s00213-005-0298-7

Kirschmann, E. K., Pollock, M. W., Nagarajan, V., and Torregrossa, M. M. (2017). Effects of adolescent cannabinoid self-administration in rats on addiction-related behaviors and working memory. *Neuropsychopharmacology* 42, 989–1000. doi: 10.1038/npp.2016.178

Lee, B. R., Ma, Y.-Y., Huang, Y. H., Wang, X., Otaka, M., Ishikawa, M., et al. (2013). Maturation of silent synapses in amygdala-accumbens projection contributes to incubation of cocaine craving. *Nat. Neurosci.* 16, 1644–1651. doi: 10.1038/nn.3533

Lefever, T. W., Marusich, J. A., Antonazzo, K. R., and Wiley, J. L. (2014). Evaluation of WIN 55,212-2 self-administration in rats as a potential cannabinoid abuse liability model. *Pharmacol. Biochem. Behav.* 118, 30–35. doi: 10.1016/j.pbb.2014.01.002

Marconi, A., Di Forti, M., Lewis, C. M., Murray, R. M., and Vassos, E. (2016). Meta-analysis of the association between the level of cannabis use and risk of psychosis. *Schizophr. Bull.* 42, 1262–1269. doi: 10.1093/schbul/sbw003

Meier, M. H., Caspi, A., Ambler, A., Harrington, H., Houts, R., Keefe, R. S. E., et al. (2012). Persistent cannabis users show neuropsychological decline from childhood to midlife. *Proc. Natl. Acad. Sci. U S A* 109, E2657–E2664. doi: 10.1073/pnas.1206820109

Meyer, H. C., and Bucci, D. J. (2016). Age differences in appetitive Pavlovian conditioning and extinction in rats. *Physiol. Behav.* 167, 354–362. doi: 10.1016/j.physbeh.2016.10.004

Mokrysz, C., Landy, R., Gage, S., Munafo, M., Roiser, J., and Curran, H. (2016). Are IQ and educational outcomes in teenagers related to their cannabis use? A prospective cohort study. *J. Psychopharmacol.* 30, 159–168. doi: 10.1177/0269881115622241

Moss, H. B., Chen, C. M., and Yi, H.-Y. (2014). Early adolescent patterns of alcohol, cigarettes, and marijuana polysubstance use and young adult substance use outcomes in a nationally representative sample. *Drug Alcohol Depend.* 136, 51–62. doi: 10.1016/j.drugalcdep.2013.12.011

O'Shea, M., McGregor, I. S., and Mallet, P. E. (2006). Repeated cannabinoid exposure during perinatal, adolescent or early adult ages produces similar longlasting deficits in object recognition and reduced social interaction in rats. *J. Psychopharmacol.* 20, 611–621. doi: 10.1177/0269881106065188

O'Shea, M., Singh, M. E., McGregor, I. S., and Mallet, P. E. (2004). Chronic cannabinoid exposure produces lasting memory impairment and increased anxiety in adolescent but not adult rats. *J. Psychopharmacol.* 18, 502–508. doi: 10.1177/026988110401800407

Pertwee, R. G. (2010). Receptors and channels targeted by synthetic cannabinoid receptor agonists and antagonists. *Curr. Med. Chem.* 17, 1360–1381. doi: 10.2174/092986710790980050

Renard, J., Rushlow, W. J., and Laviolette, S. R. (2016). What can rats tell us about adolescent cannabis exposure? Insights from preclinical research. *Can. J. Psychiatry* 61, 328–334. doi: 10.1177/0706743716645288

Salas-Wright, C. P., Vaughn, M. G., Perron, B. E., Gonzalez, J. M. R., and Goings, T. C. (2016). Changing perspectives on marijuana use during early adolescence and young adulthood: evidence from a panel of cross-sectional surveys. *Drug Alcohol Depend.* 169, 5–10. doi: 10.1016/j.drugalcdep.2016.09.026

Schneider, M. (2008). Puberty as a highly vulnerable developmental period for the consequences of cannabis exposure. *Addict. Biol.* 13, 253–263. doi: 10.1111/j.1369-1600.2008.00110.x

Schneider, M., and Koch, M. (2003). Chronic pubertal, but not adult chronic cannabinoid treatment impairs sensorimotor gating, recognition memory and the performance in a progressive ratio task in adult rats. *Neuropsychopharmacology* 28, 1760–1769. doi: 10.1038/sj.npp.1300225

Schneider, M., and Koch, M. (2007). The effect of chronic peripubertal cannabinoid treatment on deficient object recognition memory in rats after neonatal mPFC lesion. *Eur. Neuropsychopharmacol.* 17, 180–186. doi: 10.1016/j.euroneuro.2006.03.009

See, R. E., Grimm, J. W., Kruzich, P. J., and Rustay, N. (1999). The Importance of a compound stimulus in conditioned drug-seeking behavior following one week of extinction from self-administered cocaine in rats. *Drug Alcohol Depend.* 57, 41–49. doi: 10.1016/s0376-8716(99)00043-5

Spear, L. P. (2000). The Adolescent brain and age-related behavioral manisfestations. *Neurosci. Biobehav. Rev.* 24, 417–463. doi: 10.1016/s0149-7634(00)00014-2

Takahashi, R. N., and Singer, G. (1979). Self-administration of delta 9-tetrahydrocannabinol by rats. *Pharmacol. Biochem. Behav.* 11, 737–740. doi: 10.1016/0091-3057(79)90274-0

Werner, C. T., Milovanovic, M., Christian, D. T., Loweth, J. A., and Wolf, M. E. (2015). Response of the ubiquitin-proteasome system to memory retrieval after extended-access cocaine or saline self-administration. *Curr. Vasc. Pharmacol.* 40, 3006–3014. doi: 10.1038/npp.2015.156

8

Explicit and Implicit Positive Alcohol Expectancies in Problem and Non-Problem Drinkers: Differences Across Age Groups from Young Adolescence to Adulthood

Aurélie Vilenne and Etienne Quertemont*

Département Psychologie, Cognition et Comportement, Université de Liège, Liège, Belgium

Edited by:
Ofir Turel,
California State University, Fullerton and University of Southern California, USA

Reviewed by:
Martin S. Hagger,
Curtin University, Australia
Alexander Serenko,
Lakehead University, Canada
Qinghua He,
Southwest University, China

***Correspondence:**
Etienne Quertemont
equertemont@ulg.ac.be

Aims: Recent studies with animal models showed that the stimulant and sedative effects of alcohol change during the adolescent period. In humans, the stimulant effects of ethanol are most often indirectly recorded through the measurement of explicit and implicit alcohol effect expectancies. However, it is unknown how such implicit and explicit expectancies evolve with age in humans during adolescence.

Methods: Adolescent (13–16 year old), young adult (17–18 year old), and adult (35–55 year old) participants were recruited. On the basis of their score on the Alcohol Use Disorder Identification Test (AUDIT), they were classified as non-problem (AUDIT ≤ 7) or problem (AUDIT ≥ 11) drinkers. The participants completed the Alcohol Expectancy Questionnaire (AEQ) and performed two unipolar Implicit Association Test (IAT) to assess implicit associations between alcohol and the concepts of "stimulation" and "sedation".

Results: Problem drinkers from the three age groups reported significantly higher positive alcohol expectancies than non-problem drinkers on all AEQ subscales. Positive alcohol explicit expectancies also gradually decreased with age, with adolescent problem drinkers reporting especially high positive expectancies. This effect was statistically significant for all positive expectancies, with the exception of relaxation expectancies that were only close to statistical significance. In contrast, stimulation and sedation alcohol implicit associations were not significantly different between problem and non-problem drinkers and did not change with age.

Conclusion: These results indicate that explicit positive alcohol effect expectancies predict current alcohol consumption levels, especially in adolescents. Positive alcohol expectancies also gradually decrease with age in the three cross-sectional groups of adolescents, young adults, and adults. This effect might be related to changes in the physiological response to alcohol.

Keywords: age differences, alcohol expectancies, implicit associations, adolescence, stimulation, sedation

INTRODUCTION

Recent studies with animal models indicated that the stimulant and sedative effects of alcohol are age-dependent. During development, the stimulant effects of alcohol gradually decrease from weaning to adulthood, whereas the sedative effects of alcohol increase with age during the same developmental period (Silveri and Spear, 1998; Stevenson et al., 2008; Quoilin et al., 2010). In humans, this would suggest that young adolescents are more likely to feel the stimulant effects of alcohol, whereas they are less likely to experience its sedative effects, making alcohol even more enjoyable than in adults. Such effects might contribute to promote heavy alcohol drinking in young people, leading to alcohol problems later in life. Unfortunately, very few human studies attempted to directly measure the stimulant and sedative effects of ethanol (Davidson et al., 2002; van den Wildenberg et al., 2006; Addicott et al., 2007) and to our knowledge none of those studies compared participants of various ages including young adolescents. In human studies, it is much more common to measure alcohol effect expectancies through questionnaires than directly recording the behavioral effects of alcohol after consumption. Typically, alcohol drinkers are asked to fill in a questionnaire about how they think alcohol affects the behavior. In these questionnaires, some of the questions pertain to the stimulant and depressant effects of alcohol. One example is the Alcohol Expectancy Questionnaire (AEQ; Brown et al., 1987). For example, in this questionnaire, participants are asked to state how much they agree with the following item: "alcohol increases arousal; it makes people feel stronger and more powerful". Of course, one of the problems with such expectancy questionnaires is that general expectancies about alcohol consumption may differ from the actual behavioral responses after alcohol consumption. However, probably due to their ease of use, many human studies use alcohol effect expectancies to indirectly infer the stimulant and depressant effects of alcohol.

Many previous studies were interested in explicit positive alcohol effect expectancies as explanatory factors for alcohol-related problems both in adults (Jones et al., 2001) and in adolescents (Baer, 2002). In particular, alcohol explicit expectancies of arousal measured with questionnaires such as the AEQ were shown to predict current alcohol consumption (Kreusch et al., 2013). These expectancies appear to contribute both to the initiation and maintenance of drinking behaviors. Indeed, positive alcohol expectancies predict current alcohol consumption and to a smaller extent future alcohol consumption and alcohol-related problems. They also show consistent associations with problem drinking behaviors in young adults (Cameron et al., 2003; Ham and Hope, 2003). According to the alcohol expectancy theory, individuals who expect positive outcomes to occur as a result of alcohol use are more likely to drink than those who do not endorse such beliefs. As a consequence, positive expectancies, such as arousal expectancies, assessed with the AEQ (Brown et al., 1987) are associated with a higher prevalence of alcohol-related problems, whereas negative expectancies tend to limit alcohol consumption, leading to the opposite effect (for review, Jones et al., 2001). Indeed, heavier drinkers in general report more positive expectancies than light drinkers (Southwick et al., 1981). In a recent study, it was shown that heavy drinkers endorse more positive and arousing alcohol effect expectancies than light drinkers, although heavy and light drinkers do not differ in their endorsement of negative alcohol expectancies (Field and Wiers, 2012). Although all alcohol consumers show positive alcohol expectancies, high arousal expectancies were reported especially in heavy drinkers (Wiers et al., 2002; Field and Wiers, 2012). Therefore, explicit expectancies of alcohol stimulation seem to differentiate low drinkers from high drinkers (Goldman et al., 1999).

One caveat with explicit alcohol effect expectancies is that their measurement relies on self-reports and therefore are associated with many potential biases such as self-representation, limits in introspection aptitudes, and social desirability (Edwards, 1958; Arnold and Feldman, 1981; Fisher, 1993; Greenwald et al., 2002). For these reasons, more indirect assessment of expectancies were developed using a variety of tasks, most of them relying on the measurement of reaction times. For example, the Implicit Association Test (IAT) has been modified to assess the strength of alcohol implicit cognitions. The IAT is a categorization task used to assess automatic associations between concepts. Recent studies used the IAT to measure implicit alcohol associations on two dimensions: valence (positive–negative) and arousal (arousal–sedation). Whereas both light and heavy drinkers showed negative implicit associations with alcohol, the arousal dimension discriminated heavy drinkers from light drinkers. Strong associations between arousal/stimulation and alcohol were found in heavy drinkers but not in light drinkers (Wiers et al., 2002; Field and Wiers, 2012). However, another recent study, while also finding an implicit association between alcohol and arousal with the IAT, failed to show a correlation between such an implicit association and the current levels of alcohol consumption in young adults (Kreusch et al., 2013). As alcohol stimulant effects are expected to decrease with age, the age of participants might explain such a failure to find a correlation between alcohol consumption and IAT implicit alcohol associations.

Alcohol use behaviors typically change over time, especially during the transition period from adolescence to adulthood, with peak years for the initiation of drinking near 13–14 years old (Faden, 2006). Rates of alcohol use and intoxication increase during adolescence and continue to rise in the years after high school (O'Malley et al., 1998; Brown et al., 2008). Alcohol use during adolescence, particularly heavy drinking, has been associated with alcohol misuse and dependence later in life (Grant and Dawson, 1997; Cable and Sacker, 2008). These changes in alcohol drinking behaviors might be associated with changes in alcohol effect expectancies, which might in turn affect subsequent alcohol consumption. Expectations about the effects of alcohol were reported in children even before they begin to drink alcohol (Miller et al., 1990; Field and Wiers, 2012), suggesting that such expectations might influence the initiation of alcohol consumption. In young adolescents, both explicit and implicit alcohol-related cognitions were reported to influence drinking behaviors (Thush and Wiers, 2007). Furthermore, positive alcohol expectancies predicted all types of adolescent alcohol use in young men and women (Cable and Sacker, 2008). Positive expectancies were related more strongly than negative expectancies to drinking in younger age groups, while in the older groups, positive and negative expectancies were both influential (Leigh and Stacy, 2004). However, the ability of alcohol expectancies to predict subsequent drinking seems to diminish with age. Although they are robust predictors of subsequent alcohol drinking in young subjects, their predictive value is reduced in older age groups. Together, these results suggest that the role of alcohol expectancies in alcohol drinking and abuse may fluctuate with age.

The aim of the present cross-sectional study was to assess how implicit and explicit alcohol expectancies differ in various age groups from adolescence to adulthood, with a special focus on arousal expectancies that were previously shown to discriminate heavy from light drinkers (Goldman et al., 1999; Wiers et al., 2002). Participants were also classified as problem and non-problem drinkers in order to see how alcohol expectancies predict current levels of alcohol consumption in participants and whether this relationship changes across age groups. Alcohol explicit expectancies were measured with the AEQ questionnaire (Vautier and Moncany, 2008), whereas alcohol implicit associations were tested with the IAT (Greenwald et al., 2003). In order to avoid a multiplication of IAT tests, the assessment of alcohol implicit associations were limited to the arousal–sedation dimension that was previously shown to discriminate light and heavy drinkers.

MATERIALS AND METHODS

Participants

A total of 105 participants (53 women and 52 men) from three age groups were recruited for the study among university students and their relatives at the University of Liège, Belgium. Adolescent, young adult and adult participants were, respectively, 13–16, 17–18, and 35–55 years old. Adolescents were selected at the age of 13–16 because this age range includes the peak years for the initiation of alcohol drinking (Faden, 2006). The participants were first invited to fill in the Alcohol Use Disorders Identification Test (AUDIT; Saunders et al., 1993). On the basis of their AUDIT score, they were classified as non-problem drinkers (AUDIT score of maximum 7) or problem drinkers (AUDIT score of 11 or above). Additionally, in order to exclude total abstainers or adolescents who had never drunk alcohol, only participants who consumed at least one alcohol drink per week were included in the non-problem drinker group. An appointment for the experiment was made with participants meeting these inclusion criteria. The Symptom Checklist-90 (SCL-90; Derogatis, 1977), assessing psychiatric symptoms, was also used for exclusion of participants with scores of 70 or higher on any SCL-90 subscale. Regular use of other psychoactive substances (except nicotine) was also used as an exclusion criterion. Demographic data are shown in **Table 1**.

Design and Procedure

Participants were tested one by one in a small and quiet room. They first signed a consent form prior to their participation and filled in some of the questionnaires, i.e., demographic data, and alcohol consumption questionnaires. Then, they performed the IAT. At the end of the task, they filled in the rest of the questionnaires, i.e., the AEQ and the SCL-90. The procedure was approved by the Ethical Committee of the Psychology Faculty from the University of Liège.

Recent Alcohol Consumption

Recent alcohol consumption was assessed with a self-reported measure based on the timeline follow-back method (Sobell and Sobell, 1992). Participants reported how many standard alcohol drinks (=10 g) they had consumed during the previous week by indicating how many alcoholic drinks they had drunk on each day of the week. Furthermore, the number of days they drank more than six drinks of alcohol (=60 g) on a single occasion during the past 2 weeks was recorded (Wiers et al., 1997). This self-reported assessment of recent alcohol use is a complement to the measurement of habitual alcohol consumption provided by the AUDIT.

Implicit Association Test (IAT)

The IAT (Greenwald et al., 2003) was used to assess implicit associations between alcohol and two concepts: stimulation and sedation (Kreusch et al., 2013). Participants performed two unipolar variants of the test during which they had to classify

TABLE 1 | Mean age and Alcohol Use Disorder Identification Test (AUDIT) score and number of binges on the last 2 weeks (SD) for each condition.

	Age		
Consumption level	**Adolescents**	**Young adults**	**Adults**
Low drinkers	$N = 19$ (7 women) Age: 14.89 (0.994) AUDIT: 3.37 (1.862) Binge: 0.26 (0.45)	$N = 18$ (14 women) Age: 17.33 (0.485) AUDIT: 3.33 (2.058) Binge: 0.56 (0.7)	$N = 17$ (10 women) Age: 44.64 (4.859) AUDIT: 4.47 (2.095) Binge: 0.76 (1.2)
High drinkers	$N = 11$ (6 women) Age: 15.54 (0.687) AUDIT: 15.72 (4.36) Binge: 1.27 (1.1)	$N = 24$ (10 women) Age: 17.5 (0.51) AUDIT: 13.13 (2.332) Binge: 1.67 (1.2)	$N = 16$ (6 women) Age: 46.94 (4.626) AUDIT: 13.63 (3.096) Binge: 1.5 (1.8)

stimuli in two categories (i.e., alcohol and soft drinks) and two attribute categories (i.e., stimulation/sedation and neutral), using a left and a right response key. The items used for each category are listed in **Table 2**. An IAT effect is observed when the participants are faster to respond when highly associated categories are assigned the same response key. Each IAT session consisted of seven blocks. In the first and second blocks (24 trials), participants, respectively, practiced classifying target stimuli as "alcohol drink" or "soft drink" and attributed stimuli into the categories "neutral" or "stimulant" ("sedation" for the sedation IAT). In the third (practice, 12 trials) and fourth (test, 48 trials) blocks, participants had to classify stimuli belonging to one target category and one attribute category (e.g., "alcohol drink" and "neutral") with one response key and stimuli belonging to the other target category and attribute category (e.g., "soft drink" and "stimulant") with the other response key. In the fifth block (24 trials), participants practiced the reversed response assignment of the target categories. In the sixth (practice, 12 trials) and seventh (test, 48 trials) blocks, participants had to classify stimuli belonging to one target category and one attribute category in the reverse order (e.g., "soft drink" and "neutral") with one response key and stimuli belonging to the other target category and attribute category (e.g., "alcohol drink" and "stimulant") with the other response key. The assignment of the categories to the left and the right response keys and the order of the combined sorting conditions were counterbalanced across participants. Stimuli were shown in the middle of the computer screen, and the labels of the categories were presented in the upper corners, consistent with the response assignment of the categories. The stimulus word remained on the screen until a response was generated. Categorization errors were signaled with the word "*error*" appearing in front of the stimulus item. All IATs were programmed in E-Prime 2.0 (Psychology Software Tools, Inc., Sharpsburg, PA, USA). To assess the IAT effect, we used the *D*-score as recommended by Lane et al. (2007). Internal consistencies were tested by calculating the correlation between two *D*-scores (from the third training and the fourth test blocks). The internal consistency was 0.79 for the alcohol-stimulation IAT and 0.67 for the alcohol-sedation IAT.

Alcohol Use Disorders Identification Test (AUDIT)

The French version of the AUDIT questionnaire (Gache et al., 2005) includes ten multiple-choice items measuring alcohol consumption (questions one to three), dependence (questions four to six) and alcohol-related problems (questions seven to ten; Saunders et al., 1993). Questions one to eight are scored from zero to four and questions nine and ten are scored zero, two, or four. The maximum score on the AUDIT is 40. In the present study, a cut-off score of 11 was set for the recruitment of problem drinkers (Fleming et al., 1991) and a cut-off score of maximum 7 for non-problem drinkers, who are also usually qualified as low risk drinkers (Saunders et al., 1993).

Alcohol Expectancy Questionnaire (AEQ)

We used a validated French version of the AEQ (Vautier and Moncany, 2008), which included 55 self-reported items measuring positive alcohol expectancies. The AEQ includes six subscales: global positive changes, sexual enhancement, social and physical pleasure, arousal/power, social assertiveness, and relaxation. The score on each subscale was calculated by summing the scores obtained on each item (from 0 "*I do not agree*" to 10 "*I totally agree*"). An example of item of the AEQ looks like: "*Alcohol makes me worry less*".

Symptom Checklist-90 – Revised (SCL-90-R)

The French version of the SCL-90-R (Fortin and Coutu-Wakulczyk, 1985) is a 90-item self-administered psychopathological assessment questionnaire. The SCL-90-R includes nine subscales: somatization, obsessive–compulsive, interpersonal sensitivity, depression, anxiety, hostility, phobic anxiety, paranoid ideation, and psychoticism. It includes 90 items with five alternatives for each item ranging from 0 (none) to 4 (very much). The SCL-90-R scores are converted to standard *T*-scores.

Data Analysis

To control for the homogeneity of psychopathological symptoms in the six groups, a two-way analysis of variance (ANOVA; Age group × Consumption group) was computed on the SCL-90 subscale scores. The gender distribution of participants in the six experimental groups was checked using Pearson chi-square tests. The AEQ scores were tested using a multivariate analysis of variance (MANOVA) with Age and Consumption groups (problem vs. non-problem drinkers) as between-subject independent variables and the AEQ subscales as dependent variables. A statistically significant MANOVA was followed by independent two-way (Age × Consumption group) ANOVAs for each AEQ subscale separately. In order to test whether there is an IAT effect for alcohol stimulation and sedation in the whole sample, IAT results were first analyzed with student *t*-tests.

TABLE 2 | Items (in French) used for each Implicit Association Test (IAT) target and attribute category.

Soft drink	Alcohol drink	Stimulation	Sedation	Neutral
Jus d'orange	Tequila	Vigoureux	Passif	Normal
Cacao	Whisky	Excité	Tranquille	Indéfini
Coca	Vodka	Agité	Détendu	Général
Limonade	Vin	Energique	Apaisé	Ordinaire
Soda	Bière	Actif	Relaxé	Indifférent
Orangeade	Rhum	Eveillé	Endormi	Moyen

The IAT scores on both subscales were then tested using two-way (Age × Consumption group) ANOVAs. Simple eta-squared (η^2) were reported as effect sizes in the ANOVAs. All statistical analyses were performed using the software package Statistica 10 (StatSoft, Inc., Maisons-Alfort, France). Statistical significance was set at $p < 0.05$.

RESULTS

Group Homogeneity

The two-way ANOVA computed on the SCL-90 scores showed no significant main effect of the consumption group (problem vs. non-problem drinkers) and no significant interaction Age × Group for any of the SCL-90 subscales. These results confirm that the problem and non-problem drinkers did not differ on mean levels of psychopathology symptoms in the present study. In addition, there was no significant main effect of age on any of the SCL-90 subscale scores, except for hostility and phobia. Indeed, adolescents globally showed higher mean scores than young adults and adults on these two SCL-90 subscales. As there was an effect of age on hostility and phobia subscales, the two-way ANOVA computed on AEQ and IAT scores (see below) were followed by analyses of covariance in which hostility and phobia scores were included as covariates. These covariance analyses led to identical effects and conclusions than the ANOVAs, confirming that hostility and phobia differences do not explain the effects of age in these analyses. Additionally, experimental groups did not significantly differ regarding gender, $\chi^2(5) = 9.15, p = 0.10$.

Effects of Age and Alcohol Consumption on AEQ Scores

The MANOVA computed on AEQ scores showed a significant main effect of the consumption group [$F(6,94) = 3.69$; $p = 0.0025$] and a significant main effect of age [$F(12,188) = 2.48$; $p = 0.005$], whereas the interaction was not significant [$F(12,188) = 0.74$; $p = 0.71$]. Two-way ANOVAs were then computed on AEQ subscale scores. There were significant main effects of the consumption group and age for most of the subscales except for the relaxation scale, whereas none of the interactions were statistically significant. The details of these analyzes are given in **Table 3**. As shown on **Figure 1**, problem drinkers reported higher mean positive expectancies about the effects of alcohol than non-problem drinkers on all AEQ subscales. Additionally, mean positive expectancies gradually decreased with age on all AEQ subscales, although the effect of age failed to reach statistical significance on the relaxation subscale.

Effect of Age and Alcohol Consumption on IAT Scores

Implicit Association Test results were first analyzed with Student t-tests in order to test whether there is an IAT effect for alcohol stimulation and sedation in the whole sample. Significant IAT effects were found for both stimulation, $t(104) = 9.99, p < 0.01$, and sedation, $t(104) = 7.72, p < 0.01$. Participants were faster to associate stimulation and sedation concepts with alcohol than with soft drinks.

However, the two-way ANOVA computed on the stimulation scores of the IAT (**Figure 2**) failed to show significant main effects of either age [$F(2,99) = 0.77, p = 0.46, \eta^2 = 0.02$] or the consumption group [$F(1,99) = 2.95, p = 0.09, \eta^2 = 0.03$]. Moreover, no significant interaction was observed, $F(2,99) = 1.35, p = 0.26, \eta^2 = 0.03$. Similarly, the two-way ANOVA computed on the sedation scores of the IAT (**Figure 3**) showed no significant main effects of either age [$F(2,99) = 0.66, p = 0.52, \eta^2 = 0.01$] or consumption group [$F(1,99) = 0.56, p = 0.45, \eta^2 = 0.006$] and no significant interaction [$F(2,99) = 0.25, p = 0.77, \eta^2 = 0.005$].

DISCUSSION

The results of the present study show that positive alcohol explicit expectancies gradually decrease with age. Adolescents aged 13 to 16 report especially high positive alcohol effect expectancies. This effect is statistically significant for all kinds of positive expectancies, with the exception of relaxation expectancies that only show a statistical trend ($p = 0.07$). The results also show that problem drinkers from all age groups report higher positive explicit alcohol expectancies than non-problem drinkers. This

TABLE 3 | Results of the two-way ANOVA computed on the Alcohol Expectancy Questionnaire (AEQ) subscale scores.

AEQ subscale	Age	Alcohol group	Interaction
Positive changes	$F(2,99) = 4.08; p = 0.020, \eta^2 = 0.07$	$F(1,99) = 14.61; p = 0.00023, \eta^2 = 0.12$	$F(2,99) = 0.92; p = 0.40, \eta^2 = 0.02$
Sexual enhancement	$F(2,99) = 3.81; p = 0.026, \eta^2 = 0.07$	$F(1,99) = 6.89; p = 0.010, \eta^2 = 0.06$	$F(2,99) = 1.60; p = 0.21, \eta^2 = 0.03$
Social and physical pleasure	$F(2,99) = 4.17; p = 0.018, \eta^2 = 0.06$	$F(1,99) = 22.23; p = 0.000008, \eta^2 = 0.17$	$F(2,99) = 1.92; p = 0.15, \eta^2 = 0.03$
Arousal/power	$F(2,99) = 6.77; p = 0.002, \eta^2 = 0.10$	$F(1,99) = 12.65; p = 0.0006, \eta^2 = 0.10$	$F(2,99) = 2.40; p = 0.096, \eta^2 = 0.07$
Social assertiveness	$F(2,99) = 11.8; p = 0.000025, \eta^2 = 0.17$	$F(1,99) = 14.44; p = 0.00025, \eta^2 = 0.10$	$F(2,99) = 1.12; p = 0.33, \eta^2 = 0.02$
Relaxation	$F(2,99) = 2.67; p = 0.07, \eta^2 = 0.05$	$F(1,99) = 13.55; p = 0.00040, \eta^2 = 0.11$	$F(2,99) = 0.87; p = 0.42, \eta^2 = 0.02$

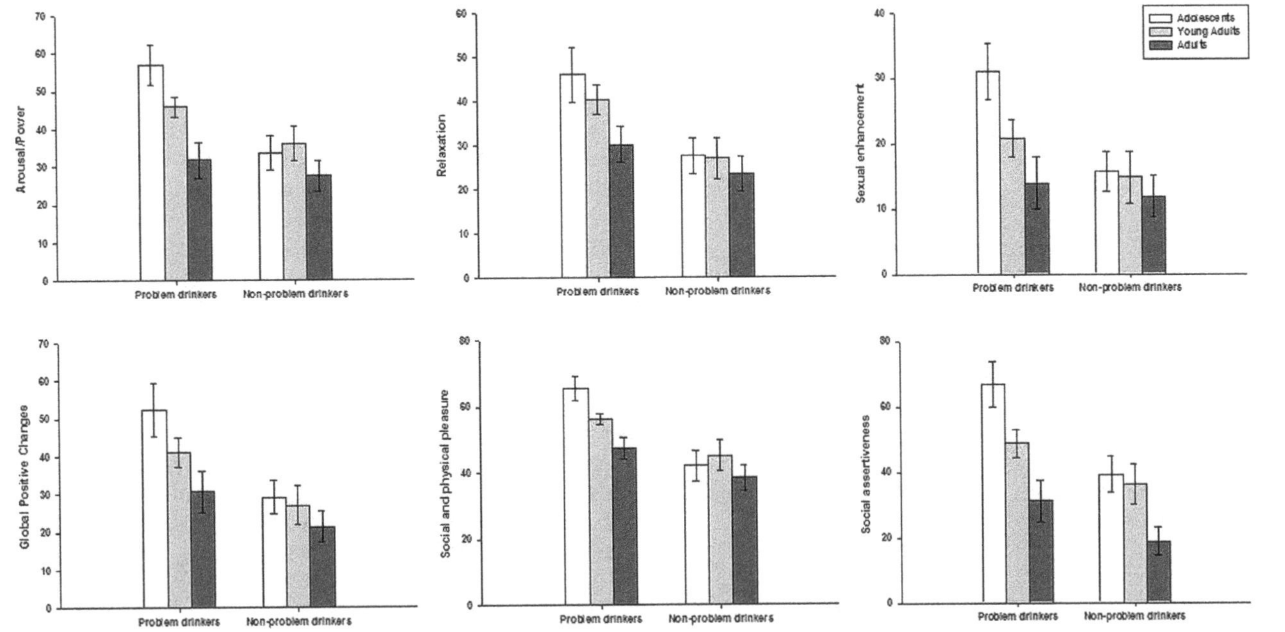

FIGURE 1 | Mean scores (±SEM) on the Alcohol Expectancy Questionnaire (AEQ) subscales according to age (adolescents, young adults, and adults) and alcohol consumption groups (problem and non-problem drinkers).

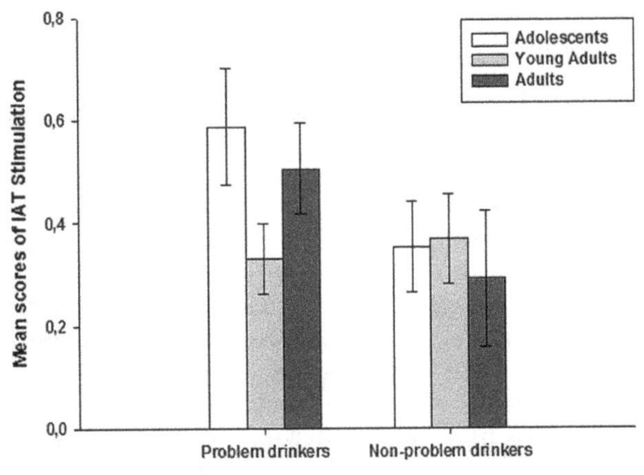

FIGURE 2 | Mean scores (±SEM) on the Implicit Association Test (IAT) stimulation subscales according to age (adolescents, young adults, and adults) and alcohol consumption groups (problem and non-problem drinkers).

effect is similar for all kinds of explicit positive expectancies. A very different pattern of results was obtained with implicit alcohol associations measured with the IAT. While implicit associations between alcohol and stimulation and sedation concepts were found in the whole sample, the present study did not find significant differences between age groups and between problem and non-problem drinkers on those measures.

The results of the present study confirm previous studies showing differences between low and high alcohol drinkers in positive explicit alcohol expectancies (Goldman et al., 1999). However, in contrast to some of those studies, the present results did no show selective differences in some specific positive expectancies. In fact, all positive alcohol explicit expectancies, except relaxation, were significant predictors of alcohol consumption behaviors. As this is a transversal study, the present study cannot solve the question of the causality direction between alcohol positive expectancies and alcohol-related behaviors. One possible explanation is that positive alcohol expectancies exert a causal influence on alcohol drinking, leading to a higher frequency of alcohol consumption and therefore to a higher prevalence of potential alcohol-related problems. Initial positive expectancies about the effects of alcohol may come from family or peer attitudes toward alcohol consumption (Lang and Stritzke, 1993; Zucker et al., 1995; Brown et al., 1999). Previous studies showed that children hold alcohol effect expectancies before they initiate alcohol drinking (Miller et al., 1990; Dunn and Goldman, 1996), confirming that alcohol expectancies are transmitted from other people outside alcohol drinking experiences. The first experiences with alcohol drinking may also contribute to develop various degrees of positive alcohol expectancies. It is well known that people differ in their initial physiological reactions to alcohol and this effect is partially determined by genetic factors (Grant, 1998). Such early acquired positive alcohol expectancies may then influence subsequent alcohol drinking behaviors. However, the causal direction of the relationship between alcohol expectancies and drinking behaviors may be the other way round. It is quite possible that repeated alcohol consumption gradually increases positive expectancies about its effects, eventually leading high drinkers to develop stronger positive expectancies than low drinkers. Such an effect may develop through a self-justification process or as

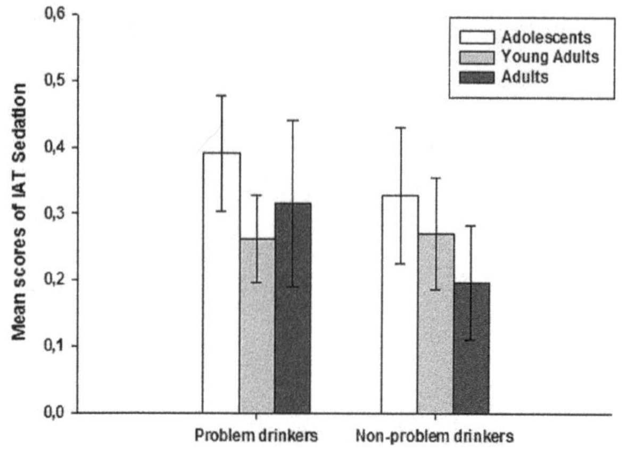

FIGURE 3 | Mean scores (±SEM) on the IAT sedation subscales according to age (adolescents, young adults, and adults) and alcohol consumption groups (problem and non-problem drinkers).

a consequence of the sensitization of the actual positive effects of alcohol consumption. Animal studies clearly showed that some of the positive effects of alcohol, especially its stimulant effects, gradually increase with repeated alcohol administrations (Kayir and Uzbay, 2002; Correa et al., 2003; Didone et al., 2008). This phenomenon is called sensitization and plays a key role is some current addiction theories, such as the incentive-sensitization theory of addiction (Robinson and Berridge, 1993, 2008). It is therefore possible that the stronger positive alcohol expectancies reported by high alcohol drinkers relate to actual "sensitized" positive effects of alcohol they experience when drinking. In the high drinker group of the present study, positive alcohol expectancies are of higher magnitude in the younger participants, which might suggest that such expectancies do not sensitize with further alcohol drinking during aging. However, only longitudinal studies following young participants before they start drinking alcohol will allow testing such hypotheses. Such studies should be able to test whether alcohol expectancies change after the initiation of alcohol consumption and following repeated alcohol consumption episodes, or whether they preexist to the first experience with alcohol.

One important result of the present study is that explicit positive expectancies gradually decrease with age from young adolescence to adulthood. In a previous study on college students aged from 17 to 35, it was shown that subjects under the age of 20 reported more positive expectancies than subjects above the age of 20 (Lundahl et al., 1997). The present study further shows that subjects under the age of 17 report even higher explicit positive alcohol effect expectancies, especially high drinkers. There are several possible explanations to such a decrease in positive alcohol expectancies with age. First, the actual physiological reactions to alcohol may change with age, translating into a more positive experience in young adolescents. To our knowledge, no studies investigated whether the actual positive effects of alcohol consumption decrease with age throughout adolescence in humans. However, results from animal research indicate that alcohol stimulant effects and alcohol reinforcing effects decrease from weaning to adulthood (Stevenson et al., 2008; Quoilin et al., 2010), whereas the sedative effects gradually increase during the same developmental period (Silveri and Spear, 1998; Spear and Varlinskaya, 2005; Quoilin et al., 2010). It is therefore possible that similar effects occur in humans, leading to changes in alcohol effect expectancies. A decrease in alcohol positive effect expectancies with age might also indirectly result from the growing awareness of the adverse effects of alcohol. With the end of adolescence, the pattern of alcohol consumption tends to change with changes in role obligations (family and employment responsibilities; Leonard and Eiden, 2007). Such changes might also indirectly impact on the positive alcohol effect expectancies. Finally, it should be remembered that this is a cross-sectional study. Therefore, we cannot rule out that age differences in positive alcohol effect expectancies result from a cohort effect rather than from developmental changes. Only future longitudinal studies can confirm that positive alcohol effect expectancies evolve with age in the same subjects in a similar way as the behavioral effects of alcohol change with age in animal models (Quoilin et al., 2010).

In contrast to explicit expectancies, implicit alcohol associations were not significantly associated with either alcohol consumption behaviors or age in the present study. As alcohol exerts both stimulant and sedative effects according to the ingested alcohol dose and to the time post-ingestion (Pohorecky, 1977; King et al., 2002), implicit alcohol associations were not tested on the arousal–sedation dimension using a single bipolar IAT task. In contrast, we used two unipolar IAT tasks to separately assess arousal and sedation implicit alcohol associations. This allowed recording the co-existence of arousal and sedation implicit associations in the same participants. For the whole sample, there is a positive and statistically significant correlation ($r = 0.29$; $p = 0.004$) between D statistics for stimulation and sedation alcohol implicit associations. This confirms that participants from the whole sample hold statistically significant implicit alcohol associations for both stimulation and sedation. Such a positive correlation also does not support the idea that sedation and stimulation are two endpoints of a single bipolar dimension of alcohol implicit associations, which would imply a strong negative correlation between both measures. In a study from Wiers et al. (2002), it was shown that heavy and light drinkers differ in their implicit arousal association as measured with the IAT. However, in a previous study from our laboratory, we found no correlation between alcohol implicit arousal association and the levels of current alcohol drinking in a non-selected sample of undergraduate students (Kreusch et al., 2013). A possible explanation to the discrepancies between the results of those studies was that the latter study did not select a sample of heavy alcohol drinkers. However, the present study also did not find significant differences in implicit alcohol stimulation associations between problem and non-problem drinkers from various age groups. Whereas the present study focused on current alcohol consumption, Thush and Wiers (2007) showed that implicit measures predicted future alcohol use over a short period of 1 month. Therefore we cannot rule out that implicit alcohol associations predict future alcohol consumption. However, the present study shows that explicit positive effect expectancies, including arousal expectancies, better predict current levels of alcohol consumption than implicit arousal alcohol associations measured through the IAT. Kreusch et al. (2013) also found that implicit alcohol arousal associations did not correlate with either explicit alcohol arousal expectancies measured through the AEQ or with the subjective stimulant experience reported after alcohol consumption and measured with the biphasic alcohol effects scale (BAES). It was argued that implicit and explicit processes are distinct and differentially influence behavior (Stacy, 1997). According to this view, implicit and explicit measures should predict unique variance in alcohol drinking behaviors. Although explicit expectancies indeed explained a part of the current alcohol drinking variance in the present study, we failed to find a significant contribution of implicit arousal and sedation alcohol associations measured with the IAT in any of the tested age groups.

In summary, the present results show higher positive alcohol explicit expectancies in problem drinkers relative to non-problem drinkers. They also show that such explicit expectancies gradually decrease with age in the three cross-sectional groups of adolescents, young adults, and adults. In contrast implicit alcohol arousal and sedation associations measured with the IAT were not significantly associated with either age or current alcohol drinking behaviors. Explicit alcohol positive expectancies may therefore be used as predictors of current alcohol consumption, especially in young adolescents.

ACKNOWLEDGMENT

This work was supported by grants from the Fonds Spéciaux pour la Recherche de l'Université de Liège obtained by EQ.

REFERENCES

Addicott, M. A., Marsh-Richard, D. M., Mathias, C. W., and Dougherty, D. M. (2007). The biphasic effects of alcohol: comparisons of subjective and objective measures of stimulation, sedation, and physical activity. *Alcohol. Clin. Exp. Res.* 31, 1883–1890. doi: 10.1111/j.1530-0277.2007.00518.x

Arnold, H. J., and Feldman, D. C. (1981). Social desirability response bias in self-report choice situations. *Acad. Manag. J.* 24, 377–385. doi: 10.2307/255848

Baer, J. S. (2002). Student factors: understanding individual variation in college drinking. *J. Stud. Alcohol. Suppl.* 14, 40–53. doi: 10.15288/jsas.2002.s14.40

Brown, S. A., Christiansen, B. A., and Goldman, M. S. (1987). The alcohol expectancy questionnaire: an instrument for the assessment of adolescent and adult alcohol expectancies. *J. Stud. Alcohol.* 48, 483–491. doi: 10.15288/jsa.1987.48.483

Brown, S. A., McGue, M., Maggs, J., Schulenberg, J., Hingson, R., Swartzwelder, S., et al. (2008). A developmental perspective on alcohol and youths 16 to 20 years of age. *Pediatrics* 121, S290–S310. doi: 10.1542/peds2007-2243D

Brown, S. A., Tate, S. R., Vik, P. W., Haas, A. L., and Aarons, G. A. (1999). Modeling of alcohol use mediates the effect of family history of alcoholism on adolescent alcohol expectancies. *Exp. Clin. Psychopharmacol.* 7, 20–27. doi: 10.1037/1064-1297.7.1.20

Cable, N., and Sacker, A. (2008). Typologies of alcohol consumption in adolescence: predictors and adult outcomes. *Alcohol Alcohol.* 43, 81–90. doi: 10.1093/alcalc/agm146

Cameron, C. A., Stritzke, W. G. K., and Durkin, K. (2003). Alcohol expectancies in late childhood: an ambivalence perspective on transitions toward alcohol use. *J. Child Psychol. Psychiatry* 44, 687–698. doi: 10.1111/1469-7610.00155

Correa, M., Arizzi, M. N., Betz, A., Mingote, S., and Salamone, J. D. (2003). Locomotor stimulant effects of intraventricular injections of low doses of ethanol in rats: acute and repeated administration. *Psychopharmacology (Berl.)* 170, 368–375. doi: 10.1007/s00213-003-1557-0

Davidson, D., Hutchison, K., Dagon, C., and Swift, R. (2002). Assessing the stimulant effects of alcohol in humans. *Pharmacol. Biochem. Behav.* 72, 151–156. doi: 10.1016/S0091-3057(01)00758-4

Derogatis, L. R. (1977). *Symptom Check List-90 Revised.* Seattle, WA: Alcohol and Drug Abuse Institute Library.

Didone, V., Quoilin, C., Tirelli, E., and Quertemont, E. (2008). Parametric analysis of the development and expression of ethanol-induced behavioral sensitization in female Swiss mice: effects of dose, injection schedule, and test context. *Psychopharmacology (Berl.)* 201, 249–260. doi: 10.1007/s00213-008-1266-9

Dunn, M. E., and Goldman, M. S. (1996). Empirical modeling of an alcohol expectancy memory network in elementary school children as a function of grade. *Exp. Clin. Psychopharmacol.* 4, 209–217. doi: 10.1037/1064-1297.4.2.209

Edwards, A. L. (1958). The social desirability variable in personality assessment and research. *Acad. Med.* 33, 610–611.

Faden, V. B. (2006). Trends in initiation of alcohol use in the United States 1975 to 2003. *Alcohol. Clin. Exp. Res.* 30, 1011–1022. doi: 10.1111/j.1530-0277.2006.00115.x

Field, M., and Wiers, R. (2012). "Automatic and controlled processes in the pathway from drug abuse to addiction," in *Drug Abuse and Addiction in Medical Illness*, eds J. C. Verster, K. Brady, M. Galanter, and P. Conrod (New York, NY: Springer), 35–45.

Fisher, R. J. (1993). Social desirability bias and the validity of indirect questioning. *J. Consum. Res.* 20, 303–315. doi: 10.2307/2489277

Fleming, M. F., Barry, K. L., and Macdonald, R. (1991). The alcohol use disorders identification test (AUDIT) in a college sample. *Int. J. Addict.* 26, 1173–1185. doi: 10.3109/10826089109062153

Fortin, M., and Coutu-Wakulczyk, G. (1985). *Validation et Normalisation d'une Mesure de Santé Mentale: le SCL-90-R.* Rapport Présenté au Conseil Québécois de la Recherche Sociale (CQRS). Montreal, QC: Université de Montréal.

Gache, P., Michaud, P., Landry, U., Accietto, C., Arfaoui, S., Wenger, O., et al. (2005). The alcohol use disorders identification test (AUDIT) as a screening tool for excessive drinking in primary care: reliability and validity of a French version. *Alcohol. Clin. Exp. Res.* 29, 2001–2007. doi: 10.1097/01.alc.0000187034.58955.64

Goldman, M. S., Del Boca, F. K., and Darkes, J. (1999). "Alcohol expectancy theory: the application of cognitive neuroscience," in *Psychological Theories of Drinking and Alcoholism: The Guilford Substance Abuse Series*, 2nd Edn, eds K. E. Leonard and H. T. Blane (New York, NY: Guilford Press), 203–246.

Grant, B. F. (1998). The impact of a family history of alcoholism on the relationship between age at onset of alcohol use and DSM-IV alcohol dependence: results from the National Longitudinal Alcohol Epidemiologic Survey. *Alcohol Health Res. World* 22, 144–147.

Grant, B. F., and Dawson, D. A. (1997). Age at onset of alcohol use and its association with DSM-IV alcohol abuse and dependence: results from the national longitudinal alcohol epidemiologic survey. *J. Subst. Abuse* 9, 103–110. doi: 10.1016/S0899-3289(97)90009-2

Greenwald, A. G., Banaji, M. R., Rudman, L. A., Farnham, S. D., Nosek, B. A., and Mellott, D. S. (2002). A unified theory of implicit attitudes, stereotypes, self-esteem, and self-concept. *Psychol. Rev.* 109, 3–25. doi: 10.1037/0033-295X.109.1.3

Greenwald, A. G., Nosek, B. A., and Banaji, M. R. (2003). Understanding and using the Implicit Association Test: I. An improved scoring algorithm. *J. Soc. Psychol.* 85, 197–216.

Ham, L. S., and Hope, D. A. (2003). College students and problematic drinking: a review of the literature. *Clin. Psychol. Rev.* 23, 719–759. doi: 10.1016/S0272-7358(03)00071-0

Jones, B. T., Corbin, W., and Fromme, K. (2001). A review of expectancy theory and alcohol consumption. *Addiction* 96, 57–72. doi: 10.1046/j.1360-0443.2001.961575.x

Kayir, H., and Uzbay, I. T. (2002). Investigation of a possible sensitization development to a challenge dose of ethanol after 2 weeks following the single injection in mice. *Pharmacol. Biochem. Behav.* 73, 551–556. doi: 10.1016/S0091-3057(02)00808-0

King, A. C., Houle, T., de Wit, H., Holdstock, L., and Schuster, A. (2002). Biphasic alcohol response differs in heavy versus light drinkers. *Alcohol. Clin. Exp. Res.* 26, 827–835. doi: 10.1111/j.1530-0277.2002.tb02611.x

Kreusch, F., Vilenne, A., and Quertemont, E. (2013). Assessing the stimulant and sedative effects of alcohol with explicit and implicit measures in a balanced placebo design. *J. Stud. Alcohol Drugs* 74, 923–930. doi: 10.15288/jsad.2013.74.923

Lane, K. A., Banaji, M. R., Nosek, B. A., and Greenwald, A. G. (2007). "Understanding and using the implicit association test: IV," in *Implicit Measures of Attitudes: Procedures and Controversies*, eds B. Wittenbrink and N. S. Schwarz (New York, NY: Guilford Press), 59–102.

Lang, A. R., and Stritzke, W. G. K. (1993). "Children and alcohol," in *Recent Developments in Alcoholism Recent Developments in Alcoholism*, ed. M. Galanter (New York, NY: Springer), 73–85.

Leigh, B. C., and Stacy, A. W. (2004). Alcohol expectancies and drinking in different age groups. *Addiction* 99, 215–227. doi: 10.1111/j.1360-0443.2003.00641.x

Leonard, K. E., and Eiden, R. D. (2007). Marital and family processes in the context of alcohol use and alcohol disorders. *Annu. Rev. Clin. Psychol.* 3, 285–310. doi: 10.1146/annurev.clinpsy.3.022806.091424

Lundahl, L. H., Davis, T. M., Adesso, V. J., and Lukas, S. E. (1997). Alcohol expectancies: effects of gender, age, and family history of alcoholism. *Addict. Behav.* 22, 115–125. doi: 10.1016/S0306-4603(96)00022-6

Miller, P. M., Smith, G. T., and Goldman, M. S. (1990). Emergence of alcohol expectancies in childhood: a possible critical period. *J. Stud. Alcohol* 51, 343–349. doi: 10.15288/jsa.1990.51.343

O'Malley, P. M., Johnston, L. D., and Bachman, J. G. (1998). Alcohol use among adolescents. *Alcohol Health Res. World* 22, 85–93.

Pohorecky, L. A. (1977). Biphasic action of ethanol. *Biobehav. Rev.* 1, 231–240. doi: 10.1016/0147-7552(77)90025-0

Quoilin, C., Didone, V., Tirelli, E., and Quertemont, E. (2010). Ontogeny of the stimulant and sedative effects of ethanol in male and female Swiss mice: gradual changes from weaning to adulthood. *Psychopharmacology* (*Berl.*) 212, 501–512. doi: 10.1007/s00213-010-1971-z

Robinson, T. E., and Berridge, K. C. (1993). The neural basis of drug craving: an incentive-sensitization theory of addiction. *Brain Res. Rev.* 18, 247–291. doi: 10.1016/0165-0173(93)90013-P

Robinson, T. E., and Berridge, K. C. (2008). The incentive sensitization theory of addiction: some current issues. *Philos. Trans. R. Soc. B Biol. Sci.* 363, 3137–3146. doi: 10.1098/rstb.2008.0093

Saunders, J. B., Aasland, O. G., Babor, T. F., De La Fuente, J. R., and Grant, M. (1993). Development of the alcohol use disorders identification test (AUDIT): WHO collaborative project on early detection of persons with harmful alcohol consumption-II. *Addiction* 88, 791–804. doi: 10.1111/j.1360-0443.1993.tb00822.x

Silveri, M. M., and Spear, L. P. (1998). Decreased sensitivity to the hypnotic effects of ethanol early in ontogeny. *Alcohol. Clin. Exp. Res.* 22, 670–676. doi: 10.1111/j.1530-0277.1998.tb04310.x

Sobell, L. C., and Sobell, M. B. (1992). "Time-line follow back: a technique for assessing selfreported alcohol consumption," in *Measuring Alcohol Consumption: Psychosocial and Biological Methods*, eds R. Z. Litten and J. Allen (Clifton, NJ: Humana Press), 41–72.

Southwick, L. L., Steele, C. M., Alan, G., and Lindell, M. K. (1981). Alcohol-related expectancies: defined by phase of intoxication and drinking experience. *J. Consult. Clin. Psychol.* 49, 713–721. doi: 10.1037/0022-006X.49.5.713

Spear, L. P., and Varlinskaya, E. I. (2005). "Adolescence," in *Recent Developments in Alcoholism Recent Developments in Alcoholism*, eds M. Galanter, C. Lowman, G. M. Boyd, V. B. Faden, E. Witt, and D. Lagressa (New York, NY: Springer), 143–159.

Stacy, A. W. (1997). Memory activation and expectancy as prospective predictors of alcohol and marijuana use. *J. Abnorm. Psychol.* 106, 61–73. doi: 10.1037/0021-843X.106.1.61

Stevenson, R. A., Besheer, J., and Hodge, C. W. (2008). Comparison of ethanol locomotor sensitization in adolescent and adult DBA/2J mice. *Psychopharmacology (Berl.)* 197, 361–370. doi: 10.1007/s00213-007-1038-y

Thush, C., and Wiers, R. W. (2007). Explicit and implicit alcohol-related cognitions and the prediction of future drinking in adolescents. *Addict. Behav.* 32, 1367–1383. doi: 10.1016/j.addbeh.2006.09.011

van den Wildenberg, E., Beckers, M., van Lambaart, F., Conrod, P. J., and Wiers, R. W. (2006). Is the strength of implicit alcohol associations correlated with alcohol-induced heart-rate acceleration? *Alcohol. Clin. Exp. Res.* 30, 1336–1348. doi: 10.1111/j.1530-0277.2006.00161.x

Vautier, S., and Moncany, D. (2008). Positive alcohol expectancies in the French context: factorial properties of data from a large sample of alcohol drinkers. *Rev. Eur. Psychol. Appl.* 58, 133–144. doi: 10.1016/j.erap.2007.02.002

Wiers, R. W., Hoogeveen, K. J., Sergeant, J. A., and Boudewijn Gunning, W. (1997). High- and low-dose alcohol-related expectancies and the differential associations with drinking in male and female adolescents and young adults. *Addiction* 92, 871–888. doi: 10.1111/j.1360-0443.1997.tb02956.x

Wiers, R. W., Van Woerden, N., Smulders, F. T. Y., and De Jong, P. J. (2002). Implicit and explicit alcohol-related cognitions in heavy and light drinkers. *J. Abnorm. Psychol.* 111, 648–658. doi: 10.1037/0021-843X.111.4.648

Zucker, R. A., Kincaid, S. B., Fitzgerald, H. E., and Bingham, C. R. (1995). Alcohol schema acquisition in preschoolers: differences between children of alcoholics and children of nonalcoholics. *Alcohol. Clin. Exp. Res.* 19, 1011–1017. doi: 10.1111/j.1530-0277.1995.tb00982.x

9

Adolescent Corticosterone and TrkB Pharmaco-Manipulations Sex-Dependently Impact Instrumental Reversal Learning Later in Life

Elizabeth T. Barfield[1,2,3,4] *and Shannon L. Gourley*[1,2,3,4]*

[1]Department of Pediatrics, Emory University, Atlanta, GA, United States, [2]Graduate Program in Neuroscience, Emory University, Atlanta, GA, United States, [3]Yerkes National Primate Research Center, Emory University, Atlanta, GA, United States, [4]Department of Psychiatry and Behavioral Sciences, Emory University, Atlanta, GA, United States

Edited by:
Nuno Sousa,
Instituto de Pesquisa em Ciências da Vida e da Saúde (ICVS), Portugal

Reviewed by:
Alicia Izquierdo,
University of California, Los Angeles, United States
Nicholas W. Simon,
University of Pittsburgh, United States
Caitlin Anne Orsini,
University of Florida, United States

***Correspondence:**
Shannon L. Gourley
shannon.l.gourley@emory.edu

Early-life trauma can increase the risk for, and severity of, several psychiatric illnesses. These include drug use disorders, and some correlations appear to be stronger in women. Understanding the long-term consequences of developmental stressor or stress hormone exposure and possible sex differences is critically important. So-called "reversal learning" tasks are commonly used in rodents to model cognitive deficits in stress- and addiction-related illnesses in humans. Here, we exposed mice to the primary stress hormone corticosterone (CORT) during early adolescence (postnatal days 31–42), then tested behavioral flexibility in adulthood using an instrumental reversal learning task. CORT-exposed female, but not male, mice developed perseverative errors. Despite resilience to subchronic CORT exposure, males developed reversal performance impairments following exposure to physical stressors. Administration of a putative tyrosine kinase receptor B (trkB) agonist, 7,8-dihydroxyflavone (7,8-DHF), during adolescence blocked CORT-induced errors in females and improved performance in males. Conversely, blockade of trkB by ANA-12 impaired performance. These data suggest that trkB-based interventions could have certain protective benefits in the context of early-life stressor exposure. We consider the implications of our findings in an extended "Discussion" section.

Keywords: juvenile, impulsivity, BDNF, tropomyosin receptor kinase B, 7,8-dihydroxyflavone

INTRODUCTION

Reversal tasks assess the ability of mice or rats to flexibly modify behaviors when reinforcement contingencies change. These tasks are commonly used to model behavioral inflexibility associated with addiction and other disorders in humans (for recent review Izquierdo et al., 2017). Typically, animals are trained to associate specific actions or stimuli with reward (e.g., food), then, the association is modified such that a previously non-predictive contingency could be used to obtain reinforcement, while the original contingency is no longer predictive. Thus, these tasks require animals to inhibit a familiar response strategy and deploy a new strategy to obtain reinforcement.

Behavioral inflexibility in these tasks may result from (Ersche et al., 2008; Jentsch et al., 2002; Schoenbaum et al., 2004) and also *predispose* organisms to (Dalley et al., 2007; Belin et al., 2008; Groman et al., 2009) drug-seeking behaviors. For example, in humans, deficits in reversal learning correlate with the severity of cocaine use (Moreno-López et al., 2015), and a "behavioral disinhibition" trait is associated with later substance use disorders (Tarter et al., 2004; Nigg et al., 2006). Further, rats or mice exhibiting low inhibitory control over impulsive responding more rapidly escalate rates of cocaine self-administration and are more prone to developing drug taking characterized as compulsive (Dalley et al., 2007; Belin et al., 2008; Cervantes et al., 2013). Thus, individual differences in behavioral flexibility and inhibitory control may influence the progression from initial drug use to habitual or compulsive drug-seeking (Cervantes et al., 2013).

Adverse experiences early in life are linked with negative psychiatric outcomes in adulthood, including increased risk for drug use disorders (Fergusson et al., 1996; Kessler et al., 1997; Dube et al., 2003; Green et al., 2010; Afifi et al., 2012) and greater lifetime severity of substance abuse (Hyman et al., 2006; Sacks et al., 2008; Enoch, 2011). Furthermore, several studies report that this association is stronger in women (Widom and White, 1997; MacMillan et al., 2001; Simpson and Miller, 2002; Hyman et al., 2008). The neurobehavioral processes that translate developmental stressor exposure into psychiatric vulnerabilities later in life are incompletely understood, but may involve disruption of prefrontal cortex (PFC)-dependent executive functions, such as behavioral flexibility and inhibitory control (Elton et al., 2014). Indeed, early-life trauma is associated with deficits in inhibitory control (Lewis et al., 2007; Mueller et al., 2010; Skowron et al., 2014; Marshall et al., 2016), and in at least one study, trait impulsivity mediated the relationship between childhood trauma and substance dependence severity in adulthood (Schwandt et al., 2013). Comparing susceptibility to early-life stress-induced inhibitory control deficits between males and females may provide insight into mechanisms of sex differences in risk for stress-related psychopathology.

In the present study, we manipulated levels of the primary glucocorticoid, corticosterone (CORT), and determined long-term consequences in an instrumental reversal task. We exposed mice to exogenous CORT from postnatal day (P) 31–42, corresponding to early adolescence in rodents (Spear, 2000), and a period of considerable structural maturation in the PFC (Shapiro et al., 2017b). Mice were then trained as adults to perform food-reinforced nose poke responses. We found that subchronic CORT exposure induced habit-biased behavior, despite the cessation of CORT exposure, and these findings are reported in Barfield et al. (in press). We then tested mice in an instrumental reversal task, and the results of those tests are reported here.

In some groups, we stimulated tyrosine kinase receptor B (trkB), the high-affinity receptor for brain-derived neurotrophic factor (BDNF), which regulates dendritic spine structure and function (Yoshii and Constantine-Paton, 2010). BDNF-trkB systems are impacted by stress (Gray et al., 2013; Numakawa et al., 2013), implicated in addiction-related behaviors (Li and Wolf, 2015), and significantly modify reward-related decision making (Pitts et al., 2016). Loss of neurotrophic support following prolonged exposure to elevated glucocorticoids is thought to contribute to structural and functional alterations in the PFC that are associated with stress-related psychopathology (Duman et al., 1997). Moreover, recent findings implicate down-regulation of BDNF-trkB signaling in the long-term behavioral consequences of adolescent stress exposure (Xu et al., 2016; Zhang et al., 2017; Barfield et al., in press). Thus, we hypothesized that stimulating trkB may have protective benefits in animals exposed to CORT during adolescence, blocking enduring behavioral deficits.

We report sex-dependent long-term consequences of both CORT and trkB manipulations in an instrumental reversal task. Namely, a history of early-adolescent CORT exposure in females, but not males, induced perseverative responding. Despite apparent resilience to early-adolescent CORT, males developed behavioral inflexibilities following repeated stressor exposure or trkB blockade during early adolescence. Further, a putative trkB agonist improved performance in both sexes. We consider the implications of our findings in an extended "Discussion" section.

MATERIALS AND METHODS

Subjects

Subjects were male and female wild-type C57BL/6 mice (Jackson Labs, Bar Harbor, ME, USA) or mice expressing *thy1*-derived yellow fluorescent protein (YFP; Feng et al., 2000) that were fully back-crossed onto a C57BL/6 background. Mice were not handled, other than for routine veterinary care, until P31. Mice were group-housed, maintained on a 12-h light cycle (0700 on) and provided food and water *ad libitum* except during instrumental conditioning when body weights were maintained at 90%–93% of baseline to motivate responding. Animal numbers for each experiment are indicated in the respective figure captions. This study was carried out in accordance with the recommendations of the Guide for the Care and Use of Laboratory Animals. The protocol was approved by the Emory University IACUC.

CORT Exposure

CORT hemisuccinate (4-pregnen-11β 21-DIOL-3 20-DIONE 21-hemisuccinate; Steraloids) was dissolved in tap water (25 μg/mL free base; Gourley et al., 2008a,b, 2012b). CORT-exposed mice were given CORT in place of normal drinking water, while control mice consumed tap water. CORT solutions were changed every 3 days. Water bottles were weighed daily, and mice weighed every other day to calculate average doses (~5–9 mg/kg/day) of CORT. Mice were exposed to CORT or water from P31 to 42, corresponding to early adolescence in rodents (Spear, 2000). After a 2-week washout period, when mice reached young adulthood (P56), instrumental conditioning began. Timelines are in the figures.

Forced Swim Stress

Mice were exposed to forced swim stress daily from P31 to 42. Mice were placed in a glass cylinder (24 cm × 15.5 cm diameter) filled with 25°C water in a dimly lit room. After 6 min, mice were dried in a warm cage lined with paper towels, then returned to the home cage. Water was changed between mice. Control mice were handled but not exposed to swim stress.

Instrumental Conditioning

Mice were trained to nose poke for food reinforcement (20 mg grain-based pellets; Bio-Serv, Flemington, NJ, USA) using Med Associates conditioning chambers equipped with two nose-poke recesses, a retractable lever, and a food magazine. Responding on each of two nose-poke recesses was reinforced using a fixed ratio 1 (FR1) schedule of reinforcement; 30 reinforcers were available for responding on each aperture, resulting in 60 reinforcers/session. Sessions ended when mice acquired all 60 reinforcers or at 70 min. Five to seven daily training sessions were conducted. Response acquisition curves represent both nose poke responses/min. Mice were then tested in an instrumental contingency degradation task, followed by a reversal task (see timeline in **Figure 1A**). Given our focus on reversal conditioning here, only reversal performance is shown.

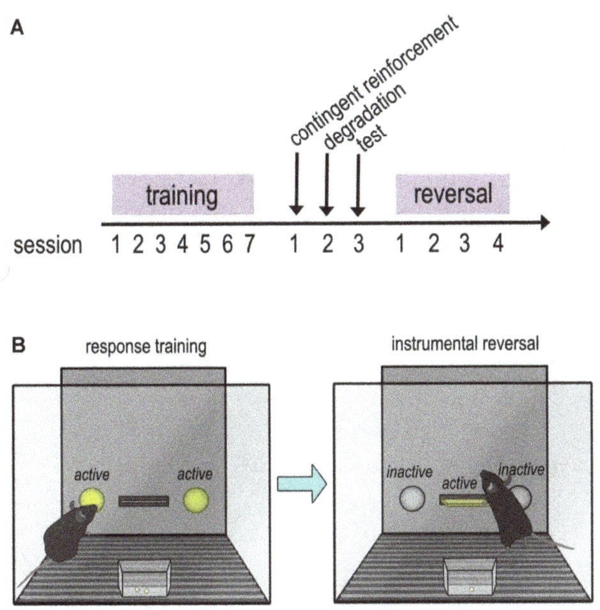

FIGURE 1 | Timeline and schematic of instrumental training and reversal task. **(A)** Timeline of training and tasks. Mice were trained to nose poke in operant conditioning chambers for food reinforcers. Next, an action-outcome contingency degradation task was performed, in which the contingency between an action and outcome are "degraded" by providing food pellets independently of the mouse's actions. The data from these tests are reported in Barfield et al. (in press). An instrumental reversal task followed, and the data from these tests are reported in the present manuscript. **(B)** Schematic of response training and instrumental reversal. In the instrumental reversal task, the reinforced response was "reversed" from a nose poke on the sides of the chamber to a lever press located in the center of the chamber that had not previously been available. Acquisition of the newly reinforced response (lever press) and inhibition of the previously reinforced response (nose poke) were measured over multiple sessions.

Instrumental Reversal Test

In this task, the reinforced response was "reversed" to a lever press; there were no consequences for generating the previously reinforced nose poke response (**Figure 1B**). Lever pressing was reinforced using an FR1 schedule, with one 25-min session/day for four consecutive days. Lever press rates reflect acquisition of a new response, while nose poke rates reflect inhibition of the previously reinforced response. The percent of correct responses made during session 1 was calculated by dividing total lever presses by total responses (lever presses + nose pokes).

Drugs (Dosing and Timing)

Male and female mice were administered (*i.p.*) the putative trkB agonist, 7,8-dihydroxyflavone (7,8-DHF; Sigma; 3 mg/kg; dissolved in 17% DMSO and saline; Zhang et al., 2014), or vehicle daily from P39 to 47, overlapping with the end of the adolescent CORT exposure period. This period is marked by significant pruning of dendritic spines on excitatory pyramidal neurons in the mouse orbital PFC (oPFC; Shapiro et al., 2017b). Additionally, expression levels of trkB in the oPFC increase during this time (Shapiro et al., 2017b), potentially facilitating activity-dependent refinement of synaptic connections and stabilizing synapses that are not pruned. This period was also determined based on prior work (Barfield et al., in press).

The trkB antagonist, ANA-12 (Sigma; 0.5 mg/kg, 1% DMSO), or vehicle was administered (*i.p.*) daily from P31 to 42, to match the period of adolescent CORT exposure.

Statistical Analyses

Two-tailed statistical analyses with $\alpha \leq 0.05$ were performed using SPSS. Response rates were compared by two-factor (group × session) or three-factor (CORT × 7,8-DHF × session) mixed analysis of variance (ANOVA) with session as a within-subjects (repeated measure) factor. Tukey's *post hoc* tests were used following interactions or main effects between greater than two groups, and results are indicated graphically. The percent of responses that were reinforced ("correct") were compared by one-factor or two-factor (CORT × 7,8-DHF) ANOVA or Student's *t*-tests. In additional comparisons, CORT-exposed mice were split into "vulnerable" and "non-vulnerable" groups based on a median split of percent correct values from session 1 of the instrumental reversal task. Throughout, values >2 SDs from the mean were excluded.

RESULTS

Early-Adolescent Corticosteroid Exposure in Females Impairs Response Inhibition in Adulthood

We exposed female and male mice to CORT in the drinking water from P31 to 42, equivalent to early adolescence in humans (Spear, 2000). Some mice also received daily *i.p.* injections of vehicle (17% DMSO and saline) or 7,8-DHF (3 mg/kg) from P39 to P47. In the interest of clarity, only vehicle-treated and non-injected mice are shown in **Figure 2**, and then all injected groups are represented in **Figures 3, 4**, respectively.

As adults, female mice acquired the nose poke responses without group differences (main effect and interaction *Fs* < 1; **Figure 2A**). When the response requirement was "reversed" to a lever press, females with a history of adolescent CORT exposure made more perseverative errors than control mice—responding on the previously reinforced nose poke apertures despite non-reinforcement—during session 1 (interaction $F_{(3,69)} = 4.0$, $p = 0.01$; **Figure 2B**). Meanwhile, acquisition of the newly reinforced lever response was unaffected (main effect and interaction *Fs* < 1; **Figure 2C**).

We also calculated the percentage of total responses that were reinforced during session 1. While this measure did not significantly differ between groups ($t_{(23)} = 1.3$, $p = 0.2$; **Figure 2D**), mice with a history of CORT exposure qualitatively appeared to segregate into two groups. As an exploratory analysis, we applied a median split to CORT mice. CORT-exposed "vulnerable" mice made significantly fewer correct responses relative to both control and CORT-exposed "non-vulnerable" mice (main effect group $F_{(2,22)} = 11.1$, $p < 0.001$; **Figure 2E**). Thus, in females, a history of CORT exposure during early adolescence increases perseverative errors, and considerable individual differences are noted.

We repeated this experiment in male mice. Mice acquired the food-reinforced nose poke responses in adulthood, without group differences (main effect and interaction *Fs* < 1; **Figure 2F**). In contrast to females, early-adolescent CORT exposure in males did not impact response reversal (errors, main effect and interaction *Fs* < 1; **Figure 2G**; lever response acquisition, main effect and interaction *Fs* < 1; **Figure 2H**). There were no differences in the percentage of responses that were reinforced ($t_{(12)} = 0.8$, $p = 0.5$; **Figure 2I**), and a median split of values revealed no differences between control mice and either of the two CORT-exposed subgroups (main effect group $F_{(2,11)} = 2.0$, $p = 0.2$; **Figure 2J**). Thus, females may be especially vulnerable to the long-term effects of CORT exposure during early adolescence on response inhibition.

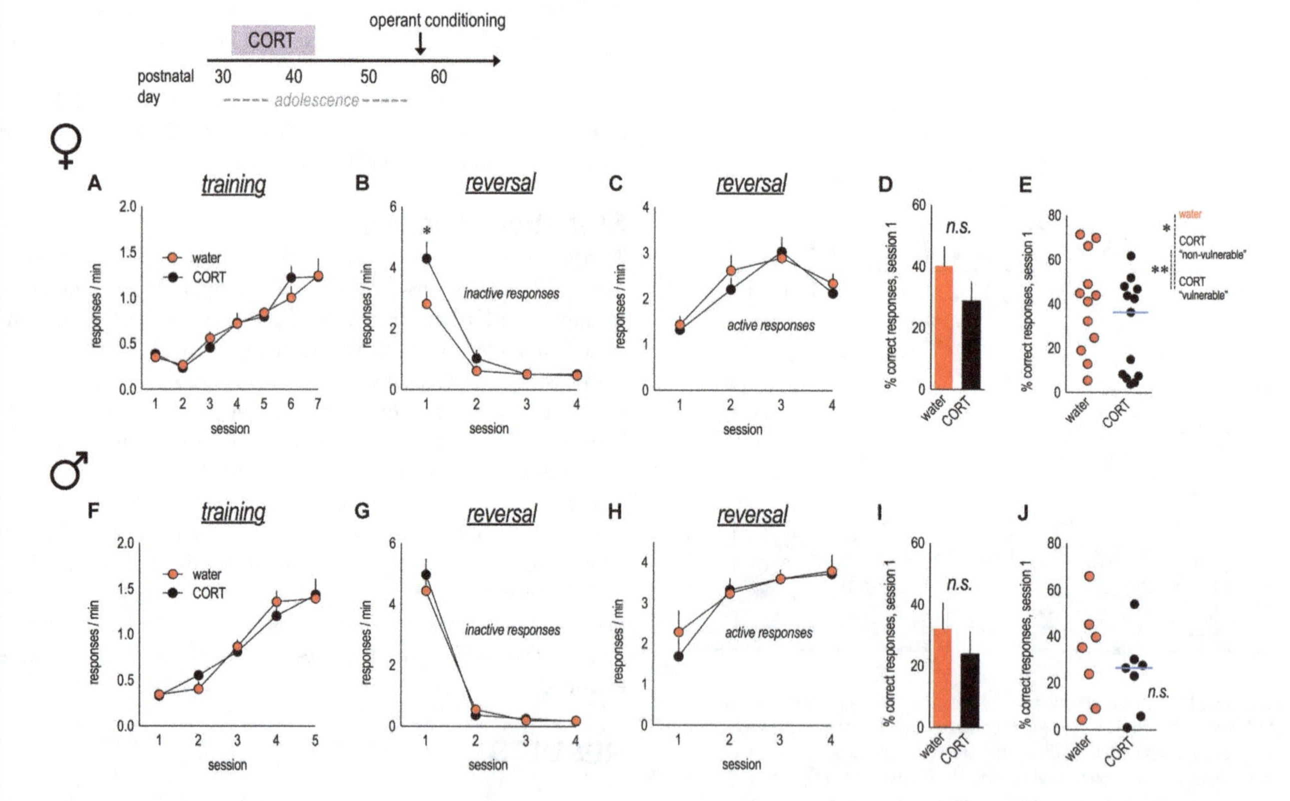

FIGURE 2 | Corticosterone (CORT) exposure in adolescent females induces reversal errors in adulthood. An experimental timeline is at top. **(A)** Female mice with a history of CORT exposure were trained to nose poke for food reinforcers, with no group differences. **(B)** In an instrumental reversal task, CORT-exposed mice made more perseverative errors, generating the previously-reinforced response. **(C)** CORT did not impact the acquisition of the new lever press response. **(D)** The percent of correct responses made during session 1 did not differ between groups. **(E)** However, a median split revealed that CORT-exposed females separated into two distinct subgroups; the "vulnerable" group made significantly fewer correct responses. $n = 12–13$/group. **(F)** Male mice exposed to CORT during adolescence acquired the nose poke responses without group differences. **(G)** A history of early-adolescent CORT exposure did not impact inhibition of the previously reinforced, now-inactive, response. **(H)** Acquisition of the newly reinforced response was also not impacted. **(I,J)** The percent of correct responses made during session 1 also did not differ between groups. $n = 7$/group. Symbols and bars represent means + SEMs, except for scatter plots, where symbols represent individual mice, and blue lines indicate the median. $^{*}p \leq 0.05$. $^{**}p \leq 0.001$.

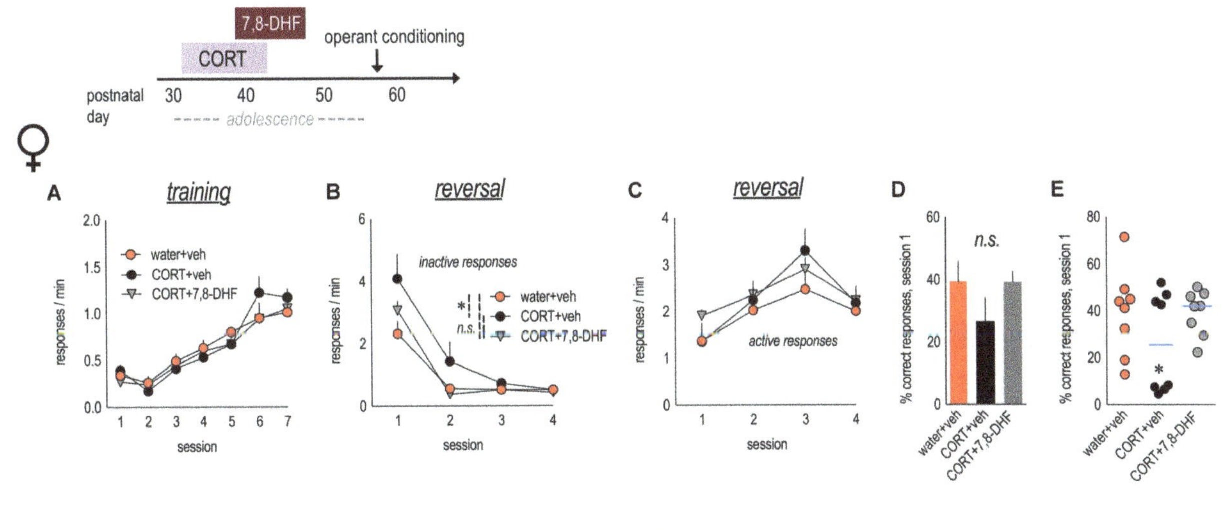

FIGURE 3 | Tyrosine kinase receptor B (TrkB) stimulation blocks perseverative errors in CORT-exposed female mice. Experimental timeline is at top. Female mice were exposed to CORT from P31 to 42 and administered the trkB agonist, 7,8-dihydroxyflavone (7,8-DHF), from P39 to 47. **(A)** As adults, mice were trained to nose poke for food reinforcers, with no differences between groups. **(B)** CORT-exposed mice made more perseverative errors, and 7,8-DHF mitigated this effect. **(C)** Groups generated the newly reinforced response at similar rates. **(D)** There were no gross effects on the percent of correct responses made during session 1. **(E)** CORT-exposed mice were divided into two subgroups on the basis of a median split of percent values, revealing two populations, including a subgroup that made significantly fewer correct responses. 7,8-DHF eliminated these differences. $n = 8$/group. Symbols and bars represent means + SEMs. *$p \leq 0.05$.

TrkB Stimulation Blocks CORT-Induced Errors

We attempted to block the long-term behavioral consequences of adolescent CORT exposure in females by administering 7,8-DHF (3 mg/kg) during mid-adolescence (P39–47). A 7,8-DHF-only group was omitted to conserve animal usage. We found no group differences in response acquisition (main effect and interaction $Fs < 1$; **Figure 3A**). As before, mice with a history of adolescent CORT exposure generated more non-reinforced responses in reversal (main effect group $F_{(2,21)} = 3.6, p = 0.046$; session × group interaction $F_{(6,63)} = 2.1, p = 0.07$), and treatment with 7,8-DHF mitigated this impairment in response inhibition (**Figure 3B**). Acquisition of the newly reinforced lever press did not differ (main effect and interaction $Fs \leq 1$; **Figure 3C**). Groups did not differ in the percentage of responses that were reinforced during session 1 (main effect group $F_{(2,21)} = 1.5$, $p = 0.3$; **Figure 3D**). Further, treatment with 7,8-DHF eliminated the existence of "vulnerable" and "non-vulnerable" populations within the CORT-exposed group (ANOVA with CORT+vehicle and CORT+7,8-DHF mice separated into two subgroups based on a median split (five groups total): main effect group $F_{(4,19)} = 7.9, p = 0.001$; **Figure 3E**). Thus, a trkB agonist occludes long-term deficits in response inhibition following early-life CORT exposure.

TrkB Stimulation in Adolescence Improves Behavioral Flexibility in Adulthood

Male mice exposed to water or CORT during early adolescence were also administered either vehicle or 7,8-DHF. As adults, all mice acquired the nose poke responses for food reinforcement, without group differences (main effect and interaction $Fs \leq 1.2$; **Figure 4A**). In instrumental reversal, a history of CORT exposure did not impact response inhibition ($Fs < 1$) or acquisition of the newly reinforced response ($Fs < 1$), as described above. Nevertheless, 7,8-DHF reduced perseverative responding during session 1 in both control and CORT-exposed animals (session × 7,8-DHF interaction $F_{(3,72)} = 7.1, p < 0.001$; **Figure 4B**) and increased responding on the newly reinforced lever in session 1 (session × 7,8-DHF interaction $F_{(3,72)} = 6.6$, $p = 0.001$; **Figure 4C**). 7,8-DHF also increased the percentage of responses that were correct during session 1 (main effect $F_{(1,24)} = 7.7, p = 0.01$; CORT × 7,8-DHF interaction $F_{(1,24)} = 1.8$, $p = 0.2$; **Figure 4D**), further indicating that stimulation of trkB during adolescence enhances behavioral flexibility in adulthood, well beyond the period of drug treatment.

Adolescent Stressor Exposure and TrkB Inhibition Impair Reversal Performance

The apparent resilience of male mice to early-adolescent CORT exposure was somewhat surprising, so we exposed another group of males to swim stress during early adolescence (daily from P31 to 42). In adulthood, we detected no group differences in the acquisition of the nose poke responses (main effect $F < 1$; interaction $F_{(4,68)} = 1.8, p = 0.1$; **Figure 5A**). When mice were required to shift responding to a previously non-reinforced lever, control and stressor-exposed mice did not differ in responding on the previously reinforced nose poke apertures (main effect $F_{(1,16)} = 1.3, p = 0.3$; interaction $F_{(3,48)} = 1.3, p = 0.3$; **Figure 5B**). However, mice with a history of adolescent stressor exposure responded less on the newly reinforced lever (main effect $F_{(1,16)} = 8.1$, $p = 0.01$; session × group interaction $F_{(3,48)} = 1.2$, $p = 0.3$; **Figure 5C**), making fewer reinforced responses during

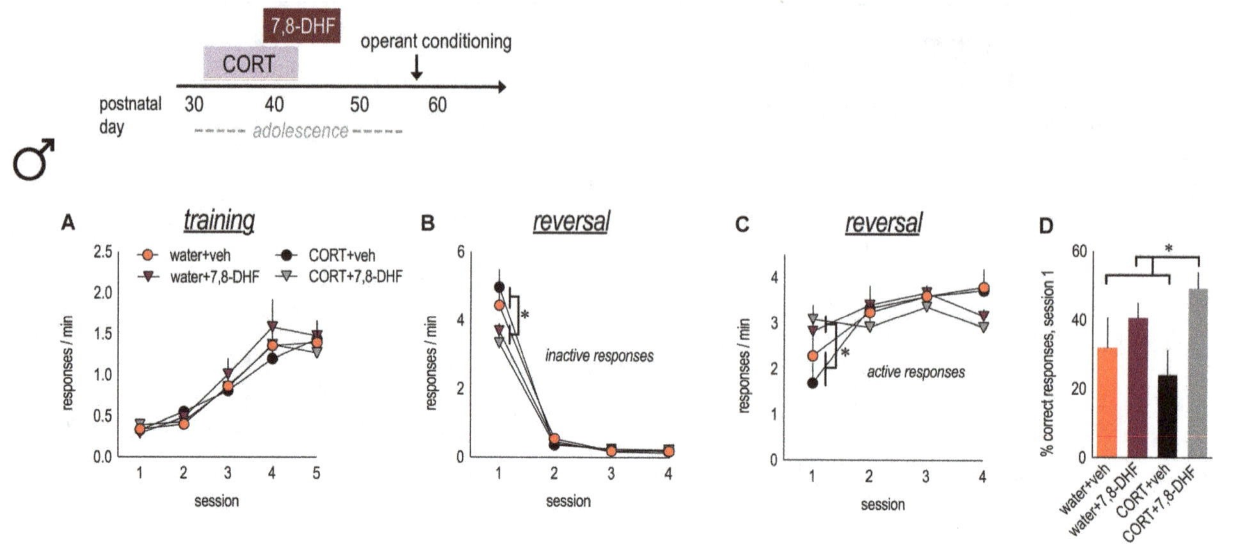

FIGURE 4 | TrkB stimulation during adolescence enhances behavioral flexibility in adulthood. Experimental timeline is at top. Male mice were exposed to CORT from P31 to 42 and administered the trkB agonist, 7,8-DHF, from P39 to 47. **(A)** Mice acquired the nose poke responses in adulthood, with no group differences. **(B)** In both water and CORT-exposed mice, 7,8-DHF reduced perseverative errors in the first reversal session. **(C)** Further, 7,8-DHF increased active response rates on the first day of reversal. **(D)** 7,8-DHF also increased the percent of correct responses made during session 1 (asterisk signifies a main effect of 7,8-DHF). $n = 7$/group. Symbols and bars represent means + SEMs. $^*p \leq 0.05$.

session 1 ($t_{(17)} = 2.3$, $p = 0.04$; **Figure 5D**). Thus, stressor exposure in early adolescence impairs the ability of male mice to develop novel response strategies in adulthood. This deficiency is similar to those following lateral oPFC (loPFC) ablation (Gourley et al., 2010; summarized in **Table 1**).

Prolonged stressor or glucocorticoid exposure can down-regulate *Bdnf* or BDNF-trkB signaling in the PFC, and these alterations are associated with impairments in PFC-dependent behavioral tasks (Gourley et al., 2009a, 2012b; Xu et al., 2016; Zhang et al., 2017). Thus, we also tested whether inhibiting trkB during early adolescence would induce reversal deficits in male mice.

Male mice received the trkB antagonist, ANA-12 (0.5 mg/kg), daily from P31 to 42, matching the period of early-adolescent CORT exposure. As adults, mice acquired the nose poke responses for food reinforcement, without group differences (main effect $F_{(1,12)} = 3.6$, $p = 0.08$; interaction $F_{(4,48)} = 2.2$, $p = 0.09$; **Figure 5E**). ANA-12 impaired response inhibition (interaction $F_{(3,33)} = 10.4$, $p < 0.001$; **Figure 5F**) and also acquisition (interaction $F_{(3,30)} = 4.1$, $p = 0.01$; **Figure 5G**) during session 1. ANA-12-treated mice made fewer correct responses overall during session 1 ($t_{(12)} = 3.1$, $p = 0.01$; **Figure 5H**). Thus, trkB inhibition during adolescence recapitulated the effects of CORT exposure in females (perseverative responding) and also stressor exposure in males (response acquisition impairments). Our findings are summarized in **Table 1**.

DISCUSSION

Adolescents who experience chronic stress have higher incidences of stress-related psychiatric illnesses and behaviors associated with addiction as adults. These behaviors may result in part from disruption of the PFC-dependent ability to flexibly modify behavior when environmental contingencies change (Elton et al., 2014; Zhang et al., 2016; see for review Watt et al., 2017). BDNF signaling through trkB regulates cellular maturational processes occurring in the PFC during adolescence (Xu et al., 2000; Shapiro et al., 2017b), and is disrupted by exposure to stress or elevated glucocorticoids (Bath et al., 2013; Numakawa et al., 2013; Suri and Vaidya, 2013). Using an oPFC-dependent instrumental reversal task in mice (see Gourley et al., 2010), we evaluated the long-term consequences of adolescent exposure to CORT, physical stress, trkB stimulation, or trkB inhibition, on behavioral flexibility. In females, adolescent CORT exposure increased perseverative errors in adulthood, and this was blocked by a trkB agonist. By contrast, behavioral flexibility was not impacted by CORT exposure in males, but was enhanced by trkB stimulation, as in females. Males did, however, develop reversal deficits in adulthood following repeated stressor exposure or trkB antagonism during adolescence. These findings add to evidence that adverse events or elevated glucocorticoid levels during adolescence can impair behavioral flexibility later in life. Moreover, our data suggest that trkB-based interventions may prevent adolescent stress-related behavioral impairments later in life.

Long-Term, Sex-Dependent Behavioral Consequences of Adolescent CORT Exposure

The majority of rodent studies examining the long-term neurobehavioral effects of early-life adversity have utilized male subjects, despite evidence for sex differences in the

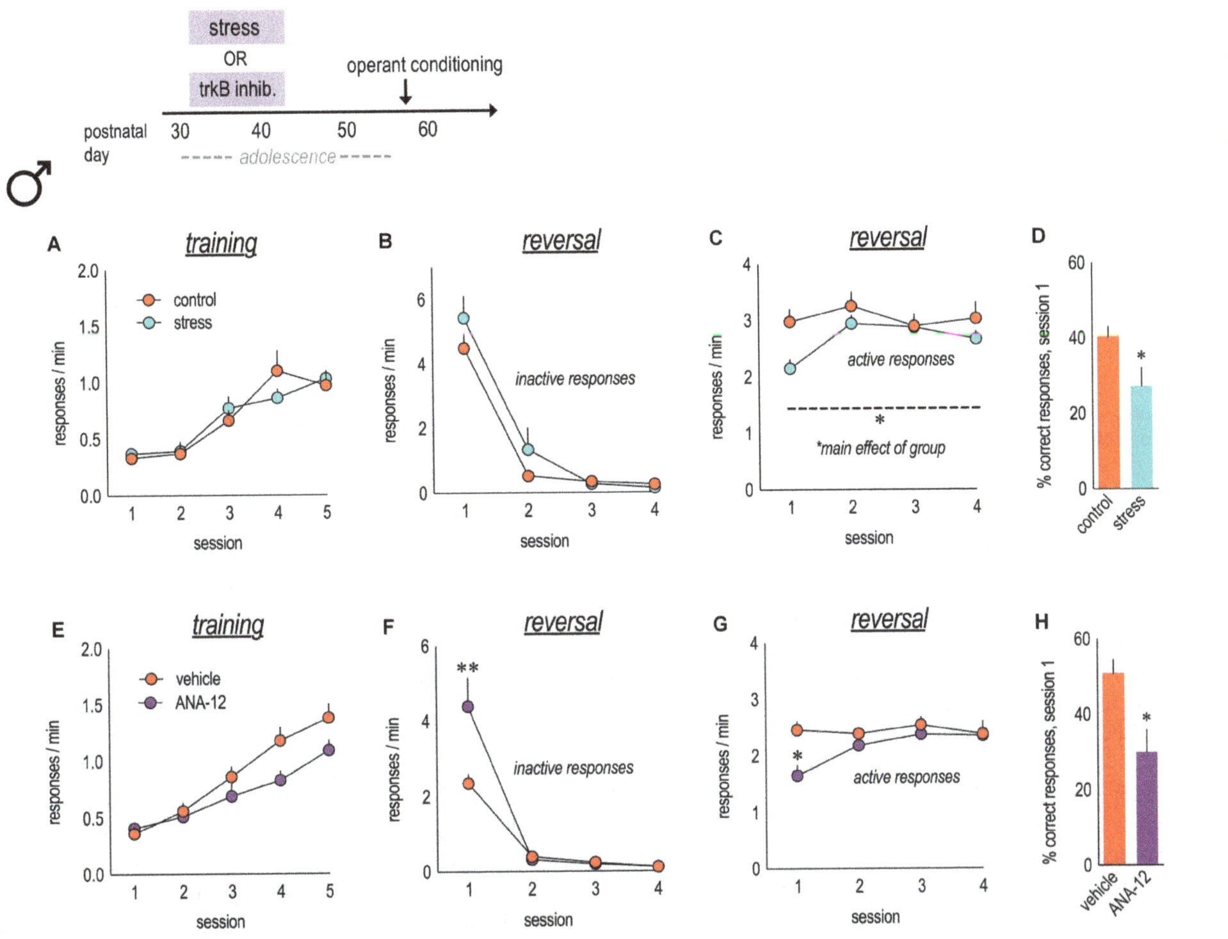

FIGURE 5 | Physical stressors and pharmacological inhibition of trkB in adolescence impair instrumental reversal in adulthood. Experimental timeline is at top. **(A)** A history of stressor exposure did not impact responding for food reinforcement during training in adulthood. **(B)** In an instrumental reversal task, both groups performed the now-inactive nose poke response at similar rates. **(C)** By contrast, stressor-exposed mice performed the now-active lever press response at lower rates. **(D)** Adolescent stressor exposure also reduced the percent of correct responses made during session 1. n = 9–10/group. **(E)** In parallel experiments, mice received daily injections of the trkB antagonist, ANA-12, from P31 to 42. Mice learned to nose poke for food reinforcement in adulthood, with no group differences. **(F)** TrkB blockade during adolescence increased perseverative errors during the first reversal session. **(G)** ANA-12 also reduced responding on the now-active lever during session 1. **(H)** ANA-12-treated mice made fewer correct responses during session 1. n = 7/group. Symbols and bars represent means + SEMs. $^*p \leq 0.05$. $^{**}p \leq 0.001$.

prevalence and severity of stress-related psychiatric illnesses (Kessler et al., 1993; MacMillan et al., 2001; Holbrook et al., 2002; Kuehner, 2003; Becker et al., 2012; Fattore et al., 2014). We report that CORT dissolved in the drinking water of mice during a period equivalent to early adolescence in humans (P31–42; Spear, 2000) impaired performance in an instrumental reversal task in adulthood in female mice, but not males. Specifically, adolescent CORT impaired the inhibition of a previously reinforced response, increasing perseverative errors. Similarly, exposure to stress-level cortisol in young-adult or older-adult female squirrel monkeys increases response inhibition errors in a detour-reaching task that assesses the ability to inhibit prepotent responses when reinforcement contingencies change (Lyons et al., 2000).

We also calculated the percent of responses that were reinforced ("correct") during the first reversal session, revealing a "CORT vulnerable" subgroup (approximately half of the group) with significantly impaired behavioral flexibility relative to a CORT-exposed "non-vulnerable" group and control mice. What mediates this vulnerability is unclear, but one factor may be dopamine D2-family receptors (D2, D3, D4). D2/3 antagonists disrupt reversal performance in monkeys and rodents (Ridley et al., 1981; Kruzich and Grandy, 2004; Floresco et al., 2006; Lee et al., 2007; De Steno and Schmauss, 2009), and variation in D2 receptor density in the ventral PFC (including oPFC; Gourley et al., 2009b) and midbrain (Laughlin et al., 2011) correlates with behavioral flexibility. Furthermore, adolescent stress exposure decreases PFC D2 expression in adulthood (Wright et al., 2008). Whether vulnerabilities to

TABLE 1 | Failures in response acquisition and errors of perseveration in an instrumental reversal task can be dissociated.

Manipulation	Region	Sex	Reference
Impairments of response acquisition			
Early-adolescent forced swim stress	n/a	M	**Figure 5C**
Early-adolescent trkB antagonism	n/a	M	**Figure 5G**
Lesion	loPFC	M	Gourley et al. (2010)
Inhibition of Abl-family kinases	loPFC	M	Gourley et al. (2012a)
Bdnf knockdown	loPFC	M	Gourley et al. (2013a)
Disconnection of the loPFC and striatum	loPFC	M	Gourley et al. (2013a)
Impairments of response inhibition			
Early-adolescent CORT exposure	n/a	F	**Figure 2B**
Early-adolescent trkB antagonism	n/a	M	**Figure 5F**
Lesion	moPFC+loPFC	M	Boulougouris et al. (2007)
Lesion	moPFC	M	Gourley et al. (2010)

Errors of perseveration (repeatedly performing an "old" response, despite reversal) or response acquisition (failing to develop a new strategy) can be dissociated in reversal tasks that rely on spatial or instrumental learning and memory. Here we detected failures in response acquisition and errors of perseveration (highlighted in blue). These deficits are associated with manipulations of the lateral oPFC (loPFC) and medial oPFC (moPFC), respectively (highlighted in gray).

corticosteroid-related modifications in dopamine D2 levels influence the behavioral patterns reported here could be tested in future experiments.

In contrast to females, males exposed to early-adolescent CORT failed to develop instrumental reversal impairments in adulthood. However, some studies report long-term deficits in reversal learning and extradimensional set-shifting (EDS; a medial PFC (mPFC)-dependent function) in male rodents following social stress during early adolescence (Snyder et al., 2015; Zhang et al., 2016). Accordingly, daily forced swim stress during early adolescence (P31–42) impaired the acquisition of the "reversed" response contingency here, resembling the effects of loPFC lesions (Gourley et al., 2010). These findings suggest that in males exposed to repeated stress during adolescence, components of the stress response besides elevations in CORT (e.g., increased noradrenergic tone) may be responsible for response acquisition deficiencies. Indeed, under conditions of chronic stress in adult rats, stress-induced release of norepinephrine in the mPFC impairs certain forms of behavioral flexibility, while noradrenergic receptor blockade in the mPFC prevents stress-induced deficits (Jett and Morilak, 2013). On the other hand, 3 weeks of CORT exposure in adolescent male mice causes errors in a similar instrumental reversal task (Shapiro et al., 2017a), indicating that males are not entirely resilient to CORT.

One possibility is that higher concentrations of CORT would have triggered reversal deficiencies in males. Females have higher basal CORT levels than males, an effect that develops during puberty (Netherton et al., 2004; McCormick and Mathews, 2007; Stroud et al., 2011). Because puberty in rodents typically occurs around P35 in females and P40 in males (Korenbrot et al., 1977; Evans, 1986), administering exogenous CORT during a time when endogenous levels in females are increasing may result in higher total CORT levels in females. While we did not measure blood serum CORT in these experiments, it is possible that recapitulating "female-like" CORT levels in males may have induced comparable behavioral inflexibility.

Because the PFC undergoes significant structural remodeling during adolescence, and PFC-dependent cognitive functions continue to develop throughout this period, prolonged stressor or CORT exposure during adolescence may be more impactful than exposure in adulthood. Consistent with this possibility, male rats exposed to 5 days of social defeat stress during early adolescence (P28–32), then housed in isolation, exhibit deficits in EDS and reversal learning in an attentional set-shifting task 6 weeks later. However, rats exposed to the same stress in mid-adolescence (P38–47) or adulthood (P70–79) do not show these cognitive impairments (Zhang et al., 2016). Furthermore, adolescent stress- or CORT-induced alterations in PFC neuronal morphology, like behavioral deficits, can persist into adulthood. For example, social isolation stress during early adolescence (P30–35) in male rats reduces synaptic density in the mPFC in adulthood (Leussis et al., 2008), suggestive of a long-term loss of dendritic spines, which house the majority of excitatory synapses in the brain. Gourley et al. (2013b) also reported dendritic spine loss on pyramidal neurons in the oPFC immediately following CORT exposure during adolescence (P35–56) that is still evident 1 week after the cessation of CORT. Meanwhile, CORT-induced spine changes in the infralimbic mPFC, hippocampus, and amygdala recover. Consistent with these findings in rodents, early-life adversity in humans is associated with reduced oPFC volume and morphological alterations in adulthood (Holz et al., 2015; Teicher and Samson, 2016). Our findings add to these and other studies reporting long-term consequences of stressor or CORT exposure during early adolescence.

TrkB Manipulations in Adolescence Influence Behavioral Flexibility in Adulthood

One mechanism by which CORT or stressor exposure during adolescence may impact PFC-dependent behaviors later in life is by reducing BDNF-dependent stimulation of trkB (Duman et al., 1997; Blugeot et al., 2011). Consistent with this possibility, the trkB agonist 7,8-DHF blocked perseverative responding in females with a history of adolescent CORT exposure. Additionally, while a subgroup of vehicle-treated CORT-exposed females was especially vulnerable to impairments in behavioral flexibility, 7,8-DHF eliminated these individual differences, and in males, 7,8-DHF improved performance above control levels.

How might 7,8-DHF have long-term behavioral consequences? One possibility is that it prevents CORT-induced disruptions in PFC synaptic maturation by augmenting or restoring trkB activity. BDNF and trkB increase in adolescence/young adulthood (Webster et al., 2002; Shapiro et al., 2017b), and BDNF-trkB signaling is critical for the maintenance of stabile dendritic spines in the postnatal brain (Vigers et al., 2012). Chronic stress or CORT exposure can reduce PFC BDNF and trkB (e.g., see Gourley et al., 2009a, 2012b), potentially altering the trajectory of dendritic spine maturation (Leussis and Andersen, 2008; Eiland et al., 2012) and behavioral outcomes. Consistent with this possibility, we found that administration of the trkB antagonist, ANA-12, during early adolescence impaired behavioral flexibility in adulthood.

Our trkB antagonism experiments were performed in males, but it is worth noting that prior reports indicate that knockdown of *Bdnf* beginning in the preadolescent period or in adulthood in female mice produces behavioral consequences that are comparable to, or more severe than, those in male mice. For example, Vigers et al. (2012) report that forebrain-specific knockdown of *Bdnf* (progressive knockdown begins at ~P21) induces depressive-like immobility in the forced swim test and contextual fear generalization in both male and female adult mice. However, Monteggia et al. (2007) report that this knockdown strategy results in depression-like behavior in female, but not male, mice. Similarly, inducible knockdown of *Bdnf* in adulthood increases susceptibility to stress-induced depression-like behavior in female mice only (Autry et al., 2009).

Recent findings in addition to ours interestingly implicate BDNF-trkB in the long-term behavioral consequences of early-adolescent stress. Male rats exposed to chronic mild stress (CMS) during early adolescence (P28–37) exhibit impairments in EDS and decreased levels of BDNF protein, the ratio of p-ERK42/44/ERK42/44, and p-CREB in the mPFC 6 weeks after stressor exposure (Zhang et al., 2017). Additionally, EDS is correlated with p-ERK/ERK ratios in mPFC, and the antidepressant duloxetine ameliorates stress-induced alterations in EDS and mPFC BDNF levels in tandem. *Impairing* BDNF-trkB signaling can also alter PFC-dependent functions and drug-taking behaviors. For example, mutant mice with disruption of promoter IV-driven (activity-dependent) BDNF expression are impaired in a spatial reversal task (Sakata et al., 2013). Knock-in mice expressing a homolog of the human *BDNF* gene polymorphism *Val66Met*, which decreases the activity-dependent release of BDNF (Chen et al., 2004), develop excessive and compulsive alcohol drinking despite adverse consequences, and this phenotype is reversible by a trkB agonist (Warnault et al., 2016). Furthermore, early-life stress decreases *Bdnf* exon IV mRNA in the PFC and increases cocaine-induced conditioned place preference (CPP) in periadolescent (P45) mice (Viola et al., 2016). Interestingly, higher CPP scores correlate with *Bdnf* expression, with higher place preference associated with lower *Bdnf*. Thus, by disrupting trkB signaling, early-life stress may increase vulnerability to compulsive drug taking.

Broader Considerations: Sex Differences in Reversal Performance

Here, we found that adolescent CORT-exposed females and adolescent stress-exposed males exhibited impairments in reversal performance in adulthood; however, the specific behavioral impairments were sexually dimorphic—females failed to inhibit the previously reinforced response, while males were unable to acquire a newly reinforced response (summarized in **Table 1**). In the context of addiction, poor control over perseverative behavior could modulate the progression from recreational drug use to abuse and dependence, increase relapse rates, and impair treatment response (Carroll et al., 2011). Meanwhile, deficits in the acquisition of a "reversed" response contingency could be comparable to impairments in the ability to adjust behavior according to positive feedback and potentially, to substitute new healthy behaviors for maladaptive ones.

The association between early-life trauma and the risk for, and severity of, drug dependence is stronger in women (Widom and White, 1997; MacMillan et al., 2001; Simpson and Miller, 2002; Hyman et al., 2008), and at least one study reports that a greater proportion of stimulant-dependent women, compared to men, have clinically significant "disinhibition" scores prior to stimulant abuse (Winhusen and Lewis, 2013). In that same study, physical abuse was associated with greater disinhibition in women, but not men. Thus, females may be more vulnerable to chronic stress-induced inhibitory control deficits, in line with our findings. Further, Elton et al. (2014) report that childhood maltreatment results in enduring, sex-dependent changes in the functional connectivity of a network mediating inhibitory behavioral control, also in line with sex-dependent effects of adolescent CORT exposure on perseverative responding here. Future work should examine whether adolescent CORT-induced deficits in response inhibition increase vulnerability to compulsive drug taking later in life. CORT exposure during adolescence increases cue-induced reinstatement of ethanol seeking in adult female, but not male, rats (Bertholomey et al., 2016), suggesting that females are especially vulnerable to adolescent CORT-induced neurobehavioral changes that increase susceptibility to drug relapse later in life.

Our findings may also point to sexually dimorphic stress-related vulnerabilities in specific brain regions, given that lesions of the medial oPFC (moPFC) impair response inhibition in this task (like CORT-exposed females), while loPFC lesions impair response acquisition (like stressor-exposed males; Gourley et al., 2010). These patterns are interesting when considered alongside studies reporting structural changes in the oPFC of substance-dependent males and females. For example, cocaine-dependent females and males exhibit decreased cerebral blood flow in the moPFC and loPFC, respectively (Adinoff et al., 2006). Adolescent females with substance dependence exhibit decreased cortical thickness and gray matter volume in regions involved in inhibitory control, decision-making, reward, and risk-taking, including the moPFC and dorsolateral PFC (DLPFC; Dalwani et al., 2015; Boulos et al., 2016), while substance-dependent adolescent males show decreased gray matter volume in DLPFC (Dalwani et al., 2011). Regner et al. (2015) report decreased oPFC gray matter volume in abstinent stimulant-dependent women, but not men. However, in a population of predominantly male treatment-seeking individuals with alcohol dependence, loPFC surface area and volume were smaller in individuals who subsequently relapsed in a 1-year period compared to individuals who remained abstinent (Cardenas et al., 2011; Durazzo et al., 2011). Together, these findings suggest that PFC subregions disrupted by both adolescent stress or glucocorticoid exposure and drugs of abuse may be sex-dependent (potentially: loPFC in males and both moPFC and loPFC in females; see **Table 1**).

CONCLUSION

PFC dysfunction and associated deficits in inhibitory control and behavioral flexibility are hallmarks of stress-related illnesses, including addiction. Substance-dependent individuals report loss of control over drug use and have difficulty modifying behaviors when reward contingencies change, potentially contributing to persistent drug seeking despite adverse consequences (Garavan and Hester, 2007; Everitt and Robbins, 2016). Being able to implement new strategies to promote behavioral change and control impulsive responses may be critical to treatment response—among cocaine-dependent individuals undergoing cognitive-behavioral therapy, higher impulsivity/risk-taking before treatment is associated with poorer treatment retention and higher relapse rates (Carroll et al., 2011).

Substance-dependent individuals exhibit structural and functional alterations in the oPFC, including blood flow abnormalities (London et al., 2000; Adinoff et al., 2006), decreased gray matter volume (Matochik et al., 2003; Tanabe et al., 2009; Dalwani et al., 2015), and decreased cortical thickness (Boulos et al., 2016). In animal models, adolescent CORT and cocaine exposure result in long-term changes in oPFC neuron structure (Gourley et al., 2012a, 2013b; DePoy et al., 2014, 2016, 2017) that are associated with maladaptive behaviors symptomatic of addiction (Lucantonio et al., 2012). Further, poor inhibitory control may be a *predisposing factor* for addiction (Jentsch and Taylor, 1999; Tarter et al., 2004; Groman et al., 2009; Moffitt et al., 2011), as is a history of early-life adversity (Fergusson et al., 1996; Kessler et al., 1997; Dube et al., 2003; Green et al., 2010; Afifi et al., 2012). These and other findings have led to the hypothesis that early-life adversity may affect addiction liability by impairing oPFC-mediated inhibitory control. That is, in individuals with a history of stressor exposure during sensitive developmental periods like adolescence, repeated drug use may further impair inhibitory control, exacerbating the development, persistence, and severity of addiction. Indeed, social stress during adolescence in rats causes binge-like cocaine self-administration in adulthood (Burke and Miczek, 2015).

Using an oPFC-dependent instrumental reversal task, we find that exposure to CORT during early adolescence induces perseverative errors in female, but not male, mice in adulthood. Further, intervention with a trkB agonist in mid-adolescence, when dendritic spines in the PFC undergo activity-dependent pruning or stabilization (Petanjek et al., 2011; Gourley et al., 2012a; Selemon, 2013; Chung et al., 2017) corrected decision-making strategies in CORT-exposed mice. With the caveat that the sexes were tested in independent cohorts here—precluding direct comparisons between them—we nevertheless argue that further related research may advance our understanding of how sex differences in the neurobehavioral response to adolescent adversities contribute to sex differences in vulnerability to, and clinical course of, stress-related illnesses. Our findings additionally suggest that pharmacotherapies augmenting trkB may ameliorate the enduring consequences of stressful life events occurring in adolescence.

AUTHOR CONTRIBUTIONS

ETB performed the experiments, analyzed the data and wrote the manuscript. ETB and SLG designed the experiments, interpreted the data and edited the manuscript.

ACKNOWLEDGMENTS

We thank A. Allen for assisting with injections.

REFERENCES

Adinoff, B., Williams, M. J., Best, S. E., Harris, T. S., Chandler, P., and Devous, M. D. (2006). Sex differences in medial and lateral orbitofrontal cortex hypoperfusion in cocaine-dependent men and women. *Gend. Med.* 3, 206–222. doi: 10.1016/s1550-8579(06)80209-3

Afifi, T. O., Henriksen, C. A., Asmundson, G. J., and Sareen, J. (2012). Childhood maltreatment and substance use disorders among men and women in a nationally representative sample. *Can. J. Psychiatry* 57, 677–686. doi: 10.1177/070674371205701105

Autry, A. E., Adachi, M., Cheng, P., and Monteggia, L. M. (2009). Gender specific impact of BDNF signaling on stress-induced depression-like behavior. *Biol. Psychiatry* 66, 84–90. doi: 10.1016/j.biopsych.2009.02.007

Barfield, E. T., Gerber, K. J., Zimmermann, K. S., Ressler, K. J., Parsons, R. G., and Gourley, S. L. (in press). Bidirectional regulation of actions and habits by ventral hippocampal trkB and adolescent corticosteroid exposure. *PLoS Biol.*

Bath, K. G., Schilit, A., and Lee, F. S. (2013). Stress effects on BDNF expression: effects of age, sex, and form of stress. *Neuroscience* 239, 149–156. doi: 10.1016/j.neuroscience.2013.01.074

Becker, J. B., Perry, A. N., and Westenbroek, C. (2012). Sex differences in the neural mechanisms mediating addiction: a new synthesis and hypothesis. *Biol. Sex Differ.* 3:14. doi: 10.1186/2042-6410-3-14

Belin, D., Mar, A. C., Dalley, J. W., Robbins, T. W., and Everitt, B. J. (2008). High impulsivity predicts the switch to compulsive cocaine-taking. *Science* 320, 1352–1355. doi: 10.1126/science.1158136

Bertholomey, M. L., Nagarajan, V., and Torregrossa, M. M. (2016). Sex differences in reinstatement of alcohol seeking in response to cues and yohimbine in rats with and without a history of adolescent corticosterone exposure. *Psychopharmacology* 233, 2277–2287. doi: 10.1007/s00213-016-4278-x

Blugeot, A., Rivat, C., Bouvier, E., Molet, J., Mouchard, A., Zeau, B., et al. (2011). Vulnerability to depression: from brain neuroplasticity to identification of biomarkers. *J. Neurosci.* 31, 12889–12899. doi: 10.1523/JNEUROSCI.1309-11.2011

Boulos, P. K., Dalwani, M. S., Tanabe, J., Mikulich-Gilbertson, S. K., Banich, M. T., Crowley, T. J., et al. (2016). Brain cortical thickness differences in adolescent females with substance use disorders. *PLoS One* 11:e0152983. doi: 10.1371/journal.pone.0152983

Boulougouris, V., Dalley, J. W., and Robbins, T. W. (2007). Effects of orbitofrontal, infralimbic and prelimbic cortical lesions on serial spatial reversal learning in the rat. *Behav. Brain Res.* 179, 219–228. doi: 10.1016/j.bbr.2007.02.005

Burke, A. R., and Miczek, K. A. (2015). Escalation of cocaine self-administration in adulthood after social defeat of adolescent rats: role of social experience and adaptive coping behavior. *Psychopharmacology* 232, 3067–3079. doi: 10.1007/s00213-015-3947-5

Cardenas, V. A., Durazzo, T. C., Gazdzinski, S., Mon, A., Studholme, C., and Meyerhoff, D. J. (2011). Brain morphology at entry into treatment for alcohol dependence is related to relapse propensity. *Biol. Psychiatry* 70, 561–567. doi: 10.1016/j.biopsych.2011.04.003

Carroll, K. M., Kiluk, B. D., Nich, C., Babuscio, T. A., Brewer, J. A., Potenza, M. N., et al. (2011). Cognitive function and treatment response in a randomized clinical trial of computer-based training in cognitive-behavioral therapy. *Subst. Use Misuse* 46, 23–34. doi: 10.3109/10826084.2011.521069

Cervantes, M. C., Laughlin, R. E., and Jentsch, J. D. (2013). Cocaine self-administration behavior in inbred mouse lines segregating different capacities for inhibitory control. *Psychopharmacology* 229, 515–525. doi: 10.1007/s00213-013-3135-4

Chen, Z. Y., Patel, P. D., Sant, G., Meng, C. X., Teng, K. K., Hempstead, B. L., et al. (2004). Variant brain-derived neurotrophic factor (BDNF) (Met66) alters the intracellular trafficking and activity-dependent secretion of wild-type BDNF in neurosecretory cells and cortical neurons. *J. Neurosci.* 24, 4401–4411. doi: 10.1523/JNEUROSCI.0348-04.2004

Chung, D. W., Wills, Z. P., Fish, K. N., and Lewis, D. A. (2017). Developmental pruning of excitatory synaptic inputs to parvalbumin interneurons in monkey prefrontal cortex. *Proc. Natl. Acad. Sci. U S A* 114, E629–E637. doi: 10.1073/pnas.1610077114

Dalley, J. W., Fryer, T. D., Brichard, L., Robinson, E. S., Theobald, D. E., Laane, K., et al. (2007). Nucleus accumbens D2/3 receptors predict trait impulsivity and cocaine reinforcement. *Science* 315, 1267–1270. doi: 10.1126/science.1137073

Dalwani, M., Sakai, J. T., Mikulich-Gilbertson, S. K., Tanabe, J., Raymond, K., McWilliams, S. K., et al. (2011). Reduced cortical gray matter volume in male adolescents with substance and conduct problems. *Drug Alcohol Depend.* 118, 295–305. doi: 10.1016/j.drugalcdep.2011.04.006

Dalwani, M. S., McMahon, M. A., Mikulich-Gilbertson, S. K., Young, S. E., Regner, M. F., Raymond, K. M., et al. (2015). Female adolescents with severe substance and conduct problems have substantially less brain gray matter volume. *PLoS One* 10:e0126368. doi: 10.1371/journal.pone.0126368

DePoy, L. M., Allen, A. G., and Gourley, S. L. (2016). Adolescent cocaine self-administration induces habit behavior in adulthood: sex differences and structural consequences. *Transl. Psychiatry* 6:e875. doi: 10.1038/tp.2016.150

DePoy, L. M., Perszyk, R. E., Zimmermann, K. S., Koleske, A. J., and Gourley, S. L. (2014). Adolescent cocaine exposure simplifies orbitofrontal cortical dendritic arbors. *Front. Pharmacol.* 5:228. doi: 10.3389/fphar.2014.00228

DePoy, L. M., Zimmermann, K. S., Marvar, P. J., and Gourley, S. L. (2017). Induction and blockade of adolescent cocaine-induced habits. *Biol. Psychiatry* 81, 595–605. doi: 10.1016/j.biopsych.2016.09.023

De Steno, D. A., and Schmauss, C. (2009). A role for dopamine D2 receptors in reversal learning. *Neuroscience* 162, 118–127. doi: 10.1016/j.neuroscience.2009.04.052

Dube, S. R., Felitti, V. J., Dong, M., Chapman, D. P., Giles, W. H., and Anda, R. F. (2003). Childhood abuse, neglect, and household dysfunction and the risk of illicit drug use: the adverse childhood experiences study. *Pediatrics* 111, 564–572. doi: 10.1542/peds.111.3.564

Duman, R. S., Heninger, G. R., and Nestler, E. J. (1997). A molecular and cellular theory of depression. *Arch. Gen. Psychiatry* 54, 597–606. doi: 10.1001/archpsyc.1997.01830190015002

Durazzo, T. C., Tosun, D., Buckley, S., Gazdzinski, S., Mon, A., Fryer, S. L., et al. (2011). Cortical thickness, surface area and volume of the brain reward system in alcohol dependence: relationships to relapse and extended abstinence. *Alcohol. Clin. Exp. Res.* 35, 1187–1200. doi: 10.1111/j.1530-0277.2011.01452.x

Eiland, L., Ramroop, J., Hill, M. N., Manley, J., and McEwen, B. S. (2012). Chronic juvenile stress produces corticolimbic dendritic architectural remodeling and modulates emotional behavior in male and female rats. *Psychoneuroendocrinology* 37, 39–47. doi: 10.1016/j.psyneuen.2011.04.015

Elton, A., Tripathi, S. P., Mletzko, T., Young, J., Cisler, J. M., James, A. G., et al. (2014). Childhood maltreatment is associated with a sex-dependent functional reorganization of a brain inhibitory control network. *Hum. Brain Mapp.* 35, 1654–1667. doi: 10.1002/hbm.22280

Enoch, M. A. (2011). The role of early life stress as a predictor for alcohol and drug dependence. *Psychopharmacology* 214, 17–31. doi: 10.1007/s00213-010-1916-6

Ersche, K. D., Roiser, J. P., Robbins, T. W., and Sahakian, B. J. (2008). Chronic cocaine but not chronic amphetamine use is associated with perseverative responding in humans. *Psychopharmacology* 197, 421–431. doi: 10.1007/s00213-007-1051-1

Evans, A. M. (1986). Age at puberty and first litter size in early and late paired rats. *Biol. Reprod.* 34, 322–326. doi: 10.1095/biolreprod34.2.322

Everitt, B. J., and Robbins, T. W. (2016). Drug addiction: updating actions to habits to compulsions ten years on. *Annu. Rev. Psychol.* 67, 23–50. doi: 10.1146/annurev-psych-122414-033457

Fattore, L., Melis, M., Fadda, P., and Fratta, W. (2014). Sex differences in addictive disorders. *Front. Neuroendocrinol.* 35, 272–284. doi: 10.1016/j.yfrne.2014.04.003

Feng, G., Mellor, R. H., Bernstein, M., Keller-Peck, C., Nguyen, Q. T., Wallace, M., et al. (2000). Imaging neuronal subsets in transgenic mice expressing multiple spectral variants of GFP. *Neuron* 28, 41–51. doi: 10.1016/s0896-6273(00)00084-2

Fergusson, D. M., Horwood, L. J., and Lynskey, M. T. (1996). Childhood sexual abuse and psychiatric disorder in young adulthood: II. Psychiatric outcomes of childhood sexual abuse. *J. Am. Acad. Child Adolesc. Psychiatry* 35, 1365–1374. doi: 10.1097/00004583-199610000-00024

Floresco, S. B., Magyar, O., Ghods-Sharifi, S., Vexelman, C., and Tse, M. T. (2006). Multiple dopamine receptor subtypes in the medial prefrontal cortex of the rat regulate set-shifting. *Neuropsychopharmacology* 31, 297–309. doi: 10.1038/sj.npp.1300825

Garavan, H., and Hester, R. (2007). The role of cognitive control in cocaine dependence. *Neuropsychol. Rev.* 17, 337–345. doi: 10.1007/s11065-007-9034-x

Gourley, S. L., Kedves, A. T., Olausson, P., and Taylor, J. R. (2009a). A history of corticosterone exposure regulates fear extinction and cortical NR2B, GluR2/3, and BDNF. *Neurpsychopharmacology* 34, 707–716. doi: 10.1038/npp.2008.123

Gourley, S. L., Koleske, A. J., and Taylor, J. R. (2009b). Loss of dendrite stabilization by the Abl-related gene (Arg) kinase regulates behavioral flexibility and sensitivity to cocaine. *Proc. Natl. Acad. Sci. U S A* 106, 16859–16864. doi: 10.1073/pnas.0902286106

Gourley, S. L., Kiraly, D. D., Howell, J. L., Olausson, P., and Taylor, J. R. (2008a). Acute hippocampal BDNF restores motivational and forced swim performance after corticosterone. *Biol. Psychiatry* 64, 884–890. doi: 10.1016/j.biopsych.2008.06.016

Gourley, S. L., Wu, F. J., Kiraly, D. D., Ploski, J. E., Kedves, A. T., Duman, R. S., et al. (2008b). Regionally specific regulation of ERK MAP kinase in a model of antidepressant-sensitive chronic depression. *Biol. Psychiatry* 63, 353–359. doi: 10.1016/j.biopsych.2007.07.016

Gourley, S. L., Lee, A. S., Howell, J. L., Pittenger, C., and Taylor, J. R. (2010). Dissociable regulation of instrumental action within mouse prefrontal cortex. *Eur. J. Neurosci.* 32, 1726–1734. doi: 10.1111/j.1460-9568.2010.07438.x

Gourley, S. L., Olevska, A., Warren, M. S., Taylor, J. R., and Koleske, A. J. (2012a). Arg kinase regulates prefrontal dendritic spine refinement and cocaine-induced plasticity. *J. Neurosci.* 32, 2314–2323. doi: 10.1523/JNEUROSCI.2730-11.2012

Gourley, S. L., Swanson, A. M., Jacobs, A. M., Howell, J. L., Mo, M., DiLeone, R. J., et al. (2012b). Action control is mediated by prefrontal BDNF and glucocorticoid receptor binding. *Proc. Natl. Acad. Sci. U S A* 109, 20714–20719. doi: 10.1073/pnas.1208342109

Gourley, S. L., Olevska, A., Zimmermann, K. S., Ressler, K. J., Dileone, R. J., and Taylor, J. R. (2013a). The orbitofrontal cortex regulates outcome-based decision-making via the lateral striatum. *Eur. J. Neurosci.* 38, 2382–2388. doi: 10.1111/ejn.12239

Gourley, S. L., Swanson, A. M., and Koleske, A. J. (2013b). Corticosteroid-induced neural remodeling predicts behavioral vulnerability and resilience. *J. Neurosci.* 33, 3107–3112. doi: 10.1523/JNEUROSCI.2138-12.2013

Gray, J. D., Milner, T. A., and McEwen, B. S. (2013). Dynamic plasticity: the role of glucocorticoids, brain-derived neurotrophic factor and other trophic factors. *Neuroscience* 239, 214–227. doi: 10.1016/j.neuroscience.2012.08.034

Green, J. G., McLaughlin, K. A., Berglund, P. A., Gruber, M. J., Sampson, N. A., Zaslavsky, A. M., et al. (2010). Childhood adversities and adult psychiatric disorders in the national comorbidity survey replication I: associations with first onset of DSM-IV disorders. *Arch. Gen. Psychiatry* 67, 113–123. doi: 10.1001/archgenpsychiatry.2009.186

Groman, S. M., James, A. S., and Jentsch, J. D. (2009). Poor response inhibition: at the nexus between substance abuse and attention deficit/hyperactivity disorder. *Neurosci. Biobehav. Rev.* 33, 690–698. doi: 10.1016/j.neubiorev.2008.08.008

Holbrook, T. L., Hoyt, D. B., Stein, M. B., and Sieber, W. J. (2002). Gender differences in long-term posttraumatic stress disorder outcomes after major trauma: women are at higher risk of adverse outcomes than men. *J. Trauma* 53, 882–888. doi: 10.1097/00005373-200211000-00012

Holz, N. E., Boecker, R., Hohm, E., Zohsel, K., Buchmann, A. F., Blomeyer, D., et al. (2015). The long-term impact of early life poverty on orbitofrontal cortex volume in adulthood: results from a prospective study over 25 years. *Neuropsychopharmacology* 40, 996–1004. doi: 10.1038/npp.2014.277

Hyman, S. M., Garcia, M., and Sinha, R. (2006). Gender specific associations between types of childhood maltreatment and the onset, escalation and severity of substance use in cocaine dependent adults. *Am. J. Drug Alcohol Abuse* 32, 655–664. doi: 10.1080/10623320600919193

Hyman, S. M., Paliwal, P., Chaplin, T. M., Mazure, C. M., Rounsaville, B. J., and Sinha, R. (2008). Severity of childhood trauma is predictive of cocaine relapse outcomes in women but not men. *Drug Alcohol Depend.* 92, 208–216. doi: 10.1016/j.drugalcdep.2007.08.006

Izquierdo, A., Brigman, J. L., Radke, A. K., Rudebeck, P. H., and Holmes, A. (2017). The neural basis of reversal learning: an updated perspective. *Neuroscience* 345, 12–26. doi: 10.1016/j.neuroscience.2016.03.021

Jentsch, J. D., Olausson, P., De La Garza, R. II., and Taylor, J. R. (2002). Impairments of reversal learning and response perseveration after repeated, intermittent cocaine administrations to monkeys. *Neuropsychopharmacology* 26, 183–190. doi: 10.1016/s0893-133x(01)00355-4

Jentsch, J. D., and Taylor, J. R. (1999). Impulsivity resulting from frontostriatal dysfunction in drug abuse: implications for the control of behavior by reward-related stimuli. *Psychopharmacology* 146, 373–390. doi: 10.1007/pl00005483

Jett, J. D., and Morilak, D. A. (2013). Too much of a good thing: blocking noradrenergic facilitation in medial prefrontal cortex prevents the detrimental effects of chronic stress on cognition. *Neuropsychopharmacology* 38, 585–595. doi: 10.1038/npp.2012.216

Kessler, R. C., Davis, C. G., and Kendler, K. S. (1997). Childhood adversity and adult psychiatric disorder in the US National Comorbidity Survey. *Psychol. Med.* 27, 1101–1119. doi: 10.1017/s0033291797005588

Kessler, R. C., McGonagle, K. A., Swartz, M., Blazer, D. G., and Nelson, C. B. (1993). Sex and depression in the National Comorbidity Survey. I: lifetime prevalence, chronicity and recurrence. *J. Affect. Disord.* 29, 85–96. doi: 10.1016/0165-0327(93)90026-g

Korenbrot, C. C., Huhtaniemi, I. T., and Weiner, R. I. (1977). Preputial separation as an external sign of pubertal development in the male rat. *Biol. Reprod.* 17, 298–303. doi: 10.1095/biolreprod17.2.298

Kruzich, P. J., and Grandy, D. K. (2004). Dopamine D_2 receptors mediate two-odor discrimination and reversal learning in C57BL/6 mice. *BMC Neurosci.* 5:12. doi: 10.1186/1471-2202-5-12

Kuehner, C. (2003). Gender differences in unipolar depression: an update of epidemiological findings and possible explanations. *Acta Psychiatr. Scand.* 108, 163–174. doi: 10.1034/j.1600-0447.2003.00204.x

Laughlin, R. E., Grant, T. L., Williams, R. W., and Jentsch, J. D. (2011). Genetic dissection of behavioral flexibility: reversal learning in mice. *Biol. Psychiatry* 69, 1109–1116. doi: 10.1016/j.biopsych.2011.01.014

Lee, B., Groman, S., London, E. D., and Jentsch, J. D. (2007). Dopamine D2/D3 receptors play a specific role in the reversal of a learned visual discrimination in monkeys. *Neuropsychopharmacology* 32, 2125–2134. doi: 10.1038/sj.npp.1301337

Leussis, M. P., and Andersen, S. L. (2008). Is adolescence a sensitive period for depression? Behavioral and neuroanatomical findings from a social stress model. *Synapse* 62, 22–30. doi: 10.1002/syn.20462

Leussis, M. P., Lawson, K., Stone, K., and Andersen, S. L. (2008). The enduring effects of an adolescent social stressor on synaptic density, part II: poststress reversal of synaptic loss in the cortex by adinazolam and MK-801. *Synapse* 62, 185–192. doi: 10.1002/syn.20483

Lewis, E. E., Dozier, M., Ackerman, J., and Sepulveda-Kozakowski, S. (2007). The effect of placement instability on adopted children's inhibitory control abilities and oppositional behavior. *Dev. Psychol.* 43, 1415–1427. doi: 10.1037/0012-1649.43.6.1415

Li, X., and Wolf, M. E. (2015). Multiple faces of BDNF in cocaine addiction. *Behav. Brain Res.* 0, 240–254. doi: 10.1016/j.bbr.2014.11.018

London, E. D., Ernst, M., Grant, S., Bonson, K., and Weinstein, A. (2000). Orbitofrontal cortex and human drug abuse: functional imaging. *Cereb. Cortex* 10, 334–342. doi: 10.1093/cercor/10.3.334

Lucantonio, F., Stalnaker, T. A., Shaham, Y., Niv, Y., and Schoenbaum, G. (2012). The impact of orbitofrontal dysfunction on cocaine addiction. *Nat. Neurosci.* 15, 358–366. doi: 10.1038/nn.3014

Lyons, D. M., Lopez, J. M., Yang, C., and Schatzberg, A. F. (2000). Stress-level cortisol treatment impairs inhibitory control of behavior in monkeys. *J. Neurosci.* 20, 7816–7821.

MacMillan, H. L., Fleming, J. E., Streiner, D. L., Lin, E., Boyle, M. H., Jamieson, E., et al. (2001). Childhood abuse and lifetime psychopathology in a community sample. *Am. J. Psychiatry* 158, 1878–1883. doi: 10.1176/appi.ajp.158.11.1878

Marshall, D. F., Passarotti, A. M., Ryan, K. A., Kamali, M., Saunders, E. F., Pester, B., et al. (2016). Deficient inhibitory control as an outcome of childhood trauma. *Psychiatry Res.* 235, 7–12. doi: 10.1016/j.psychres.2015.12.013

Matochik, J. A., London, E. D., Eldreth, D. A., Cadet, J. L., and Bolla, K. I. (2003). Frontal cortical tissue composition in abstinent cocaine abusers: a magnetic resonance imaging study. *Neuroimage* 19, 1095–1102. doi: 10.1016/s1053-8119(03)00244-1

McCormick, C. M., and Mathews, I. Z. (2007). HPA function in adolescence: role of sex hormones in its regulation and the enduring consequences of exposure to stressors. *Pharmacol. Biochem. Behav.* 86, 220–233. doi: 10.1016/j.pbb.2006.07.012

Moffitt, T. E., Arseneault, L., Belsky, D., Dickson, N., Hancox, R. J., Harrington, H., et al. (2011). A gradient of childhood self-control predicts health, wealth, and public safety. *Proc. Natl. Acad. Sci. U S A* 108, 2693–2698. doi: 10.1073/pnas.1010076108

Monteggia, L. M., Luikart, B., Barrot, M., Theobold, D., Malkovska, I., Nef, S., et al. (2007). Brain-derived neurotrophic factor conditional knockouts show gender differences in depression-related behaviors. *Biol. Psychiatry* 61, 187–197. doi: 10.1016/j.biopsych.2006.03.021

Moreno-López, L., Perales, J. C., van Son, D., Albein-Urios, N., Soriano-Mas, C., Martinez-Gonzalez, J. M., et al. (2015). Cocaine use severity and cerebellar gray matter are associated with reversal learning deficits in cocaine-dependent individuals. *Addict. Biol.* 20, 546–566. doi: 10.1111/adb.12143

Mueller, S. C., Maheu, F. S., Dozier, M., Peloso, E., Mandell, D., Leibenluft, E., et al. (2010). Early-life stress is associated with impairment in cognitive control in adolescence: an fMRI study. *Neuropsychologia* 48, 3037–3044. doi: 10.1016/j.neuropsychologia.2010.06.013

Netherton, C., Goodyear, I., Tamplin, A., and Herbert, J. (2004). Salivary cortisol and dehydroepiandrosterone in relation to puberty and gender. *Psychoneuroendocrinology* 29, 125–140. doi: 10.1016/S0306-4530(02)00150-6

Nigg, J. T., Wong, M. M., Martel, M. M., Jester, J. M., Puttler, L. I., Glass, J. M., et al. (2006). Poor response inhibition as a predictor of problem drinking and illicit drug use in adolescents at risk for alcoholism and other substance use disorders. *J. Am. Acad. Child Adolesc. Psychiatry* 45, 468–475. doi: 10.1097/01.chi.0000199028.76452.a9

Numakawa, T., Adachi, N., Richards, M., Chiba, S., and Kunugi, H. (2013). Brain-derived neurotrophic factor and glucocorticoids: reciprocal influence on the central nervous system. *Neuroscience* 239, 157–172. doi: 10.1016/j.neuroscience.2012.09.073

Petanjek, Z., Judaš, M., Šimic, G., Rasin, M. R., Uylings, H. B., Rakic, P., et al. (2011). Extraordinary neoteny of synaptic spines in the human prefrontal cortex. *Proc. Natl. Acad. Sci. U S A* 108, 13281–13286. doi: 10.1073/pnas.1105108108

Pitts, E. G., Taylor, J. R., and Gourley, S. L. (2016). Prefrontal cortical BDNF: a regulatory key in cocaine- and food-reinforced behaviors. *Neurobiol. Dis.* 91, 326–335. doi: 10.1016/j.nbd.2016.02.021

Regner, M. F., Dalwani, M., Yamamoto, D., Perry, R. I., Sakai, J. T., Honce, J. M., et al. (2015). Sex differences in gray matter changes and brain-behavior relationships in patients with stimulant dependence. *Radiology* 277, 801–812. doi: 10.1148/radiol.2015142541

Ridley, R. M., Haystead, T. A., and Baker, H. F. (1981). An analysis of visual object reversal learning in the marmoset after amphetamine and haloperidol. *Pharmacol. Biochem. Behav.* 14, 345–351. doi: 10.1016/0091-3057(81)90401-9

Sacks, J. Y., McKendrick, K., and Banks, S. (2008). The impact of early trauma and abuse on residential substance abuse treatment outcomes for women. *J. Subst. Abuse Treat.* 34, 90–100. doi: 10.1016/j.jsat.2007.01.010

Sakata, K., Martinowich, K., Woo, N. H., Schloesser, R. J., Jimenez, D. V., Ji, Y., et al. (2013). Role of activity-dependent BDNF expression in hippocampal-prefrontal cortical regulation of behavioral perseverance. *Proc. Natl. Acad. Sci. U S A* 110, 15103–15108. doi: 10.1073/pnas.1222872110

Schoenbaum, G., Saddoris, M. P., Ramus, S. J., Shaham, Y., and Setlow, B. (2004). Cocaine-experienced rats exhibit learning deficits in a task sensitive to orbitofrontal cortex lesions. *Eur. J. Neurosci.* 19, 1997–2002. doi: 10.1111/j.1460-9568.2004.03274.x

Schwandt, M. L., Heilig, M., Hommer, D. W., George, D. T., and Ramchandani, V. A. (2013). Childhood trauma exposure and alcohol dependence severity in adulthood: mediation by emotional abuse severity and neuroticism. *Alcohol. Clin. Exp. Res.* 37, 984–992. doi: 10.1111/acer.12053

Selemon, L. D. (2013). A role for synaptic plasticity in the adolescent development of executive function. *Transl. Psychiatry* 3:e238. doi: 10.1038/tp.2013.7

Shapiro, L. P., Omar, M. H., Koleske, A. J., and Gourley, S. L. (2017a). Corticosteroid-induced dendrite loss and behavioral deficiencies can be blocked by activation of Abl2/Arg kinase. *Mol. Cell. Neurosci.* 85, 226–234. doi: 10.1016/j.mcn.2017.10.007

Shapiro, L. P., Parsons, R. G., Koleske, A. J., and Gourley, S. L. (2017b). Differential expression of cytoskeletal regulatory factors in the adolescent prefrontal cortex: implications for cortical development. *J. Neurosci. Res.* 95, 1123–1143. doi: 10.1002/jnr.23960

Simpson, T., and Miller, W. (2002). Concomitance between childhood sexual and physical abuse and substance use problems: a review. *Clin. Psychol. Rev.* 22, 27–77. doi: 10.1016/s0272-7358(00)00088-x

Skowron, E. A., Cipriano-Essel, E., Gatzke-Kopp, L. M., Teti, D. M., and Ammerman, R. T. (2014). Early adversity, RSA, and inhibitory control: evidence of children's neurobiological sensitivity to social context. *Dev. Psychobiol.* 56, 964–978. doi: 10.1002/dev.21175

Snyder, K. P., Barry, M., and Valentino, R. J. (2015). Cognitive impact of social stress and coping strategy throughout development. *Psychopharmacology* 232, 185–195. doi: 10.1007/s00213-014-3654-7

Spear, L. P. (2000). The adolescent brain and age-related behavioral manifestations. *Neurosci. Biobehav. Rev.* 24, 417–463. doi: 10.1016/s0149-7634(00)00014-2

Stroud, L. R., Papandonatos, G. D., Williamson, D. E., and Dahl, R. E. (2011). Sex differences in cortisol response to corticotropin releasing hormone challenge over puberty: pittsburgh Pediatric Neurobehavioral Studies. *Psychoneuroendocrinology* 36, 1226–1238. doi: 10.1016/j.psyneuen.2011.02.017

Suri, D., and Vaidya, V. A. (2013). Glucocorticoid regulation of brain-derived neurotrophic factor: relevance to hippocampal structure and functional plasticity. *Neuroscience* 239, 196–213. doi: 10.1016/j.neuroscience.2012.08.065

Tanabe, J., Tregellas, J. R., Dalwani, M., Thompson, L., Owens, E., Crowley, T., et al. (2009). Medial orbitofrontal cortex gray matter is reduced in abstinent substance-dependent individuals. *Biol. Psychiatry* 65, 160–164. doi: 10.1016/j.biopsych.2008.07.030

Tarter, R. E., Kirisci, L., Habeych, M., Reynolds, M., and Vanyukov, M. (2004). Neurobehavior disinhibition in childhood predisposes boys to substance use disorder by young adulthood: direct and mediated etiologic pathways. *Drug Alcohol Depend.* 73, 121–132. doi: 10.1016/j.drugalcdep.2003.07.004

Teicher, M. H., and Samson, J. A. (2016). Annual research review: enduring neurobiological effects of childhood abuse and neglect. *J. Child Psychol. Psychiatry* 57, 241–266. doi: 10.1111/jcpp.12507

Vigers, A. J., Amin, D. S., Talley-Farnham, T., Gorski, J. A., Xu, B., and Jones, K. R. (2012). Sustained expression of brain-derived neurotrophic factor is required for the maintenance of dendritic spines and normal behavior. *Neuroscience* 212, 1–18. doi: 10.1016/j.neuroscience.2012.03.031

Viola, T. W., Wearick-Silva, L. E., De Azeredo, L. A., Centeno-Silva, A., Murphy, C., Mashall, P., et al. (2016). Increased cocaine-induced conditioned place preference during periadolescence in maternally separated male BALB/c mice: the role of cortical BDNF, microRNA-212, and MeCP2. *Psychopharmacology* 233, 3279–3288. doi: 10.1007/s00213-016-4373-z

Warnault, V., Darcq, E., Morisot, N., Phamluong, K., Wilbrecht, L., Massa, S. M., et al. (2016). The BDNF valine 68 to methionine polymorphism increases compulsive alcohol drinking in mice that is reversed by tropomyosin receptor kinase B activation. *Biol. Psychiatry* 79, 463–473. doi: 10.1016/j.biopsych.2015.06.007

Watt, M. J., Weber, M. A., Davies, S. R., and Forster, G. L. (2017). Impact of juvenile chronic stress on adult cortico-accumbal function: implications for cognition and addiction. *Prog. Neuropsychopharmacol. Biol. Psychiatry* 79, 136–154. doi: 10.1016/j.pnpbp.2017.06.015

Webster, M. J., Weickert, C. S., Herman, M. M., and Kleinman, J. E. (2002). BDNF mRNA expression during postnatal development, maturation and aging of the human prefrontal cortex. *Dev. Brain Res.* 139, 139–150. doi: 10.1016/s0165-3806(02)00540-0

Widom, C. S., and White, H. R. (1997). Problem behaviors in abused and neglected children grown-up: prevalence and co-occurrence of substance abuse, crime and violence. *Crim. Behav. Ment. Health* 7, 287–310. doi: 10.1002/cbm.191

Winhusen, T., and Lewis, D. (2013). Sex differences in disinhibition and its relationship to physical abuse in a sample of stimulant-dependent patients. *Drug Alcohol Depend.* 129, 158–162. doi: 10.1016/j.drugalcdep.2012.09.014

Wright, L. D., Hebert, K. E., and Perrot-Sinal, T. S. (2008). Periadolescent stress exposure exerts long-term effects on adult stress responding and expression of prefrontal dopamine receptors in male and female rats. *Psychoneuroendocrinology* 33, 130–142. doi: 10.1016/j.psyneuen.2007.10.009

Xu, B., Zang, K., Ruff, N. L., Zhang, Y. A., McConnell, S. K., Stryker, M. P., et al. (2000). Cortical degeneration in the absence of neurotrophin signaling: dendritic retraction and neuronal loss after removal of the receptor TrkB. *Neuron* 26, 233–245. doi: 10.1016/S0896-6273(00)81153-8

Xu, H., Zhang, Y., Zhang, F., Yuan, S. N., Shao, F., and Wang, W. (2016). Effects of duloxetine treatment on cognitive flexibility and BDNF expression in the mPFC of adult male mice exposed to social stress during adolescence. *Front. Mol. Neurosci.* 9:95. doi: 10.3389/fnmol.2016.00095

Yoshii, A., and Constantine-Paton, M. (2010). Postsynaptic BDNF-TrkB signaling in synapse maturation, plasticity, and disease. *Dev. Neurobiol.* 70, 304–322. doi: 10.1002/dneu.20765

Zhang, Y., Shao, F., Wang, Q., Xie, X., and Wang, W. (2017). Neuroplastic correlates in the mPFC underlying the impairment of stress-coping ability and cognitive flexibility in adult rats exposed to chronic mild stress during adolescence. *Neural Plast.* 2017:9382797. doi: 10.1155/2017/9382797

Zhang, J. C., Wu, J., Fujita, Y., Yao, W., Ren, Q., Yang, C., et al. (2014). Antidepressant effects of trkB ligands on depression-like behavior and dendritic changes in mice after inflammation. *Int. J. Neuropsychopharmacol.* 18:pyu077. doi: 10.1093/ijnp/pyu077

Zhang, F., Yuan, S., Shao, F., and Wang, W. (2016). Adolescent social defeat induced alterations in social behavior and cognitive flexibility in adult mice: effects of developmental stage and social condition. *Front. Behav. Neurosci.* 10:149. doi: 10.3389/fnbeh.2016.00149

10

Maladaptive Decision Making in Adults with a History of Adolescent Alcohol use, in a Preclinical Model, is Attributable to the Compromised Assignment of Incentive Value during Stimulus-Reward Learning

Lauren C. Kruse[1], *Abigail G. Schindler*[1,2], *Rapheal G. Williams*[3], *Sophia J. Weber*[1] *and Jeremy J. Clark*[1]*

[1]Department of Psychiatry and Behavioral Sciences, University of Washington, Seattle, WA, United States, [2]Geriatric Research Education and Clinical Center, VA Puget Sound Health Care System, Seattle, WA, United States, [3]Graduate Program in Neuroscience, University of Washington, Seattle, WA, United States

Edited by:
Jacqueline M. Barker,
Medical University of South Carolina,
United States

Reviewed by:
Jocelyn M. Richard,
Johns Hopkins University,
United States
Alicia Izquierdo,
University of California, Los Angeles,
United States

***Correspondence:**
Jeremy J. Clark
jjc1@uw.edu

According to recent WHO reports, alcohol remains the number one substance used and abused by adolescents, despite public health efforts to curb its use. Adolescence is a critical period of biological maturation where brain development, particularly the mesocorticolimbic dopamine system, undergoes substantial remodeling. These circuits are implicated in complex decision making, incentive learning and reinforcement during substance use and abuse. An appealing theoretical approach has been to suggest that alcohol alters the normal development of these processes to promote deficits in reinforcement learning and decision making, which together make individuals vulnerable to developing substance use disorders in adulthood. Previously we have used a preclinical model of voluntary alcohol intake in rats to show that use in adolescence promotes risky decision making in adulthood that is mirrored by selective perturbations in dopamine network dynamics. Further, we have demonstrated that incentive learning processes in adulthood are also altered by adolescent alcohol use, again mirrored by changes in cue-evoked dopamine signaling. Indeed, we have proposed that these two processes, risk-based decision making and incentive learning, are fundamentally linked through dysfunction of midbrain circuitry where inputs to the dopamine system are disrupted by adolescent alcohol use. Here, we test the behavioral predictions of this model in rats and present the findings in the context of the prevailing literature with reference to the long-term consequences of early-life substance use on the vulnerability to develop substance use disorders. We utilize an impulsive choice task to assess the selectivity of alcohol's effect on decision-making profiles and conditioned reinforcement to parse out the effect of incentive value attribution, one mechanism of incentive learning. Finally, we use the differential reinforcement of low rates of responding (DRL) task to examine the degree to which behavioral disinhibition may contribute to an overall decision-making profile. The findings presented here support the proposition that early life alcohol use selectively alters risk-based choice behavior through modulation of incentive learning processes, both of which may be inexorably linked through perturbations in mesolimbic circuitry and may serve as fundamental vulnerabilities to the development of substance use disorders.

Keywords: adolescent, alcohol, decision making, incentive learning, risk taking, impulsivity

INTRODUCTION

Adolescence is characterized by risky and impulsive behaviors, often including initial experimentation with drugs of abuse and most commonly, alcohol (Casey and Jones, 2010). During development, the adolescent brain undergoes substantial maturation in cortical and limbic regions involved in impulsive behaviors, decision making and reward processing (Spear, 2000; Chambers et al., 2003; Crews et al., 2007; Bava and Tapert, 2010; Marinelli and McCutcheon, 2014). Given the high vulnerability of these developing regions to the damaging effects of alcohol (Chambers et al., 2003; Pascual et al., 2009; Bava and Tapert, 2010), exposure during this critical time period can produce long-term neurobiological and behavioral changes that increase risk for chronic alcohol problems later in adulthood. In clinical work, alcohol use has been associated with deficits in adaptive decision making strategies, impulsivity and reward valuation (Goudriaan et al., 2007; Johnson et al., 2008; Brevers et al., 2014).

Using a probability discounting task coupled with a preclinical model of voluntary adolescent alcohol use, our laboratory previously demonstrated that rats with a history of adolescent alcohol use opt for more risky decision-making strategies when they are adults, consistent with findings in humans (Brevers et al., 2014; Schindler et al., 2014). This increase in risk preference is specific to adolescent alcohol use as adult animals with identical alcohol exposure do not differ in the probability discounting task (Schindler et al., 2014). Subsequent reports have demonstrated that this behavioral phenotype following adolescent alcohol use is robust (Nasrallah et al., 2011; Clark et al., 2012; Schindler et al., 2014), reproducible (Boutros et al., 2014; McMurray et al., 2014), and translates to the human condition (Brevers et al., 2014). These three core features: robust, reproducible and translational make up the fundamental elements of a successful pre-clinical model of attributes that may correspond to vulnerabilities to the development of substance abuse and alcohol use disorders (Collins and Tabak, 2014).

In addition, we have identified a neural correlate of maladaptive decision making in the mesolimbic dopamine system that is promoted by early life alcohol use. Adult animals with a history of alcohol use in adolescence show increased phasic dopamine release in the nucleus accumbens core in response to risky options and pavlovian incentive cues when compared to controls (Nasrallah et al., 2011; Spoelder et al., 2015). The mesolimbic dopamine system is implicated in reinforcement learning, goal-directed behavior and motivational processes, and may be particularly critical when these behaviors are associated with the craving and seeking of abused substances (Kelley, 2004; Everitt and Robbins, 2005; Salamone and Correa, 2012). Further examination of this mesolimbic circuit revealed a potentiation in the excitatory drive on ventral tegmental area dopamine neurons from the pedunculopontine nucleus (PPT) in animals with a history of adolescent alcohol use (Schindler et al., 2016). This is particularly striking given the important role that this structure is thought to play in both incentive-based reinforcement learning (Pan and Hyland, 2005) and choice behavior under uncertainty (Leblond et al., 2014). Importantly, we were able to demonstrate that pharmacological mitigation of this increased PPT drive was capable of completely rescuing maladaptive risk preference in animals with a history of adolescent alcohol use (Schindler et al., 2016). We have therefore hypothesized that maladaptive decision making under risk as a result of adolescent alcohol use perturbing the mesolimbic dopamine system may result from a selective deficit in incentive learning (Clark et al., 2012; Spoelder et al., 2015).

However, both risk-seeking and risk-taking behaviors have been previously attributed to impulsivity, which is another potential underlying mechanism influencing altered decision making. The concept of impulsivity incorporates various behaviors, but is commonly separated into two important features: impulsive choice and impulsive action, both of which are linked to addiction (Evenden, 1999; Olmstead, 2006; Winstanley et al., 2010). Indeed, preclinical and clinical studies have long identified impulsivity and risky decision making as behaviors contributing to the development and perpetuation of substance use disorders, including alcohol (Littlefield and Sher, 2010; Brevers et al., 2014; Jupp and Dalley, 2014a,b). Delay discounting is commonly used as a measure of impulsive decision making and performance on this task has historically been linked with performance on probability discounting tasks (Richards et al., 1999). In addition to the temporal delay of rewards influencing decision making, the amount of effort required to receive a reward can also influence choice. Several studies have connected dopamine signaling with mediating choice in the effort discounting task, but the role of alcohol, and particularly adolescent alcohol use, on effort discounting remains unclear (Floresco et al., 2008; Day et al., 2010; Ghods-Sharifi and Floresco, 2010). Interestingly, recent reports propose that performance on delay discounting and probability discounting require different decision-making processes with separate underlying neurobiological mechanisms (van Gaalen et al., 2006; Olson et al., 2007; St Onge and Floresco, 2009; Green and Myerson, 2013). In the present studies, we examine the effect of voluntary adolescent alcohol intake on impulsivity and incentive attribution to differentiate the potential role impulsivity may play in risk preference from the role incentive learning may play.

We examined differences in incentive attribution as a result of adolescent alcohol intake using Pavlovian conditioning and conditioned reinforcement, the gold standard for examining acquired motivational properties through learning. We also examined the two primary features of impulsivity, impulsive choice and impulsive action, using delay-discounting and the differential reinforcement of low rates of responding (DRL) tasks, respectively. The purpose of these studies is to further test our hypothesis that incentive based learning and assignment of motivational value through reinforcement learning, not impulsivity, is the underlying psychological mechanism of maladaptive decision making after early life alcohol use. Our results show that adults exposed to alcohol during adolescence exhibit enhanced attribution of value to reward-predictive cues compared to controls. Alternatively, we find no significant difference between alcohol-exposed and control animals on either measure of impulsivity (impulsive choice and action). Therefore, we provide further compelling evidence that adolescent alcohol use promotes disadvantageous decision making by altering a learning-based incentive attribution process and not through a general mechanism of impulsivity.

MATERIALS AND METHODS

Animals and Housing

Male Sprague-Dawley rats (Charles River, Hollister, CA, USA) were weaned at postnatal day (PND) 21 and aged PND 27 at the start of experiments. All animals were housed individually in polycarbonate tubs on a 12-h light/dark cycle (lights on at 06:00). Animals were housed individually for accurate assessment of alcohol gel consumption. Water and Teklad (Harlan, Kent, WA, USA) rodent chow was available *ad libitum* except as noted. Rats were weighed and handled daily throughout the course of the experiment. All work in this manuscript was conducted under the guidance and permission of the Institutional Animal Care and Use Committee at the University of Washington and pursuant to federal regulations regarding work with animals.

Alcohol Preparation, Administration and Withdrawal

Alcohol was presented to adolescent (PND 30–49) rats in a gel matrix consisting of distilled water, Knox gelatin, polycose (10%) and 190-proof ethanol (10%). Control gels had ethanol replaced with distilled water. Preparation was as previously described (Rowland et al., 2005; Nasrallah et al., 2011; Schindler et al., 2014). The gels were made available 24 h/day, unless otherwise noted, in addition to *ad libitum* water and chow. Alcohol gel intake levels were monitored daily and expressed in g/kg of body weight using individual gel consumption and body weights measured daily. Rats failing to consume gel during the control gel pre-exposure, exhibiting three consecutive days of no consumption, or burying of the gel in bedding once the alcohol gel exposure began were excluded from the study. Experiments began with 3 days of pre-exposure to control gel. Subsequently, adolescent rats were each split into alcohol gel and control gel groups matched by weight and baseline intake. Twenty days of 24 h/day gel exposure followed. Upon completion of the 20-day exposure to ethanol rats were monitored daily for withdrawal symptoms (e.g., seizures, weight loss and anxious behavior) for the following 20 days. No overt signs of withdrawal were observed.

Instrumental Training

All behavioral experiments were conducted in standard Med Associates chambers (St. Albans, VT, USA). For all tasks, prior to the beginning of training, animals were food restricted to maintain them at $\sim 90 \pm 2\%$ free-feeding weight. Free-feeding weight was based on pre-restriction weights. The rewards for instrumental responses and during Pavlovian conditioning were 45-mg sucrose pellets (Bio Serve, Prospect, CT, USA). Rats underwent magazine training before all tasks where 10 sucrose pellets were delivered over 15 min. For delay discounting and DRL, rats were trained on a fixed ratio 1 schedule to a criterion of ≥ 24 responses in a 30-min session. For delay discounting, once criterion was met, rats were auto-shaped over the course of 5 days (day 1 of auto-shaping required rats to perform a nosepoke into the food tray for trial initiation; day 2 increased the inter-trial interval (ITI) from 0 s to 15 s; day 3 reduced the time to perform trial-initiating nosepoke to 10 s; day 4 increased the ITI from 15 s to 30 s; day 5 increased the ITI from 30 s to 45 s).

Pavlovian Conditioned Approach and Conditioned Reinforcement

Following magazine training, rats underwent 7 days of pavlovian training with 25 trials per day. For each training session, a trial consisted of the extension of a lever (left or right, counterbalanced between animals) into the chamber along with illumination of a cue light above the lever (conditioned stimulus, CS) for 8 s, followed immediately by the delivery of two sucrose pellets (unconditioned stimulus, US) into the food tray and illumination of the tray light. The CS-US presentations occurred on a 60 s variable ITI schedule for each session. Lever presses and cup entries during lever presentation were recorded as measures of pavlovian conditioned approach. Total number of lever presses and food tray head entries during lever presentation were recorded but had no programmable response.

After 7 days of pavlovian training, all animals underwent a test for conditioned reinforcement. The chambers were rearranged such that the left and right retractable levers flanking the food tray were replaced with nosepoke ports and the food tray was replaced with a single retractable lever. The conditioned reinforcement session lasted a total of 40 min and the houselight was on for the full duration. During the session, nosepokes into the designated "active" port (located on the opposite side of wall as the lever-CS) resulted in insertion of the illuminated lever for 2 s. Nosepokes into the "inactive" port had no programmable consequences. Total number of lever presses, nosepokes into the active port, and nosepokes into the inactive port were recorded.

Delay Discounting

Following instrumental training as outlined above, animals were tested on a concurrent instrumental task involving the presentation of two levers. Each daily session consisted of 24 forced trials followed by 24 free-choice trials, with a total of seven testing sessions. At the start of each session, the chamber was in the ITI state, completely dark with no light cues. All trials began with illumination of the house light and a light in the food tray cueing the animal to make a nosepoke into the food tray within 10 s. Failure to nosepoke resulted in trial termination, and the chamber returned to the ITI state. During training, animals were exposed to forced trials wherein a successful nosepoke led to the extension of a single lever, presented pseudo-randomly. These trials served to expose the animal to each option and its associated expected value. During each session, forced choice trials were followed by free-choice trials with the same contingency for each lever. Free-choice trials follow the guidelines described above, but each successful nosepoke resulted in the extension of both levers, and the animal was free to choose between the two levers within 10 s. During both forced- and free-choice trials, one lever was associated with the delivery two sucrose pellets after 1 s and the other lever associated with the delivery of four sucrose pellets after an increasing delay of time (either 1, 2, 4, 8, 16, 32 and 64 s). Increasing delay times were tested in separate testing sessions (days) with a 1 s delay on the first day of testing, a 2 s delay on the second day of testing, and so on for all animals. This method of testing the different delay times on separate days was done in order to be kept consistent with our previous studies using the probability discounting task where the different probabilistic deliveries of reward were also tested on separate, subsequent days. Each session assessed the animal's preference between the two levers. Choice of the high reward lever was recorded during free-choice trials.

DRL

Following instrumental training as described above, animals were tested on the DRL task as a measure of impulsive action. Each 45 min session began with illumination of the house light and lever presentation. Each animal was assigned an active lever (left or right) counterbalanced between rats, which remained extended throughout the duration of the sessions. For the first 5 days, rats were tested using a 5 s DRL interval, in which a lever press resulted in pellet delivery only if at least 5 s elapsed since the previous press. Each lever press that occurred before the required 5 s wait period resulted in a resetting of the 5 s criteria, during which animals would have to wait another 5 s before pressing the lever to receive a pellet. Following five consecutive days of the 5 s DRL, the schedule was then switched to a 10 s DRL interval for 5 days, then to a 20 s DRL interval for 5 days, and finally to a 30 s DRL interval for 5 days. The total number of lever presses and the total number of reinforcers received were recorded. Percent of effective lever presses was also determined by dividing the total number of pellets received by total number of lever presses.

Statistical Analyses

All statistical analyses were conducted using GraphPad Prism 6. Behavioral data for the pavlovian training sessions were binned into five-trial epochs. A response bias score, which is a measure of the relative allocation of behavioral responses between the lever and food tray during pavlovian training, was calculated by subtracting the number of food tray entries from the number of lever presses divided by the sum of both responses: (lever press − food tray entries/(lever presses + food tray entries), resulting in a number ranging from −1 (goal-tracking response) to +1 (sign-tracking response; Meyer et al., 2012). Animals with a response bias >+0.70 were defined as animals with a strong sign-tracking bias and animals with a response bias <−0.70 were defined as having a strong goal-tracking bias, consistent with previous work (Flagel et al., 2011; Meyer et al., 2012; Spoelder et al., 2015). Conditioned responses (lever presses and food tray entries) from all phases of training were analyzed using repeated measures two-way analysis of variance (ANOVA) with treatment (alcohol and control) and trial bin treated as independent variables. Performance on the conditioned reinforcement test was analyzed using a two-way ANOVA with treatment (alcohol vs. control) and port (active vs. inactive) as the independent variables and the number of nosepokes as the dependent variable. A *t*-test was used to analyze total number of lever presses during the conditioned reinforcement test. Performance on the delay-discounting and DRL tasks were analyzed using repeated measures two-way ANOVA with treatment (alcohol vs. control) and delay (1 s, 2 s, 4 s, 8 s, 16 s, 32 s, and 64 s) or DRL interval (5, 10, 20, 30 s) as the independent variables, and preference for the high reward lever or lever presses, reinforcers and effective lever presses, respectively, as the dependent variables. Bonferroni *post hoc* analyses were used and were corrected for multiple comparisons. All data are presented as mean ± SEM and threshold for statistical significance was set at $p < 0.05$.

RESULTS

Adolescent Alcohol Intake

For the conditioned reinforcement, delay-discounting and DRL animals, average alcohol intake across the 20-day exposure period was 11.3 ± 1.6 g/kg, 12.0 ± 2.3 g/kg, and 15.4 ± 1.5 g/kg, respectively, and intake did not differ across behavior groups ($F_{(2,30)\ group} = 2.1$, NS). Across all three behavioral experiments, a total of 10% of rats did not consume the alcohol gelatin during the 20 exposure days and thus were not run in the behavioral studies. These intake levels are comparable to our previous studies further supporting this method of alcohol intake as a consistent model of moderate/recreational alcohol use (Nasrallah et al., 2011; Schindler et al., 2014; Spoelder et al., 2015). Blood alcohol levels were not obtained but have been assessed previously (Schindler et al., 2014).

The Effect of Adolescent Alcohol Intake on Acquisition of Pavlovian Conditioned Approach Behavior in Adulthood

Consistent with previously published data (Spoelder et al., 2015), pavlovian conditioned responses to either the reward-predicting lever (sign tracking) or the food tray (goal tracking) during CS presentation developed differently for alcohol-exposed and control animals over the 7 days of pavlovian training. Although both groups developed a response bias towards sign-tracking over the course of training ($F_{(34,986)\ trial\ bin} = 57.2$

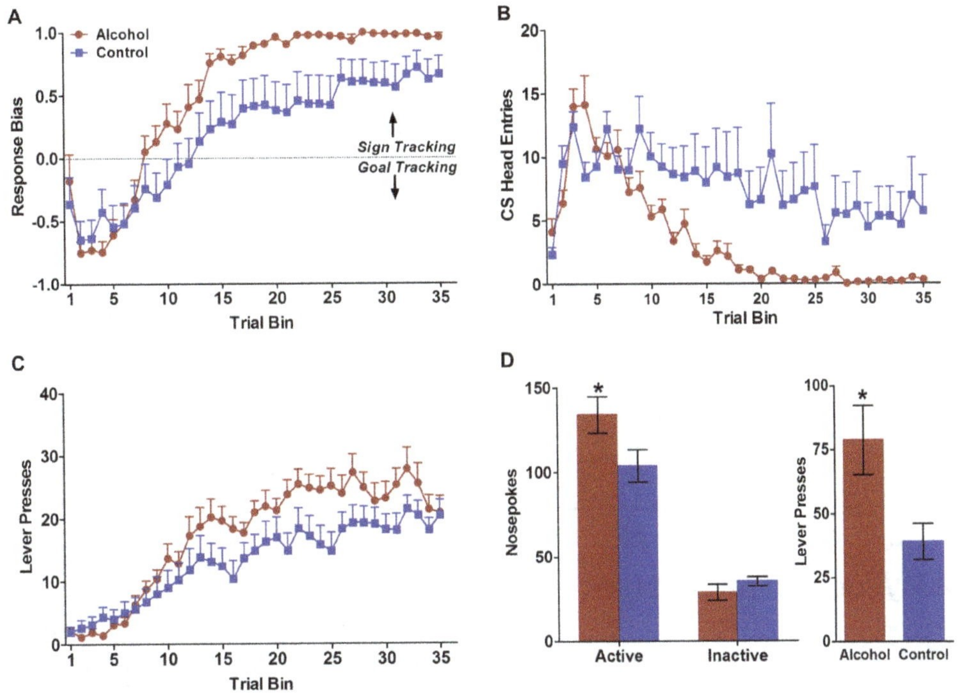

FIGURE 1 | Behavioral responses during pavlovian conditioned approach and test for conditioned reinforcement. **(A)** Alcohol-exposed (n = 16) animals reduced their conditioned responses to the food tray, whereas control (n = 15) animals continued to approach the food tray throughout the course of learning. **(B)** Both alcohol-exposed and control animals increased their conditioned responses to the reward-predicting lever over the course of learning but alcohol-exposed animals demonstrated a stronger conditioned response to the lever throughout the course of learning. **(C)** Both alcohol-exposed and control animals developed a response-bias toward sign tracking over the course of learning, but alcohol-exposed animals developed a stronger sign-tracker response bias. **(D)** In the test for conditioned reinforcement alcohol-exposed animals designated as sign trackers (n = 12) made significantly more active nosepokes compared to controls (n = 9). Alcohol-exposed and control animals did not differ in inactive nosepokes. All data are presented as mean ± SEM. *$P < 0.05$.

$p < 0.0001$; **Figure 1A**), the alcohol-exposed animals showed a stronger sign-tracking bias relative to controls later in the conditioning trials ($F_{(34,986)\ \text{trial bin} \times \text{treatment}} = 2.6$, $p < 0.001$; $F_{(1,986)\ \text{treatment}} = 4.3$, $p < 0.05$; **Figure 1A**). Further, both alcohol-exposed and control animals demonstrated reduced conditioned responding to the food tray over trials ($F_{(34,986)\ \text{trial bin}} = 14.0$, $p < 0.0001$; **Figure 1B**), but alcohol-exposed animals largely stopped responding to the food tray by trial bin 20 ($F_{(34,986)\ \text{trial bin} \times \text{treatment}} = 3.9$, $p < 0.0001$; $F_{(1,986)\ \text{treatment}} = 4.6$, $p < 0.05$ **Figure 1B**). Both alcohol-exposed animals and controls showed increased responses towards the lever over trials ($F_{(34,986)\ \text{trial bin}} = 40.6$, $p < 0.0001$; **Figure 1C**), but a greater number of contacts upon cue presentation in alcohol-exposed animals compared to controls developed over trial bins ($F_{(34,986)\ \text{trial bin} \times \text{treatment}} = 2.0$, $p < 0.001$; **Figure 1C**). Response-bias scores were also calculated as described above in the methods section. Animals with scores greater than +0.70 were designated as sign trackers and animals with scores less than −0.70 were designated as goal trackers. Based on these criteria, 13 out of 16 alcohol-exposed animals were sign trackers and 10 out of 15 control animals were sign trackers. Of the remaining eight animals, three alcohol-exposed and five controls had response bias scores that fell between −0.70 and +0.70 and therefore did not show a strong enough response to be classified as sign or goal trackers.

The Effect of Adolescent Alcohol Intake on Conditioned Reinforcement in Adulthood

All animals underwent the test of conditioned reinforcement following pavlovian training. However, given that this task measures the effectiveness of the lever-CS as a reinforcer (defining a strong sign-tracker bias), we were primarily interested in the behavior of sign-tracking animals. Therefore, only the 23 animals designated as sign trackers based on the above mentioned criterion (>+0.70 response bias score) were kept in the analyses. One sign tracker from each treatment group was dropped because the incorrect active port was assigned for the conditioned reinforcement test yielding n = 12 alcohol sign-trackers and n = 9 control sign-trackers for the final analyses. During the test of conditioned reinforcement, alcohol rats displayed more incentive attribution to the lever-CS compared to control rats. Specifically, both treatment groups made more active than inactive nosepokes ($F_{(1,38)\ \text{port}} = 116.4$, $p < 0.0001$; **Figure 1D**), but sign trackers with a history of adolescent alcohol intake demonstrated significantly more nosepokes in the active port compared to controls ($F_{(1,38)\ \text{treatment} \times \text{port}} = 5.2$, $p < 0.05$; **Figure 1D**), with no difference between alcohol and control animals in the inactive port confirmed by follow-up tests ($p < 0.05$). Further, during the 2-s lever extension period following a poke in the active port, alcohol animals also had significantly more

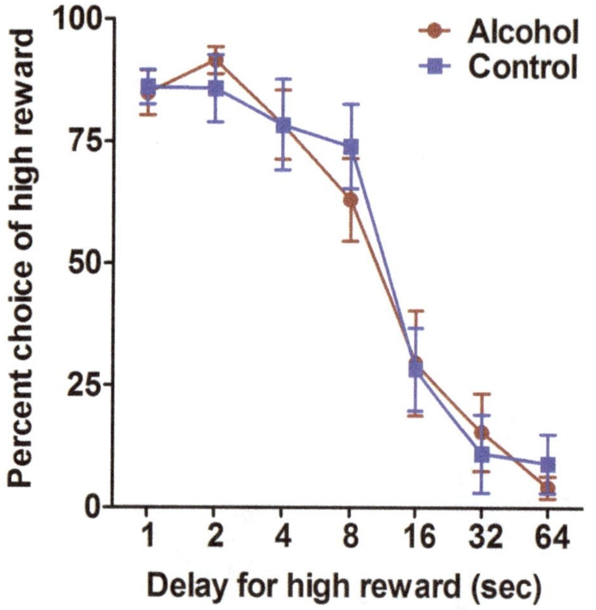

FIGURE 2 | Impulsive choice as measured by performance on the delay-discounting task. Alcohol-exposed ($n = 7$) and control ($n = 6$) animals both demonstrated a decrease in choice of the large reward option with increasing delay. Alcohol-exposed and control animals did not differ in choice behavior over delay conditions. All data are presented as mean ± SEM for the percent of trials on which the larger delayed reward was chosen for 1, 2, 4, 8, 16, 32 and 64 s delay intervals.

lever presses than control animals ($t_{(1,19)} = 2.4$, $p < 0.05$; **Figure 3**). As expected, the alcohol ($n = 3$) and control ($n = 5$) rats that were not classified as sign trackers (response bias scores between −0.70 and +0.70) did not differ in total number of active or inactive nosepokes ($F_{(1,4)\ \text{treatment}} = 0.2$, NS; $F_{(1,4)\ \text{treatment} \times \text{port}} = 0.02$, NS; **Figure 1**). Taken together with the results from Pavlovian conditioned approach, our data indicate that the lever-CS acquired both the attractiveness and wanting properties of an incentive stimulus to a greater extent in the alcohol-exposed animals compared to controls.

The Effect of Adolescent Alcohol Intake on Impulsive Choice in Adulthood

The delay-discounting task was used to assess the effect of adolescent alcohol intake on impulsive choice in adulthood. Analysis of choice behavior on the delay-discounting task generated standard discounting curves for choice of the larger but delayed reward option over all conditions, with increasing delay of the large reward resulting in decreased choice of the large reward option for both alcohol-exposed and control animals ($F_{(6,66)\ \text{delay}} = 62.1$, $p < 0.0001$; **Figure 2**). Alcohol-exposed and control animals did not differ in choice behavior over any of the delay conditions ($F_{(1,66)\ \text{treatment}} = 0.02$, NS; $F_{(6,66)\ \text{delay} \times \text{treatment}} = 0.4$, NS; **Figure 2**). These data indicate that moderate adolescent alcohol intake does not appear to alter impulsive choice in adulthood compared to animals without a history of adolescent alcohol.

The Effect of Adolescent Alcohol Intake on Impulsive Action in Adulthood

The DRL task was used to assess the effect of adolescent alcohol intake on impulsive action in adulthood, as measured by the ability of the animals to withhold responding for reinforcers during 5, 10, 20, and 30 s DRL intervals. Alcohol-exposed animals did not differ from controls on total number of lever presses ($F_{(3,54)\ \text{DRL} \times \text{treatment}} = 0.6$, NS; $F_{(1,54)\ \text{treatment}} = 0.01$, NS; **Figure 3A**) or total number of reinforces received ($F_{(3,54)\ \text{DRL} \times \text{treatment}} = 0.4$, NS; $F_{(1,54)\ \text{treatment}} = 0.02$, NS; **Figure 3B**) at any of the DRL intervals. Effective lever presses were also analyzed as a measure of the percent of lever presses that resulted in delivery of the reward. Alcohol treatment during adolescence did not alter the percent of effective lever presses ($F_{(3,54)\ \text{DRL} \times \text{treatment}} = 0.7$, NS; $F_{(1,54)\ \text{treatment}} = 0.01$, NS; **Figure 3C**) at any of the DRL intervals. Total lever presses ($F_{(3,54)\ \text{treatment}} = 24.9$, $p < 0.0001$; **Figure 3A**), reinforcers ($F_{(3,54)\ \text{treatment}} = 246.8$, $p < 0.0001$; **Figure 3B**), and effective

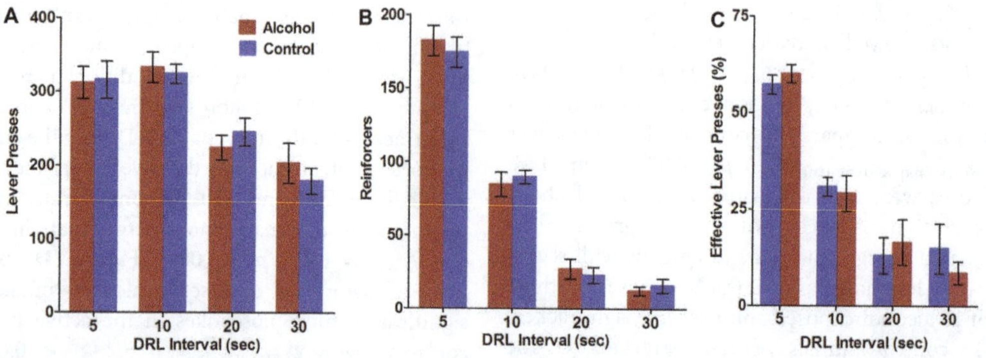

FIGURE 3 | Impulsive action as measured by performance on the differential reinforcement of low rates of responding (DRL) task. Alcohol-exposed ($n = 9$) animals did not differ from controls ($n = 11$) on **(A)** the total number of lever presses performed, **(B)** the total number of reinforcers received, or **(C)** the percentage of lever presses that resulted in reward delivery. All data are presented as mean ± SEM averaged across all 5-day blocks for the 5, 10, 20 and 30 s DRL intervals.

lever presses ($F_{(3,54)\ \text{treatment}}$ = 63.9, $p < 0.0001$; **Figure 3C**) decreased with increasing DRL intervals, in both groups, suggesting animals in both groups were less able to withhold responding as the time to wait before responding increased. Thus, using our model of voluntary alcohol intake, adolescent alcohol use does not appear to differentially affect the ability of animals to withhold responding for a reward compared to controls.

DISCUSSION

Alcohol is the most commonly abused substance among adolescents and use during this sensitive developmental period is one of the best predictors of risk for development of alcohol use disorder (Grant et al., 2001). Maladaptive decision making strategies and altered reinforcement learning processes are two long-term consequences of adolescent alcohol use that may be contributing factors for alcohol problems later in life. Using a preclinical model of moderate voluntary adolescent alcohol intake, our laboratory has shown that alcohol use during this sensitive developmental period promotes risky decision making and alterations in incentive learning processes in adulthood, both of which are mirrored by perturbations in cue-evoked dopamine signaling (Nasrallah et al., 2011; Schindler et al., 2014; Spoelder et al., 2015). We have proposed that these two processes, risk-based decision making and incentive learning, are fundamentally linked through dysfunction of midbrain circuitry where inputs to the dopamine system are disrupted by adolescent alcohol use; with the latter potentially influencing performance on the former. The present work supports the behavioral predictions of this model. We show that alcohol-exposed animals attribute greater incentive value to a reward-predicting cue, demonstrated by increased approach to the cue and a greater willingness to work to receive the cue even in the absence of reward. Further, we show that animals exposed to alcohol during adolescence did not differ from controls in impulsive choice, impulsive action, or effortful choice. The findings presented here, in combination with previous work from our laboratory, support the proposition that early life alcohol use selectively modulates incentive learning processes and alters risk-based choice behavior (Clark et al., 2012; Schindler et al., 2014; Spoelder et al., 2015), but not other aspects of decision making including impulsive choice and behavioral inhibition.

Cues in an environment that repeatedly predict reward can attain value through a Pavlovian process referred to as stimulus-reward learning. In the realm of addiction, cues associated with drugs often attain enhanced incentive value and play a critical role in promoting drug craving, seeking and relapse following periods of abstinence (O'Brien et al., 1998; Shaham et al., 2003; Milton and Everitt, 2012). In preclinical research, animals classified as sign trackers show enhanced attribution of value to reward predicting cues, are more prone to display behaviors associated with drug-abuse, and are thought to model addiction-vulnerable populations in humans (Flagel et al., 2009, 2010; Spoelder et al., 2015). The value attributed to incentive stimuli can be defined by attractiveness, measured by approach to the stimulus, and wanting, measured by the animal's willingness to work to obtain the stimulus (Berridge et al., 2009). Consistent with our previous work (Spoelder et al., 2015), we confirm that voluntary adolescent alcohol exposure results in adult animals finding the reward-predicting cue more attractive, compared to control animals, as evidenced by a greater sign-tracking bias and increased approach to the lever-CS. Greater sign-tracking behavior in adulthood following a history of adolescent alcohol has also been shown with non-voluntary models of alcohol administration (McClory and Spear, 2014). Thus, exposure to alcohol during adolescence appears to consistently produce a phenotype associated with addiction-vulnerability. Further, we have previously shown that this greater attribution of value to reward-predictive cues may be dopamine dependent (Spoelder et al., 2015). We show that sign trackers with a history of adolescent alcohol use demonstrated a greater wanting of the cue by working harder than control sign trackers to obtain the lever-CS even in the absence of reward delivery. Alcohol-exposed animals also made significantly more lever presses following an active nosepoke during the 40 min conditioned reinforcement test, further demonstrating the greater attraction of the lever-CS for alcohol-exposed animals compared to controls. These data support evidence in both clinical and preclinical literature that alcohol use during adolescence, whether moderate or heavy, leads to alterations in incentive learning processes producing behaviors often apparent in addiction-prone individuals.

These findings further lend support to our hypothesis that maladaptive decision making under risk, a consequence of adolescent alcohol use, is a result of altered incentive learning. However, other underlying constructs such as altered valuation of primary rewards, deficits in reinforcement learning where corrupted value is assigned to specific cues and actions, and/or increased impulsivity, could also influence the risk-seeking phenotype. Thus, in a series of experiments begun in Clark et al., 2012 and completed in the current work we have attempted to parse the specific contribution of these constructs to maladaptive decision making in adults with a history of adolescent alcohol use. First, we asked if increased risk preference was due to altered reward valuation where the shape of an individual's utility curve is thought to determine choice under uncertainty (Clark et al., 2012). Indeed, in economic theory, risk attitude is attributed to this relationship between the objective value of a reward and its desirability (subjective value; Glimcher and Rustichini, 2004). Reward valuation was assessed by conducting progressive ratio experiments at different reward levels to estimate each subject's utility curve, and no differences between alcohol and control groups were found (Clark et al., 2012). We hypothesized, therefore, that increased risk preference can be attributed to a selective deficit in reward learning as probability discounting is a special case where subjects are asked to constantly alter the value they assign to a probabilistic option trial by trial through reinforcement learning. We showed this in a simple computational model and supported this hypothesis in further studies where we demonstrated that alcohol animals, consistent with human alcoholics, are more prone to risky choices in the gain domain and after wins rather than losses (Clark et al., 2012; Brevers et al., 2014; Schindler et al., 2016). Finally, in the current work, we explore impulsivity as a potential contributor to the risk-seeking phenotype.

Deficits in impulse control are a key feature of alcohol use disorders, with higher levels of impulsivity predisposing to the development of alcohol problems later in life and increased likelihood of relapse following abstinence (Mitchell et al., 2005; Jupp and Dalley, 2014b; Stevens et al., 2014). Impulsive choice reflects a more cognitive aspect of impulsivity thought of as impulsive decision making, whereas impulsive action reflects an inability to inhibit a motor response thought of as behavioral inhibition (Evenden, 1999; Olmstead, 2006; Winstanley et al., 2010). Using delay discounting, we show that voluntary alcohol intake during adolescence had no effect on impulsive choice in adulthood, evidenced by similar discounting curves between alcohol-exposed and control animals across delay sessions. These results are consistent with another study that used a non-voluntary model of alcohol administration and found no effect of chronic intermittent ethanol exposure during adolescence on impulsive choice when tested later in adulthood (Mejia-Toiber et al., 2014). Adolescent alcohol exposure also did not alter the ability to withhold responding for a reward in the DRL task, indicating that moderate adolescent alcohol intake does not alter impulsive action in adulthood. Finally, the amount of work required to obtain a reward could also influence decision making under risk. Less is known about the relationship between effortful decision making and alcohol use disorders, but our data show that moderate alcohol use during adolescence does not appear to influence effortful decision making in adulthood (Supplementary Figure S1).

Previous studies have explored the relationship between probability discounting, delay discounting, incentive learning, sign-tracking behavior and addiction-prone phenotypes with varying results on how these behaviors cluster (Flagel et al., 2010; Lovic et al., 2011). For instance, Lovic et al. (2011) found that sign trackers displayed greater impulsive action, but not choice, compared to goal trackers. (Flagel et al. (2010); Flagel et al. (2011)) found that rats selectively bred for response to novelty, a phenotype associated with addiction, are sign trackers that also show greater impulsive action but not choice, and greater incentive value attribution but no difference in risky decision making. Our work demonstrates that alterations in decision making under risk and incentive value attribution cluster together as a result of alcohol use during adolescence. Given that we have shown the pharmacological attenuation of risky behavior (Schindler et al., 2016), future studies examining if this same drug attenuates the enhanced attribution of value to reward-predicting cues would confirm an overlapping mechanism between these behaviors that appear to cluster. Together with our previous work, we can begin to outline an emerging profile of the selective effects of moderate adolescent alcohol use on decision making, with apparent perturbations in risk-based, but not delay- or effort-based, decision making.

In addition to delay discounting, the probability-discounting task has also been used as a measure of impulsive choice (Flagel et al., 2010), with some researchers attributing performance on tasks involving decision making under risk to features of impulsivity (Richards et al., 1999). However, emerging clinical and preclinical data indicate that performance on probability-discounting and delay-discounting tasks are dissociable neurobiologically (van Gaalen et al., 2006; St Onge and Floresco, 2009), genetically (Flagel et al., 2010) and by age (Olson et al., 2007). Our data are consistent with and add to this emerging literature by showing that moderate adolescent alcohol use alters probability but not delay discounting in adulthood. It is interesting to speculate how these results may support a differential sensitivity of the underlying neurobiological mechanisms of probability and delay discounting, to alcohol during development. The pathway that mediates decision making under risk appears to be sensitive to moderate levels of alcohol during the adolescent time period, whereas the pathway that mediates either feature of impulsivity is not (Schindler et al., 2014, 2016). We should consider that impulsivity later in life could be altered by adolescent exposure, but heavy or excessive alcohol use may be required to see an effect. Nevertheless, the system that mediates risky behavior appears to be highly sensitive to even moderate levels of alcohol during development identifying it as an important target. Future studies examining the role of impulsivity and risk in substance use disorders should therefore treat delay and probability discounting as separable tasks that can provide unique information about the relationship between adolescent drug use and later decision making deficits.

Taken together with our previous work, the findings presented here support our hypothesis that the compromised encoding of Pavlovian cues following alcohol exposure in adolescence may underlie suboptimal decision making strategies in adulthood. Our data additionally support delay- and probability-discounting as dissociable decision-making paradigms, and confirm that impulsivity is not likely an explanation for maladaptive decision making under risk in adulthood seen following adolescent alcohol use. One limitation of the present set of experiments is that only the effect of adolescent alcohol intake, but not adult alcohol intake, on incentive value attribution and impulsivity in adulthood was assessed. Thus, we cannot state that the results are specific to adolescent intake. However, we have previously demonstrated that moderate alcohol intake during adulthood does not alter risky decision making (Schindler et al., 2014). Taken together with our previous work (Nasrallah et al., 2011; Spoelder et al., 2015; Schindler et al., 2016), we believe these effects are a result of alcohol on the developing mesolimbic dopamine system and would not expect those changes to occur with adult alcohol exposure. Aberrant changes in risk-based decision making and incentive learning following adolescent alcohol use are associated with perturbations in mesolimbic dopamine neurotransmission enduring into adulthood and the combination of such neurobiological and behavioral deficits may serve as critical vulnerabilities to the development of substance use disorders later in life.

AUTHOR CONTRIBUTIONS

LCK performed most of the studies, analyzed the data. LCK and JJC wrote the manuscript. JJC, AGS and LCK conceived the studies and edited the manuscript. RGW performed the delay discounting study. SJW performed analyses for the delay data.

alcohol use and abuse, a major public health concern throughout the world.

REFERENCES

Bava, S., and Tapert, S. F. (2010). Adolescent brain development and the risk for alcohol and other drug problems. *Neuropsychol. Rev.* 20, 398–413. doi: 10.1007/s11065-010-9146-6

Berridge, K. C., Robinson, T. E., and Aldridge, J. W. (2009). Dissecting components of reward: 'liking', 'wanting' and learning. *Curr. Opin. Pharmacol.* 9, 65–73. doi: 10.1016/j.coph.2008.12.014

Boutros, N., Semenova, S., Liu, W., Crews, F. T., and Markou, A. (2014). Adolescent intermittent ethanol exposure is associated with increased risky choice and decreased dopaminergic and cholinergic neuron markers in adult rats. *Int. J. Neuropsychopharmacol.* 18:pyu003. doi: 10.1093/ijnp/pyu003

Brevers, D., Bechara, A., Cleeremans, A., Kornreich, C., Verbanck, P., and Noël, X. (2014). Impaired decision-making under risk in individuals with alcohol dependence. *Alcohol. Clin. Exp. Res.* 38, 1924–1931. doi: 10.1111/acer.12447

Casey, B. J., and Jones, R. M. (2010). Neurobiology of the adolescent brain and behavior: implications for substance use disorders. *J. Am. Acad. Child Adolesc. Psychiatry* 49, 1189–1201; quiz 1285. doi: 10.1016/j.jaac.2010.08.017

Chambers, R. A., Taylor, J. R., and Potenza, M. N. (2003). Developmental neurocircuitry of motivation in adolescence: a critical period of addiction vulnerability. *Am. J. Psychiatry* 160, 1041–1052. doi: 10.1176/appi.ajp.160.6.1041

Clark, J. J., Nasrallah, N. A., Hart, A. S., Collins, A. L., Bernstein, I. L., and Phillips, P. E. (2012). Altered risk-based decision making following adolescent alcohol use results from an imbalance in reinforcement learning in rats. *PLoS One* 7:e37357. doi: 10.1371/journal.pone.0037357

Collins, F. S., and Tabak, L. A. (2014). Policy: NIH plans to enhance reproducibility. *Nature* 505, 612–613. doi: 10.1038/505612a

Crews, F., He, J., and Hodge, C. (2007). Adolescent cortical development: a critical period of vulnerability for addiction. *Pharmacol. Biochem. Behav.* 86, 189–199. doi: 10.1016/j.pbb.2006.12.001

Day, J. J., Jones, J. L., Wightman, R. M., and Carelli, R. M. (2010). Phasic nucleus accumbens dopamine release encodes effort- and delay-related costs. *Biol. Psychiatry* 68, 306–309. doi: 10.1016/j.biopsych.2010.03.026

Evenden, J. L. (1999). Varieties of impulsivity. *Psychopharmacology* 146, 348–361. doi: 10.1007/pl00005481

Everitt, B. J., and Robbins, T. W. (2005). Neural systems of reinforcement for drug addiction: from actions to habits to compulsion. *Nat. Neurosci.* 8, 1481–1489. doi: 10.1038/nn1579

Flagel, S. B., Akil, H., and Robinson, T. E. (2009). Individual differences in the attribution of incentive salience to reward-related cues: implications for addiction. *Neuropharmacology* 56, 139–148. doi: 10.1016/j.neuropharm.2008.06.027

Flagel, S. B., Clark, J. J., Robinson, T. E., Mayo, L., Czuj, A., Willuhn, I., et al. (2011). A selective role for dopamine in stimulus-reward learning. *Nature* 469, 53–57. doi: 10.1038/nature09588

Flagel, S. B., Robinson, T. E., Clark, J. J., Clinton, S. M., Watson, S. J., Seeman, P., et al. (2010). An animal model of genetic vulnerability to behavioral disinhibition and responsiveness to reward-related cues: implications for addiction. *Neuropsychopharmacology* 35, 388–400. doi: 10.1038/npp.2009.142

Floresco, S. B., Tse, M. T., and Ghods-Sharifi, S. (2008). Dopaminergic and glutamatergic regulation of effort- and delay-based decision making. *Neuropsychopharmacology* 33, 1966–1979. doi: 10.1038/sj.npp.1301565

Ghods-Sharifi, S., and Floresco, S. B. (2010). Differential effects on effort discounting induced by inactivations of the nucleus accumbens core or shell. *Behav. Neurosci.* 124, 179–191. doi: 10.1037/a0018932

Glimcher, P. W., and Rustichini, A. (2004). Neuroeconomics: the consilience of brain and decision. *Science* 306, 447–452. doi: 10.1126/science.1102566

Goudriaan, A. E., Grekin, E. R., and Sher, K. J. (2007). Decision making and binge drinking: a longitudinal study. *Alcohol. Clin. Exp. Res.* 31, 928–938. doi: 10.1111/j.1530-0277.2007.00378.x

Grant, B. F., Stinson, F. S., and Harford, T. C. (2001). Age at onset of alcohol use and DSM-IV alcohol abuse and dependence: a 12-year follow-up. *J. Subst. Abuse* 13, 493–504. doi: 10.1016/s0899-3289(01)00096-7

Green, L., and Myerson, J. (2013). How many impulsivities? A discounting perspective. *J. Exp. Anal. Behav.* 99, 3–13. doi: 10.1002/jeab.1

Johnson, C. A., Xiao, L., Palmer, P., Sun, P., Wang, Q., Wei, Y., et al. (2008). Affective decision-making deficits, linked to a dysfunctional ventromedial prefrontal cortex, revealed in 10th grade Chinese adolescent binge drinkers. *Neuropsychologia* 46, 714–726. doi: 10.1016/j.neuropsychologia.2007.09.012

Jupp, B., and Dalley, J. W. (2014a). Behavioral endophenotypes of drug addiction: etiological insights from neuroimaging studies. *Neuropharmacology* 76, 487–497. doi: 10.1016/j.neuropharm.2013.05.041

Jupp, B., and Dalley, J. W. (2014b). Convergent pharmacological mechanisms in impulsivity and addiction: insights from rodent models. *Br. J. Pharmacol.* 171, 4729–4766. doi: 10.1111/bph.12787

Kelley, A. E. (2004). Memory and addiction: shared neural circuitry and molecular mechanisms. *Neuron* 44, 161–179. doi: 10.1016/j.neuron.2004.09.016

Leblond, M., Sukharnikova, T., Yu, C., Rossi, M. A., and Yin, H. H. (2014). The role of pedunculopontine nucleus in choice behavior under risk. *Eur. J. Neurosci.* 39, 1664–1670. doi: 10.1111/ejn.12529

Littlefield, A. K., and Sher, K. J. (2010). The multiple, distinct ways that personality contributes to alcohol use disorders. *Soc. Personal. Psychol. Compass* 4, 767–782. doi: 10.1111/j.1751-9004.2010.00296.x

Lovic, V., Saunders, B. T., Yager, L. M., and Robinson, T. E. (2011). Rats prone to attribute incentive salience to reward cues are also prone to impulsive action. *Behav. Brain Res.* 223, 255–261. doi: 10.1016/j.bbr.2011.04.006

Marinelli, M., and McCutcheon, J. E. (2014). Heterogeneity of dopamine neuron activity across traits and states. *Neuroscience* 282, 176–197. doi: 10.1016/j.neuroscience.2014.07.034

McClory, A. J., and Spear, L. P. (2014). Effects of ethanol exposure during adolescence or in adulthood on Pavlovian conditioned approach in Sprague-Dawley rats. *Alcohol* 48, 755–763. doi: 10.1016/j.alcohol.2014.05.006

McMurray, M. S., Amodeo, L. R., and Roitman, J. D. (2014). Effects of voluntary alcohol intake on risk preference and behavioral flexibility during rat adolescence. *PLoS One* 9:e100697. doi: 10.1371/journal.pone.0100697

Mejia-Toiber, J., Boutros, N., Markou, A., and Semenova, S. (2014). Impulsive choice and anxiety-like behavior in adult rats exposed to chronic intermittent ethanol during adolescence and adulthood. *Behav. Brain Res.* 266, 19–28. doi: 10.1016/j.bbr.2014.02.019

Meyer, P. J., Lovic, V., Saunders, B. T., Yager, L. M., Flagel, S. B., Morrow, J. D., et al. (2012). Quantifying individual variation in the propensity to attribute incentive salience to reward cues. *PLoS One* 7:e38987. doi: 10.1371/journal.pone.0038987

Milton, A. L., and Everitt, B. J. (2012). The persistence of maladaptive memory: addiction, drug memories and anti-relapse treatments. *Neurosci. Biobehav. Rev.* 36, 1119–1139. doi: 10.1016/j.neubiorev.2012.01.002

Mitchell, J. M., Fields, H. L., D'Esposito, M., and Boettiger, C. A. (2005). Impulsive responding in alcoholics. *Alcohol. Clin. Exp. Res.* 29, 2158–2169. doi: 10.1097/01.alc.0000191755.63639.4a

Nasrallah, N. A., Clark, J. J., Collins, A. L., Akers, C. A., Phillips, P. E., and Bernstein, I. L. (2011). Risk preference following adolescent alcohol use is associated with corrupted encoding of costs but not rewards by mesolimbic dopamine. *Proc. Natl. Acad. Sci. U S A* 108, 5466–5471. doi: 10.1073/pnas.1017732108

O'Brien, C. P., Childress, A. R., Ehrman, R., and Robbins, S. J. (1998). Conditioning factors in drug abuse: can they explain compulsion? *J. Psychopharmacol.* 12, 15–22. doi: 10.1177/026988119801200103

Olmstead, M. C. (2006). Animal models of drug addiction: where do we go from here? *Q. J. Exp. Psychol.* 59, 625–653. doi: 10.1080/17470210500356308

Olson, E. A., Hooper, C. J., Collins, P., and Luciana, M. (2007). Adolescents' performance on delay and probability discounting tasks: contributions of age, intelligence, executive functioning, and self-reported externalizing behavior. *Pers. Individ. Dif.* 43, 1886–1897. doi: 10.1016/j.paid.2007.06.016

Pan, W. X., and Hyland, B. I. (2005). Pedunculopontine tegmental nucleus controls conditioned responses of midbrain dopamine neurons in behaving rats. *J. Neurosci.* 25, 4725–4732. doi: 10.1523/JNEUROSCI.0277-05.2005

Pascual, M., Boix, J., Felipo, V., and Guerri, C. (2009). Repeated alcohol administration during adolescence causes changes in the mesolimbic dopaminergic and glutamatergic systems and promotes alcohol intake in the adult rat. *J. Neurochem.* 108, 920–931. doi: 10.1111/j.1471-4159.2008.05835.x

Richards, J. B., Zhang, L., Mitchell, S. H., and de Wit, H. (1999). Delay or probability discounting in a model of impulsive behavior: effect of alcohol. *J. Exp. Anal. Behav.* 71, 121–143. doi: 10.1901/jeab.1999.71-121

Rowland, N. E., Nasrallah, N., and Robertson, K. L. (2005). Accurate caloric compensation in rats for electively consumed ethanol-beer or ethanol-polycose mixtures. *Pharmacol. Biochem. Behav.* 80, 109–114. doi: 10.1016/j.pbb.2004.10.010

Salamone, J. D., and Correa, M. (2012). The mysterious motivational functions of mesolimbic dopamine. *Neuron* 76, 470–485. doi: 10.1016/j.neuron.2012.10.021

Schindler, A. G., Soden, M. E., Zweifel, L. S., and Clark, J. J. (2016). Reversal of alcohol-induced dysregulation in dopamine network dynamics may rescue maladaptive decision-making. *J. Neurosci.* 36, 3698–3708. doi: 10.1523/JNEUROSCI.4394-15.2016

Schindler, A. G., Tsutsui, K. T., and Clark, J. J. (2014). Chronic alcohol intake during adolescence, but not adulthood, promotes persistent deficits in risk-based decision making. *Alcohol. Clin. Exp. Res.* 38, 1622–1629. doi: 10.1111/acer.12404

Shaham, Y., Shalev, U., Lu, L., De Wit, H., and Stewart, J. (2003). The reinstatement model of drug relapse: history, methodology and major findings. *Psychopharmacology* 168, 3–20. doi: 10.1007/s00213-002-1224-x

Spear, L. P. (2000). The adolescent brain and age-related behavioral manifestations. *Neurosci. Biobehav. Rev.* 24, 417–463. doi: 10.1016/s0149-7634(00)00014-2

Spoelder, M., Tsutsui, K. T., Lesscher, H. M., Vanderschuren, L. J., and Clark, J. J. (2015). Adolescent alcohol exposure amplifies the incentive value of reward-predictive cues through potentiation of phasic dopamine signaling. *Neuropsychopharmacology* 40, 2873–2885. doi: 10.1038/npp.2015.139

Stevens, L., Verdejo-Garcia, A., Goudriaan, A. E., Roeyers, H., Dom, G., and Vanderplasschen, W. (2014). Impulsivity as a vulnerability factor for poor addiction treatment outcomes: a review of neurocognitive findings among individuals with substance use disorders. *J. Subst. Abuse Treat.* 47, 58–72. doi: 10.1016/j.jsat.2014.01.008

St Onge, J. R., and Floresco, S. B. (2009). Dopaminergic modulation of risk-based decision making. *Neuropsychopharmacology* 34, 681–697. doi: 10.1038/npp.2008.121

van Gaalen, M. M., van Koten, R., Schoffelmeer, A. N., and Vanderschuren, L. J. (2006). Critical involvement of dopaminergic neurotransmission in impulsive decision making. *Biol. Psychiatry* 60, 66–73. doi: 10.1016/j.biopsych.2005.06.005

Winstanley, C. A., Olausson, P., Taylor, J. R., and Jentsch, J. D. (2010). Insight into the relationship between impulsivity and substance abuse from studies using animal models. *Alcohol. Clin. Exp. Res.* 34, 1306–1318. doi: 10.1111/j.1530-0277.2010.01215.x

11

Traumatic Brain Injuries during Development: Implications for Alcohol Abuse

*Zachary M. Weil * and Kate Karelina*

Behavioral Neuroendocrinology Group, Department of Neuroscience, Center for Brain and Spinal Cord Repair, Ohio State University Wexner Medical Center, Columbus, OH, United States

Edited by:
Jacqueline M. Barker,
Medical University of South Carolina,
United States

Reviewed by:
Firas H. Kobeissy,
University of Florida, United States
Aleksei Yurievich Egorov,
Institute of Evolutionary Physiology and Biochemistry (RAS), Russia

****Correspondence:***
Zachary M. Weil
zachary.weil@osumc.edu

Traumatic brain injuries are strongly related to alcohol intoxication as by some estimates half or more of all brain injuries involve at least one intoxicated individual. Additionally, there is mounting evidence that traumatic brain injuries can themselves serve as independent risk factors for the development of alcohol use disorders, particularly when injury occurs during juvenile or adolescent development. Here, we will review the epidemiological and experimental evidence for this phenomenon and discuss potential psychosocial mediators including attenuation of negative affect and impaired decision making as well as neurochemical mediators including disruption in the glutamatergic, GABAergic, and dopaminergic signaling pathways and increases in inflammation.

Keywords: alcohol, traumatic brain injury, dopamine, inflammation, adolescent

INTRODUCTION

Traumatic brain injuries (TBI) have received tremendous scientific and public attention in recent years. This attention is commensurate with the enormous societal and economic costs associated with a condition that affects millions of Americans and because of underreporting is likely even larger than current estimates. One important insight that has become clear is that TBIs are more than discrete events but are the start of a lifelong process comprising recovery, adaptation, and vulnerability to a large variety of other disease states (Masel and DeWitt, 2010; Corrigan and Hammond, 2013). In particular, children and adolescents who suffer TBI are less likely to finish school and maintain employment and suffer a greater risk of neurological and psychiatric disorders (among many others; Corrigan et al., 2013).

Alcohol is a prominent component of TBI. A recent assessment of the U.S. national trauma registry revealed alcohol use to be present in as many as 50% of all TBI-related emergency department visits (Chen et al., 2012). Not surprisingly alcohol use in general and binge drinking in particular are powerful risk factors for TBI (Savola et al., 2005; Vaaramo et al., 2014) and contribute substantially to mortality of TBI patients (see reference Opreanu et al., 2010 for a review). Critically, the use of alcohol in patients recovering from TBI is highly deleterious and there is significant evidence that patients that drink after TBI have poorer cognitive, neuropsychiatric and occupational outcomes than those that do not (Corrigan, 1995; Weil et al., 2016a; Unsworth and Mathias, 2017). Drinking after TBI is associated with poor long term outcomes in a variety of domains (Corrigan, 1995). Similar results have been reported in experimental TBI, for example we recently reported that administration of binge-like levels of alcohol in adulthood produces significant functional and neuropathological impairments in mice that had experienced TBI as juveniles (Karelina et al., 2017). Given that both past TBI and drinking are risk factors for future

TBI *and* repeated TBI tend to produce much more severe damage (Guskiewicz et al., 2000; Giza et al., 2013; McCrory et al., 2013) reducing drinking behavior in this patient population will serve to both improve outcomes and reduce the possibility of devastating future injuries.

The strong epidemiological association between brain injuries and pre-injury drinking mean that the TBI population is composed disproportionately of heavy drinkers. However, there is emerging clinical and experimental evidence that TBI may serve as an independent risk factor for the development of alcohol use disorders (AUDs; Weil et al., 2016a; Merkel et al., 2017a). This is particularly apparent among patients that suffer TBIs during childhood or adolescence. The TBI-induced increase in alcohol abuse among patients that suffer injuries during development likely reflects both a greater vulnerability of the developing nervous system to disruption by injury and that children are less likely to already be problem drinkers at the time of their injuries, and thus it is easier to detect independent contributions of TBI to the development of AUDs (Weil et al., 2016a).

DRINKING IN TBI PATIENTS

The relationship between TBI and alcohol abuse is well-known but had been considered to be unidirectional, i.e., drinking was a risk factor for head injuries. The possibility that the opposite was also true, i.e., that brain injuries could under specific conditions increases drinking behavior, was obscured by several factors. First, problem drinking (particularly binge-drinking) is a key predictor and proximate cause of TBI (Corrigan and Mysiw, 2012). Therefore, the TBI population is made up disproportionately of heavy drinkers making it difficult to detect effects of TBI on later alcohol-related outcomes (Corrigan, 1995). Second, patients with the most severe injuries often reduce drinking during the first months after injury. This seems to occur because of a combination of factors but includes lack of access to alcohol because of physical disability and hospitalization (and inpatient rehabilitation; Bombardier et al., 2003). Third, most studies have examined individuals injured as adults but that represents both a relatively small proportion of the total population and includes individuals that have either already begun drinking or are past the age at which new AUD tend to emerge (Grant and Dawson, 1997). Finally, patients that begin (or resume) drinking after injury are more likely to be lost to follow up in longitudinal studies and thus the numbers of these individuals might be underestimated (Corrigan et al., 1997). Indeed, studies of post-TBI drinking in adults have most often reported that there is an initial decrease in alcohol intake followed by some patients gradually returning to problem drinking and others becoming abstainers (Kreutzer et al., 1996; Ponsford et al., 2007). Studies have produced conflicting reports as to whether adult injuries increase the rates of, or vulnerability to, AUDs (Bjork and Grant, 2009).

In contrast, early life injury has been consistently and repeatedly associated with the later development of AUDs (Weil et al., 2016a; Merkel et al., 2017a). For instance, high school students that suffered a TBI were more than twice as likely to meet the diagnostic criteria for AUDs after injury (Ilie et al., 2015). Further the earlier that injuries occur the stronger the association with substance abuse. Children injured before age five were more than 3.6 times as likely to exhibit substance abuse as teenagers than were uninjured children (McKinlay et al., 2014). Patients in an inpatient rehabilitation setting for TBI were more than twice as likely to meet the diagnostic criteria for substance abuse if they had experienced a previous injury before the age of 16 (Corrigan et al., 2013). In addition, among inmates in the South Carolina penitentiary system, age of first brain injury was associated with both severity and earlier age of onset of substance abuse (Fishbein et al., 2016).

A similar age of injury-related discrepancy in drinking after TBI has also been reported in animals. We recently reported that juvenile TBI, but not adult injury, significantly increased alcohol self-administration in a two-bottle choice paradigm in mice (Weil et al., 2016b). Other investigations of drinking behavior in animals injured as adults have produced conflicting results with some studies reporting increases and others reporting decreases (Lowing et al., 2014; Lim et al., 2015; Mayeux et al., 2015). Taken together, it seems that injuries that occur early in life are more likely to produce AUD, however, the specific mechanisms that link TBI to vulnerability to problem drinking remain unspecified.

POTENTIAL MECHANISMS OF INCREASED DRINKING AFTER TBI

In the next section we will discuss two very general classes of potential mediators that underlie the increased drinking behavior observed in pediatric brain injury patients (summarized in **Figure 1**). This is not intended to be an exhaustive discussion but rather to highlight some of the active areas of research.

PSYCHOSOCIAL FACTORS

TBI interacts with or exacerbates many of the traditional risk factors for AUD and may limit some of the moderating factors that serve to reduce AUD risk. Although, the individual contributions of these risk factors are likely relatively minor, when taken together they contribute to the increased likelihood of AUD in these patients. For example, many head injury patients have a family history of AUD, which results in both increased modeling of drinking behavior and genetic risk (Laucht et al., 2007). In addition, head injuries in pediatric populations are strongly, but often indirectly, associated with alcohol intoxication. In children and adolescents, vehicular accidents and physical violence are responsible for a substantial subset of injuries (though the exact percentages shift across age; Keenan and Bratton, 2006; Narang and Clarke, 2014) and extremely large percentages of head injuries related to assaults or incidences of physical abuse are associated with intoxication of either the injured child or more often the assailant, who is often a parent or other close relative (Kraus et al., 1989; Dube et al., 2001). A similar relationship exists for motor vehicle accidents where at least one participant is likely to be intoxicated (Stoduto et al., 1993). Further, male children are more likely to experience

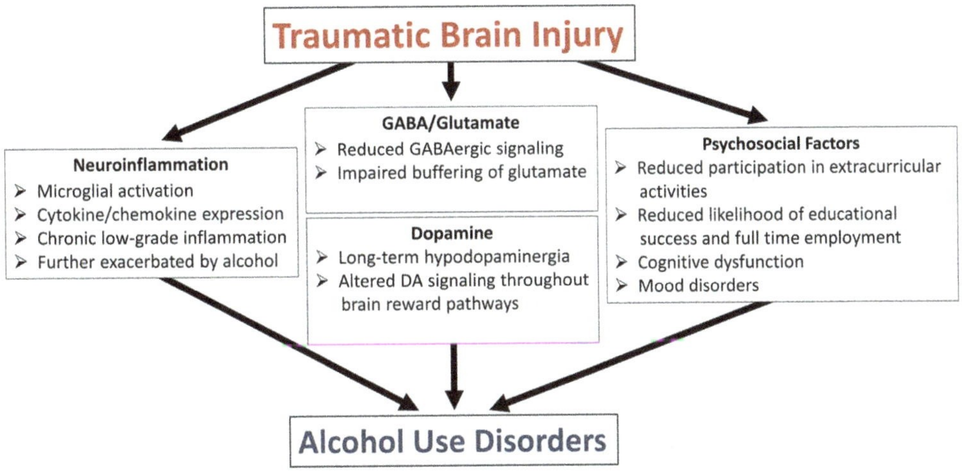

FIGURE 1 | Potential mechanisms linking traumatic brain injury to alcohol use disorders.

abuse-associated head trauma and are also at greater risk of later TBI and adolescent AUD (Costello et al., 1999; Narang and Clarke, 2014). Thus, the pediatric TBI population consists disproportionately of individuals from a family with alcohol use problems and/or a history of abuse, which are both critical risk factors for the development of AUDs (Dube et al., 2001; Barnow et al., 2002).

TBI also reduces many of the negative predictors of substance abuse. For instance, participation in extracurricular activities, forming stable romantic relationships, educational success, and full time employment are associated with reduced risk of alcohol abuse, yet all are less likely in brain injury survivors (Stewart-Scott and Douglas, 1998; Corrigan et al., 2013). Further, more severe TBI is often associated with prolonged absence from school and long-term disability, which often results in alienation from peer groups and increased alcohol use (Glang et al., 1997; Maggs et al., 2008).

The decision to drink has been proposed to reflect a balance between potential negative consequences (hangover, relationship issues, health consequences etc.) and perceived gains (reducing social inhibitions, negative mood states etc.) (Goldman, 1994). TBI can influence both sides of that equation by both reducing the ability to perceive negative consequences and increasing the perception of gains to be derived from drinking. For instance, that framework, termed the incentive motivation theory (Goldman, 1994), would predict that individuals less able to foresee the future consequences of their actions would be more likely to elect to drink. Indeed, TBI survivors show deficits in delay discounting and other cognitive tasks that require evaluation of delayed consequences (Bechara et al., 1994; Kolitz et al., 2003; Graham and Cardon, 2008). Finally, TBI results in more general executive dysfunction that can manifest itself as impulsivity and reduced inhibition, which can serve as predictors of AUD (Laucht et al., 2007; Iacono et al., 2008).

The other component of the incentive motivation theory is that individuals perceive a benefit to drinking. This perceived benefit could be in the form of increasing mood state, or reducing negative emotions or pain, and thus serves as a form of self-medication (King et al., 2004; Bolton et al., 2009). TBI survivors suffer from psychiatric sequelae including anxiety, depression and in a large subset of cases, post-traumatic stress disorder (PTSD; Breslau et al., 1991, 1997; Jorge et al., 2004). TBI often damages corticolimbic structures that regulate mood states, and endocrine and autonomic physiology as well as inducing long-term inflammatory responses, which can all increase the symptoms of affective disorders (Juengst et al., 2015). Even beyond direct damage to the nervous system, patients that acquire long-term cognitive or physical disabilities after brain injury often undergo a significant and prolonged period of adjustment to living with a disability (Smedema and Ebener, 2010). Thus, the very real possibility exists that brain injured patients are drinking to reduce the negative emotional states that are promoted by brain injury (Beresford et al., 2005).

NEUROINFLAMMATORY SIGNALING

The psychosocial and genetic risk factors associated with pediatric TBI also occur in the context of damage to the developing nervous system and likely disruptions of normal brain development. TBI is a complex pathophysiological process that can involve neuronal death, axon disconnection and degeneration, metabolic dysfunction, and aberrant neuroplasticity among other processes depending on the exact type and severity of the injury, comorbidities and age of the patient (Werner and Engelhard, 2007). However, one feature nearly universal to TBI is inflammation (Kelley et al., 2007; Ziebell and Morganti-Kossmann, 2010; Johnson et al., 2013). TBI both directly activates immune cells in the brain and primes cells such that future inflammatory stimuli produce exaggerated inflammatory responses (Fenn et al., 2014) and this is particularly true when inflammatory events occur early in life (Bilbo and Schwarz, 2009). The enhanced basal and stimulus-evoked immune responsiveness of the injured nervous system is important because there is a bidirectional relationship between neuroinflammation and alcohol intake (Kelley and Dantzer, 2011).

Alcohol produces a central inflammatory response characterized by activation of microglia and induction of inflammatory signaling and cytokines (Valles et al., 2004; Crews et al., 2011). Indeed the brains of long-term alcoholics exhibit evidence of prolonged low-grade inflammatory responses that may contribute to cognitive decline (He and Crews, 2008; Leclercq et al., 2014; Yen et al., 2017). The specific mechanism through which alcohol induces inflammatory responses is not fully understood but likely includes activation of the danger signal detecting molecules toll-like receptors (TLR; Alfonso-Loeches et al., 2010; Pascual et al., 2011). Critically, inflammation and components of inflammatory signaling drive drinking behavior (Crews et al., 2011). Mice treated with the bacterial cell wall component lipopolysaccharide (a molecule that induces a potent inflammatory response) self-administer significantly more alcohol (Blednov et al., 2011). Further, treatment with minocycline, a semisynthetic antibiotic with potent central anti-inflammatory activity produces a prolonged reduction in spontaneous alcohol self-administration (Agrawal et al., 2011). Mice lacking various components of inflammatory signaling cascades also drink less under basal conditions (Blednov et al., 2012).

Thus, TBI produces both acute inflammatory responses *and* primes immune cells like microglia to exhibit exaggerated inflammatory responses to other stimuli later in life. In this manner, TBI can establish a vicious cycle wherein inflammatory responses promote drinking behavior and subsequent drinking further exacerbates inflammatory responses (Mayeux et al., 2015). Critically, the alteration in inflammatory responses from alcohol occur in a brain already impacted by TBI and thus in addition to the deleterious consequences of heavy drinking that occur in otherwise healthy individuals, TBI patients face the potential of enhanced and chronic neuroinflammatory responses.

NEUROCHEMICAL ABNORMALITIES

Dysfunction in neuronal signaling after TBI, during development, can be roughly categorized into several etiologies. First, there is some (although often minimal) frank loss of neurons and associated axonal degeneration that directly disconnects or otherwise impairs neuronal connections. Additionally, as many critical neurodevelopmental events are occurring during these developmental epochs, TBI can result in disruption in the establishment of, or homeostasis in, neurochemical systems.

For instance, the ascending dopaminergic system undergoes significant functional and anatomical plasticity during late childhood and early adolescence (Philpot et al., 2009). This is characterized by changing tonic and stimulus evoked firing, alterations in synthetic machinery, transporter expression, and receptor distribution (Wahlstrom et al., 2010; McCutcheon et al., 2012). Importantly, this period of rapid neurodevelopment coincides temporally with vulnerability to substance abuse (Grant and Dawson, 1998). Early experience with drugs of abuse is a key risk factor for the development of substance abuse disorders and has been shown experimentally to alter the long-term function of the dopamine system (Guerri and Pascual, 2010).

Similarly, dysfunction in dopaminergic signaling is both a common consequence of TBI and a risk factor for the development of AUD (Martinez et al., 2005). There is a large body of experimental animal work indicating that dopamine physiology is significantly altered by TBI, with most studies reporting an acute hyperdopaminergia that resolves into a long-term hypodopaminergic state (Yan et al., 2001, 2002; Wagner et al., 2005a,b, 2009; Hutson et al., 2011).

Although, there is little direct evidence of dopaminergic dysfunction in human TBI patients (Donnemiller et al., 2000), drugs that enhance dopaminergic signaling (either by increasing synaptic dopamine or directly agonizing dopamine receptors) are relatively effective and part of the standard of care for reducing the cognitive deficits experienced by TBI patients (Neurobehavioral Guidelines Working et al., 2006; Bales et al., 2009; Huang et al., 2016). The utility of these drugs does not necessarily indicate that the dopamine system is hypofunctional in human patients (i.e., more dopamine may be helpful to improve cognitive outcomes in patients because of other neurological deficits) but the preponderance of evidence from clinical and experimental sources suggest some level of long term dysfunction in this system (Bales et al., 2009).

Critically, the alterations in dopamine signaling appear to occur beyond what would be expected from frank axonal degeneration or neuronal death (although damage to the ventral tegmental area and striatal targets have been reported following TBI; Dunn-Meynell and Levin, 1997; Ding et al., 2001; Hutson et al., 2011). Rather the alterations in dopamine signaling likely include alterations in network regulation and ongoing inflammation (Merkel et al., 2017a,b). Inflammatory signaling also serves to impair dopaminergic signaling and likely plays a role in the vulnerability to substance abuse in the brain-injured population (Felger and Miller, 2012). For instance, tyrosine hydroxylase production of L-Dopa is the rate-limiting step in dopamine biosynthesis. This enzymatic reaction requires the cofactor, tetrahydrobiopterin (BH4), which is also required for the synthesis of nitric oxide by nitric oxide synthases which are strongly upregulated by inflammatory signals meaning that BH4 can be shunted away from tyrosine hydroxylase when the brain is inflamed (Cunnington and Channon, 2010; Ono et al., 2010; Felger and Miller, 2012).

In contrast, surprisingly little is known about long-term adjustments in the glutamatergic and GABAergic systems after TBI. Acutely, TBI is associated with large, uncontrolled glutamate release that is a key factor in the damage associated with trauma (Katayama et al., 1990; Bullock et al., 1998). Further GABAergic neurons may be disproportionately likely to die and are overall less effective at balancing excitation. Finally, there is often persistent dysfunction in glial cells that typically buffer extracellular glutamate concentrations by expressing transporter proteins. Together, these lead to a net increase in excitatory signaling (Cantu et al., 2015) and the dysregulation in excitatory-inhibitory balance is very often associated with the development of post-traumatic epilepsy, particularly after pediatric injury (Ates et al., 2006; Pavlov et al., 2011). Over the long term there are compensatory changes that seem to buffer excess excitation but as a consequence of limiting excitatory neurotransmission may limit cognitive recovery (De Beaumont et al., 2012). This is evidenced by the consistent finding that TBI impairs the expression of long-term potentiation (Giza and Prins, 2006; Schwarzbach et al., 2006; Dorsett et al., 2017).

Like TBI, AUD are associated with disruption in the balance in excitatory-inhibitory balance and dysregulation of both glutamatergic and GABAergic signaling (Koob and Volkow, 2016). Alcohol both directly modulates activity of glutamate and GABA receptors, and can induce compensatory adjustments in these systems that perpetuate problem drinking (Chandler, 2003; Fitzgerald et al., 2012). The dynamic role of GABA:glutamate dysregulation and the interaction with normal development of this system in the evolution of drinking after TBI remains unspecified but deserves further attention.

CONCLUDING REMARKS

Alcohol use among adolescents is exceptionally common in western societies. Many individuals can drink heavily during this developmental period without developing AUD. However, patients with a history of TBI are much more likely to develop AUD. This is a major and critical public health problem because drinking after TBI can increase the risk of post-traumatic seizures, impair the efficacy of rehabilitation programs and increase the likelihood of subsequent TBI. The specific mechanisms that link TBI to AUD remain unspecified but it seems highly likely that it involves the coincidence of key psychosocial and neurochemical risk factors with important periods of neurological development. Targeting AUD in this population has the potential to significantly improve long-term outcomes.

AUTHOR CONTRIBUTIONS

All authors listed have made a substantial, direct and intellectual contribution to the work, and approved it for publication.

REFERENCES

Agrawal, R. G., Hewetson, A., George, C. M., Syapin, P. J., and Bergeson, S. E. (2011). Minocycline reduces ethanol drinking. *Brain Behav. Immun.* 25(Suppl. 1), S165–S169. doi: 10.1016/j.bbi.2011.03.002

Alfonso-Loeches, S., Pascual-Lucas, M., Blanco, A. M., Sanchez-Vera, I., and Guerri, C. (2010). Pivotal role of TLR4 receptors in alcohol-induced neuroinflammation and brain damage. *J. Neurosci.* 30, 8285–8295. doi: 10.1523/JNEUROSCI.0976-10.2010

Ates, O., Ondul, S., Onal, C., Buyukkiraz, M., Somay, H., Cayli, S. R., et al. (2006). Post-traumatic early epilepsy in pediatric age group with emphasis on influential factors. *Child Nerv. Syst.* 22, 279–284. doi: 10.1007/s00381-006-0171-y

Bales, J. W., Wagner, A. K., Kline, A. E., and Dixon, C. E. (2009). Persistent cognitive dysfunction after traumatic brain injury: a dopamine hypothesis. *Neurosci. Biobehav. Rev.* 33, 981–1003. doi: 10.1016/j.neubiorev.2009.03.011

Barnow, S., Schuckit, M. A., Lucht, M., John, U., and Freyberger, H. J. (2002). The importance of a positive family history of alcoholism, parental rejection and emotional warmth, behavioral problems and peer substance use for alcohol problems in teenagers: a path analysis. *J. Stud. Alcohol* 63, 305–315. doi: 10.15288/jsa.2002.63.305

Bechara, A., Damasio, A. R., Damasio, H., and Anderson, S. W. (1994). Insensitivity to future consequences following damage to human prefrontal cortex. *Cognition* 50, 7–15. doi: 10.1016/0010-0277(94)90018-3

Beresford, T. P., Arciniegas, D., Clapp, L., Martin, B., and Alfers, J. (2005). Reduction of affective lability and alcohol use following traumatic brain injury: a clinical pilot study of anti-convulsant medications. *Brain Inj.* 19, 309–313. doi: 10.1080/02699050410001720121

Bilbo, S. D., and Schwarz, J. M. (2009). Early-life programming of later-life brain and behavior: a critical role for the immune system. *Front. Behav. Neurosci.* 3:14. doi: 10.3389/neuro.08.014.2009

Bjork, J. M., and Grant, S. J. (2009). Does traumatic brain injury increase risk for substance abuse? *J. Neurotrauma* 26, 1077–1082. doi: 10.1089/neu.2008.0849

Blednov, Y. A., Benavidez, J. M., Geil, C., Perra, S., Morikawa, H., and Harris, R. A. (2011). Activation of inflammatory signaling by lipopolysaccharide produces a prolonged increase of voluntary alcohol intake in mice. *Brain Behav. Immun.* 25(Suppl. 1), S92–S105. doi: 10.1016/j.bbi.2011.01.008

Blednov, Y. A., Ponomarev, I., Geil, C., Bergeson, S., Koob, G. F., and Harris, R. A. (2012). Neuroimmune regulation of alcohol consumption: behavioral validation of genes obtained from genomic studies. *Addict. Biol.* 17, 108–120. doi: 10.1111/j.1369-1600.2010.00284.x

Bolton, J. M., Robinson, J., and Sareen, J. (2009). Self-medication of mood disorders with alcohol and drugs in the National Epidemiologic Survey on Alcohol and Related Conditions. *J. Affect. Disord.* 115, 367–375. doi: 10.1016/j.jad.2008.10.003

Bombardier, C. H., Temkin, N. R., Machamer, J., and Dikmen, S. S. (2003). The natural history of drinking and alcohol-related problems after traumatic brain injury. *Arch. Phys. Med. Rehabil.* 84, 185–191. doi: 10.1053/apmr.2003.50002

Breslau, N., Davis, G. C., Andreski, P., and Peterson, E. (1991). Traumatic events and posttraumatic stress disorder in an urban population of young adults. *Arch. Gen. Psychiatry* 48, 216–222. doi: 10.1001/archpsyc.1991.01810270028003

Breslau, N., Davis, G. C., Peterson, E. L., and Schultz, L. (1997). Psychiatric sequelae of posttraumatic stress disorder in women. *Arch. Gen. Psychiatry* 54, 81–87. doi: 10.1001/archpsyc.1997.01830130087016

Bullock, R., Zauner, A., Woodward, J. J., Myseros, J., Choi, S. C., Ward, J. D., et al. (1998). Factors affecting excitatory amino acid release following severe human head injury. *J. Neurosurg.* 89, 507–518. doi: 10.3171/jns.1998.89.4.0507

Cantu, D., Walker, K., Andresen, L., Taylor-Weiner, A., Hampton, D., Tesco, G., et al. (2015). Traumatic brain injury increases cortical glutamate network activity by compromising GABAergic control. *Cereb. Cortex* 25, 2306–2320. doi: 10.1093/cercor/bhu041

Chandler, L. J. (2003). Ethanol and brain plasticity: receptors and molecular networks of the postsynaptic density as targets of ethanol. *Pharmacol. Ther.* 99, 311–326. doi: 10.1016/S0163-7258(03)00096-2

Chen, C. M., Yi, H.-Y., Yoon, Y.-H., and Dong, C. (2012). Alcohol use at time of injury and survival following traumatic brain injury: results from the National Trauma Data Bank. *J. Stud. Alcohol Drugs* 73, 531–541. doi: 10.15288/jsad.2012.73.531

Corrigan, J. D. (1995). Substance abuse as a mediating factor in outcome from traumatic brain injury. *Arch. Phys. Med. Rehabil.* 76, 302–309. doi: 10.1016/S0003-9993(95)80654-7

Corrigan, J. D., Bogner, J. A., Mysiw, W. J., Clinchot, D., and Fugate, L. (1997). Systematic bias in outcome studies of persons with traumatic brain injury. *Arch. Phys. Med. Rehabil.* 78, 132–137. doi: 10.1016/S0003-9993(97)90253-7

Corrigan, J. D., Bogner, J., Mellick, D., Bushnik, T., Dams-O'Connor, K., Hammond, F. M., et al. (2013). Prior history of traumatic brain injury among persons in the traumatic brain injury model systems national database. *Arch. Phys. Med. Rehabil.* 94, 1940–1950. doi: 10.1016/j.apmr.2013.05.018

Corrigan, J. D., and Hammond, F. M. (2013). Traumatic brain injury as a chronic health condition. *Arch. Phys. Med. Rehabil.* 94, 1199–1201. doi: 10.1016/j.apmr.2013.01.023

Corrigan, J. D., and Mysiw, W. J. (2012). "Substance abuse among persons with TBI," in *Brain Injury Medicine: Principles and Practice, 2nd Edn*, eds N. D. Zasler, D. I. Katz, R. D. Zafonte, D. B. Arciniegas, M. R. Bullock, and J. S. Kreutzer (New York, NY: Demos Medical Publishing), 1315–1328.

Costello, E. J., Erkanli, A., Federman, E., and Angold, A. (1999). Development of psychiatric comorbidity with substance abuse in adolescents: effects of timing and sex. *J. Clin. Child Psychol.* 28, 298–311. doi: 10.1207/S15374424jccp280302

Crews, F. T., Zou, J., and Qin, L. (2011). Induction of innate immune genes in brain create the neurobiology of addiction. *Brain Behav. Immun.* 25, S4–S12. doi: 10.1016/j.bbi.2011.03.003

Cunnington, C., and Channon, K. M. (2010). Tetrahydrobiopterin: pleiotropic roles in cardiovascular pathophysiology. *Heart* 96, 1872–1877. doi: 10.1136/hrt.2009.180430

De Beaumont, L., Tremblay, S., Poirier, J., Lassonde, M., and Theoret, H. (2012). Altered bidirectional plasticity and reduced implicit motor learning in concussed athletes. *Cereb. Cortex* 22, 112–121. doi: 10.1093/cercor/bhr096

Ding, Y., Yao, B., Lai, Q., and McAllister, J. P. (2001). Impaired motor learning and diffuse axonal damage in motor and visual systems of the rat following traumatic brain injury. *Neurol. Res.* 23, 193–202. doi: 10.1179/016164101101198334

Donnemiller, E., Brenneis, C., Wissel, J., Scherfler, C., Poewe, W., Riccabona, G., et al. (2000). Impaired dopaminergic neurotransmission in patients with traumatic brain injury: a SPECT study using 123I-beta-CIT and 123I-IBZM. *Eur. J. Nucl. Med.* 27, 1410–1414. doi: 10.1007/s002590000308

Dorsett, C. R., McGuire, J. L., DePasquale, E. A., Gardner, A. E., Floyd, C. L., and McCullumsmith, R. E. (2017). Glutamate neurotransmission in rodent models of traumatic brain injury. *J. Neurotrauma* 34, 263–272. doi: 10.1089/neu.2015.4373

Dube, S. R., Anda, R. F., Felitti, V. J., Croft, J. B., Edwards, V. J., and Giles, W. H. (2001). Growing up with parental alcohol abuse: exposure to childhood abuse, neglect, and household dysfunction. *Child Abuse Negl.* 25, 1627–1640. doi: 10.1016/S0145-2134(01)00293-9

Dunn-Meynell, A. A., and Levin, B. E. (1997). Histological markers of neuronal, axonal and astrocytic changes after lateral rigid impact traumatic brain injury. *Brain Res.* 761, 25–41. doi: 10.1016/S0006-8993(97)00210-2

Felger, J. C., and Miller, A. H. (2012). Cytokine effects on the basal ganglia and dopamine function: the subcortical source of inflammatory malaise. *Front. Neuroendocrinol.* 33, 315–327. doi: 10.1016/j.yfrne.2012.09.003

Fenn, A. M., Gensel, J. C., Huang, Y., Popovich, P. G., Lifshitz, J., and Godbout, J. P. (2014). Immune activation promotes depression 1 month after diffuse brain injury: a role for primed microglia. *Biol. Psychiatry* 76, 575–584. doi: 10.1016/j.biopsych.2013.10.014

Fishbein, D., Dariotis, J. K., Ferguson, P. L., and Pickelsimer, E. E. (2016). Relationships between traumatic brain injury and illicit drug use and their association with aggression in inmates. *Int. J. Offender Ther. Comp. Criminol.* 60, 575–597. doi: 10.1177/0306624X14554778

Fitzgerald, G. J., Liu, H., and Morzorati, S. L. (2012). Decreased sensitivity of NMDA receptors on dopaminergic neurons from the posterior ventral tegmental area following chronic nondependent alcohol consumption. *Alcohol. Clin. Exp. Res.* 36, 1710–1719. doi: 10.1111/j.1530-0277.2012.01762.x

Giza, C. C., Kutcher, J. S., Ashwal, S., Barth, J., Getchius, T. S., Gioia, G. A., et al. (2013). Summary of evidence-based guideline update: evaluation and management of concussion in sports: report of the Guideline Development Subcommittee of the American Academy of Neurology. *Neurology* 80, 2250–2257. doi: 10.1212/WNL.0b013e31828d57dd

Giza, C. C., and Prins, M. L. (2006). Is being plastic fantastic? Mechanisms of altered plasticity after developmental traumatic brain injury. *Dev Neurosci.* 28, 364–379. doi: 10.1159/000094163

Glang, A., Todis, B., Cooley, E., Wells, J., and Voss, J. (1997). Building social networks for children and adolescents with traumatic brain injury: a school-based intervention. *J. Head Trauma Rehabil.* 12, 32–47. doi: 10.1097/00001199-199704000-00005

Goldman, M. S. (1994). The alcohol expectancy concept: applications to assessment, prevention, and treatment of alcohol abuse. *Appl. Prevent. Psychol.* 3, 131–144. doi: 10.1016/S0962-1849(05)80066-6

Graham, D. P., and Cardon, A. L. (2008). An update on substance use and treatment following traumatic brain injury. *Ann. N.Y. Acad. Sci.* 1141, 148–162. doi: 10.1196/annals.1441.029

Grant, B. F., and Dawson, D. A. (1997). Age at onset of alcohol use and its association with DSM-IV alcohol abuse and dependence: results from the national longitudinal alcohol epidemiologic survey. *J. Subst. Abuse* 9, 103–110. doi: 10.1016/S0899-3289(97)90009-2

Grant, B. F., and Dawson, D. A. (1998). Age of onset of drug use and its association with DSM-IV drug abuse and dependence: results from the National Longitudinal Alcohol Epidemiologic Survey. *J. Subst. Abuse* 10, 163–173. doi: 10.1016/S0899-3289(99)80131-X

Guerri, C., and Pascual, M. (2010). Mechanisms involved in the neurotoxic, cognitive, and neurobehavioral effects of alcohol consumption during adolescence. *Alcohol* 44, 15–26. doi: 10.1016/j.alcohol.2009.10.003

Guskiewicz, K. M., Weaver, N. L., Padua, D. A., and Garrett, W. E. Jr. (2000). Epidemiology of concussion in collegiate and high school football players. *Am. J. Sports Med.* 28, 643–650. doi: 10.1177/03635465000280050401

He, J., and Crews, F. T. (2008). Increased MCP-1 and microglia in various regions of the human alcoholic brain. *Exp. Neurol.* 210, 349–358. doi: 10.1016/j.expneurol.2007.11.017

Huang, C. H., Huang, C. C., Sun, C. K., Lin, G. H., and Hou, W. H. (2016). Methylphenidate on cognitive improvement in patients with traumatic brain injury: a meta-analysis. *Curr. Neuropharmacol.* 14, 272–281. doi: 10.2174/1570159X13666150514233033

Hutson, C. B., Lazo, C. R., Mortazavi, F., Giza, C. C., Hovda, D., and Chesselet, M. F. (2011). Traumatic brain injury in adult rats causes progressive nigrostriatal dopaminergic cell loss and enhanced vulnerability to the pesticide paraquat. *J. Neurotrauma* 28, 1783–1801. doi: 10.1089/neu.2010.1723

Iacono, W. G., Malone, S. M., and McGue, M. (2008). Behavioral disinhibition and the development of early-onset addiction: common and specific influences. *Annu. Rev. Clin. Psychol.* 4, 325–348. doi: 10.1146/annurev.clinpsy.4.022007.141157

Ilie, G., Mann, R. E., Hamilton, H., Adlaf, E. M., Boak, A., Asbridge, M., et al. (2015). Substance use and related harms among adolescents with and without traumatic brain injury. *J. Head Trauma Rehabil.* 30, 293–301. doi: 10.1097/HTR.0000000000000101

Johnson, V. E., Stewart, J. E., Begbie, F. D., Trojanowski, J. Q., Smith, D. H., and Stewart, W. (2013). Inflammation and white matter degeneration persist for years after a single traumatic brain injury. *Brain* 136(Pt 1), 28–42. doi: 10.1093/brain/aws322

Jorge, R. E., Robinson, R. G., Moser, D., Tateno, A., Crespo-Facorro, B., and Arndt, S. (2004). Major depression following traumatic brain injury. *Arch. Gen. Psychiatry* 61, 42–50. doi: 10.1001/archpsyc.61.1.42

Juengst, S. B., Kumar, R. G., Failla, M. D., Goyal, A., and Wagner, A. K. (2015). Acute inflammatory biomarker profiles predict depression risk following moderate to severe traumatic brain injury. *J. Head Trauma Rehabil.* 30, 207–218. doi: 10.1097/HTR.0000000000000031

Karelina, K., Gaier, K. R., Prabhu, M., Wenger, V., Corrigan, T. E., and Weil, Z. M. (2017). Binge ethanol in adulthood exacerbates negative outcomes following juvenile traumatic brain injury. *Brain Behav. Immun.* 60, 304–311. doi: 10.1016/j.bbi.2016.11.009

Katayama, Y., Becker, D. P., Tamura, T., and Hovda, D. A. (1990). Massive increases in extracellular potassium and the indiscriminate release of glutamate following concussive brain injury. *J. Neurosurg.* 73, 889–900. doi: 10.3171/jns.1990.73.6.0889

Keenan, H. T., and Bratton, S. L. (2006). Epidemiology and outcomes of pediatric traumatic brain injury. *Dev. Neurosci.* 28, 256–263. doi: 10.1159/000094152

Kelley, B. J., Lifshitz, J., and Povlishock, J. T. (2007). Neuroinflammatory responses after experimental diffuse traumatic brain injury. *J. Neuropathol. Exp. Neurol.* 66, 989–1001. doi: 10.1097/NEN.0b013e3181588245

Kelley, K. W., and Dantzer, R. (2011). Alcoholism and inflammation: neuroimmunology of behavioral and mood disorders. *Brain Behav. Immun.* 25(Suppl. 1), S13–S20. doi: 10.1016/j.bbi.2010.12.013

King, S. M., Iacono, W. G., and McGue, M. (2004). Childhood externalizing and internalizing psychopathology in the prediction of early substance use. *Addiction* 99, 1548–1559. doi: 10.1111/j.1360-0443.2004.00893.x

Kolitz, B. P., Vanderploeg, R. D., and Curtiss, G. (2003). Development of the Key Behaviors Change Inventory: a traumatic brain injury behavioral outcome assessment instrument. *Arch. Phys. Med. Rehabil.* 84, 277–284. doi: 10.1053/apmr.2003.50100

Koob, G. F., and Volkow, N. D. (2016). Neurobiology of addiction: a neurocircuitry analysis. *Lancet Psychiatry* 3, 760–773. doi: 10.1016/S2215-0366(16)00104-8

Kraus, J. F., Morgenstern, H., Fife, D., Conroy, C., and Nourjah, P. (1989). Blood-alcohol tests, prevalence of involvement, and outcomes following brain injury. *Am. J. Public Health* 79, 294–299. doi: 10.2105/AJPH.79.3.294

Kreutzer, J. S., Witol, A. D., and Marwitz, J. H. (1996). Alcohol and drug use among young persons with traumatic brain injury. *J. Learn. Disabil.* 29, 643–651. doi: 10.1177/002221949602900608

Laucht, M., Becker, K., Blomeyer, D., and Schmidt, M. H. (2007). Novelty seeking involved in mediating the association between the dopamine D4 receptor gene exon III polymorphism and heavy drinking in male adolescents: results from a high-risk community sample. *Biol. Psychiatry* 61, 87–92. doi: 10.1016/j.biopsych.2006.05.025

Leclercq, S., De Saeger, C., Delzenne, N., de Timary, P., and Starkel, P. (2014). Role of inflammatory pathways, blood mononuclear cells, and gut-derived bacterial products in alcohol dependence. *Biol. Psychiatry* 76, 725–733. doi: 10.1016/j.biopsych.2014.02.003

Lim, Y. W., Meyer, N. P., Shah, A. S., Budde, M. D., Stemper, B. D., and Olsen, C. M. (2015). Voluntary alcohol intake following blast exposure in a rat model of mild traumatic brain injury. *PLoS ONE* 10:e0125130. doi: 10.1371/journal.pone.0125130

Lowing, J. L., Susick, L. L., Caruso, J. P., Provenzano, A. M., Raghupathi, R., and Conti, A. C. (2014). Experimental traumatic brain injury alters ethanol consumption and sensitivity. *J. Neurotrauma* 31, 1700–1710. doi: 10.1089/neu.2013.3286

Maggs, J. L., Patrick, M. E., and Feinstein, L. (2008). Childhood and adolescent predictors of alcohol use and problems in adolescence and adulthood in the National Child Development Study. *Addiction* 103, 7–22. doi: 10.1111/j.1360-0443.2008.02173.x

Martinez, D., Gil, R., Slifstein, M., Hwang, D.-R., Huang, Y., Perez, A., et al. (2005). Alcohol dependence is associated with blunted dopamine transmission in the ventral striatum. *Biol. Psychiatry* 58, 779–786. doi: 10.1016/j.biopsych.2005.04.044

Masel, B. E., and DeWitt, D. S. (2010). Traumatic brain injury: a disease process, not an event. *J. Neurotrauma* 27, 1529–1540. doi: 10.1089/neu.2010.1358

Mayeux, J. P., Teng, S. X., Katz, P. S., Gilpin, N. W., and Molina, P. E. (2015). Traumatic brain injury induces neuroinflammation and neuronal degeneration that is associated with escalated alcohol self-administration in rats. *Behav. Brain Res.* 279, 22–30. doi: 10.1016/j.bbr.2014.10.053

McCrory, P., Meeuwisse, W. H., Aubry, M., Cantu, B., Dvorak, J., Echemendia, R. J., et al. (2013). Consensus statement on concussion in sport: the 4th International Conference on Concussion in Sport held in Zurich, November 2012. *Br. J. Sports Med.* 47, 250–258. doi: 10.1136/bjsports-2013-092313

McCutcheon, J. E., Conrad, K. L., Carr, S. B., Ford, K. A., McGehee, D. S., and Marinelli, M. (2012). Dopamine neurons in the ventral tegmental area fire faster in adolescent rats than in adults. *J. Neurophysiol.* 108, 1620–1630. doi: 10.1152/jn.00077.2012

McKinlay, A., Corrigan, J., Horwood, L. J., and Fergusson, D. M. (2014). Substance abuse and criminal activities following traumatic brain injury in childhood, adolescence, and early adulthood. *J. Head Trauma Rehabil.* 29, 498–506. doi: 10.1097/HTR.0000000000000001

Merkel, S. F., Cannella, L. A., Razmpour, R., Lutton, E., Raghupathi, R., Rawls, S. M., et al. (2017a). Factors affecting increased risk for substance use disorders following traumatic brain injury: what we can learn from animal models. *Neurosci. Biobehav. Rev.* 77, 209–218. doi: 10.1016/j.neubiorev.2017.03.015

Merkel, S. F., Razmpour, R., Lutton, E. M., Tallarida, C. S., Heldt, N. A., Cannella, L. A., et al. (2017b). Adolescent traumatic brain injury induces chronic mesolimbic neuroinflammation with concurrent enhancement in the rewarding effects of cocaine in mice during adulthood. *J. Neurotrauma* 34, 165–181. doi: 10.1089/neu.2015.4275

Narang, S., and Clarke, J. (2014). Abusive head trauma: past, present, and future. *J. Child Neurol.* 29, 1747–1756. doi: 10.1177/0883073814549995

Neurobehavioral Guidelines Working, G., Warden, D. L., Gordon, B., McAllister, T. W., Silver, J. M., Barth, J. T., et al. (2006). Guidelines for the pharmacologic treatment of neurobehavioral sequelae of traumatic brain injury. *J. Neurotrauma* 23, 1468–1501. doi: 10.1089/neu.2006.23.1468

Ono, K., Suzuki, H., and Sawada, M. (2010). Delayed neural damage is induced by iNOS-expressing microglia in a brain injury model. *Neurosci. Lett.* 473, 146–150. doi: 10.1016/j.neulet.2010.02.041

Opreanu, R. C., Kuhn, D., and Basson, M. D. (2010). Influence of alcohol on mortality in traumatic brain injury. *J. Am. Coll. Surg.* 210, 997–1007. doi: 10.1016/j.jamcollsurg.2010.01.036

Pascual, M., Fernandez-Lizarbe, S., and Guerri, C. (2011). Role of TLR4 in ethanol effects on innate and adaptive immune responses in peritoneal macrophages. *Immunol. Cell Biol.* 89, 716–727. doi: 10.1038/icb.2010.163

Pavlov, I., Huusko, N., Drexel, M., Kirchmair, E., Sperk, G., Pitkanen, A., et al. (2011). Progressive loss of phasic, but not tonic, gaba(a) receptor-mediated inhibition in dentate granule cells in a model of post-traumatic epilepsy in rats. *Neuroscience* 194, 208–219. doi: 10.1016/j.neuroscience.2011.07.074

Philpot, R. M., Wecker, L., and Kirstein, C. L. (2009). Repeated ethanol exposure during adolescence alters the developmental trajectory of dopaminergic output from the nucleus accumbens septi. *Int. J. Dev. Neurosci.* 27, 805–815. doi: 10.1016/j.ijdevneu.2009.08.009

Ponsford, J., Whelan-Goodinson, R., and Bahar-Fuchs, A. (2007). Alcohol and drug use following traumatic brain injury: a prospective study. *Brain Inj.* 21, 1385–1392. doi: 10.1080/02699050701796960

Savola, O., Niemela, O., and Hillbom, M. (2005). Alcohol intake and the pattern of trauma in young adults and working aged people admitted after trauma. *Alcohol Alcohol.* 40, 269–273. doi: 10.1093/alcalc/agh159

Schwarzbach, E., Bonislawski, D. P., Xiong, G., and Cohen, A. S. (2006). Mechanisms underlying the inability to induce area CA1 LTP in the mouse after traumatic brain injury. *Hippocampus* 16, 541–550. doi: 10.1002/hipo.20183

Smedema, S. M., and Ebener, D. (2010). Substance abuse and psychosocial adaptation to physical disability: analysis of the literature and future directions. *Disabil. Rehabil.* 32, 1311–1319. doi: 10.3109/09638280903514721

Stewart-Scott, A. M., and Douglas, J. M. (1998). Educational outcome for secondary and postsecondary students following traumatic brain injury. *Brain Inj.* 12, 317–331. doi: 10.1080/026990598122629

Stoduto, G., Vingilis, E., Kapur, B. M., Sheu, W. J., Mclellan, B. A., and Liban, C. B. (1993). Alcohol and drug-use among motor-vehicle collision victims admitted to a regional trauma unit - demographic, injury, and crash characteristics. *Accid. Anal. Prev.* 25, 411–420. doi: 10.1016/0001-4575(93)90070-D

Unsworth, D. J., and Mathias, J. L. (2017). Traumatic brain injury and alcohol/substance abuse: a Bayesian meta-analysis comparing the outcomes of people with and without a history of abuse. *J. Clin. Exp. Neuropsychol.* 39, 547–562. doi: 10.1080/13803395.2016.1248812

Vaaramo, K., Puljula, J., Tetri, S., Juvela, S., and Hillbom, M. (2014). Head trauma sustained under the influence of alcohol is a predictor for future traumatic brain injury: a long-term follow-up study. *Eur. J. Neurol.* 21, 293–298. doi: 10.1111/ene.12302

Valles, S. L., Blanco, A. M., Pascual, M., and Guerri, C. (2004). Chronic ethanol treatment enhances inflammatory mediators and cell death in the brain and in astrocytes. *Brain Pathol.* 14, 365–371. doi: 10.1111/j.1750-3639.2004.tb00079.x

Wagner, A. K., Chen, X., Kline, A. E., Li, Y., Zafonte, R. D., and Dixon, C. E. (2005a). Gender and environmental enrichment impact dopamine transporter expression after experimental traumatic brain injury. *Exp. Neurol.* 195, 475–483. doi: 10.1016/j.expneurol.2005.06.009

Wagner, A. K., Drewencki, L. L., Chen, X., Santos, F. R., Khan, A. S., Harun, R., et al. (2009). Chronic methylphenidate treatment enhances striatal dopamine neurotransmission after experimental traumatic brain injury. *J. Neurochem.* 108, 986–997. doi: 10.1111/j.1471-4159.2008.05840.x

Wagner, A. K., Sokoloski, J. E., Ren, D., Chen, X., Khan, A. S., Zafonte, R. D., et al. (2005b). Controlled cortical impact injury affects dopaminergic transmission in the rat striatum. *J. Neurochem.* 95, 457–465. doi: 10.1111/j.1471-4159.2005.03382.x

Wahlstrom, D., Collins, P., White, T., and Luciana, M. (2010). Developmental changes in dopamine neurotransmission in adolescence: behavioral implications and issues in assessment. *Brain Cogn.* 72, 146–159. doi: 10.1016/j.bandc.2009.10.013

Weil, Z. M., Corrigan, J. D., and Karelina, K. (2016a). Alcohol abuse after traumatic brain injury: experimental and clinical evidence. *Neurosci. Biobehav. Rev.* 62, 89–99. doi: 10.1016/j.neubiorev.2016.01.005

Weil, Z. M., Karelina, K., Gaier, K. R., Corrigan, T. E., and Corrigan, J. D. (2016b). Juvenile traumatic brain injury increases alcohol consumption and reward in female mice. *J. Neurotrauma* 33, 895–903. doi: 10.1089/neu.2015.3953

Werner, C., and Engelhard, K. (2007). Pathophysiology of traumatic brain injury. *Br. J. Anaesth.* 99, 4–9. doi: 10.1093/bja/aem131

Yan, H. Q., Kline, A. E., Ma, X., Hooghe-Peters, E. L., Marion, D. W., and Dixon, C. E. (2001). Tyrosine hydroxylase, but not dopamine beta-hydroxylase, is increased in rat frontal cortex after traumatic brain injury. *Neuroreport* 12, 2323–2327. doi: 10.1097/00001756-200108080-00009

Yan, H. Q., Kline, A. E., Ma, X., Li, Y., and Dixon, C. E. (2002). Traumatic brain injury reduces dopamine transporter protein expression in the rat frontal cortex. *Neuroreport* 13, 1899–1901. doi: 10.1097/00001756-200210280-00013

Yen, C. H., Ho, P. S., Yeh, Y. W., Liang, C. S., Kuo, S. C., Huang, C. C., et al. (2017). Differential cytokine levels between early withdrawal and remission states in patients with alcohol dependence. *Psychoneuroendocrinology* 76, 183–191. doi: 10.1016/j.psyneuen.2016.10.015

Ziebell, J. M., and Morganti-Kossmann, M. C. (2010). Involvement of pro- and anti-inflammatory cytokines and chemokines in the pathophysiology of traumatic brain injury. *Neurotherapeutics* 7, 22–30. doi: 10.1016/j.nurt.2009.10.016

12

Chronic Ketamine Exposure Causes White Matter Microstructural Abnormalities in Adolescent Cynomolgus Monkeys

Qi Li[1,2,3†], Lin Shi[4,5†], Gang Lu[6], Hong-Luan Yu[7], Fu-Ki Yeung[8], Nai-Kei Wong[9], Lin Sun[10], Kai Liu[8], David Yew[11], Fang Pan[12], De-Feng Wang[8] and Pak C. Sham[1,2,13*]*

[1] Department of Psychiatry, The University of Hong Kong, Hong Kong, Hong Kong, [2] State Key Laboratory for Cognitive and Brain Sciences, The University of Hong Kong, Hong Kong, Hong Kong, [3] The University of Hong Kong Shenzhen Institute of Research and Innovation (HKU-SIRI), The University of Hong Kong, Hong Kong, Hong Kong, [4] Department of Medicine and Therapeutics, Chinese University of Hong Kong, Hong Kong, Hong Kong, [5] Chow Yuk Ho Center of Innovative Technology for Medicine, Chinese University of Hong Kong, Hong Kong, Hong Kong, [6] School of Biomedical Sciences, Chinese University of Hong Kong, Hong Kong, Hong Kong, [7] Department of Psychology, Qilu Hospital of Shandong University, Jinan, China, [8] Research Center for Medical Image Computing, Department of Imaging and Interventional Radiology, Chinese University of Hong Kong, Hong Kong, Hong Kong, [9] Chemical Biology Laboratory for Infectious Diseases, Shenzhen Institute of Hepatology, The Third People's Hospital of Shenzhen, Shenzhen, China, [10] Department of Psychology, Weifang Medical University, Weifang, China, [11] School of Chinese Medicine, Chinese University of Hong Kong, Hong Kong, Hong Kong, [12] Department of Medical Psychology, Shandong University School of Medicine, Jinan, China, [13] Genome Research Centre, The University of Hong Kong, Hong Kong, Hong Kong

Edited by:
Jacqueline M. Barker,
Medical University of South Carolina,
United States

Reviewed by:
Philip R. Corlett,
Yale University, United States
Marco Grados,
Johns Hopkins School of Medicine,
United States

***Correspondence:**
De-Feng Wang
dfwang@cuhk.edu.hk
Pak C. Sham
pcsham@hku.hk

† These authors have contributed equally to this work.

Acute and repeated exposures to ketamine mimic aspects of positive, negative, and cognitive symptoms of schizophrenia in humans. Recent studies by our group and others have shown that chronicity of ketamine use may be a key element for establishing a more valid model of cognitive symptoms of schizophrenia. However, current understanding on the long-term consequences of ketamine exposure on brain circuits has remained incomplete, particularly with regard to microstructural changes of white matter tracts that underpin the neuropathology of schizophrenia. Thus, the present study aimed to expand on previous investigations by examining causal effects of repeated ketamine exposure on white matter integrity in a non-human primate model. Ketamine or saline (control) was administered intravenously for 3 months to male adolescent cynomolgus monkeys (n = 5/group). Diffusion tensor imaging (DTI) experiments were performed and tract-based spatial statistics (TBSS) was used for data analysis. Fractional anisotropy (FA) was quantified across the whole brain. Profoundly reduced FA on the right side of sagittal striatum, posterior thalamic radiation (PTR), retrolenticular limb of the internal capsule (RLIC) and superior longitudinal fasciculus (SLF), and on the left side of PTR, middle temporal gyrus and inferior frontal gyrus were observed in the ketamine group compared to controls. Diminished white matter integrity found in either fronto-thalamo-temporal or striato-thalamic connections with tracts including the SLF, PTR, and RLIC lends support to similar findings from DTI studies on schizophrenia in humans. This study suggests that chronic ketamine exposure is a useful pharmacological paradigm that might provide translational insights into the pathophysiology and treatment of schizophrenia.

Keywords: ketamine, diffusion tensor imaging (DTI), thalamus, frontal gyrus, cynomologus monkeys

INTRODUCTION

Acute and repeated exposures to ketamine, an *N*-methyl-*D*-aspartate (NMDA) receptor antagonist, can be used to model aspects of positive, negative, and cognitive symptoms of schizophrenia in humans (Krystal et al., 1994; Newcomer et al., 1999; Dawson et al., 2013; Stone et al., 2014). A growing body of neuroimaging studies have demonstrated that acute administration of ketamine induces symptoms in healthy individuals comparable to an acute psychotic state, which include delusions (Abel et al., 2003a; Corlett et al., 2013), dissociative sensation (Deakin et al., 2008; De Simoni et al., 2013) and emotion blunting (Abel et al., 2003b; Daumann et al., 2008). However, a number of studies have indicated that acute ketamine administration does not significantly impair cognitive functions such as working memory, verbal fluency, and attention (Honey et al., 2004, 2005; Fu et al., 2005; Daumann et al., 2008). Furthermore, acute ketamine exposure has yielded inconsistent findings on resting-state functional connectivity particularly prefrontal cortex functional connectivity with subcortical brain regions (Scheidegger et al., 2012; Driesen et al., 2013), and these regions play an important role in executive functions (Bonelli and Cummings, 2007). Recently, it has been postulated that the most-reported short-term psychological effects of ketamine dependence were "floating or circling" sensation, while the long-term effects of ketamine dependence were memory impairment, personality changes, and slowed reactions (Curran and Morgan, 2000; Morgan et al., 2004; Fan et al., 2015). Thus, chronic ketamine use may provide a more valid model of cognitive symptoms of schizophrenia. Improved mechanistic characterization of the effects of long-term ketamine exposure on brain circuits is likewise crucial to a better understanding of the etiology of cognitive symptoms of schizophrenia.

Moreover, compelling phenotypic similarity between chronic ketamine use and schizophrenia exists in functional neural activity or white matter alterations, particularly, in light of disconnections involving the prefrontal cortex. In a recent functional magnetic resonance imaging (*f*MRI) study, it was reported that effects of chronic ketamine use on resting-state functional connectivity are coupled to increased activity in the frontal gyrus and decreased activity in the anterior cingulate cortex (ACC; Liao et al., 2012). Our previous study has also demonstrated that repeated exposure to ketamine in non-human primates reduced functional neural activity in the midbrain, posterior cingulate cortex (PCC), and visual cortex, but increased activity in the striatum (Yu et al., 2012). Diffusion tensor imaging (DTI) is an MRI-based neuroimaging technique that provides information about white matter microstructure *in vivo*. Damages in frontal white matter and corpus callosum have been reported in human cocaine addicts (Moeller et al., 2007; Wang et al., 2013). UP until now, only two clinical DTI findings have reported that chronic ketamine exposure disrupts white matter integrity in the frontal cortex (Liao et al., 2010; Edward Roberts et al., 2014). Liao et al. also reported reduced bilateral frontal gray matter volume in chronic ketamine users (Liao et al., 2011). However, exposure to other psychoactive substances of patients with ketamine dependence may confound interpretation of these results. In view of a paucity of knowledge about the long-term consequences of ketamine administration in brain structures, along with ethical concerns and technical difficulties in addressing this issue in humans, investigation on chronic ketamine exposure in preclinical animal models is clearly warranted.

Adolescents are socially vulnerable to drugs of abuse and display susceptibility to the development of drug dependence (Anthony and Petronis, 1995; Chambers et al., 2003). Despite the high prevalence of ketamine use among adolescents and young adults in Hong Kong and internationally (Lankenau and Clatts, 2004; Tang et al., 2015), disproportionately little is known about its impact on the developing brain. Again, it is particularly challenging to evaluate the drug effects on this age group in clinic. Non-human primates represent an excellent animal model because they share high similarity with humans in the pharmacokinetics and metabolism of several drugs and more importantly their prefrontal cortex is evolutionarily closely aligned with human counterparts (Preuss, 1995; Innocenti et al., 2016). Given the well-established role of prefrontal cortex in cognitive symptoms of psychosis, the aim of the present study was to expand on previous DTI investigations by examining potential causal effects of repeated ketamine exposure on white matter integrity and connectivity profiles between prefrontal cortex and subcortical brain regions in an adolescent non-human primate model. We predicted that chronic ketamine exposure perturbs the integrity of prefrontal cortex and its connectivity with subcortical regions.

MATERIALS AND METHODS

Animals and Ketamine Administration

Male adolescent cynomolgus monkeys (*Macaca fascicularis*) were purchased from Yunnan Laboratory Primate Inc. and all experiments were conducted in full compliance with license from the Ethics Committee of Shandong University. The animals were bred from a colony of natural-habitat-reared *M. fascicularis* and were kept at Hongli Animal Center (approval ID for use of non-human primates in this study: SYXK, 20050041) in a room maintained at temperature of 25°C with a 12:12 h light-dark cycle. Monkeys were individually housed in stainless steel cages (90 × 90 × 70 cm, SCXK Su 2003-0006) with water available *ad libitum* and were allowed to have visual and auditory contact with each other. They were fed twice daily with whole grains diet (Military Medical Animal Center of the Chinese Liberation Army, SCXK), supplemented with fresh fruits each day. Rearing procedures had been reviewed and approved by the Animal Care Committee of Shandong University.

Ten monkeys were randomly divided into two groups: Ketamine (1 mg/kg) or saline (control) was administered intravenously for 3 months to male adolescent *M. fascicularis* at 4.12 ± 0.65 (mean ± standard deviation) years old (ketamine group = 5, control group = 5). Based on studies by our group and others (Stoet and Snyder, 2006; Yu et al., 2012; Sun et al., 2014), ketamine dose of 1 mg/kg in an injection volume of 1 mL in saline was chosen and freshly prepared on the day of injection. Ketamine was given daily intravenously via arm vein under mild physical constraints for 13 weeks (i.e., ~3 months), while control monkeys were given sterile saline 1 mL. Ketamine was not given to the monkeys 24 h before the day of DTI scanning. No other pharmacological agents were administered to monkeys throughout the whole experiments. Animal body weights were recorded monthly to monitor the monkeys' well-being.

Diffusion Tensor Imaging (DTI)

DTI experiments were performed on a 3-T Signa Magnetic Resonance System (GE Company). Briefly, monkeys were anesthetized by intramuscular injection with ketamine (10 mg/kg) and xylazine hydrochloride (Sumianxin, 0.1 mL/kg; China Institute of Military Veterinary, Academy of Military Medical Sciences, Changchun, China; Feng et al., 2013). Anesthetized animals were immediately transferred to the MRI room. Anesthesia was sustained throughout the whole scanning period with no extra anesthetic doses being required. The monkeys were kept in place with sponges and sand bags and were oriented in a head-forward sphinx position. Respiration rate and body temperature were continuously monitored during the scan. DTI scanning was performed by using an EP/S sequence with the following parameters: repetition time = 6 s; echo time = 89.8 ms; field of view = 14 cm; flip angle = 90°; matrix = 256 × 256; slice thickness = 2.6 mm. Diffusion weighted imaging (b = 1,000 s/mm^2) was performed in 25 non-collinear directions with 1 non-diffusion weighted image.

Data Analysis

Fractional anisotropy (FA) was derived from diffusion data which quantifies how strongly directional a local tract structure is. In order to localize brain changes, group comparison of FA-value was performed between control group and ketamine group ($p < 0.005$, uncorrected). Tract-based spatial statistics (TBSS; Smith et al., 2006) part of FSL (Smith et al., 2004) was used in data processing. First, the raw diffusion data were preprocessed and corrected to eliminate the effects of head movement and eddy currents by using FMRIB Diffusion Toolbox (FDT). Then, a binary brain mask was created by brain-extracting the no diffusion weighting (b = 0) image by using Brain Extraction Tool (BET; Smith, 2002) and mean FA images were created by fitting a tensor model to the corrected diffusion data with its brain mask. Before group comparison, all FA images were aligned onto the MNI152 standard space by non-linear registration and resliced into 1 × 1 × 1 mm^3 resolution by TBSS software for later accurate cluster quantification. A mean FA skeleton was created such that it most represents the centers of all tracts common to the group. The voxel-wise group statistical comparison was performed to show which voxels on the mean FA skeleton mask had significant difference between control group and ketamine group. The analysis statistics was based on TBSS with threshold-free cluster enhancement (TFCE) algorithm. TFCE method was adopted with a non-parametric approach of permutation test of 500 permutations (Smith and Nichols, 2009). Results were generated based on significant threshold at uncorrected one-tailed TFCE $p < 0.005$.The quantification of voxel size within a cluster was then performed by using Xjview toolbox (http://www.alivelearn.net/xjview). To locate the actual anatomical regions of those significant clusters in monkey, a diffusion tensor based white matter brain atlas for rhesus macaques was applied (Adluru et al., 2012) onto the results as anatomical underlay.

RESULTS

Regions of Significant Difference in Fractional Anisotropy (FA) between Groups

Group comparison between chronic ketamine administration group and controls revealed seven different anatomical regions, where the ketamine group had FA-values significantly lower than that of the control group. The anatomic location and size of these clusters with peak t-values for ketamine group and controls are as shown in **Table 1**. In this table, statistical analysis found significant FA changes ($p < 0.005$) between ketamine group and controls in the right side of sagittal striatum (SS; $t = 4.3829$), posterior thalamic radiation (PTR, right side, $t = 3.9214$; left side, $t = 7.1843$), middle temporal gyrus white matter (MTG-WM, left side, $t = 4.3206$), inferior frontal gyrus WM (IFG-WM, left side, $t = 3.8225$), retrolenticular limb of the internal capsule (RLIC, right side, $t = 2.5386$), and superior longitudinal fasciculus (SLF, right side, $t = 4.9845$).

Figure 1 showed spatial distribution of the brain regions indicating a reduction of FA ($p < 0.005$, TFCE-uncorrected) in right SS in the ketamine administration group when compared with controls. In addition, the significant regions were located in the posterior region of the thalamic radiation. Both right and left PTR showed reduced FA ($p < 0.005$) in the ketamine administration group (**Figures 2, 3**). The RLIC comes from the thalamus and more posteriorly this becomes the optical radiation (Larry et al., 2012). **Figure 6** indicated a reduction of FA ($p < 0.005$) in the right RLIC in the ketamine group compared with controls. SLF, the largest association bundles, connects to the cortex of the frontal, parietal, occipital and temporal lobes (Larry et al., 2012). We found reduced FA in the right SLF in ketamine administration group ($p < 0.005$; **Figure 7**). Consistent with a ground-breaking finding reported by Liao et al. (2010), the present study showed decreased FA ($p < 0.005$) in left side of IFG (**Figure 5**) and MTG (**Figure 4**) in chronic ketamine administration group compared with controls. Moreover, our previous functional image study on the same model showed hypofunctions in the PCC and visual cortex (Yu et al., 2012).

There were no cluster areas where the ketamine group had FA-values higher than that of controls.

DISCUSSION

The present study provides direct experimental evidence that chronic ketamine exposure significantly disrupts white matter microstructures across a number of critical brain circuits. We found that repeated ketamine exposure elicits bidirectional reduced FA of PTR, left side of middle temporal gyrus WM (MTG-WM) and inferior frontal gyrus WM (IFG-WM), and also reduced FA in the right side of sagittal striatum (SS), RLIC, and SLF. More importantly, reduced integrity of fronto-thalamo-temporal or striato-thalamic white matter connectivity observed in this study is consistent with, and extend the previous clinical findings in chronic ketamine users.

TABLE 1 | Regions with significant FA differences between chronic ketamine exposure group and controls.

Region of significant clusters	Hemisphere	Cluster size (voxels)	Peak coordinates [*x*, *y*, *z*]	Peak *t*-value
Sagittal striatum (SS)	Right	7	[52, 27, 33]	4.3829
Posterior thalamic radiation (PTR)	Right	27	[54, 23, 35]	3.9214
Posterior thalamic radiation (PTR)	Left	12	[20, 27, 35]	7.1843
Middle temporal gyrus WM (MTG-WM)	Left	4	[15, 37, 37]	4.3206
Inferior frontal gyrus WM (IFG-WM)	Left	3	[23, 61, 43]	3.8225
Retrolenticular limb of the internal capsule (RLIC)	Right	4	[52, 38, 38]	2.5386
Superior longitudinal fasciculus (SLF)	Right	21	[54, 27, 42]	4.9845

x, y, z are co-ordinates based on the reference DTI monkey brain template FA map (Adluru et al., 2012) with its atlas (http://www.nitrc.org/projects/rmdtitemplate/). z indicates the vertical distance from the lowest axial plane of reference image in mm, x refers to sagittal plane, y refers to coronal plane. The uncorrected p-value of all the voxels in the cluster are p < 0.005. WM, white matter.

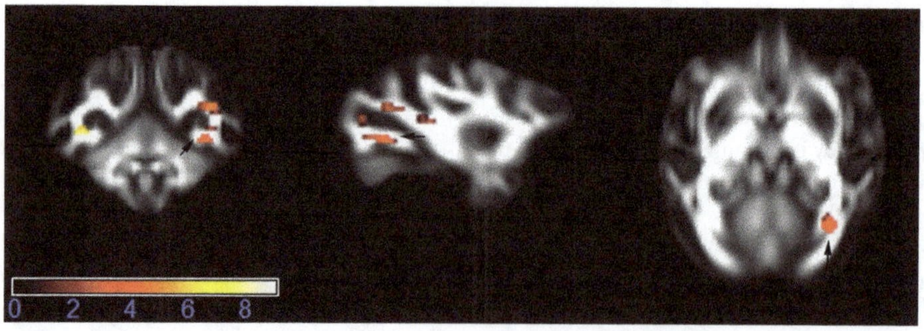

FIGURE 1 | Areas in sagittal striatum (SS, right side) with reduced fractional anisotropy values in the chronic ketamine exposure group compared to controls at $p < 0.005$ (in red; uncorrected). The anatomical underlay is DTI-based monkey brain image template (UWRMAC-DTI271) FA map with white matter atlas. Figure from left to right side is coronal view, sagittal view, and axial view of the images, respectively. The color bar represents the *t*-value.

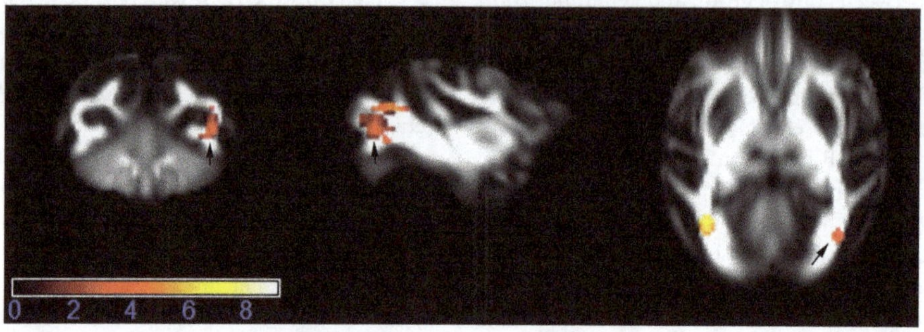

FIGURE 2 | Areas in posterior thalamic radiation (PTR, right side) with reduced fractional anisotropy values in the chronic ketamine exposure group compared to controls at $p < 0.005$ (in red; uncorrected). The anatomical underlay is DTI-based monkey brain image template (UWRMAC-DTI271) FA map with white matter atlas. Figure from left to right side is coronal view, sagittal view, and axial view of the images, respectively. The color bar represents the *t*-value.

Our current DTI findings of abnormality in the IFG-WM and MTG-WM with chronic ketamine exposure in non-human primate are largely consistent with white matter tract patterns observed in previous clinical imaging studies of schizophrenia in humans (Thompson et al., 2001; Kyriakopoulos et al., 2008; Ellison-Wright and Bullmore, 2009). In a comprehensive meta-analysis of DTI studies on schizophrenia, Ellison-Wright et al. (Ellison-Wright and Bullmore, 2009) summarized two locations of FA reductions in the deep white matter of the left frontal and temporal lobes. Disruption of fronto-temporal white matter network may contribute to cognitive deficits in schizophrenia (Kubicki et al., 2007). Even though abnormalities in the white matter have not been found consistently in schizophrenia patients in methodologically varied studies, the frontal white matter seems to be commonly affected. Recently, Zalesky et al. (2011) showed that a fronto-parietal/occipital network may represent the key macro-circuit affected in schizophrenia, while an aberrant network structure of bilateral inferior frontal cortex and temporal has been reported in schizophrenia patients (van den Heuvel et al., 2010). These findings suggest that

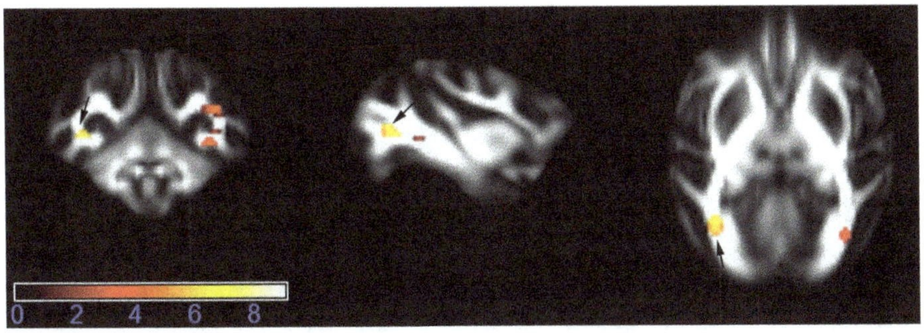

FIGURE 3 | Areas in posterior thalamic radiation (PTR, left side) with reduced fractional anisotropy values in the chronic ketamine exposure group compared to controls at $p < 0.005$ (in red; uncorrected). The anatomical underlay is DTI-based monkey brain image template (UWRMAC-DTI271) FA map with white matter atlas. Figure from left to right side is coronal view, sagittal view, and axial view of the images, respectively. The color bar represents the *t*-value.

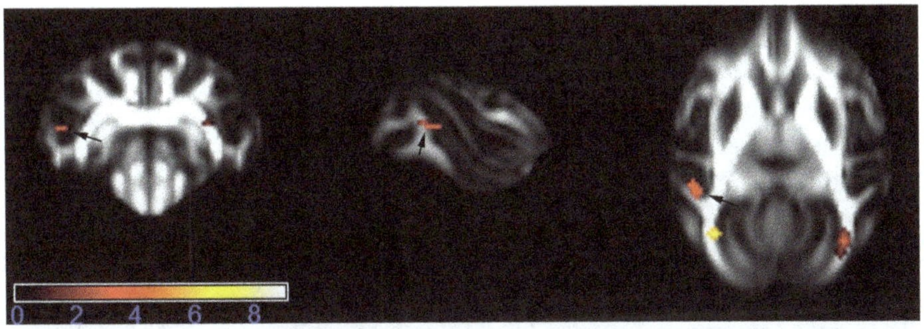

FIGURE 4 | Areas in middle temporal gyrus WM (MTG-WM, left side) with reduced fractional anisotropy values in the chronic ketamine exposure group compared to controls at $p < 0.005$ (in red; uncorrected). The anatomical underlay is DTI-based monkey brain image template (UWRMAC-DTI271) FA map with white matter atlas. Figure from left to right side is coronal view, sagittal view, and axial view of the images, respectively. The color bar represents the *t*-value.

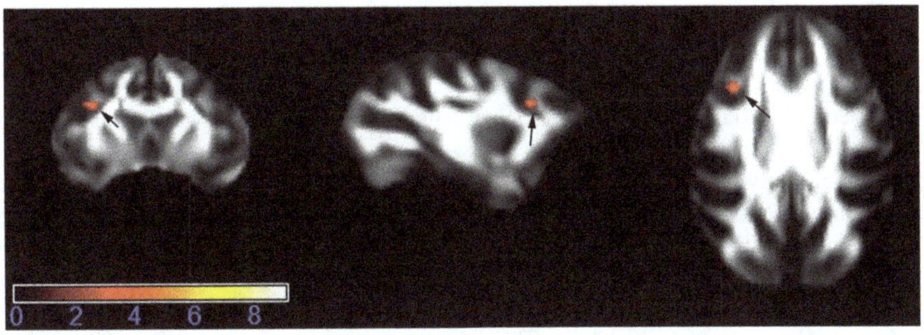

FIGURE 5 | Areas in inferior frontal gyrus WM (IFG-WM, left side) with reduced fractional anisotropy values in the chronic ketamine exposure group compared to controls at $p < 0.005$ (in red; uncorrected). The anatomical underlay is DTI-based monkey brain image template (UWRMAC-DTI271) FA map with white matter atlas. Figure from left to right side is coronal view, sagittal view, and axial view of the images, respectively. The color bar represents the *t*-value.

schizophrenia patients have a less organized brain networks with a reduced central role for the key frontal hub, which results in limited integration of information between brain regions.

Consistent with the view of "hypofrontality" in schizophrenia (Wolkin et al., 1992), a growing number of brain imaging studies have shown that the frontal white matter abnormalities may be as a fundamental change in patients with chronic drug dependence (Nestler, 2005; Wang et al., 2013). Animal studies by our group and others have shown that apoptosis of neuronal cells in the frontal cortex is induced by chronic exposure to ketamine (Zou et al., 2009; Yeung et al., 2010; Sun et al., 2014). To date, however, there have been only two clinical studies examining white matter integrity in chronic ketamine users (Liao et al., 2010; Edward Roberts et al., 2014). Liao et al. (2010) first reported that white matter changes with reduced FA in the bilateral frontal and left temporo-parietal cortices are

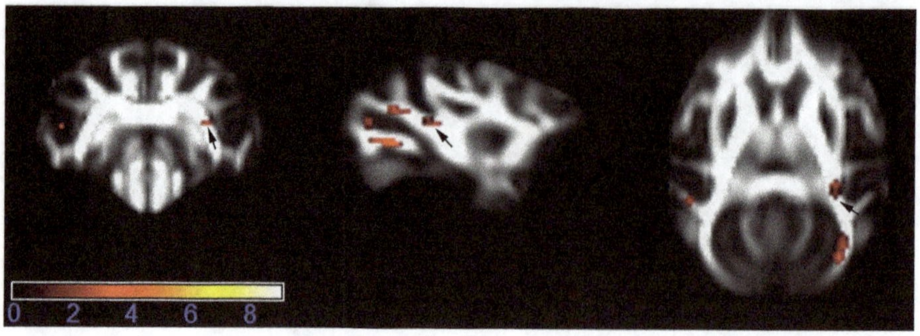

FIGURE 6 | Areas in retrolenticular limb of the internal capsule (RLIC, right side) with reduced fractional anisotropy values in the chronic ketamine exposure group compared to controls at $p < 0.005$ (in red; uncorrected). The anatomical underlay is DTI-based monkey brain image template (UWRMAC-DTI271) FA map with white matter atlas. Figure from left to right side is coronal view, sagittal view, and axial view of the images, respectively. The color bar represents the *t*-value.

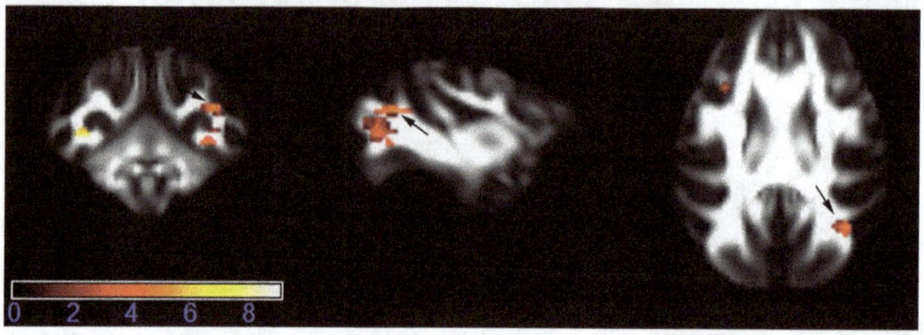

FIGURE 7 | Areas in superior longitudinal fasciculus (SLF, right side) with reduced fractional anisotropy values in the chronic ketamine exposure group compared to controls at $p < 0.005$ (in red; uncorrected). The anatomical underlay is DTI-based monkey brain image template (UWRMAC-DTI271) FA map with white matter atlas. Figure from left to right side is coronal view, sagittal view, and axial view of the images, respectively. The color bar represents the *t*-value.

associated with chronic ketamine use. Later, Edward Roberts et al. (2014) partially replicated the findings reported by Liao et al., which revealed a reduction in axial diffusivity in the right side of prefrontal white matter in chronic ketamine users. They further observed that the connectivity between caudate nucleus and lateral prefrontal cortex pathway was positively associated with dissociative experiences in ketamine users (Edward Roberts et al., 2014). Our findings are also in partial agreement with those studies, as the brain areas of abnormality observed in this study were also located in the left side of frontal lobe (IFG-WM) and temporal lobe (MTG-WM). The absence of an effect of ketamine on right side of frontal lobe in this study may be because a shorter duration of ketamine exposure or the use of only male animals in our experiment. A second consideration is that all the subjects in our study started to receive ketamine during adolescence, which is a stage of development known to involve brain plasticity (Blakemore and Choudhury, 2006). In addition, frontal lobe deficits may well be associated with the ketamine-related memory defects and cognitive symptoms in schizophrenia patients. Our research group have demonstrated that chronic exposure to ketamine impaired working memory in mice, which was correlated with dysfunction of GABA signaling system in the prefrontal cortex (Tan et al., 2011). However, further investigation including studies on working memory symptoms combined with neuroimaging is needed to better understand the neuropathological roles of the frontal lobe in chronic ketamine users.

Both IFG-WM and MTG-WM lie laterally to the SLF (Adluru et al., 2012), the major white matter connection between the prefrontal and parietal/temporal cortices, which are functionally related to verbal working memory performance (Hazlett et al., 2008; Karlsgodt et al., 2008). Edward Roberts et al. (2014) reported reduced axial diffusivity in the right side of SLF in ketamine users. In addition, recent evidence has demonstrated that activities in the right IFG network connected by SLF, especially in the right hemisphere, play prominent roles in corporeal awareness during illusion (Amemiya and Naito, 2016). Patients with first-episode paranoid schizophrenia exhibited reduced FA in the right SLF and right internal capsule (Guo et al., 2012). In line with these findings, decreased FA in the right SLF in our study may implicate fronto-parietal white matter disconnectivity in symptoms associated with chronic ketamine exposure in monkeys.

White matter FA in bilateral PTR, a region encompassing fiber pathways that connects the caudal parts of thalamus with the occipital and parietal lobes, was reduced in monkeys chronically exposed to ketamine. This association tract is of interest because it plays a key role connecting visual and motor processes, and is an integral part of neural network regulating cognitive performance (Cremers et al., 2016). Bilateral FA reduction in the PTR has been reported in patients with schizophrenia (Peters et al., 2010; Melonakos et al., 2011; Melicher et al., 2015). However, Edward Roberts et al. (2014) found impairment only on the right side of PTR in chronic ketamine users. Our results encourage further investigation into the role of this projection in ketamine use.

The sagittal striatum, which includes a large part of both the inferior longitudinal fasciculus and inferior fronto-occipital fasciculus, projects to the frontal and limbic cortices (Adluru et al., 2012). Striatum and its cortical connections are critical in the pathogenesis of the complex cognitive symptoms of schizophrenia (Simpson et al., 2010). There is corroborative evidence from animal models and clinical investigations that sensorimotor gating function is modulated by cortico-striato-thalamic circuitry (Hazlett et al., 2008; Li et al., 2009, 2010). In the present study, compromised white matter tract integrity seen on right side of striato-thalamic connections, specifically tracts including RLIC and PTR, supports white matter alterations in the brain of chronic ketamine users as reported by Edward Roberts et al. (2014). These white matter alterations in the brain may also contribute to the dissociative experiences reported by chronic ketamine users (Edward Roberts et al., 2014). Moreover, reduced FA in RLIC was reported to be associated with negative symptoms in patients with schizophrenia (Arnedo et al., 2015).

CONCLUSION

The results of the present study confirm chronic ketamine use during adolescence causes brain damage in areas known to be involved in neurodevelopment during adolescence, in particular, fronto-thalamo-temporal white matter connection (Alcauter et al., 2014; Xiao et al., 2016). Based on clinical findings on chronic ketamine exposure, our study has systematically surveyed major brain regions posited to have reductions in white matter integrity. More importantly, the current observations of reduced white matter in eitherfronto-thalamo-temporal or striato-thalamic networks involving white matter tracts including the SLF, PTR, and RLIC echo findings in human DTI studies on schizophrenia. These results furnish a rational basis for studying chronic ketamine exposure of adolescent brain as a pharmacological paradigm and may yield translational insights into the pathophysiology and treatment of schizophrenia.

LIMITATIONS

Firstly, we acknowledge that the sample size of the current study was modest. Our findings are nonetheless promising, being the first direct evidence for establishing the casual effects of chronic ketamine exposure on microstructure integrity of white matter tracts in adolescent non-human primates. Secondly, we examined only male adolescent monkeys in this study. A decision to dedicate finite experimental resources to males was made because male subjects are generally more vulnerable to drug addiction (DePoy et al., 2016), and there is evidence that males experiencing neurodevelopmental perturbations associated with schizophrenia were inferior to females in memory performance (Goldstein et al., 1998).

AUTHOR CONTRIBUTIONS

QL, LS (2nd author), GL, DY, FP, DW, and PS contributed to design, acquisition, analysis, and interpretation of data for this work. QL wrote the draft for the manuscript. GL, HY, LS (7th author), and FP performed the experiments. LS (2nd author), FY, KL, QL, and DW prepared all figures and image analysis. NW, GL, HY, LS (2nd author), and PS revised and edited the manuscript. PS approved the final draft of the manuscript. All authors reviewed the manuscript for intellectual content and approved submission.

REFERENCES

Abel, K. M., Allin, M. P., Kucharska-Pietura, K., Andrew, C., Williams, S., David, A. S., et al. (2003a). Ketamine and fMRI BOLD signal: distinguishing between effects mediated by change in blood flow versus change in cognitive state. *Hum. Brain Mapp.* 18, 135–145. doi: 10.1002/hbm.10064

Abel, K. M., Allin, M. P., Kucharska-Pietura, K., David, A., Andrew, C., Williams, S., et al. (2003b). Ketamine alters neural processing of facial emotion recognition in healthy men: an fMRI study. *Neuroreport* 14, 387–391. doi: 10.1097/00001756-200303030-00018

Adluru, N., Zhang, H., Fox, A. S., Shelton, S. E., Ennis, C. M., Bartosic, A. M., et al. (2012). A diffusion tensor brain template for rhesus macaques. *Neuroimage* 59, 306–318. doi: 10.1016/j.neuroimage.2011.07.029

Alcauter, S., Lin, W., Smith, J. K., Short, S. J., Goldman, B. D., Reznick, J. S., et al. (2014). Development of thalamocortical connectivity during infancy and its cognitive correlations. *J. Neurosci.* 34, 9067–9075. doi: 10.1523/JNEUROSCI.0796-14.2014

Amemiya, K., and Naito, E. (2016). Importance of human right inferior frontoparietal network connected by inferior branch of superior longitudinal fasciculus tract in corporeal awareness of kinesthetic illusory movement. *Cortex* 78, 15–30. doi: 10.1016/j.cortex.2016.01.017

Anthony, J. C., and Petronis, K. R. (1995). Early-onset drug use and risk of later drug problems. *Drug Alcohol Depend.* 40, 9–15. doi: 10.1016/0376-8716(95)01194-3

Arnedo, J., Mamah, D., Baranger, D. A., Harms, M. P., Barch, D. M., Svrakic, D. M., et al. (2015). Decomposition of brain diffusion imaging data uncovers latent schizophrenias with distinct patterns of white matter anisotropy. *Neuroimage* 120, 43–54. doi: 10.1016/j.neuroimage.2015.06.083

Blakemore, S. J., and Choudhury, S. (2006). Development of the adolescent brain: implications for executive function and social cognition. *J. Child Psychol. Psychiatry* 47, 296–312. doi: 10.1111/j.1469-7610.2006.01611.x

Bonelli, R. M., and Cummings, J. L. (2007). Frontal-subcortical circuitry and behavior. *Dialogues Clin. Neurosci.* 9, 141–151.

Chambers, R. A., Taylor, J. R., and Potenza, M. N. (2003). Developmental neurocircuitry of motivation in adolescence: a critical period of addiction vulnerability. *Am. J. Psychiatry* 160, 1041–1052. doi: 10.1176/appi.ajp.160.6.1041

Corlett, P. R., Cambridge, V., Gardner, J. M., Piggot, J. S., Turner, D. C., Everitt, J. C., et al. (2013). Ketamine effects on memory reconsolidation favor a learning model of delusions. *PLoS ONE* 8:e65088. doi: 10.1371/journal.pone.0065088

Cremers, L. G. M., de Groot, M., Hofman, A., Krestin, G. P., van der Lugt, A., Niessen, W. J., et al. (2016). Altered tract-specific white matter microstructure is related to poorer cognitive performance: the Rotterdam Study. *Neurobiol. Aging* 39, 108–117. doi: 10.1016/j.neurobiolaging.2015.11.021

Curran, H. V., and Morgan, C. (2000). Cognitive, dissociative and psychotogenic effects of ketamine in recreational users on the night of drug use and 3 days later. *Addiction* 95, 575–590. doi: 10.1046/j.1360-0443.2000.9545759.x

Daumann, J., Heekeren, K., Neukirch, A., Thiel, C. M., Moller-Hartmann, W., and Gouzoulis-Mayfrank, E. (2008). Pharmacological modulation of the neural basis underlying inhibition of return (IOR) in the human 5-HT2A agonist and NMDA antagonist model of psychosis. *Psychopharmacology* 200, 573–583. doi: 10.1007/s00213-008-1237-1

Dawson, N., Morris, B. J., and Pratt, J. A. (2013). Subanaesthetic ketamine treatment alters prefrontal cortex connectivity with thalamus and ascending subcortical systems. *Schizophr. Bull.* 39, 366–377. doi: 10.1093/schbul/sbr144

De Simoni, S., Schwarz, A. J., O'Daly, O. G., Marquand, A. F., Brittain, C., Gonzales, C., et al. (2013). Test-retest reliability of the BOLD pharmacological MRI response to ketamine in healthy volunteers. *Neuroimage* 64, 75–90. doi: 10.1016/j.neuroimage.2012.09.037

Deakin, J. F., Lees, J., McKie, S., Hallak, J. E., Williams, S. R., and Dursun, S. M. (2008). Glutamate and the neural basis of the subjective effects of ketamine: a pharmaco-magnetic resonance imaging study. *Arch. Gen. Psychiatry* 65, 154–164. doi: 10.1001/archgenpsychiatry.2007.37

DePoy, L. M., Allen, A. G., and Gourley, S. L. (2016). Adolescent cocaine self-administration induces habit behavior in adulthood: sex differences and structural consequences. *Transl. Psychiatry* 6:e875. doi: 10.1038/tp.2016.150

Driesen, N. R., McCarthy, G., Bhagwagar, Z., Bloch, M., Calhoun, V., D'Souza, D. C., et al. (2013). Relationship of resting brain hyperconnectivity and schizophrenia-like symptoms produced by the NMDA receptor antagonist ketamine in humans. *Mol. Psychiatry* 18, 1199–1204. doi: 10.1038/mp.2012.194

Edward Roberts, R., Curran, H. V., Friston, K. J., and Morgan, C. J. (2014). Abnormalities in white matter microstructure associated with chronic ketamine use. *Neuropsychopharmacology* 39, 329–338. doi: 10.1038/npp.2013.195

Ellison-Wright, I., and Bullmore, E. (2009). Meta-analysis of diffusion tensor imaging studies in schizophrenia. *Schizophr. Res.* 108, 3–10. doi: 10.1016/j.schres.2008.11.021

Fan, N., Xu, K., Ning, Y., Wang, D., Ke, X., Ding, Y., et al. (2015). Development of a checklist of short-term and long-term psychological symptoms associated with ketamine use. *Shanghai Arch. Psychiatry* 27, 186–194. doi: 10.11919/j.issn.1002-0829.214158

Feng, Y., Chai, J., Chu, W., Ma, L., Zhang, P., and Duan, H. (2013). Combination of ketamine and xylazine exacerbates cardiac dysfunction in severely scalded rats during the shock stage. *Exp. Ther. Med.* 6, 641–648. doi: 10.3892/etm.2013.1213

Fu, C. H., Abel, K. M., Allin, M. P., Gasston, D., Costafreda, S. G., Suckling, J., et al. (2005). Effects of ketamine on prefrontal and striatal regions in an overt verbal fluency task: a functional magnetic resonance imaging study. *Psychopharmacology* 183, 92–102. doi: 10.1007/s00213-005-0154-9

Goldstein, J. M., Seidman, L. J., Goodman, J. M., Koren, D., Lee, H., Weintraub, S., et al. (1998). Are there sex differences in neuropsychological functions among patients with schizophrenia? *Am. J. Psychiatry* 155, 1358–1364. doi: 10.1176/ajp.155.10.1358

Guo, W., Liu, F., Liu, Z., Gao, K., Xiao, C., Chen, H., et al. (2012). Right lateralized white matter abnormalities in first-episode, drug-naive paranoid schizophrenia. *Neurosci. Lett.* 531, 5–9. doi: 10.1016/j.neulet.2012.09.033

Hazlett, E. A., Buchsbaum, M. S., Zhang, J., Newmark, R. E., Glanton, C. F., Zelmanova, Y., et al. (2008). Frontal-striatal-thalamic mediodorsal nucleus dysfunction in schizophrenia-spectrum patients during sensorimotor gating. *Neuroimage* 42, 1164–1177. doi: 10.1016/j.neuroimage.2008.05.039

Honey, G. D., Honey, R. A., O'Loughlin, C., Sharar, S. R., Kumaran, D., Suckling, J., et al. (2005). Ketamine disrupts frontal and hippocampal contribution to encoding and retrieval of episodic memory: an fMRI study. *Cereb. Cortex* 15, 749–759. doi: 10.1093/cercor/bhh176

Honey, R. A., Honey, G. D., O'Loughlin, C., Sharar, S. R., Kumaran, D., Bullmore, E. T., et al. (2004). Acute ketamine administration alters the brain responses to executive demands in a verbal working memory task: an FMRI study. *Neuropsychopharmacology* 29, 1203–1214. doi: 10.1038/sj.npp.1300438

Innocenti, G. M., Dyrby, T. B., Andersen, K. W., Rouiller, E. M., and Caminiti, R. (2016). The crossed projection to the striatum in two species of monkey and in humans: behavioral and evolutionary significance. *Cereb. Cortex.* doi: 10.1093/cercor/bhw161. [Epub ahead of print].

Karlsgodt, K. H., van Erp, T. G., Poldrack, R. A., Bearden, C. E., Nuechterlein, K. H., and Cannon, T. D. (2008). Diffusion tensor imaging of the superior longitudinal fasciculus and working memory in recent-onset schizophrenia. *Biol. Psychiatry* 63, 512–518. doi: 10.1016/j.biopsych.2007.06.017

Krystal, J. H., Karper, L. P., Seibyl, J. P., Freeman, G. K., Delaney, R., Bremner, J. D., et al. (1994). Subanesthetic effects of the noncompetitive NMDA antagonist, ketamine, in humans. Psychotomimetic, perceptual, cognitive, and neuroendocrine responses. *Arch. Gen. Psychiatry* 51, 199–214. doi: 10.1001/archpsyc.1994.03950030035004

Kubicki, M., McCarley, R., Westin, C. F., Park, H. J., Maier, S., Kikinis, R., et al. (2007). A review of diffusion tensor imaging studies in schizophrenia. *J. Psychiatr. Res.* 41, 15–30. doi: 10.1016/j.jpsychires.2005.05.005

Kyriakopoulos, M., Bargiotas, T., Barker, G. J., and Frangou, S. (2008). Diffusion tensor imaging in schizophrenia. *Eur. Psychiatry* 23, 255–273. doi: 10.1016/j.eurpsy.2007.12.004

Lankenau, S. E., and Clatts, M. C. (2004). Drug injection practices among high-risk youths: the first shot of ketamine. *J. Urban Health* 81, 232–248. doi: 10.1093/jurban/jth110

Larry, R. S., Berg, D., Bloom, F. E., Sascha, D. L., Anirvan, G., and Nicholas, C. S. (2012). *Fundamental Neuroscience, 4th Edn.* Waltham, MA: Elsevier.

Li, Q., Cheung, C., Wei, R., Cheung, V., Hui, E. S., You, Y., et al. (2010). Voxel-based analysis of postnatal white matter microstructure in mice exposed to immune challenge in early or late pregnancy. *Neuroimage* 52, 1–8. doi: 10.1016/j.neuroimage.2010.04.015

Li, Q., Cheung, C., Wei, R., Hui, E. S., Feldon, J., Meyer, U., et al. (2009). Prenatal immune challenge is an environmental risk factor for brain and behavior change relevant to schizophrenia: evidence from MRI in a mouse model. *PLoS ONE* 4:e6354. doi: 10.1371/journal.pone.0006354

Liao, Y., Tang, J., Corlett, P. R., Wang, X., Yang, M., Chen, H., et al. (2011). Reduced dorsal prefrontal gray matter after chronic ketamine use. *Biol. Psychiatry* 69, 42–48. doi: 10.1016/j.biopsych.2010.08.030

Liao, Y., Tang, J., Fornito, A., Liu, T., Chen, X., Chen, H., et al. (2012). Alterations in regional homogeneity of resting-state brain activity in ketamine addicts. *Neurosci. Lett.* 522, 36–40. doi: 10.1016/j.neulet.2012.06.009

Liao, Y., Tang, J., Ma, M., Wu, Z., Yang, M., Wang, X., et al. (2010). Frontal white matter abnormalities following chronic ketamine use: a diffusion tensor imaging study. *Brain* 133(Pt 7), 2115–2122. doi: 10.1093/brain/awq131

Melicher, T., Horacek, J., Hlinka, J., Spaniel, F., Tintera, J., Ibrahim, I., et al. (2015). White matter changes in first episode psychosis and their relation to the size of sample studied: a DTI study. *Schizophr. Res.* 162, 22–28. doi: 10.1016/j.schres.2015.01.029

Melonakos, E. D., Shenton, M. E., Rathi, Y., Terry, D. P., Bouix, S., and Kubicki, M. (2011). Voxel-based morphometry (VBM) studies in schizophrenia-can white matter changes be reliably detected with VBM? *Psychiatry Res.* 193, 65–70. doi: 10.1016/j.pscychresns.2011.01.009

Moeller, F. G., Hasan, K. M., Steinberg, J. L., Kramer, L. A., Valdes, I., Lai, L. Y., et al. (2007). Diffusion tensor imaging eigenvalues: preliminary evidence for altered myelin in cocaine dependence. *Psychiatry Res.* 154, 253–258. doi: 10.1016/j.pscychresns.2006.11.004

Morgan, C. J., Monaghan, L., and Curran, H. V. (2004). Beyond the K-hole: a 3-year longitudinal investigation of the cognitive and subjective effects of ketamine in recreational users who have substantially reduced their use of the drug. *Addiction* 99, 1450–1461. doi: 10.1111/j.1360-0443.2004.00879.x

Nestler, E. J. (2005). Is there a common molecular pathway for addiction? *Nat. Neurosci.* 8, 1445–1449. doi: 10.1038/nn1578

Newcomer, J. W., Farber, N. B., Jevtovic-Todorovic, V., Selke, G., Melson, A. K., Hershey, T., et al. (1999). Ketamine-induced NMDA receptor hypofunction as a model of memory impairment and psychosis. *Neuropsychopharmacology* 20, 106–118. doi: 10.1016/S0893-133X(98)00067-0

Peters, B. D., Blaas, J., and de Haan, L. (2010). Diffusion tensor imaging in the early phase of schizophrenia: what have we learned? *J. Psychiatr. Res.* 44, 993–1004. doi: 10.1016/j.jpsychires.2010.05.003

Preuss, T. M. (1995). Do rats have prefrontal cortex? The rose-woolsey-akert program reconsidered. *J. Cogn. Neurosci.* 7, 1–24. doi: 10.1162/jocn.1995.7.1.1

Scheidegger, M., Walter, M., Lehmann, M., Metzger, C., Grimm, S., Boeker, H., et al. (2012). Ketamine decreases resting state functional network connectivity in healthy subjects: implications for antidepressant drug action. *PLoS ONE* 7:e44799. doi: 10.1371/journal.pone.0044799

Simpson, E. H., Kellendonk, C., and Kandel, E. (2010). A possible role for the striatum in the pathogenesis of the cognitive symptoms of schizophrenia. *Neuron* 65, 585–596. doi: 10.1016/j.neuron.2010.02.014

Smith, S. M. (2002). Fast robust automated brain extraction. *Hum. Brain Mapp.* 17, 143–155. doi: 10.1002/hbm.10062

Smith, S. M., and Nichols, T. E. (2009). Threshold-free cluster enhancement: addressing problems of smoothing, threshold dependence and localisation in cluster inference. *Neuroimage* 44, 83–98. doi: 10.1016/j.neuroimage.2008.03.061

Smith, S. M., Jenkinson, M., Johansen-Berg, H., Rueckert, D., Nichols, T. E., Mackay, C. E., et al. (2006). Tract-based spatial statistics: voxelwise analysis of multi-subject diffusion data. *Neuroimage* 31, 1487–1505. doi: 10.1016/j.neuroimage.2006.02.024

Smith, S. M., Jenkinson, M., Woolrich, M. W., Beckmann, C. F., Behrens, T. E., Johansen-Berg, H., et al. (2004). Advances in functional and structural MR image analysis and implementation as FSL. *Neuroimage* 23(Suppl. 1), S208–S219. doi: 10.1016/j.neuroimage.2004.07.051

Stoet, G., and Snyder, L. H. (2006). Effects of the NMDA antagonist ketamine on task-switching performance: evidence for specific impairments of executive control. *Neuropsychopharmacology* 31, 1675–1681. doi: 10.1038/sj.npp.1300930

Stone, J. M., Pepper, F., Fam, J., Furby, H., Hughes, E., Morgan, C., et al. (2014). Glutamate, N-acetyl aspartate and psychotic symptoms in chronic ketamine users. *Psychopharmacology* 231, 2107–2116. doi: 10.1007/s00213-013-3354-8

Sun, L., Li, Q., Li, Q., Zhang, Y., Liu, D., Jiang, H., et al. (2014). Chronic ketamine exposure induces permanent impairment of brain functions in adolescent cynomolgus monkeys. *Addict. Biol.* 19, 185–194. doi: 10.1111/adb.12004

Tan, S., Rudd, J. A., and Yew, D. T. (2011). Gene expression changes in GABA(A) receptors and cognition following chronic ketamine administration in mice. *PLoS ONE* 6:e21328. doi: 10.1371/journal.pone.0021328

Tang, M., Ching, C. K., Tse, M. L., Ng, C., Lee, C., Chong, Y. K., et al. (2015). Surveillance of emerging drugs of abuse in Hong Kong: validation of an analytical tool. *Hong Kong Med. J.* 21, 114–123. doi: 10.12809/hkmj144398

Thompson, P. M., Vidal, C., Giedd, J. N., Gochman, P., Blumenthal, J., Nicolson, R., et al. (2001). Mapping adolescent brain change reveals dynamic wave of accelerated gray matter loss in very early-onset schizophrenia. *Proc. Natl. Acad. Sci. U.S.A.* 98, 11650–11655. doi: 10.1073/pnas.201243998

van den Heuvel, M. P., Mandl, R. C., Stam, C. J., Kahn, R. S., and Hulshoff Pol, H. E. (2010). Aberrant frontal and temporal complex network structure in schizophrenia: a graph theoretical analysis. *J. Neurosci.* 30, 15915–15926. doi: 10.1523/JNEUROSCI.2874-10.2010

Wang, C., Zheng, D., Xu, J., Lam, W., and Yew, D. T. (2013). Brain damages in ketamine addicts as revealed by magnetic resonance imaging. *Front. Neuroanat.* 7:23. doi: 10.3389/fnana.2013.00023

Wolkin, A., Sanfilipo, M., Wolf, A. P., Angrist, B., Brodie, J. D., and Rotrosen, J. (1992). Negative symptoms and hypofrontality in chronic schizophrenia. *Arch. Gen. Psychiatry* 49, 959–965. doi: 10.1001/archpsyc.1992.01820120047007

Xiao, Y., Friederici, A. D., Margulies, D. S., and Brauer, J. (2016). Development of a selective left-hemispheric fronto-temporal network for processing syntactic complexity in language comprehension. *Neuropsychologia* 83, 274–282. doi: 10.1016/j.neuropsychologia.2015.09.003

Yeung, L. Y., Wai, M. S., Fan, M., Mak, Y. T., Lam, W. P., Li, Z., et al. (2010). Hyperphosphorylated tau in the brains of mice and monkeys with long-term administration of ketamine. *Toxicol. Lett.* 193, 189–193. doi: 10.1016/j.toxlet.2010.01.008

Yu, H., Li, Q., Wang, D., Shi, L., Lu, G., Sun, L., et al. (2012). Mapping the central effects of chronic ketamine administration in an adolescent primate model by functional magnetic resonance imaging (fMRI). *Neurotoxicology* 33, 70–77. doi: 10.1016/j.neuro.2011.11.001

Zalesky, A., Fornito, A., Seal, M. L., Cocchi, L., Westin, C. F., Bullmore, E. T., et al. (2011). Disrupted axonal fiber connectivity in schizophrenia. *Biol. Psychiatry* 69, 80–89. doi: 10.1016/j.biopsych.2010.08.022

Zou, X., Patterson, T. A., Sadovova, N., Twaddle, N. C., Doerge, D. R., Zhang, X., et al. (2009). Potential neurotoxicity of ketamine in the developing rat brain. *Toxicol. Sci.* 108, 149–158. doi: 10.1093/toxsci/kfn270

13

Adolescent Ethanol Exposure Leads to Stimulus-Specific Changes in Cytokine Reactivity and Hypothalamic-Pituitary-Adrenal Axis Sensitivity in Adulthood

*Andrew S. Vore[1], Tamara Doremus-Fitzwater[2], Anny Gano[1] and Terrence Deak[1]**

[1]*Behavioral Neuroscience Program, Department of Psychology, Binghamton University, Binghamton, NY, USA,* [2]*Department of Psychology, Ithaca College, Ithaca, NY, USA*

Edited by:
Mary M. Torregrossa,
University of Pittsburgh, USA

Reviewed by:
Jessica R. Barson,
Drexel University College of Medicine, USA
Heather Trantham-Davidson,
Medical University of South Carolina, USA

Correspondence:
Terrence Deak

Adolescent alcohol use comprises a significant public health concern and is often characterized by binge-like consumption patterns. While ethanol exposure in adulthood has been shown to alter the stress response, including the Hypothalamic–Pituitary–Adrenal (HPA) axis, few studies have examined whether binge-like ethanol exposure during adolescence results in enduring changes in HPA axis sensitivity in adulthood. In the present studies, adolescent Sprague-Dawley rats were given intragastric (i.g.) intubations of ethanol (4 g/kg) or vehicle once per day for three consecutive days, beginning on postnatal day (P) 30 (±1). This exposure was followed by a 2-day period of rest/withdrawal. Rats received a total of either two (Experiments 1, 2 and 3) or four (Experiment 4) cycles of ethanol exposure and were subsequently allowed to age normally until adulthood. In Experiment 1, adult, (P71–75), ethanol- or vehicle-exposed rats received a 60 min restraint stress challenge. In Experiment 2, rats received a 50 μg/kg injection of lipopolysaccharide (LPS). In Experiment 3, rats received a challenge of 2.5 g/kg ethanol (intraperitoneally; i.p.). In Experiment 4, male and female ethanol- or vehicle- exposed rats received a 50 μg/kg injection of LPS. In all experiments, blood samples were collected for later assessment of corticosterone (CORT), blood ethanol concentrations (BECs), and the cellular fraction of blood was analyzed for cytokine gene expression. As expected, all three challenges led to a time-dependent surge in CORT. Gene expression analyses of cytokines (Interleukin [IL]-6, IL-1β, and Tumor necrosis factor alpha [TNFα]) from the cellular fraction of blood revealed unique, time-dependent patterns of cytokine expression depending upon the nature of the adult challenge incurred (restraint, LPS, or EtOH). Importantly, adolescent ethanol exposure led to attenuated restraint and LPS-induced cytokine

Abbreviations: ACTH, Adrenocorticotropic hormone; AIE, Adolescent intermittent ethanol; ANOVA, Analysis of variance; AUD, Alcohol use disorder; AVP, Vasopressin; BALs, Blood alcohol levels; BECs, Blood ethanol concentrations; C, Celcius; CORT, Corticosterone; CRH, Corticotropin-releasing hormone; CTA, Conditioned taste aversion; HPA, Hypothalamic-Pituitary-Adrenal; HSF1, Heat shock factor protein 1; Hsp70, 70 kilodalton heat shock protein; IACUC, Institutional animal care and use committee; i.g., Intragastric; IκBα, Nuclear factor of kappa light polypeptide gene enhancer in B-cells inhibitor, alpha; IL, Interleukin; i.p., Intraperitoneal; LPS, Lipopolysaccharide; MYD88, Myeloid differentiation primary response gene; NFκB, Nuclear factor kappa-light-chain-enhancer of activated B cells; P, Postnatal day; PAE, Prenatal alcohol exposure; PVN, Paraventricular nucleus of the hypothalamus; RT-PCR, Real time reverse transcription polymerase chain reaction; TLR4, Toll-like receptor 4.

expression in males, whereas female rats displayed an absence of cytokine alterations, and a tendency toward heightened HPA axis reactivity. These findings suggest that adolescent ethanol exposure may cause lasting alterations in cytokine regulation and HPA axis sensitivity that (a) persist into adulthood; (b) may vary depending on the nature of the challenge incurred during adulthood; and that (c) are sex-specific.

Keywords: adolescent intermittent ethanol, rat, sex differences, HPA axis, cytokine

INTRODUCTION

Alcohol use and abuse disorders comprise a substantial public health and financial burden, resulting in an estimated 3.3 million deaths per year globally and $223.5 billion in financial burden to the United States alone (Centers for Disease Control and Prevention, 2014; World Health Organization, 2014). It has been estimated that almost 75% of this impact can be attributed to binge drinking, defined as ethanol consumption that results in Blood Ethanol Concentrations (BECs) of 0.08 mg/dL or higher (Centers for Disease Control and Prevention, 2014). Alcohol consumption is prevalent in adolescence and a large percentage of adolescent individuals that consume alcohol exhibit binge-like consumption patterns. These patterns of intake typically begin in early to late adolescence, peaking in early adulthood (21–25 years of age), with consumption tapering across adulthood in individuals that exhibit normative alcohol use. Binge-like alcohol consumption can be particularly harmful, and early, high frequency binge drinking has been shown to correlate with later alcohol use disorder (AUD) development (Grant and Dawson, 1997; Crews et al., 2016).

Adolescence is a time of unique sensitivity to the consequences of ethanol exposure. Mirroring what is seen in humans, adolescent rodents consume notably higher quantities of ethanol than adult counterparts (Doremus et al., 2005; Spear, 2016). Adolescent rats show altered reactivity to ethanol exposure with increased sensitivity to the positive effects of ethanol exposure and decreased sensitivity to the negative effects (Doremus et al., 2003; Varlinskaya and Spear, 2004a). Adolescent animals have also exhibited increased locomotor sensitization to ethanol and higher sensitivity to the motivational effects of ethanol (Pautassi et al., 2008) compared to adult counterparts that received similar quantities of ethanol. This differential reaction to a spectrum of consequences of ethanol exposure likely contributes to adolescent animals consuming higher quantities of ethanol, since insensitivity to negative consequences of high dose ethanol use (sedation, motor impairment, aversion) and hypersensitivity to various positive elements would seem to promote future ethanol consumption (Varlinskaya and Spear, 2004b).

A more concerning element of adolescent ethanol exposure is its ability to cause potentially lifelong changes in development. Adolescence is a critical time of neural refinement during which the brain undergoes a series of structural and functional changes. Increases in myelination, decreases in gray matter volumes, and a reduced total number of synapses indicate that adolescence is a time during which novel connections are being made and prior connections are being refined (Giedd, 2008). Underlying neurodevelopmental changes during adolescence may confer added potential for insult from substances such as ethanol (Guerri and Pascual, 2010). A common functional consequence of adolescent ethanol exposure is the retention of an adolescent-like phenotype into adulthood. This "locking in" of the adolescent phenotype into adulthood has been shown to occur in a variety of phenomena and is not seen in adult rats following exposure to similar quantities of ethanol. Behavioral phenomenon such as resilience to withdrawal-induced anxiety (Doremus et al., 2003), reduced sensitivity to the sedative effects of ethanol (Matthews et al., 2008), as well as reduced sensitivity to conditioned taste aversion (CTA) induction (Diaz-Granados and Graham, 2007) have all demonstrated this locking in-like effect following adolescent ethanol exposure when challenged during adulthood. This phenomenon has also been demonstrated to extend beyond just ethanol challenge effects. Observed baseline differences in impulsivity, novelty seeking, and many other phenomena have also shown to linger into adulthood following adolescent ethanol exposure (see Spear and Swartzwelder, 2014 for a recent review).

Ethanol alone is a potent stimulator of the hypothalamic-pituitary-adrenal (HPA) axis as demonstrated by dose-dependent increases in plasma adrenocorticotropic hormone (ACTH) and corticosterone (CORT; Rivier et al., 1984; Doremus-Fitzwater et al., 2014). Importantly, cross sectional studies comparing adolescent and adult rats have indicated that stressors such as hypoxia and restraint stress result in prolonged ACTH and CORT responses when compared to adult rodents (Romeo et al., 2016), though differences in peak CORT responses were not observed. A similar difference occurs following ethanol challenge as well, where adolescents exhibit delayed recovery (or shutoff) of the axis relative to adults. While this effect was more pronounced in female rats, both male and female adolescent rats have shown increased CORT at several points after ethanol when compared to adult animals challenged with the same dose of ethanol (Willey et al., 2012). In contrast, prior exposure to ethanol in adolescence has been shown to blunt the HPA-axis response to subsequent ethanol exposure up to 24 days later (Lee and Rivier, 2003). Thus, intrinsic differences in the HPA axis response to stress between adolescents and adults are now well-precedented in the literature, though the mechanisms underlying these differences remain obscure.

Beyond effects on the HPA axis, ethanol also has substantial effects on cytokine release and the immune system. Cytokines are a class of proteins that play a key role in propagation of the inflammatory response evoked by immunological threats, tissue damage, and other challenges such as stress (see Deak et al., 2015 for a recent review). In particular, the pro-inflammatory cytokines IL-1, TNF-α and IL-6 are rapidly induced by immune challenges or psychological stress, and often act synergistically with one another to influence host defense and tissue repair. These cytokines also potently induce HPA axis activation, with glucocorticoids in turn influencing subsequent cytokine expression and activity. In this way, HPA-immune interactions serve as an exemplar of bi-directional communication between the brain and the immune system.

From a longitudinal perspective, recent studies have begun to explore whether the adolescent period also represents a critical period during which ethanol exposure can produce life-long changes in HPA axis sensitivity and immune function. For instance, adolescent ethanol exposure (6 exposures to 3 g/kg intraperitoneal (i.p.)) in male rats resulted in reduced baseline CORT and sensitized CORT release following acute or repeated ethanol challenge in adulthood (Przybycien-Szymanska et al., 2010, 2011). These changes in CORT patterns correlated with decreased vasopressin (AVP) and increased corticotropin-releasing hormone (CRH) within the paraventricular nucleus of the hypothalamus (PVN) of adolescent ethanol exposed rats following acute and binge ethanol challenge, suggesting alterations in central regulation of HPA axis regulation. In contrast, a more recent study showed that adolescent ethanol exposure (daily exposure to ethanol vapor for 6 h maintaining blood alcohol levels, BALs of 200 mg/dL) blunted the HPA axis response to adult ethanol challenge (3.2–4.5 g/kg intragastric (i.g.); Allen et al., 2016). Though dose, route and frequency of ethanol exposure during adolescence are likely explanations for the differences between these studies, a more fundamental question regarding the potential for stressor-specific outcomes in adults with a history of adolescent ethanol exposure still remains.

With this in mind, our primary goal was to establish how binge-like ethanol exposure during adolescence would alter cytokine and HPA axis responses to stress challenges incurred during adulthood. In doing so, we adopted an adolescent alcohol exposure procedure that has previously been shown to produce changes lasting to adulthood in HPA axis regulation, including alterations in CORT release as well as changes in AVP and CRH following binge and acute ethanol exposure (Przybycien-Szymanska et al., 2010, 2011). Following intermittent binge ethanol exposure in adolescence, three distinct studies were executed in which rats were given different challenges in adulthood to test whether axis sensitivity may depend upon the nature/modality of the stress challenge experienced as adults. Thus, adult rats with a history of adolescent ethanol exposure were challenged by restraint, lipopolysaccharide (LPS) administration, or adult ethanol exposure (Experiments 1–3 respectively). Though our primary interest was HPA axis sensitivity indicated by plasma CORT responses, we also had a secondary interest in how adolescent intermittent ethanol (AIE) would influence the expression of cytokines within the cellular fraction of whole blood as a secondary index of stress sensitivity, and due to the potential mechanistic role that plasma cytokines might play in HPA axis responses (Rivest et al., 2000; Szelényi, 2001). In human research, analysis of peripheral cytokine levels has been shown to be useful in monitoring general immune activation and to correlate well with expected levels of neuroimmune activation (Sullivan et al., 2006). In addition, elevated levels of peripheral pro-inflammatory cytokines have been shown to correlate with psychiatric illness in a specific subset of individuals (Fillman et al., 2016). Finally, due to the literature demonstrating that male animals display profound HPA axis blunting following adolescent ethanol exposure, we examined potential sex differences in HPA axis reactivity following adolescent alcohol exposure.

MATERIALS AND METHODS

General Methods

Subjects

In the first three studies, male Sprague-Dawley rats ($N = 50$) were purchased from Harlan Laboratories and shipped at postnatal day (P) 22 ± 1. In the fourth study, male and female Sprague-Dawley rats ($N = 30$) were bred in-house using breeders originally derived from Harlan (Envigo). With day of birth being deemed postnatal day (P) 0, rats were allowed to develop normally until P21 at which point animals were weaned and pair-housed with a same-sex partner from a different litter in standard Plexiglas bins. In all cases, rats were given 1 week to acclimate to colony conditions and were then handled (P29) for 2–3 min to acclimate them to human contact prior to experimentation. Colony conditions were maintained at 22 ± 1°C on a 12:12 light:dark cycle. Animals were pair-housed in standard Plexiglas bins with *ad libitum* access to food and water. Rats housed in pairs were always assigned to the same experimental group. In all experiments, rats were treated in accordance with Public Health Service (PHS) policy and all experimental protocols were approved by the Institutional Animal Care and Use Committee (IACUC) at Binghamton University.

Adolescent Alcohol Exposure Procedure

Starting at early adolescence (P30–32) rats received 4.0 g/kg intragastric (i.g.) intubations of ethanol or an equivolume dose of vehicle (tap water) once per day at approximately 1000 h. When administered i.g., ethanol solution was prepared daily using 95% ethanol stock diluted to a final working concentration of 20% in tap water. Weights were taken daily at least 90 min prior to intubations. Animals received three consecutive days of intubations followed by a 2-day period of rest/withdrawal during which animals remained undisturbed in their home cage. This cycle of intubations (3 days on, 2 days off) was then repeated a second time (Experiments 1–3), reaching its conclusion on P40–42. In Experiment 4, this cycle was administered four times, spanning ages of approximately P30–P50. Rats were then reared to adulthood without further manipulation until weights were again collected on P73–75.

At this time, rats were randomly divided into cohorts for independent experiments.

Drug Preparations

When injected i.p., ethanol was prepared in a 20% solution mixed fresh daily using 95% ethanol stock with sterile physiological saline used as the vehicle. LPS (from serotype E0111:B4; Sigma Chemical Co.) solution was initially diluted 1.0 mg/mL using sterile (pyrogen-free) physiological saline and stored in frozen aliquots at −20°C until needed. On the day of experimentation, an aliquot of LPS was thawed and mixed fresh daily to the working concentration of 50 μg/mL LPS and delivered on a 1 mL/kg basis, also in pyrogen free physiological saline.

Blood Sampling and Processing Procedure

In each experiment, rats were removed from their home cage and briefly placed into restraint tubes for the acquisition of blood samples. Blood samples were collected using the tail clip method in which the last 0.5–1.0 mm of the tail was transected. The tail was then stroked until whole blood was obtained as previously described (Hueston and Deak, 2014b). Rats were immediately returned to their home cage following each time point except in conditions where rats were assigned to the restraint stress condition. Animals were returned to their home cage within 2 min after first intrusion. Following collection, plasma was immediately separated through refrigerated centrifugation and stored at −20°C until analysis. RNA was extracted from the remaining fractionated layers of leukocytes and erythrocytes. Prior studies have shown that RNA extraction of whole blood is possible (Schwochow et al., 2012). Due to elimination of the plasma fraction and the lack of nuclei or cell organelles such as mitochondria in erythrocytes, it was reasoned that extraction on the combined buffy layer and erythrocyte fractions would largely reflect gene expression changes in leukocytes. The combined layers were stored at −80°C until analysis of expression of blood cytokine levels using Real Time Reverse Transcription Polymerase Chain Reaction (RT-PCR).

Corticosterone Measures

Quantitative determinations of plasma CORT levels were assessed using a CORT EIA kit (Cat No: ADI-901-097; Enzo Life Sciences, Farmingdale, NY, USA) as described in Hueston and Deak (2014a) with an inter-assay variability of 7.616% and an assay sensitivity of 27.0 pg/mL. Manufacturer's instructions were followed for all steps except that samples were heat inactivated by immersion in 75°C water for a period of 60 min to denature endogenous CBG.

Reverse-Transcription Polymerase Chain Reaction

All RT-PCR was conducted using procedures described in previous work (Hueston and Deak, 2014a). Blood pellets were stored at −80°C until the time of RNA extraction. Total RNA in the sample was homogenized in Trizol RNA reagent (Invitrogen) using a TissueLyser and 5 mm stainless steel beads (Qiagen). Total RNA was then extracted through the use of RNeasy mini columns (Qiagen) following manufacturer's instructions. RNA yield and purity were evaluated using a Nanodrop system (ThermoScientific) and cDNA was synthesized using a QuantiTect reverse transcription kit (Qiagen). All RT-PCR was run using a CFX384 real-time PCR detection system (Bio-Rad). All results were normalized to β-Actin as a housekeeper gene. Primer sequences for all targets run can be found in **Table 1**.

Blood Ethanol Concentrations

BECs were determined from 5 μL samples of plasma using an Analox AM-1 alcohol analyzer (Analox Instruments, Lunenburg, MA, USA; as described in Doremus-Fitzwater et al., 2015). The machine was calibrated using a 200 mg/dL standard and tested every 15 samples using an alcohol quality control standard of known concentration purchased from Analox Instruments. Samples below 10–15 mg/dL were within a range considered to be noise and as such were interpreted as 0 values.

Statistical Analyses

All analyses of CORT levels, BECs and cytokine expression were analyzed using a mixed factorial ANOVA ($p < 0.05$). Fisher's Least Significant Difference ($p < 0.05$) was used as a *post hoc* examination in instances where two way interactions were noted to identify loci of significant difference. Outliers were defined as data points that were more extreme than ±2 standard deviations from a given experimental group's mean. If an outlier was identified within a given PCR reaction, it was excluded from that specific analysis but not across the remainder of the gene targets. Before analyzing individual cytokine data, β-Actin was examined to determine differences that may exist between groups in expression of this target gene of reference. All gene expression was reported quantified relative to expression of this reference gene.

TABLE 1 | Primer sequences and accession numbers.

Primer	Accession number	Oligo	Sequence
β-Actin	NM_031144.3	Forward	5′-GTCGTACCACTGGCATTGTG-3′
		Reverse	5′-GCCATCTCTTGCTCGAAGTC-3′
IL-6	NM_012589	Forward	5′-TAGTCCTTCCTACCCCAACTTCC-3′
		Reverse	5′-TTGGTCCTTAGCCACTCCTTC-3′
IL-1β	NM_031512	Forward	5′-AGGACCCAAGCACCTTCTTT-3′
		Reverse	5′-AGACAGCACGAGGCATTTTT-3′
TNF-α	NM_012675	Forward	5′-GGGGCCACCACGCTCTTCTG-3′
		Reverse	5′-CGACGTGGGCTACGGGTTG-3′
IκBα	NM_080899	Forward	5′-CTGTTGAAGTGTGGGGCTGA-3′
		Reverse	5′-AGGGCAACTCATCTTCCGTG-3′

Experiment 1: Axis Reactivity to Restraint Stress Challenge Following Adolescent Ethanol Exposure

In the first experiment, restraint stress was chosen as a challenge due to its ability to reliably produce activation of the HPA axis and for reported differences between adolescent and adult CORT responses to restraint stress (Romeo et al., 2016). Male rats (n = 6–8 per group; N = 14) were given two cycles of intermittent ethanol exposure or vehicle intubations as described above. At adulthood (P73–75), rats from both groups were placed into clear Plexiglas restraint tubes and a baseline blood sample was collected immediately. Rats remained in restraint and subsequent blood samples were collected at 15, 30 and 60 min time points. Immediately after the 60 min time point, rats were returned to their home cage and a final recovery sample was collected 60 min later (i.e., 120 min following stress onset; see **Figure 1A**).

Experiment 2: Axis Reactivity to Lipopolysaccharide Challenge Following Adolescent Ethanol Exposure

In the second experiment, LPS challenge was chosen as a representative, immune-based challenge that is known to activate the HPA axis through cytokine-mediated mechanisms. Male rats (n = 8 per group; N = 16) were given two cycles of intermittent ethanol exposure or vehicle intubations as described above. During adulthood (P73–75) rats were injected with 50 μg/kg (i.p.) LPS or equivolume vehicle. Blood was collected at baseline, 45, 90 and 180 min post injection.

Experiment 3: Axis Reactivity to Ethanol Challenge Following Adolescent Ethanol Exposure

In the third experiment, rats were given an acute ethanol challenge during adulthood to test for durable changes in HPA axis sensitivity to the same challenge(s) utilized during adolescence, and to provide a referent to other published studies (Przybycien-Szymanska et al., 2010, 2011; Allen et al., 2016). Male rats (n = 8–10 per group; N = 18) were given two cycles of intermittent ethanol exposure or vehicle intubations as described above. During adulthood (P73–75), the test day began with collection of a baseline blood sample, after which rats were given a 2.5 g/kg i.p. ethanol or equivolume vehicle. Subsequent blood samples were collected 30, 60, 120 and 240 min post injection (see **Figure 1A**).

Experiment 4: Sex-Differences in the Consequences of Adult LPS Challenge Following Adolescent Ethanol Exposure

The goals of the fourth experiment were to: (a) replicate the initial effect of reduced CORT and cytokine responses observed in adults with a history of adolescent alcohol exposure; (b) extend the period of alcohol exposure more broadly across the adolescent period; and (c) determine whether the impact of adolescent alcohol exposure on adult stress sensitivity would be sex-specific. Because early life shipping can produce variations in stress history and thereby influence stress reactivity (Laroche et al., 2009a,b; Vargas et al., 2016), rats for Experiment 4 were bred in house. Thus, in Experiment 4, rats (n = 6–8 per group; N = 30) were given four cycles of vehicle or ethanol intubations utilizing the procedure described above. After reaching adulthood, all rats received a 50 μg/kg i.p. LPS injection. Blood was collected at baseline, 45, 90, 180 and 360 min post injection.

RESULTS

Experiments 1–3

Plasma Corticosterone Response to Challenges

Data were analyzed using a mixed between-subjects (adolescent Ethanol or Vehicle exposure) and repeated-measures (time course) analysis of variance (ANOVA). Restraint challenge showed significant CORT elevation peaking around 30 min and CORT levels returning to baseline by 120 min ($F_{(4,48)} = 62.07$, $p < 0.001$; **Figure 1B**). LPS challenge produced comparable increases in CORT across the 45 and 90 min time points, which then decreased by the 180 min time point ($F_{(3,42)} = 22.64$, $p < 0.001$; **Figure 1C**). Adult ethanol challenge increased CORT within 30 min and sustained high CORT levels through the 120 min time point ($F_{(4,64)} = 70.65$, $p < 0.001$). CORT still showed notable elevation at 240 min (**Figure 1D**), though the response was clearly resolving at this time point. Although no statistically significant effects of adolescent ethanol history on CORT response were observed on in response to the adult challenges, visual inspection of the data suggested a moderate attenuation of CORT in response to LPS challenge.

Blood Ethanol Concentrations Following Ethanol Challenge

As expected, rats injected with ethanol exhibited a marked and time-dependent elevation in BECs that peaked at 30–60 min and tapered over the remainder of the time course ($F_{(4,64)} = 200.15$, $p < 0.001$; **Figure 1E**). Rats with a history of adolescent alcohol exposure showed trended higher mean BECs at both 30 and 60 min after ethanol, though this effect was not statistically significant. It should be noted that mean peak BECs were approximately 25 mg/dL higher at both time points relative to rats that received vehicle during adolescence. Potential differences in alcohol pharmacokinetics in adolescent-exposed rats could therefore be an area worth examining in more targeted studies.

Blood Pellet mRNA Expression Levels Following Restraint Challenge

While restraint challenge produced no significant alterations in IL-6 expression (**Figure 2A**), significantly increased IL-1β expression was noted at 30 min ($F_{(4,48)} = 10.16$, $p < 0.001$) and IL-1β remained elevated throughout the remainder of the time course (**Figure 2D**). No alterations in TNF-α expression

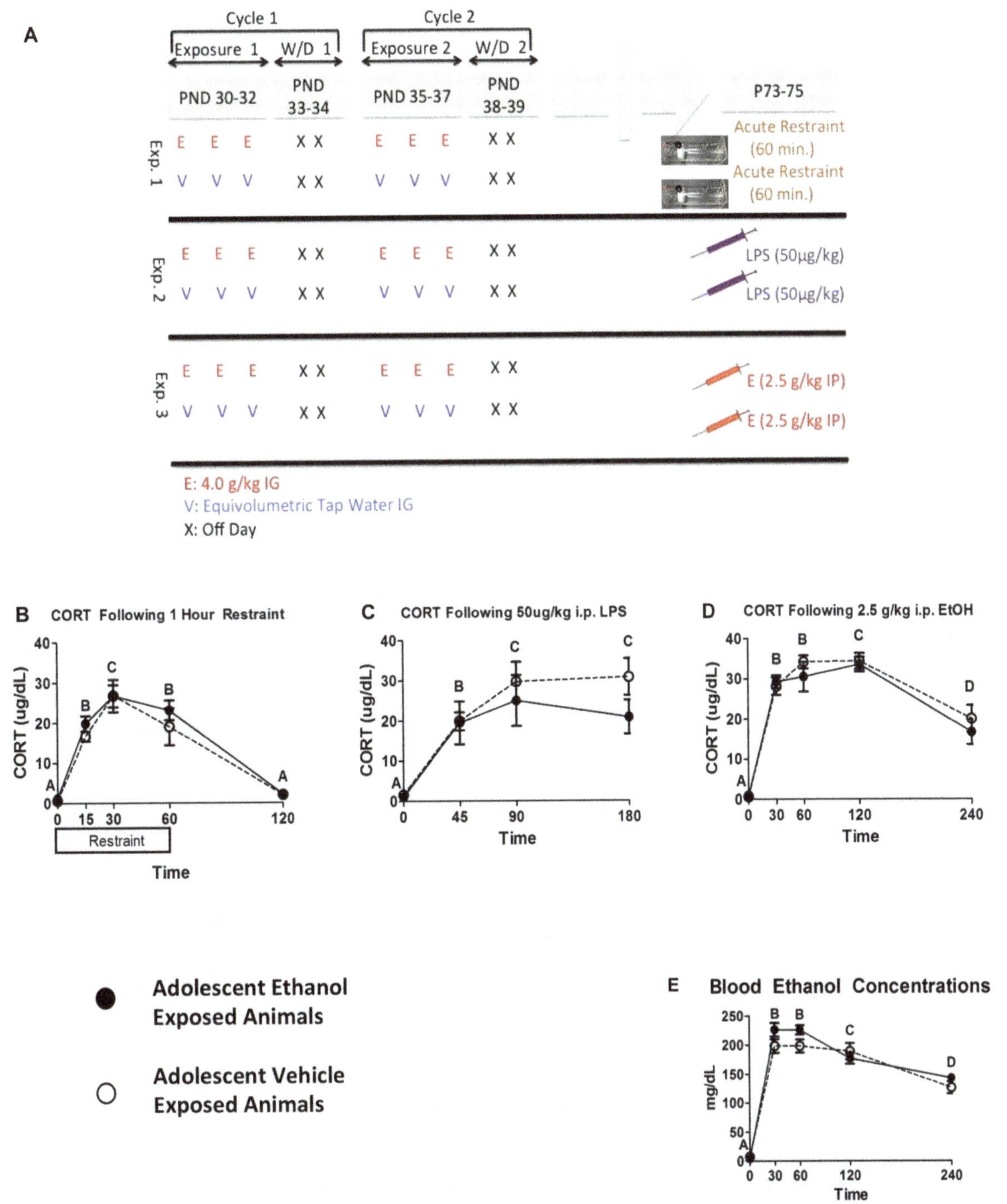

FIGURE 1 | Plasma Data from Experiments 1–3. This figure shows a schematic diagramming Experiments 1–3 **(A)**. It also shows plasma corticosterone (CORT) levels following 1 h of restraint **(B)**, 50 μg/kg i.p. lipopolysaccharide (LPS) injection **(C)**, and 2.5 g/kg i.p. EtOH injection **(D)** and corresponding blood ethanol concentrations (BECs) in the ethanol challenge group **(E)**. Plasma was sampled 0, 15, 30, 60 and 120 min following restraint, 0, 45, 90 and 180 min following LPS challenge, and 0, 30, 60, 120 and 240 min following ethanol challenge. A significant main effect of time point is denoted by a lettering system in which time points that differ in letter are significantly different.

were noted (**Figure 2G**) however; significant increases in Nuclear factor of kappa light polypeptide gene enhancer in B-cells inhibitor, alpha (IκBα) expression at 30 and 60 min ($F_{(4,48)} = 13.53$, $p < 0.001$) were seen that had returned to baseline levels by the 120 min time point (**Figure 2J**). A pattern showing that adolescent exposure to ethanol

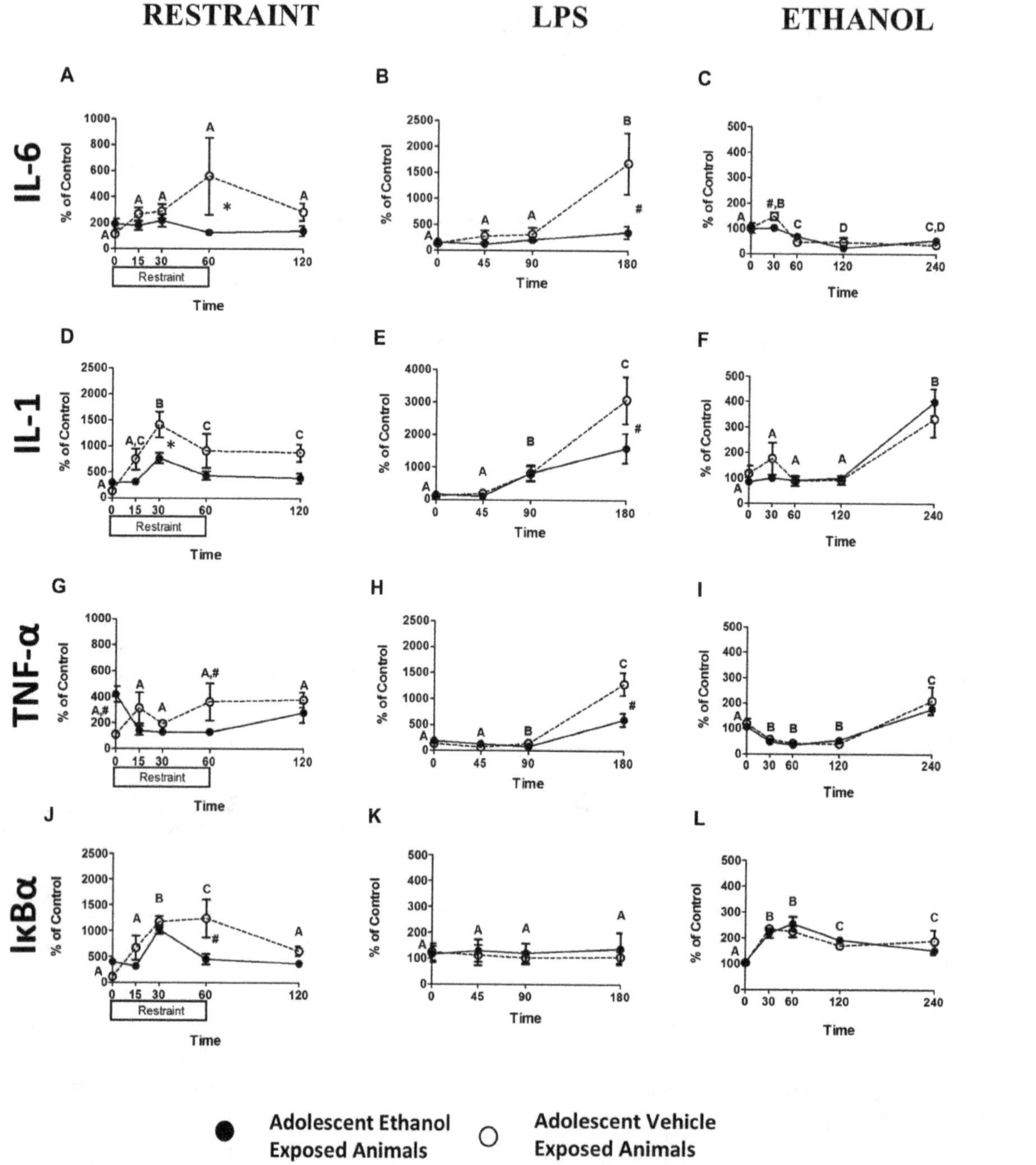

FIGURE 2 | Cytokine Expression from Experiments 1–3. This figure shows mRNA expression changes following restraint, LPS and ethanol challenge in IL-6 (**A–C** respectively), IL-1 (**D–F** respectively), TNF-α (**G–I** respectively), IκBα (**J–L** respectively). Samples were collected at 0, 15, 30, 60 and 120 min following restraint, 0, 45, 90 and 180 min following LPS challenge, and 0, 30, 60, 120 and 240 min following ethanol challenge. Data is expressed relative to ultimate control (vehicle animals at the baseline time point) normalized to β-Actin. A significant main effect of time point is denoted by a lettering system in which time points that differ in letter are significantly different. A pound sign indicates a significant interaction between adolescent exposure and challenge stimulus at a given time point. An asterisk indicates a trend interaction between adolescent exposure and challenge stimulus at a given time point. All *post hoc* comparisons were made using Fisher's Least Significant Difference *post hoc* test ($p < 0.05$).

attenuated response to adult restraint challenge was seen in IL-6, IL-1β, TNF- α, and IκBα expression. A trend showing attenuation of IL-6 expression in the adolescent ethanol exposed rats was seen at the 60-min time point ($F_{(4,48)} = 2.55$, $p = 0.051$; **Figure 2A**). A similar trend showed that IL-1β expression was attenuated in the adolescent ethanol exposed rats at the 30-min time point ($F_{(4,48)} = 2.44$, $p = 0.06$; **Figure 2D**). Finally, a similar reduction was seen at the 60-min time point in both TNF-α ($F_{(4,48)} = 5.49$, $p < 0.005$; **Figure 2G**) and IκBα ($F_{(4,48)} = 4.77$, $p < 0.005$; **Figure 2J**) expression.

Blood Pellet mRNA Expression Levels Following LPS Challenge

Blood analysis revealed significant changes in expression of IL-6, IL-1β and TNF-α following LPS challenge. An increase in IL-6 expression at 180 min ($F_{(3,42)} = 9.33$, $p < 0.001$) as well as an overall decrease in IL-6 expression in rats exposed to ethanol in adolescence ($F_{(1,14)} = 4.96$, $p < 0.05$) was noted (**Figure 2B**). A distinct increase in IL-1β expression ($F_{(3,42)} = 23.94$, $p < 0.001$) occurred at 90 min and appeared to still be escalating at 180 min (**Figure 2E**). A similar pattern of results was found for TNF-α expression ($F_{(3,42)} = 56.27$, $p < 0.001$) with a profound increase occurring at 180 min and a decrease in overall expression in the adolescent exposed animals ($F_{(1,14)} = 6.09$, $p < 0.05$; **Figure 2H**). It was also found that adolescent ethanol exposure resulted in significant attenuation of IL-6 ($F_{(3,42)} = 5.55$, $p < 0.05$; **Figure 2B**), IL-1β ($F_{(3,42)} = 3.07$, $p < 0.05$; **Figure 2E**), and TNF-α ($F_{(3,42)} = 10.60$, $p < 0.001$; **Figure 2H**) expression at the 180 min time point in contrast to vehicle-exposed counterparts. Neither alterations in IκBα expression resultant from LPS challenge nor any significant effects of AIE were noted (**Figure 2K**).

Blood Pellet mRNA Expression Levels Following Ethanol Challenge

Data were analyzed using a mixed between subjects (adolescent Ethanol or Vehicle exposure) and repeated measures (0, 30, 60, 120 and 240 min post-injection) ANOVA. Analysis revealed significant changes in overall IL-6, IL-1β, TNF-α and IκBα expression across time. A significant decrease in overall IL-6 expression ($F_{(4,64)} = 21.89$, $p < 0.001$) was noted from 60 min post-challenge to 240 min (**Figure 2C**). Significant increases in IL-1β expression did not begin to occur until after 120 min showing continued escalation at the 240 min time point ($F_{(4,64)} = 27.40$, $p < 0.001$; **Figure 2F**). TNF-α also showed a significant reduction in expression ($F_{(4,64)} = 39.58$, $p < 0.001$) during the 30, 60 and 120 min time points and began to show rebound elevation at 240 min (**Figure 2I**). IκBα showed an increase in expression through the 60 min time point that had begun to taper by the 240 min time point ($F_{(4,64)} = 17.27$, $p < 0.001$; **Figure 2L**). Rats that received ethanol exposure during adolescence demonstrated significantly reduced IL-6 expression in contrast to vehicle-exposed rats ($F_{(4,64)} = 3.03$, $p < 0.05$; **Figure 2C**). No effects of adolescent ethanol exposure on IL-1β, TNF-α, or IκBα were observed.

Experiment 4 Results

Corticosterone Response to Challenge

Data were analyzed using a mixed between-subjects (adolescent Ethanol or Vehicle exposure; male or female) and repeated-measures (time course) ANOVA. Sex-specific analyses were then run using a mixed between subjects (adolescent Ethanol or Vehicle exposure) and repeated measures (time course) ANOVA. When ANOVAs for each sex were run separately, LPS challenge produced significant increases in both male and female CORT release with female animals showing overall higher levels of CORT than males. A significant main effect of time point was found in both females ($F_{(4,48)} = 40.86$, $p < 0.001$; **Figure 3C**) as well as in males ($F_{(4,56)} = 22.58$, $p < 0.001$; **Figure 3B**). CORT increased at the 45-min time point and remained at peak through the 360-min time point in both males ($F_{(4,56)} = 22.58$, $p < 0.001$; **Figure 3B**) and females ($F_{(4,48)} = 40.86$, $p < 0.001$; **Figure 3C**). Although there was a trend indicating that adolescent ethanol exposure increased CORT release following LPS challenge in female rats ($F_{(4,48)} = 1.68$, $p = 0.17$), no such effect was seen in male rats (**Figures 3B,C**). A planned comparison examining CORT in female adolescent ethanol and vehicle exposed animals at the 90 min timepoint revealed a significant sensitization of LPS induced CORT in adolescent ethanol exposed animals when compared to vehicle exposed animals at the same timepoint ($t_{(12)} = 2.34$, $p < 0.05$).

Blood Pellet mRNA Expression Levels Following LPS Challenge

When the data were analyzed using an omnibus ANOVA including sex as a variable, a significant sex by adolescent interaction was noted ($F_{(1,26)} = 7.20$, $p < 0.05$; **Figures 4A,B**). When ANOVAs for each sex were run separately, IL-6 showed a trend in the male adolescent ethanol exposed rats showing attenuation of expression in contrast to vehicle exposed animals ($F_{(4,56)} = 2.04$, $p = 0.10$; **Figure 4A**). No such effects were noted in female animals (**Figure 4B**). While adolescent ethanol exposure visibily reduced IL-6 expression in male rats it had little recognizable effect on IL-6 expression in the females.

When data were analyzed using an omnibus ANOVA including sex as a variable, rats that received adolescent ethanol exposure showed significantly reduced levels of IL-1β expression when compared to vehicle exposed counterparts ($F_{(4,104)} = 2.95$, $p < 0.05$) however, this appears to be largely a result of the differences noted in the male animals (**Figures 4C,D**). When ANOVAs for each sex were run separately, a significant attenuation of IL-1β expression was replicated in the male, adolescent ethanol exposed rats at the 180 min time point ($F_{(4,56)} = 3.44$, $p < 0.05$; **Figure 4C**). Interestingly, no such interaction was noted for the female animals although a significant increase in overall expression was noted at the 90 and 180 min time points ($F_{(4,48)} = 14.63$, $p < 0.001$; **Figure 4D**).

When data were analyzed using an omnibus ANOVA including sex as a variable, males showed much greater TNF-α increase in expression over the time course in contrast to female counterparts, regardless of adolescent exposure ($F_{(4,104)} = 2.71$, $p < 0.05$; **Figures 4E,F**). Regardless of sex, TNF-α expression increased with peak levels being reached by the 360 min time point ($F_{(4,104)} = 11.06$, $p < 0.001$; **Figures 4E,F**). When ANOVAs for each sex were run separately, TNF-α expression in males

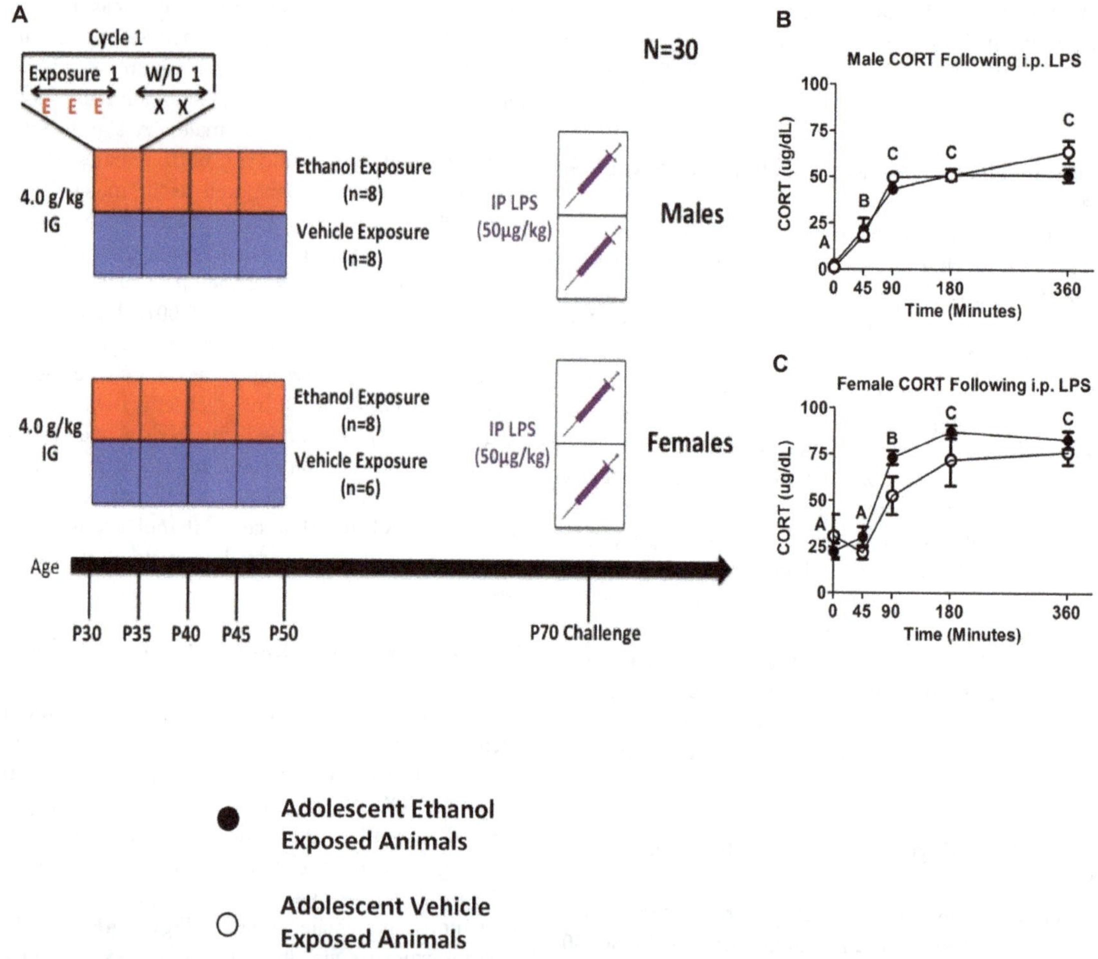

FIGURE 3 | Plasma CORT from Experiment 4. The figure shows a schematic diagramming Experiment 4 **(A)**. It also shows plasma CORT levels in male and female rodents following 50 μg/kg i.p. LPS injection at 0, 45, 90, 180 and 360 min time points **(B, C)**. A significant main effect of time point is denoted by a lettering system in which time points that differ in letter are significantly different.

showed a similar pattern of expression as in the previous experiment with a noticeable but not significant attenuation of expression developing in the adolescent ethanol exposed animals. Males showed much higher overall levels of expression than females ($F_{(1,26)} = 5.07$, $p < 0.05$; **Figures 4E,F**). Females also showed a significant increase in overall TNF-α expression at the 360 min time point ($F_{(4,48)} = 4.90765$, $p < 0.05$; **Figure 4F**).

IκBα closely mirrored the pattern of expression observed in Experiment 1. When data were analyzed using an omnibus ANOVA including sex as a variable, a significant three way interaction between adolescent exposure, sex and treatment ($F_{(4,104)} = 3.60$, $p < 0.01$) revealed that again adolescent ethanol exposure resulted in significant attenuation of IκBα exposure but exclusively in the male animals (**Figures 4G,H**). Female animals showed little to no consequence of adolescent ethanol exposure. Interestingly while in both female and male rats IκBα expression peaked at approximately the 1500% mark in the vehicle exposed male rats expression continued to escalate until the 360 min time point reaching almost double the magnitude of expression seen in the remaining three groups (**Figures 4G,H**).

DISCUSSION

Our primary goal in these studies was to examine how AIE would alter the HPA axis response to different types of challenge in adulthood. This set of studies shows that not only does adolescent ethanol exposure produce lasting changes in HPA axis sensitivity into adulthood, but that these changes are both sexually dimorphic and stimulus specific. Whereas adolescent ethanol exposed male rats showed blunting of peripheral cytokine expression in several key pro-inflammatory cytokines in response to restraint and LPS administered during adulthood, minimal differences were observed in response to ethanol challenge. These findings suggest that the HPA axis is not debilitated by adolescent ethanol challenge and

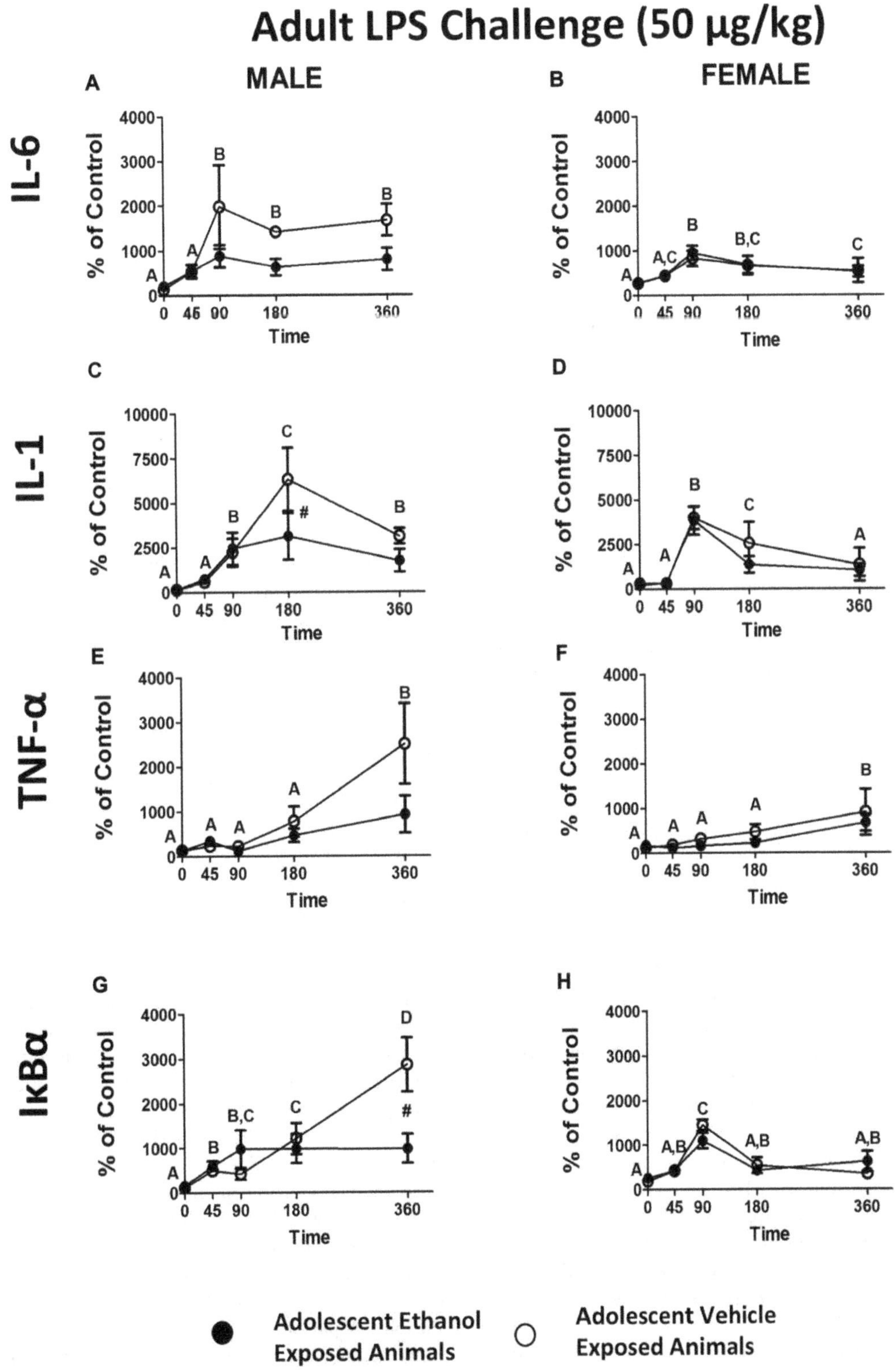

FIGURE 4 | Cytokine expression in male and female rats from experiment 4. This figure shows mRNA expression changes in male and female rats following i.p. LPS injection in IL-6 **(A,B)**, IL-1 **(C,D)**, TNF-α **(E,F)** and IκBα **(G,H)**. Samples were collected at 0, 45, 90, 180 and 360 min following LPS injection. Data is expressed relative to ultimate control (Vehicle animals at the baseline time point) normalized to β-Actin. A significant main effect of time point is denoted by a lettering system in which time points that differ in letter are significantly different. A pound sign indicates a significant interaction between adolescent exposure and challenge stimulus at a given time point. All *post hoc* comparisons were made using Fisher's Least Significant Difference *post hoc* test ($p < 0.05$).

might suggest adaptations that occur extrinsic to the axis. The three challenges used in the study each represent unique modalities for stimulating the HPA axis, restraint being psychological, LPS being immune, and ethanol being the same stimulus used to invoke the changes. Each stimulus produced a unique profile of cytokine expression in blood and the effects of AIE were different between challenge modality.

Alcohol is known to produce immune dysfunction. However, unlike other illnesses, the immune dysfunction that occurs is rarely at a level that would be considered clinical, rather it becomes notable following exposure to a subsequent challenge (Szabo and Saha, 2015). One example of this is the increased susceptibility to bacterial infections such as pneumonia and tuberculosis that occurs in heavy drinkers and alcohol dependent individuals (Cook, 1998; Ogunsakin et al., 2016). In addition, evidence from both human and animal studies has shown that prenatal ethanol exposure can result in increased vulnerability to infection and disease that may persist across the lifespan (Gauthier, 2015). In this study, a pronounced immunosuppressive effect of AIE in response to subsequent LPS challenge was seen in male rats while no difference was noted in females. In contrast, no effect of AIE on the CORT response in male rats was noted, yet a sensitization was observed in females. Although the functional significance for males and females with a history of adolescent ethanol exposure remains unclear, these divergent outcomes suggest that males may be more prone to infection, whereas females may be more prone to stress-related disorders (depression, anxiety) that are often co-morbid with HPA axis dysregulation (Weinberg et al., 2008). In this way, adolescent ethanol exposure may contribute to sex differences in specific disease vulnerabilities that emerge later in life.

Prenatal Alcohol Exposure (PAE) has also been shown to alter HPA axis reactivity in adulthood, suggesting there may be multiple developmental windows during which ethanol can impact later stress sensitivity. For instance, PAE-exposed animals show hyperactivity of the CORT response to restraint stress imposed later in life (Weinberg, 1992; Wieczorek et al., 2015). This hyperactivity has also been shown in response to LPS challenge, IL-1β challenge, local inflammatory challenge probed via turpentine injection, and other types of stressors (Lee and Rivier, 1996; Raineki et al., 2014). The consequences of PAE on adult challenge also appear to be sexually dimorphic as well as stimulus specific. PAE has led to an enhanced HPA axis response in adults to stressors such as acute restraint and forced swim in female rats but not in males (Weinberg et al., 2008). In contrast, solely PAE-exposed male rodents have shown a hyper-reactive HPA response to prolonged restraint and exposure to cold (Kim et al., 1999; Weinberg et al., 2008). Both sexes have shown hyper-reactivity of the axis to immune challenges such as LPS and IL-1β challenge (Weinberg et al., 2008). The results of the present studies clearly demonstrate that adolescent ethanol exposure is capable of causing changes in HPA axis reactivity lasting into adulthood. Based on the results of this study, the effects of adolescent ethanol exposure on later adult challenge appear to be stimulus specific and show sex specific effects, much like has been shown in studies involving PAE.

Prior work from our lab demonstrated that male adolescent rats displayed a blunted cytokine response in the CNS following either LPS challenge or ethanol challenge relative to adult comparators (Doremus-Fitzwater et al., 2015). One potential interpretation of the blunted cytokine responses observed in adolescent-exposed males in the present studies is that this may represent a "locking-in-like" effect. It is noteworthy, however, that, circulating concentrations of endotoxin following LPS challenge were substantially reduced in adolescents compared to adults, suggesting that adolescents may not process LPS in the same way as their adult counterparts. Whether this effect is through differential uptake and transit of LPS into the bloodstream, enhanced clearance of LPS from blood, or other immunological differences between adolescents and adults remains unclear. Nevertheless, plasma endotoxin concentrations were predictive of the HPA axis response (Doremus-Fitzwater et al., 2015). Unfortunately, it was not possible to measure plasma endotoxin concentrations in the present studies due to the limited available sample. Future studies will be necessary to test whether adolescent alcohol exposure impacts subsequent immune processing of LPS in a manner consistent with a "locking in-like" effect. The lack of AIE effects on cytokine expression in female rodents could suggest that female adolescent and adults would not demonstrate the previously noted differences in response to LPS challenge or that females displayed some form of resiliency to the changes that resulted in the "locking-in-like" effect.

Future studies should further probe the mechanisms by which adolescent alcohol exposure influences adult cytokine reactivity and stress sensitivity. LPS invokes an inflammatory response at least in part through its effects on Toll-like receptor 4 (TLR4), activating the NFKB pathway, and ultimately stimulating inflammatory cytokine expression and release (Doremus-Fitzwater et al., 2015). Female rodents have shown an enhanced ethanol-induced inflammatory response during adolescence, as exhibited by increased inflammatory cytokine levels in serum and in brain, however, this effect was not observed in male rats (Pascual et al., 2016). This difference may be mediated by up-regulated TLR4 expression during intoxication that are more pronounced in female rodents than in males, as supported by the fact that TLR4 KO mice do not exhibit these cytokine differences (Pascual et al., 2016). Binge ethanol expression has also been shown to interfere with LPS induced NFKB activity. Ethanol induces Heat shock factor protein 1 (HSF1) and 70 kilodalton heat shock protein (hsp70), two enzymes that ultimately inhibit TLR4/Myeloid differentiation primary response gene (MYD88) signaling via inhibition of the NFKB pathway (Muralidharan et al., 2014). This results in something akin to endotoxin tolerance in monocytes and macrophages pretreated with ethanol (Muralidharan et al., 2014). Lingering inhibition of TLR4/MYD88 signaling resulting from binge ethanol exposure could lead to a reduced cytokine response in male rats that could be normalized in females through sensitized TLR4 expression in female rats following AIE. While this is just one potential explanation for the effects seen in this study, future studies should address the mechanism of these changes and TLR4 signaling pathways might be a good place to start.

Although the results of this study showed few consequences of adolescent ethanol exposure on the response to adult ethanol challenge, the existing literature examining similar manipulations is conflicting. The work of Pak using a similar model of ethanol administration has shown sensitization of the axis response in males following adult ethanol challenge (Przybycien-Szymanska et al., 2010, 2011). In contrast, a different study in which male adolescent rats received AIE and were challenged with ethanol in adulthood showed blunting of the axis response to later ethanol challenge (Allen et al., 2016). There are a number of factors that could account for this disparity. In the first set of studies, the number of ethanol cycles as well as the challenge dose was different, and the experiments were conducted using Wistar rats. In the second set of studies the method of adolescent administration was via daily vapor inhalation, whereas our studies utilized an intermittent, intragastric administration procedure. This could suggest that the dose, route, and schedule of ethanol exposure during adolescence may be critical determinants of long-term changes in HPA axis reactivity and cytokine gene induction.

One important question to address in future studies will be the mechanisms underlying the apparent HPA axis sensitization observed in females as a result of adolescent ethanol exposure. In particular, it will be important to identify whether these changes reflect altered function of neural circuits that govern HPA axis regulation, or intrinsic differences in sensitivity of endocrine glands comprising the HPA axis. This can be readily tested through a systematic series of hormonal challenges (CRH or ACTH injection) as we have done under other circumstances (Hueston and Deak, 2014b; also see Spencer and Deak, 2016 for an overview). Such studies are planned for the near future. It will also be important to extend these physiological findings to behavioral circumstances as well. For instance, the suppressed cytokine response evoked by LPS would predict that males with a history of adolescent ethanol exposure should display reduced sickness behavior under conditions of acute illness as adults. Given the HPA dysregulation observed in females with an adolescent history of ethanol, one might predict heightened anxiety and/or depression in adulthood. Given the established association between age of first alcohol use and subsequent vulnerability to addiction (Ystrom et al., 2014), it will also be important to assess whether adolescent ethanol exposure might increase vulnerability to addiction, particularly in females since stress dysregulation has been posited as one pathway towards addiction (Miller and Spear, 2006; Koob, 2008). These and many other issues will need to be explored in future studies.

As with any pre-clinical model of ethanol exposure, the mode of ethanol delivery and subsequent BECs achieved require careful consideration. We elected to utilize intragastric intubation for these studies because it mimics the normal route of administration for ethanol, and allows for binge-like doses to be achieved consistently and reliably. Such BECs would be difficult to achieve through voluntary consumption in rat, though that may be a path for future studies. BECs during the adolescent intubation regimen were not assessed due to concerns that the blood sampling procedure might have an enduring influence on the study outcomes. However, prior studies from our lab reported peak BECs of approximately 180 mg/dl after delivery of 4 g/kg (i.g.) of ethanol, which is consistent with a binge-like range of BECs (Buck et al., 2011; Doremus-Fitzwater et al., 2015). Because BECs were not assessed in the present studies, we cannot rule out the possibility that the sex-specific outcomes observed here might be due to intrinsic differences in ethanol metabolism (or other pharmacokinetic differences) between males and females (Truxell et al., 2007). Finally, our studies did not include a group of non-intubated controls to assess the influence of the intubation procedure itself. We occasionally use non-intubated controls and have not seen any evidence emerge to demonstrate long-term effects of the intubation procedure itself thus far. For practical purposes, however, we cannot do so in every study design. Nevertheless, these issues raise a more general question regarding whether any stress challenge (not just ethanol) imposed during adolescence might lead to similar outcomes. This is an interesting question that will have to be resolved in future studies. Overall, any ethanol delivery approach has both strengths and limitations and the study outcomes should be considered within an appropriate framework.

While this study yielded several interesting results, there are several procedural differences that must be considered in the interpretation of study outcomes. For instance, Experiments 1–3 utilize rats shipped from a vendor post weaning, whereas Experiment 4 utilized rats bred in house. The use of shipped animals for developmental studies is not ideal (see Laroche et al., 2009a,b; Spencer and Deak, 2016; Vargas et al., 2016), though it remains common practice for many investigators who do not have access to a breeding facility. Despite this limitation, Experiments 2 and 4 both yielded similar, durable influences of adolescent ethanol on LPS-induced cytokines as adults, even though the overall magnitude of cytokine responses across studies varied widely. A second disparity in study design was the number of ethanol cycles that the animals received during adolescence. Two cycles of intermittent ethanol exposure were utilized in Experiments 1–3, whereas four cycles were utilized in Experiment 4. Ultimately, the increase in number of cycles did not alter the directionality of the effects seen although it did appear to increase their magnitude. The model of ethanol administration is an important consideration because other studies have suggested that it is not only the amount of ethanol that is the dominant factor in creating durable effects resulting from AIE, but also the number of periods of abstinence between ethanol exposures (Lopez and Becker, 2005; Diaz-Granados and Graham, 2007). Indeed, periods of acute withdrawal that occur throughout intermittent ethanol exposure may play a critical role in causing some of the lasting changes of ethanol (Spear, 2016). Finally, to truly attribute the results of this study to an adolescent critical period, follow up studies that incorporate an adult control (that receive the same quantity of ethanol over the same time frame) and that control for the time difference between AIE and challenge between the two studies would be needed. Despite these minor limitations, the present study yielded important and highly consistent results that warrant further investigation.

A final element of the study that affects interpretation of the results is the use of the cellular fraction of blood to study peripheral cytokine expression (Wang et al., 2016; Opstad et al., 2017). Although it is more common in contemporary studies to utilize plasma protein measures to detect cytokines, cytokines in plasma have very short half-lives and the assays to measure them require comparatively large samples. Thus, a viable alternative for procuring cytokine signals is to utilize gene expression in the cellular fraction, which can be done in very small samples, thereby allowing for the use of a within-subjects experimental design. Although there is always a question as to how such gene expression changes might align with functional protein measures, the detailed time course information gathered in the present study can be used to inform selection of more discrete time points for protein measures. Such studies are already planned in the near future. Furthermore, while the functional relationship between peripheral cytokines and central cytokines is unclear, prior studies have suggested that peripheral cytokine release may play a role in activating subsequent central action. LPS induced TNF-α in serum has been shown to play a role in triggering a proinflammatory response in the brain (Qin et al., 2007, 2008). Further research probing the relationship between these elements of the immune response would be worthwhile.

In conclusion, the effects of ethanol during adolescence appear to be mitigated by many factors. The results of this study as well as other work suggest that how the ethanol is administered, the nature/modality of the subsequent challenge stimulus, and the sex of the animals all may interact with AIE. While the rates of binge drinking in both adolescents and adults is very high, men are almost twice as likely to engage in binge drinking as women (Centers for Disease Control and Prevention, 2012). Differences in how men and women may be affected by ethanol, particularly during periods of developmental vulnerability, may contribute to the difference in AUD prevalence that exists between men and women (Nolen-Hoeksema, 2004). Despite all of this, it has been reported that women suffer more negative consequences of heavy ethanol use, including increased susceptibility to physical illness at lower levels of exposure than has been seen in men (Nolen-Hoeksema, 2004). Several drugs of abuse have been linked to weakened natural immune system function during use and at times lingering afterwards. Ethanol abuse specifically has been shown to produce a pronounced immunosuppressive effect and can increase the chances of individuals with ethanol being vulnerable to infection (Szabo, 1997; Szabo and Saha, 2015). Alterations in HPA axis reactivity and cytokine function could help to explain some of ethanol's effects on the immune system and the potential for adolescent ethanol use to cause lasting alterations in immune function. This could lead to a lifetime of heightened immune vulnerability to an array of types of challenge stimuli. Better understanding of how adolescent ethanol exposure affects the immune system and the longevity of such changes could help to better understand the risk of individuals exposed to future insults and help identify targets to reverse negative alterations.

AUTHOR CONTRIBUTIONS

ASV, TD-F, AG and TD made substantial contributions to the conception or design of the work as well as participated in the acquisition, analysis, or interpretation of data for the work. In addition, they played a significant role in drafting the work or revising it critically for important intellectual content and submitted for final approval of the version to be published. All authors agree to be accountable for all aspects of the work in ensuring that questions related to the accuracy or integrity of any part of the work are appropriately investigated and resolved.

ACKNOWLEDGMENTS

Special thanks to Dennis Lovelock, Jackie Paniccia, Amy Perkins and Maryam Sammakia for playing a critical role in the execution of these studies.

REFERENCES

Allen, C. D., Grigoleit, J. S., Hong, J., Bae, S., Vaughan, J., and Lee, S. (2016). Exposure to alcohol during adolescence exerts long-term effects on stress response and the adult brain stress circuits. *Neuroscience* 339, 64–71. doi: 10.1016/j.neuroscience.2016.09.031

Buck, H. M., Hueston, C. M., Bishop, C., and Deak, T. (2011). Enhancement of the hypothalamic-pituitary-adrenal axis but not cytokine responses to stress challenges imposed during withdrawal from acute alcohol exposure in Sprague-Dawley rats. *Psychopharmacology (Berl)* 218, 203–215. doi: 10.1007/s00213-011-2388-z

Centers for Disease Control and Prevention. (2012). Vital signs: binge drinking prevalence, frequency, and intensity among adults—U.S., 2010. *MMWR Morb. Mortal. Wkly. Rep.* 61, 14–19.

Centers for Disease Control and Prevention. (2014). Alcohol use and your health. Available online at: http://www.cdc.gov/alcohol/fact-sheets/alcohol-use.htm

Cook, R. T. (1998). Alcohol abuse, alcoholism, and damage to the immune system— a review. *Alcohol. Clin. Exp. Res.* 22, 1927–1942. doi: 10.1111/j.1530-0277.1998.tb05900.x

Crews, F. T., Vetreno, R. P., Broadwater, M. A., and Robinson, D. L. (2016). Adolescent alcohol exposure persistently impacts adult neurobiology and behavior. *Pharmacol. Rev.* 68, 1074–1109. doi: 10.1124/pr.115.012138

Deak, T., Quinn, M., Cidlowski, J. A., Victoria, N. C., Murphy, A. Z., and Sheridan, J. F. (2015). Neuroimmune mechanisms of stress: sex differences, developmental plasticity, and implications for pharmacotherapy of stress-related disease. *Stress* 18, 367–380. doi: 10.3109/10253890.2015.1053451

Diaz-Granados, J. L., and Graham, D. L. (2007). The effects of continuous and intermittent ethanol exposure in adolesence on the aversive properties of ethanol during adulthood. *Alcohol. Clin. Exp. Res.* 31, 2020–2027. doi: 10.1111/j.1530-0277.2007.00534.x

Doremus, T. L., Brunell, S. C., Rajendran, P., and Spear, L. P. (2005). Factors influencing elevated ethanol consumption in adolescent relative to adult rats. *Alcohol. Clin. Exp. Res.* 29, 1796–1808. doi: 10.1097/01.alc.0000183007.65998.aa

Doremus, T. L., Brunell, S. C., Varlinskaya, E. I., and Spear, L. P. (2003). Anxiogenic effects during withdrawal from acute ethanol in adolescent and adult rats. *Pharmacol. Biochem. Behav.* 75, 411–418. doi: 10.1016/s0091-3057(03)00134-5

Doremus-Fitzwater, T. L., Buck, H. M., Bordner, K., Richey, L., Jones, M. E., and Deak, T. (2014). Intoxication- and withdrawal-dependent expression of central and peripheral cytokines following initial ethanol exposure. *Alcohol. Clin. Exp. Res.* 38, 2186–2198. doi: 10.1111/acer.12481

Doremus-Fitzwater, T. L., Gano, A., Paniccia, J. E., and Deak, T. (2015). Male adolescent rats display blunted cytokine responses in the CNS after acute ethanol or lipopolysaccharide exposure. *Physiol. Behav.* 148, 131–144. doi: 10.1016/j.physbeh.2015.02.032

Fillman, S. G., Weickert, T. W., Lenroot, R. K., Catts, S. V., Bruggemann, J. M., Catts, V. S., et al. (2016). Elevated peripheral cytokines characterize a subgroup of people with schizophrenia displaying poor verbal fluency and reduced Broca's area volume. *Mol. Psychiatry* 21, 1090–1098. doi: 10.1038/mp.2015.90

Gauthier, T. W. (2015). Prenatal alcohol exposure and the developing immune system. *Alcohol. Res.* 37, 279–285.

Giedd, J. N. (2008). The teen brain: insights from neuroimaging. *J. Adolesc. Health* 42, 335–343. doi: 10.1016/j.jadohealth.2008.01.007

Grant, B. F., and Dawson, D. A. (1997). Age at onset of alcohol use and its association with DSM-IV alcohol abuse and dependence: results from the national longitudinal alcohol epidemiologic survey. *J. Subst. Abuse* 9, 103–110. doi: 10.1016/s0899-3289(97)90009-2

Guerri, C., and Pascual, M. (2010). Mechanisms involved in the neurotoxic, cognitive and neurobehavioral effects of alcohol consumption during adolescence. *Alcohol* 44, 15–26. doi: 10.1016/j.alcohol.2009.10.003

Hueston, C. M., and Deak, T. (2014a). The inflamed axis: the interaction between stress, hormones, and the expression of inflammatory-related genes within key structures comprising the hypothalamic-pituitary-adrenal axis. *Physiol. Behav.* 124, 77–91. doi: 10.1016/j.physbeh.2013.10.035

Hueston, C. M., and Deak, T. (2014b). On the time course, generality and regulation of plasma progesterone release in male rats by stress exposure. *Endocrinology* 155, 3527–3537. doi: 10.1210/en.2014-1060

Kim, C. K., Giberson, P. K., Yu, W., Zoeller, R. T., and Weinberg, J. (1999). Effects of prenatal ethanol exposure on hypothalamic-pituitary-adrenal responses to chronic cold stress in rats. *Alcohol. Clin. Exp. Res.* 23, 301–310. doi: 10.1111/j.1530-0277.1999.tb04114.x

Koob, G. F. (2008). A role for brain stress systems in addiction. *Neuron* 59, 11–34. doi: 10.1016/j.neuron.2008.06.012

Laroche, J., Gasbarro, L., Herman, J. P., and Blaustein, J. D. (2009a). Enduring influences of peripubertal/adolescent stressors on behavioral response to estradiol and progesterone in adult female mice. *Endocrinology* 150, 3717–3725. doi: 10.1210/en.2009-0099

Laroche, J., Gasbarro, L., Herman, J. P., and Blaustein, J. D. (2009b). Reduced behavioral response to gonadal hormones in mice shipped during the peripubertal/adolescent period. *Endocrinology* 150, 2351–2358. doi: 10.1210/en.2008-1595

Lee, S., and Rivier, C. (1996). Gender differences in the effect of prenatal alcohol exposure on the hypothalamic-pituitary-adrenal axis response to immune signals. *Psychoneuroendocrinology* 21, 145–155. doi: 10.1016/0306-4530(95)00038-0

Lee, S., and Rivier, C. (2003). Long-term influence of an initial exposure to alcohol on the rat hypothalamic-pituitary axis. *Alcohol. Clin. Exp. Res.* 27, 1463–1470. doi: 10.1097/01.alc.0000086065.06203.dd

Lopez, M. F., and Becker, H. C. (2005). Effect of pattern and number of chronic ethanol exposures on subsequent voluntary ethanol intake in C57BL/6J mice. *Psychopharmacology* 181, 688–696. doi: 10.1007/s00213-005-0026-3

Matthews, D. B., Tinsley, K. L., Diaz-Granados, J. L., Tokunaga, S., and Silvers, J. M. (2008). Chronic intermittent exposure to ethanol during adolescence produces tolerance to the hypnotic effects of ethanol in male rats: a dose-dependent analysis. *Alcohol* 42, 617–621. doi: 10.1016/j.alcohol.2008.09.001

Miller, M. W., and Spear, L. P. (2006). The alcoholism generator. *Alcohol. Clin. Exp. Res.* 30, 1466–1469. doi: 10.1111/j.1530-0277.2006.00177.x

Muralidharan, S., Ambade, A., Fulham, M. A., Deshpande, J., Catalano, D., and Mandrekar, P. (2014). Moderate alcohol induces stress proteins HSF1 and hsp70 and inhibits proinflammatory cytokines resulting in endotoxin tolerance. *J. Immunol.* 193, 1975–1987. doi: 10.4049/jimmunol.1303468

Nolen-Hoeksema, S. (2004). Gender differences in risk factors and consequences for alcohol use and problems. *Clin. Psychol. Rev.* 24, 981–1010. doi: 10.1016/j.cpr.2004.08.003

Ogunsakin, O., Hottor, T., Mehta, A., Lichtveld, M., and McCaskill, M. (2016). Chronic ethanol exposure effects on vitamin D levels among subjects with alcohol use disorder. *Environ. Health Insights* 10, 191–199. doi: 10.4137/ehi.s40335

Opstad, T. B., Brusletto, B. S., Arnesen, H., Pettersen, A. Å., and Seljeflot, I. (2017). Cigarette smoking represses expression of cytokine IL-12 and its regulator miR-21-An observational study in patients with coronary artery disease. *Immunobiology* 222, 169–175. doi: 10.1016/j.imbio.2016.10.007

Pascual, M., Montesinos, J., Marcos, M., Torres, J. L., Costa-Alba, P., Garcia-García, F., et al. (2016). Gender differences in the inflammatory cytokine and chemokine profiles induced by binge ethanol drinking in adolescence. *Addict. Biol.* doi: 10.1111/adb.12461 [Epub ahead of print].

Pautassi, R. M., Myers, M., Spear, L. P., Molina, J. C., and Spear, N. E. (2008). Adolescent but not adult rats exhibit ethanol-mediated appetitive second-order conditioning. *Alcohol. Clin. Exp. Res.* 32, 2016–2027. doi: 10.1111/j.1530-0277.2008.00789.x

Przybycien-Szymanska, M. M., Mott, N. N., Paul, C. R., Gillespie, R. A., and Pak, T. R. (2011). Binge-pattern alcohol exposure during puberty induces long-term changes in HPA axis reactivity. *PLoS One* 6:e18350. doi: 10.1371/journal.pone.0018350

Przybycien-Szymanska, M. M., Rao, Y. S., and Pak, T. R. (2010). Binge-pattern alcohol exposure during puberty induces sexually dimorphic changes in genes regulating the HPA axis. *Am. J. Physiol. Endocrinol. Metab.* 298, E320–E328. doi: 10.1152/ajpendo.00615.2009

Qin, L., He, J., Hanes, R. N., Pluzarev, O., Hong, J. S., and Crews, F. T. (2008). Increased systemic and brain cytokine production and neuroinflammation by endotoxin following ethanol treatment. *J. Neuroinflammation* 5:10. doi: 10.1186/1742-2094-5-10

Qin, L., Wu, X., Block, M. L., Liu, Y., Breese, G. R., Hong, J. S., et al. (2007). Systemic LPS causes chronic neuroinflammation and progressive neurodegeneration. *Glia* 55, 453–462. doi: 10.1002/glia.20467

Raineki, C., Hellemans, K. G., Bodnar, T., Lavigne, K. M., Ellis, L., Woodward, T. S., et al. (2014). Neurocircuitry underlying stress and emotional regulation in animals prenatally exposed to alcohol and subjected to chronic mild stress in adulthood. *Front. Endocrinol. (Lausanne)* 5:5. doi: 10.3389/fendo.2014.00005

Rivest, S., Lacroix, S., Vallières, L., Nadeau, S., Zhang, J., and Laflamme, N. (2000). How the blood talks to the brain parenchyma and the paraventricular nucleus of the hypothalamus during systemic inflammatory and infectious stimuli. *Proc. Soc. Exp. Biol. Med.* 223, 22–38. doi: 10.1111/j.1525-1373.2000.22304.x

Rivier, C., Bruhn, T., and Vale, W. (1984). Effect of ethanol on the hypothalamic-pituitary-adrenal axis in the rat: role of corticotropin-releasing factor (CRF). *J. Pharmacol. Exp. Ther.* 229, 127–131.

Romeo, R. D., Patel, R., Pham, L., and So, V. M. (2016). Adolescence and the ontogeny of the hormonal stress response in male and female rats and mice. *Neurosci. Biobehav. Rev.* 70, 206–216. doi: 10.1016/j.neubiorev.2016.05.020

Schwochow, D., Serieys, L. E., Wayne, R. K., and Thalmann, O. (2012). Efficient recovery of whole blood RNA— a comparison of commercial RNA extraction protocols for high-throughput applications in wildlife species. *BMC Biotechnol.* 12:33. doi: 10.1186/1472-6750-12-33

Spear, L. P. (2016). Consequences of adolescent use of alcohol and other drugs: studies using rodent models. *Neurosci. Biobehav. Rev.* 70, 228–243. doi: 10.1016/j.neubiorev.2016.07.026

Spear, L. P., and Swartzwelder, H. S. (2014). Adolescent alcohol exposure and persistence of adolescent-typical phenotypes into adulthood: a mini-review. *Neurosci. Biobehav. Rev.* 45, 1–8. doi: 10.1016/j.neubiorev.2014.04.012

Spencer, R. L., and Deak, T. (2016). A users guide to HPA axis research. *Physiol. Behav.* doi: 10.1016/j.physbeh.2016.11.014 [Epub ahead of print].

Sullivan, P. F., Fan, C., and Perou, C. M. (2006). Evaluating the comparability of gene expression in blood and brain. *Am. J. Med. Genet. B Neuropsychiatr. Genet.* 141b, 261–268. doi: 10.1002/ajmg.b.30272

Szabo, G. (1997). Alcohol's contribution to compromised immunity. *Alcohol Health Res. World* 21, 30–41.

Szabo, G., and Saha, B. (2015). Alcohol's effect on host defense. *Alcohol Res.* 37, 159–170.

Szelényi, J. (2001). Cytokines and the central nervous system. *Brain Res. Bull.* 54, 329–338. doi: 10.1016/S0361-9230(01)00428-2

Truxell, E. M., Molina, J. C., and Spear, N. E. (2007). Ethanol intake in the juvenile, adolescent and adult rat: effects of age and prior exposure to ethanol. *Alcohol. Clin. Exp. Res.* 31, 755–765. doi: 10.1111/j.1530-0277.2007.00358.x

Vargas, J., Junco, M., Gomez, C., and Lajud, N. (2016). Early life stress increases metabolic risk, HPA axis reactivity and depressive-like behavior when combined with postweaning social isolation in rats. *PLoS One* 11:e0162665. doi: 10.1371/journal.pone.0162665

Varlinskaya, E. I., and Spear, L. P. (2004a). Acute ethanol withdrawal (hangover) and social behavior in adolescent and adult male and female Sprague-Dawley rats. *Alcohol. Clin. Exp. Res.* 28, 40–50. doi: 10.1097/01.alc.0000108655.51087.df

Varlinskaya, E. I., and Spear, L. P. (2004b). Changes in sensitivity to ethanol-induced social facilitation and social inhibition from early to late adolescence. *Ann. N Y Acad. Sci.* 1021, 459–461. doi: 10.1196/annals.1308.064

Wang, W., Liu, Z., Su, J., Chen, W. S., Wang, X. W., Bai, S. X., et al. (2016). Macrophage micro-RNA-155 promotes lipopolysaccharide-induced acute lung injury in mice and rats. *Am. J. Physiol. Lung Cell. Mol. Physiol.* 311, L494–L506. doi: 10.1152/ajplung.00001.2016

Weinberg, J. (1992). Prenatal ethanol effects: sex difference in offspring stress responsiveness. *Alcohol* 9, 219–223. doi: 10.1016/0741-8329(92)90057-h

Weinberg, J., Sliwowska, J. H., Lan, N., and Hellemans, K. G. (2008). Prenatal alcohol exposure: foetal programming, the hypothalamic-pituitary-adrenal axis and sex differences in outcome. *J. Neuroendocrinol.* 20, 470–488. doi: 10.1111/j.1365-2826.2008.01669.x

Wieczorek, L., Fish, E. W., O'Leary-Moore, S. K., Parnell, S. E., and Sulik, K. K. (2015). Hypothalamic-pituitary-adrenal axis and behavioral dysfunction following early binge-like prenatal alcohol exposure in mice. *Alcohol* 49, 207–217. doi: 10.1016/j.alcohol.2015.01.005

Willey, A. R., Anderson, R. I., Morales, M., Ramirez, R. L., and Spear, L. P. (2012). Effects of ethanol administration on corticosterone levels in adolescent and adult rats. *Alcohol* 46, 29–36. doi: 10.1016/j.alcohol.2011.08.005

World Health Organization (2014). Global status report on alcohol and health. Available online at: http://apps.who.int/iris/bitstream/10665/112736/1/9789240692763_eng.pdf

Ystrom, E., Kendler, K. S., and Reicborn-Kjennnerud, T. (2014). Early age of alcohol initiation is not the cause of alcohol use disorders in adulthood, but is a major indicator of genetic risk. A population-based twin study. *Addiction* 109, 1824–1832. doi: 10.1111/add.12620

14

Persistent Decreases in Adult Subventricular and Hippocampal Neurogenesis Following Adolescent Intermittent Ethanol Exposure

*Wen Liu and Fulton T. Crews **

Bowles Center for Alcohol Studies, University of North Carolina at Chapel Hill, Chapel Hill, NC, United States

Edited by:
Mary M. Torregrossa, University of Pittsburgh, United States

Reviewed by:
S. Alex Marshall, High Point University, United States
Christian P. Müller, University of Erlangen-Nuremberg, Germany

***Correspondence:**
Fulton T. Crews
ftcrews@med.unc.edu

Neurogenesis in hippocampal dentate gyrus (DG) and subventricular zone (SVZ) matures during adolescence to adult levels. Binge drinking is prevalent in adolescent humans, and could alter brain neurogenesis and maturation in a manner that persists into adulthood. To determine the impact of adolescent binge drinking on adult neurogenesis, Wistar rats received adolescent intermittent ethanol (AIE) exposure (5.0 g/kg/day, i.g., 2 days on/2 days off from postnatal day, P25–P54) and sacrificed on P57 or P95. Neural progenitor cell proliferation, differentiation, survival and maturation using immunohistochemistry was determined in the DG and SVZ. We found that AIE exposure decreased neurogenesis in both brain regions in adulthood (P95). In the DG at P57, AIE exposure resulted in a significant reduction of SOX2+, Tbr2+, Prox1+ and parvalbumin (PV)+IR expression, and at P95 decreased DCX+ and PV+IR expression. AIE exposure also reduced the expression of two cell proliferation markers (Ki67+ and BrdU+IR with 300 mg/kg, 2 h) at P95. The immune signaling molecule β-2 microglobulin+ and the cell death marker activated caspase-3+IR were significantly increased in the DG by AIE exposure. In the SVZ, AIE exposure decreased SOX2+, Mash1+, DCX+ and Dlx2+IR expression at P95, but not at P57. Thus, in adulthood both brain regions have reduced neurogenesis following AIE exposure. To assess progenitor cell survival and maturation, rats were treated with BrdU (150 mg/kg/day, 14 days) to label proliferating cells and were sacrificed weeks later on P95. In the hippocampus DG, AIE exposure increased survival BrdU+ cells which differentiated into Iba1+ microglia. In contrast, SVZ had decreased BrdU+ cells similar to decreased DCX+ neurogenesis. These data indicate that AIE exposure causes a lasting decrease in both adult hippocampal DG and forebrain SVZ neurogenesis with brain regional differences in the AIE response that persist into adulthood.

Keywords: adolescent intermittent ethanol, neurogenesis, hippocampal dentate gyrus, subventricular zone, rat

Abbreviations: AIE, adolescent intermittent ethanol; ANOVA, analysis of variance; BEC, blood ethanol concentration; DCX, doublecortin; DG, dentate gyrus; HIP, hippocampus; i.g., intragastric; i.p., intraperitoneal; NPCs, neuroprogenitor cells; PBS, phosphate-buffered saline; PV, parvalbumin; Proxl, prospero homeobox protein 1; RMS, rostral migratory stream; Sox2, sex determining regions Y-box 2; SVZ, subventricular zone; Tbr2, T-box brain protein 2; TLR, Toll-like receptor.

INTRODUCTION

Adult neurogenesis involves the formation of new brain neurons that alter neurocircuits and contribute to neuroplasticity. Adult brain neurons are generated from neural stem cells and progenitor cells in two specific neurogenic niches of the brain: the hippocampal dentate gyrus (DG) subgranular zone and the lateral ventricle subventricular zone (SVZ; Eriksson et al., 1998; Spalding et al., 2013; Ernst et al., 2014). Neurons born in the hippocampal DG differentiate and integrate into existing networks as granule cells, and neurons born in the SVZ migrate to the olfactory bulbs where they become periglomerular neurons. Neurogenesis is a complex developmental process that includes neuroprogenitor cell (NPC) proliferation, migration, differentiation and survival. Emerging new findings have found that the progenitors and developmental milestones of neurogenesis in the DG and SVZ are different (Kempermann et al., 2004, 2015; Abrous et al., 2005; Ming and Song, 2005, 2011; Lledo et al., 2006; Song et al., 2016). In the DG, six stages identified by morphology and expression of markers have been defined (Kempermann et al., 2015); whereas in the SVZ progenitor stages of differentiation have been divided into five phases of adult neurogenesis (Ming and Song, 2011). In the DG, markers of NPCs that distinguish stages of neurogenesis, including sex determining regions Y-box 2 (SOX2) which is expressed in non-radial and horizontal type-1 cells, and Tbr2, a T-box transcription factor expressed by type-2a and -2b intermediate NPCs that persist to maturation into neuroblasts (type-3). Immature/mature neuron markers include doublecortin (DCX), a microtubule-associated protein expressed in migrating neuroblasts but lost after maturation to mature granule cells in DG (Brown et al., 2003; Rao and Shetty, 2004; Couillard-Despres et al., 2005), prospero homeobox protein 1 (Prox1), which is expressed in the neuroblast, immature and mature neurons (Lavado and Oliver, 2007; Lavado et al., 2010; Hodge and Hevner, 2011), and parvalbumin (PV), which labels mature γ-aminobutyric acid (GABAergic) interneurons of the nervous system. Adult SVZ neurogenesis involves different NPCs and development (Ming and Song, 2005, 2011), briefly, radial glia-like cells (type B) in the SVZ have SOX2, Mash1 is expressed in amplifying NPC (type C), and formation of neuroblasts. Dlx2 and DCX are markers of SVZ neuroblasts and immature neurons, and mature interneurons are expressed by NeuN. These NPC maturation and markers studies provide opportunities to determine sensitivity of various NPC progenitor stages in both DG and SVZ to environment, drugs and/or other factors.

New emerging evidence has suggested that altered neurogenesis and gliogenesis may contribute to drug taking and drug seeking (Mandyam and Koob, 2012). Further, studies suggest that drug-induced loss of neurogenesis contributes to addiction and recovery from a variety of drugs, including alcohol (Mandyam and Koob, 2012; Staples and Mandyam, 2016). Previous studies have found that chronic ethanol treatment of adult rats reduces NPC proliferation in the DG (Nixon and Crews, 2002; Herrera et al., 2003; He et al., 2005) and SVZ (Crews et al., 2004; Hansson et al., 2010; Campbell et al., 2014). A binge model of alcohol dependence found reduced adult hippocampal DG neurogenesis following ethanol treatment (Nixon and Crews, 2004; Hansson et al., 2010). Interestingly, abstinence after adult binge ethanol treatment results in bursts of NPC proliferation over the first week of abstinence that restore DG neurogenesis after about 30 days of abstinence (Nixon and Crews, 2004; Nixon et al., 2008). Further, stress and chronic ethanol self-administration by adult mice reduce hippocampal neurogenesis and induce depression-like behavior that are reversed by the antidepressant fluoxetine (Stevenson et al., 2009). Although hippocampal DG neurogenesis has been linked to drug dependence, SVZ neurogenesis has not been extensively studied. One study using a rat 7-week ethanol treatment model of chronic relapsing alcohol dependence that increases ethanol self-administration results in a loss of both DG and SVZ neurogenesis (Hansson et al., 2010). Interestingly, in this study DG neurogenesis recovered over weeks of abstinence similar to the binge studies noted above whereas SVZ neurogenesis was decreased after 21 days of abstinence following ethanol treatment (Hansson et al., 2010). Thus, neurogenesis in DG and SVZ differ in NPC markers, maturation and inhibition by ethanol.

Adolescence is a critical developmental stage during which brain networks that regulate cognition and emotion mature (Dahl, 2004; Crews et al., 2016). Binge drinking is also common in human adolescents (Wechsler et al., 1995; O'Malley et al., 1998). Human and animal studies suggest that alcohol exposure during adolescence alters brain development causing unique long lasting changes in adulthood (Spear, 2000). Previous studies have found hippocampal neurogenesis is greater in adolescents than adults (He and Crews, 2007) and adolescent rat hippocampal DG neurogenesis is more sensitive to ethanol inhibition than adult DG neurogenesis (Crews et al., 2006). More recent studies using adolescent intermittent ethanol (AIE) exposure have found reduced adult neurogenesis using ethanol vapor (Ehlers et al., 2013a), intragastric (i.g) ethanol exposure (Ehlers et al., 2013a; Broadwater et al., 2014; Vetreno and Crews, 2015), intraperitoneal (i.p) exposure (Sakharkar et al., 2016) or ethanol self-administration (Briones and Woods, 2013). Broadwater et al. (2014) directly compared adolescent and adulthood binge ethanol exposure on adult neurogenesis and found AIE persistently reduced adult DG neurogenesis whereas identical adult treatment only transiently reduced DG neurogenesis suggesting ethanol exposure during adolescence, but not adulthood, markedly reduced DCX expression in the hippocampal DG 4 weeks after the final ethanol exposure. Although acute adolescent binge ethanol exposure has been found to reduce both DG and SVZ neurogenesis (Crews et al., 2006), to our knowledge the impact of AIE on proliferation and maturation of NPC in SVZ neurogenesis has not been determined. This study reports for the first time the impact of AIE exposure, a model of underage binge drinking, on multiple markers across the stages of neurogenesis in both the hippocampal DG and forebrain SVZ in adulthood. We report here that AIE causes a persistent loss of both SVZ and DG neurogenesis, and that the AIE-induced changes in markers of NPC stages and cell death suggest that the mechanisms of the AIE-induced loss of new neuron formation in DG and SVZ is different for each brain region.

MATERIALS AND METHODS

Animals and AIE Exposure

Timed-pregnant Wistar rats ($n = 10$), young mothers at the same age, were ordered from Harlan Laboratories, Inc. (Indianapolis, IN, USA) under a protocol approved by the Institutional Animal Care and Use Committees at the University of North Carolina. All animals were maintained at 22°C under a 12:12-h light/dark cycles with free access to food and water. Timed-pregnant dams at embryonic day 17 (E17), were allowed to acclimate to our vivarium. On the day following birth (postnatal day 1, P1), litters were culled to 10 pups. On weaning at P21, male offspring were pair-housed with a same-gender, same-age non-littermate and body weight match assigned to two experimental groups, including control and AIE group. This study was done in all males. The AIE group was exposed intermittently (e.g., 2 days on, 2 days off) with ethanol (5 g/kg, 25% ethanol w/v, i.g., 10 ml/kg) during adolescence (P25–P54); and the control group was administered with the same volume of water as described previously (Liu and Crews, 2015). Body weight was measured every 4 days. All control and AIE rats grew normally from P25 (control: 44.0 ± 1.3 g; AIE: 45.9 ± 1.3 g) to P54 (control: 262.7 ± 3.9 g; AIE: 258.4 ± 4.8 g) during AIE exposure. As expected, there was a significant main difference of age with body weight [$F_{(1,384)} = 1298.25$, $p < 0.001$], and no significant effect on group [$F_{(7,384)} = 0.07$, $p = 0.786$], age × group interaction [$F_{(7,384)} = 0.60$, $p = 0.753$]. From P57 to P95 after final ethanol exposure, the body weight of all animals also revealed a significant main difference of age [$F_{(9,320)} = 118.28$, $p < 0.001$], and but no group effect [$F_{(1,320)} = 0.01$, $p = 0.932$] or age × group interaction [$F_{(9,320)} = 0.26$, $p = 0.985$]. All rats appeared normal throughout the experiment consistent with AIE binge exposure not causing observable changes in health. During AIE exposure, tail blood samples were collected and measured twice 1 h after ethanol exposure (5 g/kg i.g.) at P38 and 54. Blood ethanol concentrations (O'Malley et al., 1998) were measured using a GM7 Analyzer (Analox, London, UK). Their average values were 152.17 ± 11.09 at P38 and 211.86 ± 19.26 mg/dl at P54. Statistics showed that the BECs had a significant difference between at postnatal day 38 and 54 [$F_{(1,50)} = 7.21$, $p < 0.01$]. At P54, animals of both control and AIE group were randomly reassigned to three groups respectively with body weight match after the last ethanol exposure. BrdU (5′-bromo-2-deoxyuridine, Sigma; St. Louis, MO, USA) is incorporated into DNA during cell division. To assess proliferation, control and AIE groups were sacrificed on P57, 2 h after BrdU injection ($n = 8$/each group, 300 mg/kg, dissolved in 0.9% saline, i.p.). A second group of control and AIE rats were sacrificed on P95 2 h after BrdU injection($n = 8$/each group, 300 mg/kg i.p.) to assess persistent changes in progenitor proliferation. For progenitor cell survival and differentiation study, a third group of control ($n = 8$) and AIE ($n = 10$) were administered BrdU 150 mg/kg daily starting at P54 for 14 days, and were allowed to survive 4 weeks after BrdU treatment, and sacrificed on P95 (See Supplementary Figure S1 for additional details).

Animal Tissue Collection, Preparation and Immunohistochemistry

Rats were deeply anesthetized with an overdose of sodium pentobarbital, and transcardially perfused with 0.1 M phosphate-buffered saline (PBS, pH7.4) followed by 4% paraformaldehyde (in 0.1 M phosphate buffer, pH 7.4). Brains were removed, and post-fixed for 24 h in 4% paraformaldehyde at 4°C. Coronal sections were obtained at a thickness of 40 μm in 1:12 series after cryoprotection with 20% and 30% sucrose, gradually. Every 12th section was used for each of the following antigens.

For BrdU staining, DNA denaturation was performed by incubating the section in 2 N HCl for 30 min 37°C (Kuhn et al., 1996). The sections were then incubated with 0.6% hydrogen peroxide (H_2O_2) for 30 min to remove endogenous peroxidase activity. Anti-mouse BrdU (Chemicon, MAB3424, Temecula, CA, USA) was used at a dilution of 1:2000 and incubated overnight at 4°C, and sections were incubated with biotinylated horse anti-mouse secondary antibody (1:200, Vector Laboratories, Burlingame, CA, USA) at room temperature for 1 h. Then avidin-biotin-peroxidase complex (ABC Elite Kit, Vector Laboratories) was added for 1 h at room temperature. Finally, the BrdU-positive cells were visualized using DAB (nickel-enhanced diaminobenzidine). For all other antigens, sections were incubated in 0.6% H_2O_2 for 30 min, and blocked in 3% goat serum (0.1% Triton X-100) for 1 h at room temperature. In the current studies, all other primary antibodies were used with different dilutions (**Table 1**) overnight at 4°C. At the second day, sections were rinsed in PBS, and incubated with biotinylated secondary goat anti-rabbit or anti-mouse or anti-chicken antibody (1:200, Vector Laboratories, Burlingame, CA, USA) for 1 h at room temperature. Subsequently, the positive cells were visualized using DAB.

Double fluorescence staining for BrdU and Ki67 was done using a mix of mouse anti-BrdU (1:2000, MAB3424, Chemicom, Temecula, CA, USA) and rabbit anti-Ki67 (1:400, ab66155, Abcam, Inc., Cambridge, MA, USA). Then, sections were incubated in the dark for 1 h with following secondary antibodies (1:200, a mix of goat anti-mouse 594 and anti-rabbit 488, Alexa Fluors, Molecular Probes Eugene, OR, USA). For mouse anti-BrdU (1:2000, MAB3424, Chemicon) and chicken anti-Tbr2 (1:800, S-C123463/31819, Lifespan bioscience Inc., Seattle, WA, USA), the secondary antibodies were used with a mix of goat anti-mouse 488 and anti-chicken 594 (1:200, Alexa Fluors, Molecular Probes Eugene, OR, USA). For mouse anti-BrdU (1:2000, MAB3424, Chemicom) and rabbit anti-Iba1 (1:500, 019-19741, Wako/Fisher, Cambridge, MA, USA), the secondary antibodies were used with a mix of goat anti-mouse 488 and anti-rabbit 594 (1:200, Alexa Fluors, Molecular Probes Eugene, OR, USA). For mouse anti-BrdU (1:2000, MAB3424, Chemicom) and anti-rabbit NeuN (1:1000, EMB Millipore, ABN78, Billerica, MA, USA), sections were incubated in the dark for 1 h with following secondary antibodies (1:200, a mix of goat anti-mouse 594 and anti-rabbit 488 Alexa Fluors,

TABLE 1 | Primary antibodies in the present study.

Antibodies	Isotype	Source/Purification	Dilution	Source
BrdU	Mouse IgG	Monoclonal	1:2000	Chemicon, Temecula, CA, USA (MAB3424)
Ki67	Rabbit IgG	Polyclonal	1:400	Abcam Inc., Cambridge, MA, USA (ab66155)
Tbr2/EOMES	Chicken IgG	Polyclonal	1:200	Lifespan Biosciences, Inc., Seattle, WA, USA (LSC123463/31819)
Sox2	Rabbit IgG	Polyclonal	1:1000	Abcam Inc., Cambridge, MA, USA (ab97959)
DCX	Rabbit IgG	Polyclonal	1:1000	Abcam Inc., Cambridge, MA, USA (ab18723)
Prox1	Rabbit IgG	Polyclonal	1:1000	Abcam Inc., Cambridge, MA, USA (ab37128)
Parvalbumin	Rabbit IgG	Polyclonal	1:1000	Abcam Inc., Cambridge, MA, USA (ab11427)
NeuN	Rabbit IgG	Polyclonal	1:1000	EMD Millipore, Billerica, MA, USA (ABN78)
Iba1	Rabbit IgG	Polyclonal	1:500	Wako/Fisher, Cambridge, MA, USA (019-19741)
Nestin	Rabbit IgG	Polyclonal	1:400	Abcam Inc., Cambridge, MA, USA (ab27952)
Mash1	Rabbit IgG	Polyclonal	1:50	Novus Biologicals, Littleton, CO, USA (NBP1-51269)
Dlx2	Rabbit IgG	Polyclonal	1:1000	Abcam Inc., Cambridge, MA, USA (ab18188)
β-2 microglobulin	Rabbit IgG	Polyclonal	1:50	Santa Cruz Biotechnology Inc., Dallas, TX, USA (sc-15366)
Cleaved caspase-3	Rabbit IgG	Polyclonal	1:1200	Cell Signaling Technology, Danvers, MA, USA (#9661)

Molecular Probes Eugene, OR, USA). All sections were covered slips with anti-fade mounting reagent (ProLong, Molecular Probes).

Quantification

Bioquant Nova Advanced Image Analysis (R&M Biometric, Nashville, TN, USA) was used for image capture and analysis (Crews et al., 2004). Images were captured by using an Olympus BX50 Microscope and Sony DXC-390 video camera linked to a computer. In the hippocampal DG, positive cells (BrdU+, Ki67+, Tbr2+, SOX2+, Prox1+, PV+, β-2 microglobulin+ and activated caspase-3+IR) were counted using prolife counting in the granule cell layer of the dorsal DG of HIP (Bregma from −2.30 mm to −4.52 mm; Paxinos and Watson, 1997) and expressed as cells per square millimeter with both sides of 3–5 section per animals, and the average value per mm^2 was used (See Supplementary Figure S1D). For DCX+IR, the granule cell layer of the hippocampal DG was outlined and pixel density was measured for the outlined area (pixels/mm^2). In the SVZ, positive cells (Nestin+, Dlx2+, BrdU+ and activated caspase-3+IR) were counted using prolife counting similar to that described by Kuhn et al. (1996) and Crews et al. (2006) in the special regions interested and expressed as cells per square millimeter with both sides of 3–5 section per animals, and the average value per mm^2 was used. For SOX2+, Mash1+ and DCX+IR, pixel densities were measured for the outlined area (pixels/mm^2; see Supplementary Figure S1D). In the SVZ, Bregma from 1.20 mm to −0.30 mm (Paxinos and Watson, 1997), positive immunoreactivities were measured at series of three 50 μm boxes along the length of SVZ as described (Kuhn et al., 1996; Crews et al., 2006).

Confocal analyses were conducted using LesicaSP2 AOBS Upright Laser Scanning Confocal in Michael Hooker Microscopy Facility of University of North Carolina. In the granule cell layer of hippocampal DG, 50–100 BrdU positive cells per sample were analyzed for co-labeling with Tbr2 or Iba1 or NeuN. The percentages of co-label in BrdU+IR were calculated.

Statistical Analysis

All values (including body weight, positive cells and pixel values) were reported as mean ± SEM and analyzed using analysis of variance (ANOVA) (IBM SPSS Statistics 22). The change of body weight was analyzed using a mixed ANOVA (group × day) with day as the repeated measure. Significant effects of AIE exposure on the body weight at different days were used with Student's *t*-test. For the effect of AIE exposure on the expression of positive cells or pixel values, ANOVA was used to test statistical significance, and followed by comparison of each group mean with Independent-Samples *T*-Test, and the *p*-value was used for statistical significance. The significant difference were considered if $p < 0.05$ at least. In this study, the percentage of the maturational decline between P57 and P95 with marker+IR expression was (P57 − P95)/P57 * 100; and the maturational increase between P57 and P95 with marker+IR expression was (P95 − P57)/P57 * 100. The percentage of AIE-induced decrease was (Control − AIE)/Control * 100; and AIE-induced increase was (AIE − Control)/Control * 100. Pearson correlations were used to determine the correlation across all markers in either the hippocampal DG or SVZ region.

RESULTS

AIE Exposure Reduces Hippocampal Dentate Gyrus Neurogenesis

Neurogenesis in adults involves NPC proliferation followed by maturation to an integrated functional neuron over a period of several weeks. We used multiple markers of NPCs that distinguish stages of neurogenesis and neuronal maturation on P57 (3 days after last ethanol exposure) and P95 (41 days after abstinence). We first determined proliferation using two indices, Ki67 and BrdU. Ki67, an endogenous marker of cell proliferation, is a nuclear protein expressed in all phases of the cell cycle, except the resting phase. We administered BrdU 2 h before sacrifice, which marks dividing cells during S-phase of the mitotic process. We found that AIE exposure did not affect BrdU+ and Ki67+IR expression 3 days after last ethanol exposure (P57), however, 41 days later (P95) there was a difference. Control levels of both BrdU+IR (42.6 ± 5.4%) [$F_{(1,27)} = 69.31$, $p < 0.001$] and Ki67+ (42.3 ± 5.4%) [$F_{(1,27)} = 42.39$, $p < 0.001$] declined with age from P57 to P95 (**Figure 1**), consistent with the known maturational decline in hippocampal neurogenesis. Interestingly,

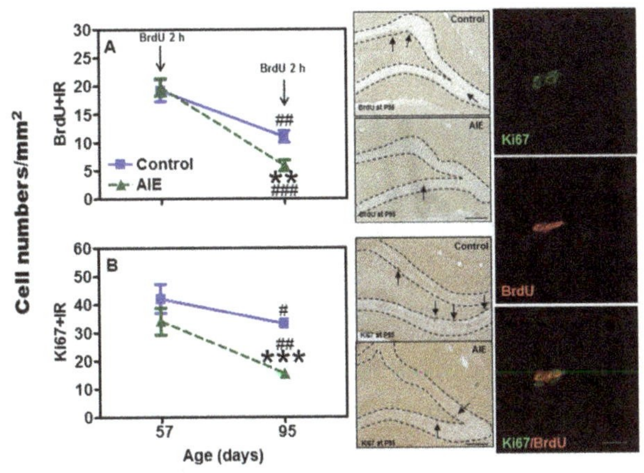

FIGURE 1 | Effects of adolescent intermittent ethanol (AIE, 5 g/kg, i.g., 2 days on/2 days off) exposure on BrdU+ (2 h, **A**) and Ki67+IR **(B)** expression in the hippocampal dentate gyrus (DG) of male rat brain at P57 and P95. Figure on left side: AIE exposure remarkably decreased BrdU+ (47%, **A**) and Ki67+IR (46%, **B**) expression at P95, but not at P57. $^{**}p < 0.01$, $^{***}p < 0.001$ compared with control group. BrdU+ **(A)** and Ki67+IR **(B)** expression had the maturational decline in both control (BrdU+IR: 43%; Ki67+IR: 42%) and AIE group (BrdU+IR: 70%; Ki67+IR: 63%) from P57 to P95. $^{\#}p < 0.05$, $^{\#\#}p < 0.01$, $^{\#\#\#}p < 0.001$ compared with control or AIE group at P57, respectively. The data were expressed as the numbers of BrdU+ **(A)** or Ki67+IR **(B)** positive cells, each point is mean ± SEM per mm^2 (n = 7~8/group). Middle panels: BrdU+ and Ki67+IR expression in the granular cell layer of the hippocampal DG at P95 (Immunohistochemical staining, Bar scale = 100 μm). Right panels: photomicrographs of confocal images in the granular cell layer of hippocampal DG, Ki67+ (green) and BrdU+ (red), Bar scale = 15 μm.

the maturational decline appeared to be accelerated in AIE (BrdU: 70.4 ± 5.0%, $p < 0.001$, Ki67: 63.3 ± 3.1%, $p < 0.001$) treated animals since at P95. AIE exposure decreased BrdU+ (46.8 ± 9.0%, $p < 0.01$, **Figure 1A**) and Ki67+IR (46.0 ± 4.6%, $p < 0.001$, **Figure 1B**) in the DG compared to control P95. For Ki67+IR study, two-way ANOVA showed that there was a main significant effect of group [$F_{(1,27)} = 10.59$, $p < 0.01$]. These findings suggest AIE exposure alters the maturation of proliferating NPCs in the DG.

To assess milestones of neurogenesis stages, we determined SOX2 and Tbr2 that mark NPCs of radial glial-like (Type-1) and intermediate progenitor cells (Type-2). Interestingly, both SOX2+ (**Figure 2**) and Tbr2+IR (**Figure 3**) show significant AIE-induced changes on P57 that are resolved by P95. AIE exposure significantly reduced SOX2+IR expression at P57 (16.9 ± 4.6%, $p < 0.05$, **Figure 2**), but not at P95. Both control and AIE group showed the maturational decline between P57 and P95 with SOX2+IR expression (control: 27.9 ± 3.4%, $p < 0.001$; AIE: 13.4 ± 1.9%, $p < 0.01$). Two-way ANOVA indicated that there was a main significant effect of group [$F_{(1,27)} = 5.14$, $p < 0.05$], age [$F_{(1,27)} = 35.99$, $p < 0.001$] and group × age interaction [$F_{(1,27)} = 4.87$, $p < 0.05$] on SOX2+IR. However, the maturational decline in AIE group was less than in control ($p < 0.01$, from P57 to P95). We determined both Tbr2+IR expression and cellular cluster size. AIE exposure significantly reduced Tbr2+IR expression

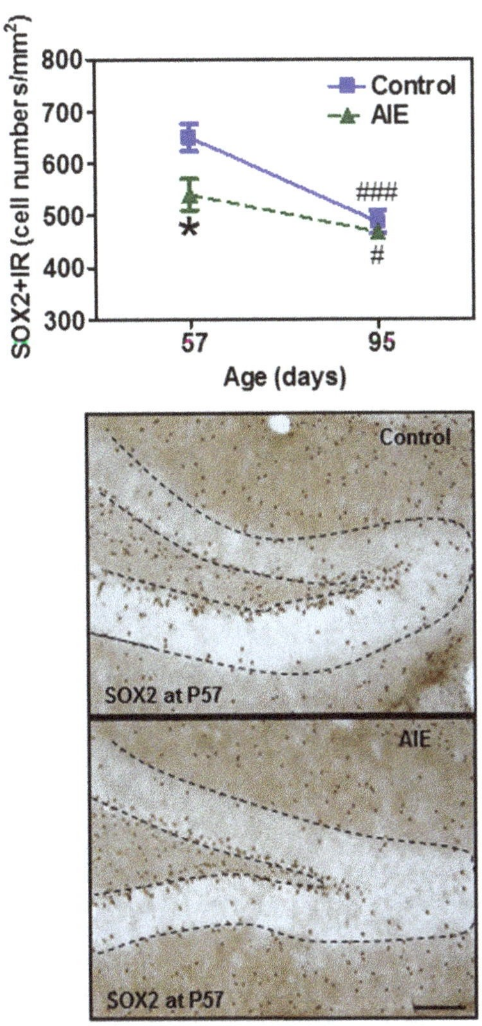

FIGURE 2 | Effects of AIE (5 g/kg, i.g., 2 days on/2 days off) exposure on SOX2+IR expression in the hippocampal DG of male rat brain at P57 and P95. Figure on the top: AIE exposure remarkably decreased SOX2+IR (17%) expression at P57, but not at P95. $^{*}p < 0.05$ compared with control group. SOX2+IR expression had the maturational decline in both control (28%) and AIE group (13%) from P57 to P95. $^{\#}p < 0.05$, $^{\#\#\#}p < 0.001$ compared with control or AIE group at P57, respectively. The data were expressed as the numbers of SOX2+IR positive cells, each point is mean ± SEM per mm^2 (n = 7~8/group). Below panels: SOX2+IR expression in the granular cell layer of the hippocampal DG at P57 (Immunohistochemical staining, Bar scale = 50 μm).

(33.5 ± 4.9%, $p < 0.01$, **Figure 3A**) on P57, but not at P95. There was maturational decline of Tbr2+IR expression in control (62.5 ± 3.0%, $p < 0.001$) and AIE (58.5 ± 6.0%, $p < 0.001$). Two-way ANOVA indicated that there was a main significant effect of group [$F_{(1,27)} = 23.72$, $p < 0.01$], age [$F_{(1,27)} = 129.95$, $p < 0.0001$), and group × age interaction [$F_{(1,27)} = 7.04$, $p < 0.05$] on Tbr2+IR (**Figure 3**). Determination of mean cluster size of Tbr2+IR cells in the AIE animals (2.8 ± 0.2 cell numbers/cluster) were significantly smaller than controls (3.5 ± 0.2 cell numbers/cluster) at P57 ($p < 0.05$),

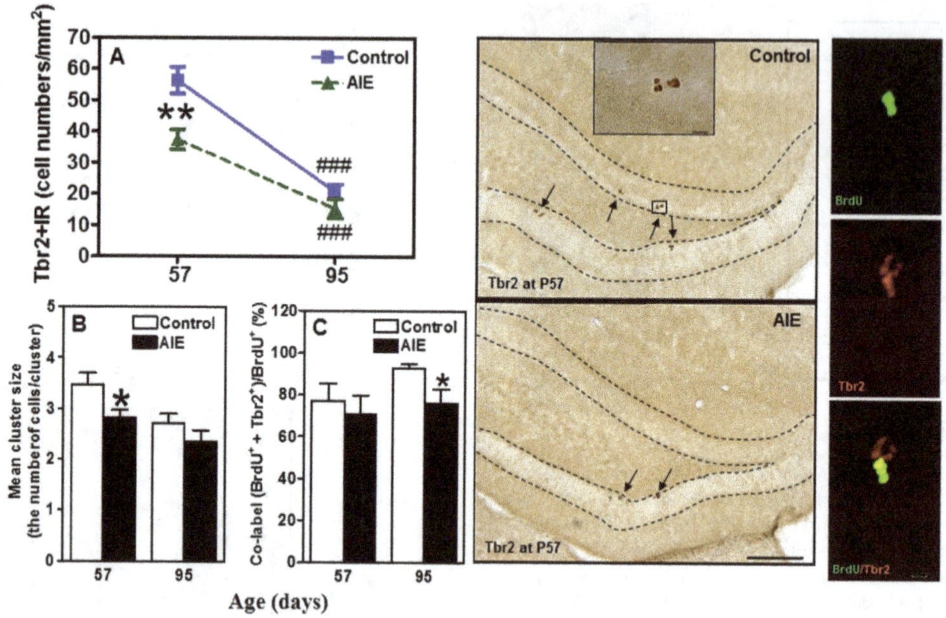

FIGURE 3 | Effects of AIE (5 g/kg, i.g., 2 days on/2 days off) exposure on Tbr2+IR expression in the hippocampal DG of male rat brain at P57 and P95. **(A)** AIE exposure remarkably decreased 34% Tbr2+IR expression at P57, but not at P95. $^{**}p < 0.01$ compared with control group. Tbr2+IR expression had the maturational decline in both control (63%) and AIE group (59%) from P57 to P95. $^{\#\#\#}p < 0.001$ compared with control or AIE group at P57, respectively. The data were expressed as the numbers of Tbr2+IR positive cells, each point is mean ± SEM per mm^2 (n = 7~8/group). **(B)** Tbr2+IR cell clusters and cell numbers per cluster were counted in the granular cell layer of the DG of control and AIE group at P57 and P95, and mean cell numbers per cluster were used. The mean cluster size of AIE group were significantly smaller than control group at P57 ($^{*}p < 0.05$). **(C)** AIE exposure resulted in a reduction of co-localization of Tbr2/BrdU+ cells in BrdU+ cells compared with control group ($^{*}p < 0.05$) at P95. Middle panels: Tbr2+IR expression in the granular cell layer of the hippocampal DG at P57 (Immunohistochemical staining, Bar scale = 100 μm, inset 10 μm). Right panels: photomicrographs of confocal images in the granular cell layer of the hippocampal DG, BrdU+ (green) and Tbr2+ (red), Bar scale = 10 μm.

however, they were not different on P95 (Control 2.7 ± 0.2 vs. AIE 2.4 ± 0.2 cell numbers/cluster, **Figure 3B**). Tbr2+/BrdU+ co-localization in controls was 77.3 ± 8.2% on P57 and 92.6 ± 2.2% on P95, with AIE animals having slightly fewer co-localized cells compared to control group at P95 (18.7 ± 5.8%, $p < 0.05$). Tbr2+/BrdU+ co-localization in AIE group was 70.9 ± 8.9% on P57 and 76.1 ± 6.0% on P95 (**Figure 3C**). These results suggest that AIE exposure reduces P57 radial glia-like and intermediate neuronal progenitor cells altering maturation of hippocampal DG.

To determine immature neuron formation, we used DCX and Prox1 markers as well as the mature GABAergic marker PV. All three markers decreased with age between P57 and P95 in the control group, DCX+ (48.6 ± 3.9%, $p < 0.001$, **Figure 4A**), Prox1+ (32.9 ± 5.0%, $p < 0.001$, **Figure 4B**) and PV+IR (28.7 ± 5.9%, $p < 0.05$, **Figure 4C**) consistent with the maturational decline in DG neurogenesis. AIE exposure resulted in a reduction with Prox1+ (15.3 ± 4.8%, $p < 0.05$) and PV+IR expression (26.8 ± 6.0%, $p < 0.05$), and had a reductive trend in DCX+IR (t = 2.069, p = 0.059) compared with P57 controls. At P95, AIE exposure reduced DCX+ (29.1 ± 5.1%, $p < 0.01$) and PV+IR (28.2 ± 5.1%, $p < 0.05$), but not Prox1+IR (**Figure 4**). These findings indicate a persistent loss of DCX+IR immature neurons and PV GABAergic neurons in adults following AIE exposure.

Survival and Differentiation of NPCs in Hippocampal Dentate Gyrus after AIE Exposure

To investigate the survival and differentiation of neurogenesis, BrdU was injected daily for 14 days to label dividing NPCs (P54-P68) and rats sacrificed weeks later allowing BrdU+ NPCs to mature. Surprisingly, we found that AIE exposure remarkably increased BrdU+IR expression 42.11 ± 6.92% [$F_{(1,16)}$ = 21.40, $p < 0.001$, **Figure 5A**]. Co-localization studies indicated that BrdU+ co-labeled with mature neuronal marker NeuN+ was 80.1 ± 1.1% in controls that was lower in the AIE group (74.4 ± 1.3%, $p < 0.05$, **Figure 5C**), suggesting slightly fewer neurons after AIE exposure. Interestingly, a small percentage of BrdU+ cells positive for microglial Iba1+ was increased by AIE from a control level of 1.5 ± 0.6% to 3.7 ± 0.3%, ($p < 0.01$) in AIE treated rats (**Figure 5B**). These findings suggest an altered differentiation of NPCs in hippocampal DG following AIE exposure.

AIE Exposure Increases β-2 Microglobulin and Activated Caspase-3 Expression in the Hippocampal Dentate Gyrus

To investigate mechanisms, we assessed immune signaling with β-2 microglobulin (β2M) and cell death using activated caspase-3

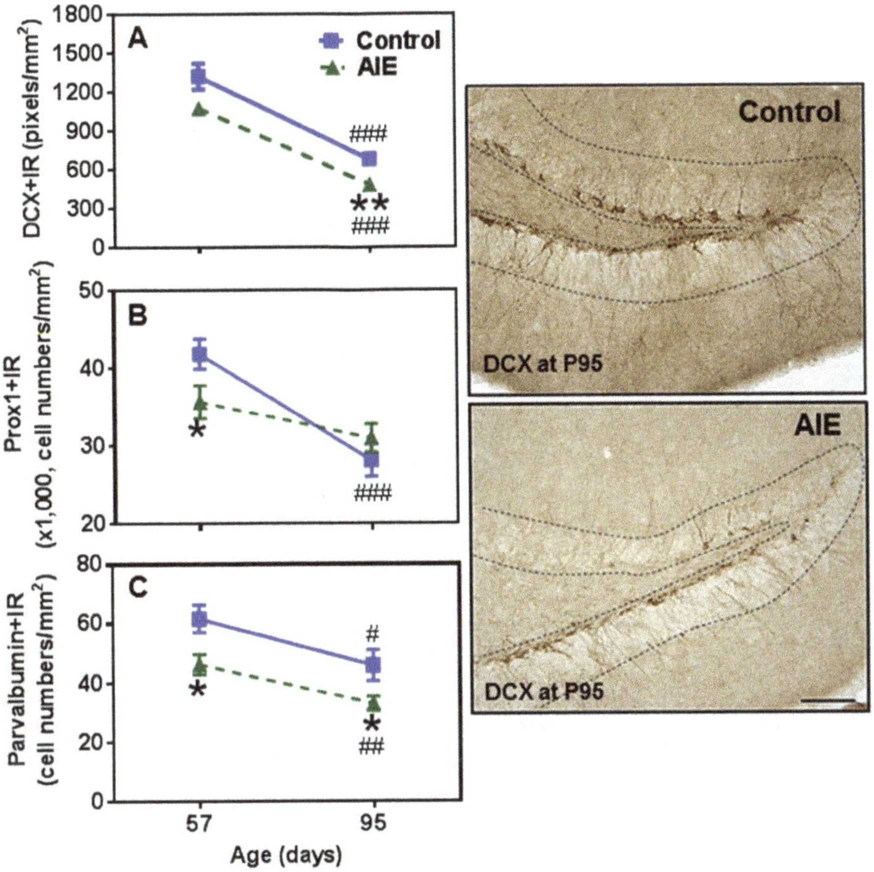

FIGURE 4 | Effects of AIE (5 g/kg, i.g., 2 days on/2 days off) exposure on DCX+ **(A)** Prox1+ **(B)** and parvalbumin (PV)+IR **(C)** expression in the hippocampal DG of male rat brain at P57 and P95. AIE exposure remarkably reduced Prox1+ (**B**, 15%) and PV+IR (**C**, 27%) expression at P57 compared with control group, and reduced DCX+ (**A**, 29%) and PV+IR (**C**, 28%) expression at P95. $^{*}p < 0.05$, $^{**}p < 0.01$ compared with control group. There was a significantly maturational decline with DCX+ (**A**, control: 49%; AIE: 56%), Prox1+ (**B**, control: 33%) or PV+IR (**C**, control: 29%; AIE: 29%) expression in control or AIE group. $^{\#}p < 0.05$, $^{\#\#}p < 0.01$, $^{\#\#\#}p < 0.001$ compared with control or AIE group at P57, respectively. The data were expressed as pixels of DCX+ **(A)** or the numbers of Prox1+ **(B)** or PV+IR **(C)** positive cells, each point is mean ± SEM per mm^2 (n = 7~8/group). Right panels: DCX+IR expression in the granular cell layer of the hippocampal DG (Immunohistochemical staining, Bar scale = 50 μm).

(as cleaved caspase-3). β2M is a major histocompatability complex 1 (MHC1) protein that is expressed on microglia and neurons, is involved in synaptic stripping and is known to inhibit hippocampal neurogenesis (Smith et al., 2015; Yousef et al., 2015). Caspase-3 is a protease which is activated during cell death, particularly apoptosis, and an antibody recognizes the active protease providing a marker of dying cells. Previous studies have found that injection of β2M into young adult mice results in loss of DG Tbr2+ and DCX+ NPCs (Smith et al., 2015), similar to our finding in young adults following AIE exposure. We found that AIE exposure did not alter DG β2M+IR expression at P57, whereas AIE-treated animals had about double the number of cells expressing β2M+IR at P95 (**Figure 6**). AIE-treated animals showed maturational increase expression from P57 to P95 (46.6 ± 11.6%, $p < 0.05$), not in control group. Two-way ANOVA of β2M+IR cells showed that there was a main effect of group [$F_{(1,27)} = 13.27$, $p < 0.001$] and age [$F_{(1,27)} = 6.82$, $p < 0.05$], but a trend effect of group × age interaction [$F_{(1,27)} = 3.59$, $p = 0.069$]. Interestingly, activated caspase-3+IR expression was slightly increased by AIE at P57 (26.7 ± 8.7%, $p < 0.05$). Maturation of controls to P95 slightly increased activated caspase-3+IR, but the increase of AIE group at P95 was about double the level of controls (**Figure 7**), e.g., increases between P57 and P95 for controls is 15.5 ± 4.4%, ($p < 0.05$) compared with AIE increases of 29.2 ± 7.0%, ($p < 0.05$). At P95, activated caspase-3+IR in DG after AIE exposure was increased 41.2 ± 8.5%, ($p < 0.01$) compared with controls (**Figure 7**). Two-way ANOVA of activated caspase-3+IR cells indicated that there was a main effect of group [$F_{(1,28)} = 16.88$, $p < 0.0001$] and age [$F_{(1,28)} = 8.54$, $p < 0.01$], but no effect of group × age interaction [$F_{(1,28)} = 1.29$, $p = 0.266$]. Interestingly, the AIE-induced increase in activated caspase-3+IR positively correlated with the AIE-induced reduction of Ki67+IR at P57 [$F_{(1,5)} = 11.5$, $r = 0.83$, $p = 0.020$], consistent with increased cell death reducing proliferating NPCs (**Table 2**). Similarly, in

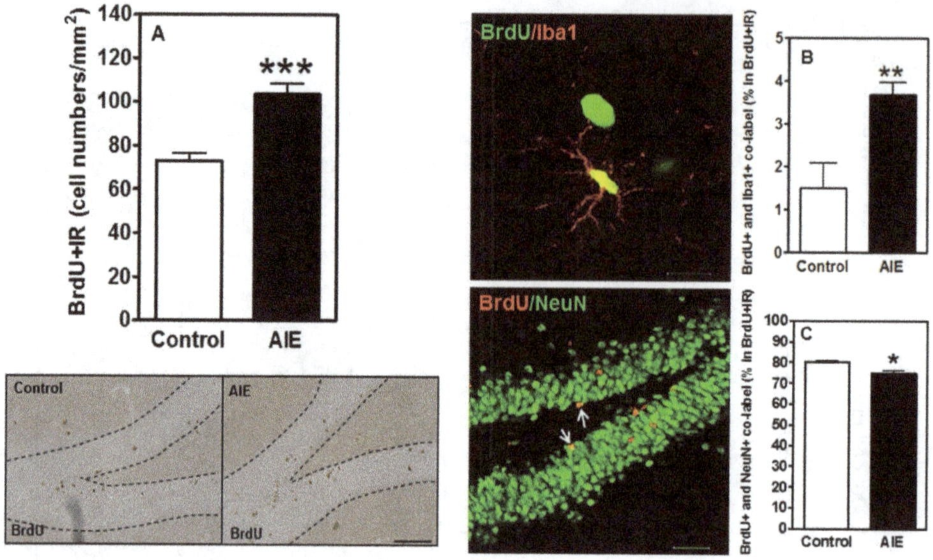

FIGURE 5 | Effects of AIE (5 g/kg, i.g., 2 days on/2 days off) exposure on survival BrdU+IR expression after abstinence in the hippocampal DG of male rat brain at P95. **(A)** BrdU+IR expression was measured after 6 weeks of abstinence, 4 weeks following labeling with BrdU (150 mg/kg, i.p. 14 days). AIE exposure significantly increased BrdU+IR expression in the DG **(A)** $^{***}p < 0.001$ compared with control group. The data were expressed as the numbers of BrdU+IR positive cells, each point is mean ± SEM per mm^2 (n = 8~10/group). Left below panels: BrdU+IR expression in the granular cell layer of the hippocampal DG (Immunohistochemical staining, Bar scale = 50 μm). Middle panels show photomicrographs of confocal images in the granular cell layer of the hippocampal DG, top one: BrdU+ (green) and Iba1+ (red) (Bar scale = 15 μm), and bottom one: BrdU+ (red) and NeuN+ (green) (Bar scale = 50 μm). **(B)** A small percentage of BrdU+ cells were positive Iba1+ 1.5% in control vs. 3.7% in AIE ($^{**}p < 0.01$). **(C)** 74% BrdU+ co-labeled with NeuN+ in AIE was less than in control group (80%, $^{*}p < 0.05$).

adulthood at P95 the AIE-induced increase in activated caspase-3+IR positively correlated with the AIE-induced reduction DCX+IR [$F_{(1,6)} = 8.3$, $r = 0.76$, $p = 0.028$] and Prox1+IR [$F_{(1,6)} = 7.5$, $r = 0.75$, $p = 0.034$], consistent with AIE-induced increases in cell death contributing to loss of adult neurogenesis (**Table 2**). Thus, DG cell death and expression of β2M+IR is increased by AIE exposure and appears to contribute to the loss of both proliferating NPCs and maturing neuron loss in adulthood.

Subventricular Zone Neurogenesis and AIE Exposure

SVZ and hippocampal DG differ in adult neuroprogenitors and neurogenesis. SOX2+ and Mash1+IR mark SVZ early progenitors, and both showed a maturational decline between P57 and P95 (**Figure 8**). SOX2+IR did not differ between groups at P57, but the maturational decline in controls was 24.5 ± 4.5% ($p < 0.05$) compared to the AIE decline of 41.1 ± 3.2% ($p < 0.001$) that resulted in reduced expression of SOX2+IR at P95 (18.3 ± 4.1%, $p < 0.05$, **Figure 8A**). Two-way ANOVA revealed that there was a main effect of age [$F_{(1,26)} = 33.92$, $p < 0.0001$], without effect of group [$F_{(1,26)} = 0.37$, $p = 0.549$], group × age interaction [$F_{(1,26)} = 3.05$, $p = 0.092$] on SOX2+IR. Similarly, Mash1+IR was not significantly decreased by AIE at P57, but by P95 AIE exposure decreased Mash1+IR to 59.2 ± 6.3% ($p < 0.05$, **Figure 8B**) of control. Two-way ANOVA showed that there was a significant effect of age [$F_{(1,27)} = 6.02$, $p < 0.05$], group [$F_{(1,27)} = 8.81$, $p < 0.01$], without effect of group × age interaction [$F_{(1,27)} = 0.79$, $p = 0.382$] on Mash1+IR.

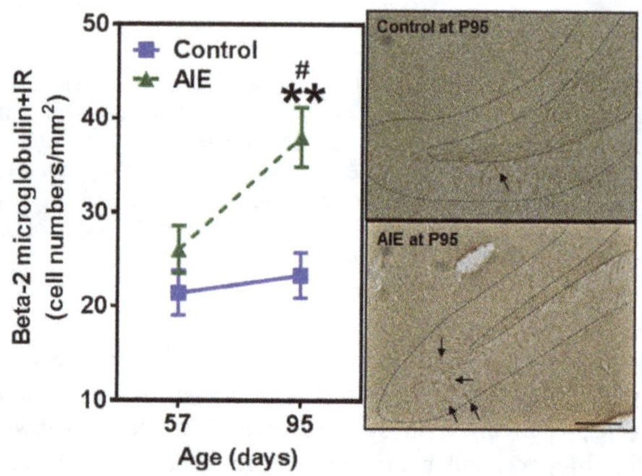

FIGURE 6 | Effects of AIE (5 g/kg, i.g., 2 days on/2 days off) exposure on β2M+IR expression in the hippocampal DG of male rat brain at P57 and P95. Figure on the left: AIE exposure remarkably increased β2M+IR expression (63%) compared with control group at P95. $^{**}p < 0.01$ compared with control group. β2M+IR expression had a significantly maturational increase in AIE group (47%). $^{\#}p < 0.05$ compared with AIE group at P57. The data were expressed as the numbers of β2M+IR positive cells, each point is mean ± SEM per mm^2 (n = 7~8/group). Right panels: β2M+IR expression in the granular cell layer of the hippocampal DG (Immunohistochemical staining, Bar scale = 50 μm).

Interestingly, no correlation of SVZ markers was found at P57 in either controls or AIE exposure animals (**Table 2**). Determination of BrdU+IR 2 h. after injection (S-phase marker

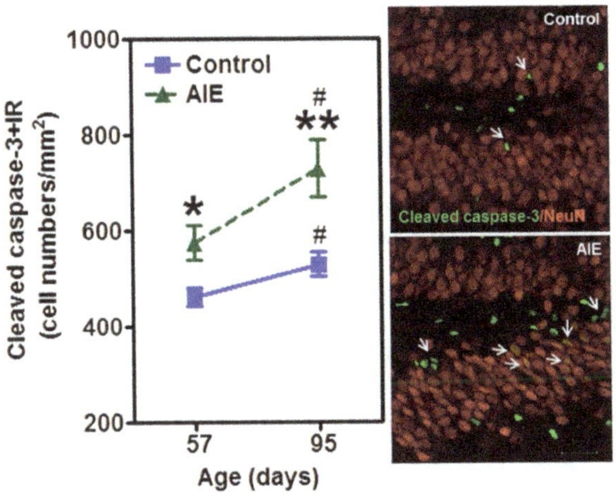

FIGURE 7 | Effects of AIE (5 g/kg, i.g., 2 days on/2 days off) exposure on activated caspase-3+IR expression in the hippocampal DG of male rat brain at P57 and P95. Figure on the left: AIE exposure remarkably increased the apoptosis marker activated caspase-3+IR from P57 (27%) to P95 (41%) compared with control group. $^{*}p < 0.05$, $^{**}p < 0.01$ compared with control group. Activated caspase-3+IR expression had a significantly maturational increase in control (16%) and AIE group (29%). $^{\#}p < 0.05$ compared with control or AIE group at P57, respectively. The data were expressed as the numbers of activated caspase-3+IR positive cells, each point is mean ± SEM per mm^2 (n = 8/group). Right panels: photomicrographs of confocal images in the granular cell layer of the hippocampal DG, activated caspased-3+ (green) and NeuN+ (red), Bar scale = 30 μm.

of cell proliferation) did not find a change in SVZ (**Table 3**). Also nestin+IR (a marker of neural stem cell, type B) expression in the SVZ at P57 and P95 were not altered by AIE exposure (**Table 3**). These finding suggest SVZ neurogenesis does not show immediate changes following AIE exposure, but following maturation to adulthood at P95 led to an AIE induced loss of early progenitor markers Mash1 and SOX2 in the SVZ.

To further investigate SVZ neurogenesis, we determined neuroprogenitor markers Dlx2+IR and DCX+IR as well as NPC survival using BrdU+IR. Similar to the other SVZ markers studied, AIE exposure did not markedly alter neurogenesis markers at P57, just after AIE exposure, but after maturation to P95 AIE exposure was found to significantly reduce Dlx2+IR (12.7 ± 4.9% $p < 0.05$) and DCX+IR (19.6 ± 5.8%, $p < 0.05$) expression compared with controls (**Figures 9A,B**). Dlx2+IR did not show a maturational decline, but DCX+IR had maturational decline between P57 and P95 in the control (25.5 ± 5.0%, $p < 0.05$) and AIE group (32.7 ± 4.9%, $p < 0.01$) in the SVZ (**Figure 9B**), respectively. Two-way ANOVA revealed that there was a main effect of age [$F_{(1,27)} = 1.73$, $p = 0.199$], without effect of group [$F_{(1,27)} = 6.73$, $p = 0.015$] and group × age interaction [$F_{(1,27)} = 0.04$, $p = 0.853$] on Dlx2+IR. And there was a significant effect of age [$F_{(1,24)} = 20.19$, $p < 0.0001$], group [$F_{(1,24)} = 4.19$, $p = 0.05$], without effect of group × age interaction [$F_{(1,24)} = 0.19$, $p = 0.671$] on DCX+IR. The AIE-induced decrease in Dlx2+ and DCX+IR at P95 correlated across individuals (**Table 2**). SVZ progenitor survival was determined following repeated BrdU (150 mg/kg i.p.) daily injected at P54 followed by weeks of maturation to P95 as described above. We found that AIE exposure markedly decreased SVZ BrdU+IR expression 41 days after abstinence in the SVZ (20.5 ± 2.8%, $p < 0.05$). One-way ANOVA revealed that there was significant effect of group [$F_{(1,16)} = 9.25$, $p < 0.01$] (see Supplementary Figure S2). Although these findings indicate AIE exposure caused a loss of adult SVZ neurogenesis, unlike hippocampus, we did not find a change in β2M+ and activated caspase-3+IR expression in the SVZ compared with controls at P57 or P95 (**Table 3**). These findings indicate that AIE exposure alters SVZ leading to a progressive persistent loss of SVZ neurogenesis that appears to increase with age.

DISCUSSION

In this study we investigated the impact of AIE exposure, a model of human adolescent binge drinking, on hippocampal DG and SVZ neurogenesis. Neurogenesis is a dynamic self-renewal

TABLE 2 | Pearson correlations across markers in the hippocampal dentate gyrus (DG) and subventricular zone (SVZ) of male rat brain.

Markers	Markers in the DG			Markers in the SVZ	
	Ki67	DCX	Prox1	SOX2	Dlx2
BrdU	-	$F_{(1,5)} = 11.2$, $r = 0.83$ $p = 0.020$ (AIE, P57)	-	-	$F_{(1,5)} = 9.9$, $r = 0.82$ $p = 0.025$ (Control, P95)
	-	$F_{(1,6)} = 10.0$, $r = 0.79$ $p = 0.020$ (AIE, P95)	-	-	-
SOX2	$F_{(1,5)} = 13.3$, $r = 0.85$ $p = 0.015$ (AIE, P57)	-	-	N/A	-
DCX	-	N/A	-	-	$F_{(1,6)} = 6.9$, $r = 0.73$ $p = 0.04$ (AIE, P95)
Activated caspase-3	$F_{(1,5)} = 11.5$, $r = 0.83$, $p = 0.020$ (AIE, P57)	-	-	$F_{(1,6)} = 14.9$, $r = 0.85$ $p = 0.008$ (AIE, P95)	-
	-	$F_{(1,6)} = 8.3$, $r = 0.76$ $p = 0.028$ (AIE, P95)	$F_{(1,6)} = 7.5$, $r = 0.75$ $p = 0.034$ (AIE, P95)	-	-

AIE (5 g/kg, i.g., 2 days on/2 days off) group at P57 and P95 with significant F, r and p values. Only correlation of $p < 0.05$, $p < 0.01$ are shown. (-), no any correlation.

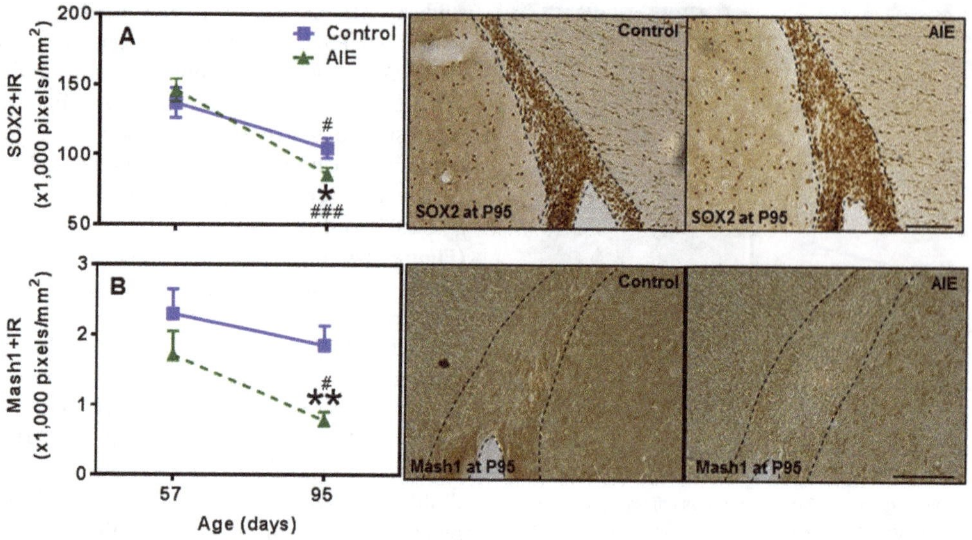

FIGURE 8 | Effects of AIE (5 g/kg, i.g., 2 days on/2 days off) exposure on SOX2+ and Mash1+IR expression in the subventricular zone (SVZ) of male rat brain at P57 and P95. AIE exposure remarkably decreased SOX2+ (18%, **A**) and Mash1+IR (59%, **B**) at P95 compared with control group. $^{*}p < 0.05$, $^{**}p < 0.01$ compared with control group. There was a significant maturational decline with SOX2+ (**A**, control: 25%; AIE: 41%), and Mash1+IR (**B**, AIE: 56%) expression in control or AIE group. $^{\#}p < 0.05$, $^{\#\#\#}p < 0.001$ compared with control or AIE group at P57, respectively. The data were expressed as pixels of SOX2+ and Mash1+IR, each point is mean ± SEM per mm² (n = 7~8/group). Right panels: SOX2+ and Mash1+IR expression in the SVZ at P95 (Immunohistochemical staining, Bar scale = 100 μm on SOX2+IR; 50 μm on Mash1+IR).

multistage process that involves the proliferation, migration, differentiation, and functional integration of new neurons into the preexisting neural circuitry that persists into adulthood in these two brain regions. We report here that AIE exposure decreases hippocampal progenitor makers SOX2+, Ki67+, Tbr2+ and BrdU+IR proliferation as well as markers of neuronal maturation, e.g., neurogenesis markers DCX+, Prox1+ and PV+IR (**Figure 10**). These finding are consistent with previous studies of hippocampal neurogenesis that AIE vapor treatment reduces adult Ki67+, DCX+ and BrdU+IR survival markers of neurogenesis in association with increased disinhibitory behavior and increased activated caspase-3+IR (Ehlers et al., 2013a). Similarly, AIE treatment with i.p injection of ethanol has been found to decrease adult hippocampal Ki67+ and DCX+IR while increasing HDAC activity and decreasing BDNF in association with increased anxiety (Sakharkar et al., 2016). Previous studies have found adolescents are more sensitive to ethanol inhibition of neurogenesis than adults (Crews et al., 2006). Studies by Nixon's group have investigated a continuous intoxication 4 day binge alcohol dependence model in adolescence and reported decreased hippocampal NPC survival 28 days after ethanol exposure, increased markers of cell death, and reduced DCX+IR, but no change in hippocampal Ki67+IR just after alcohol exposure ended (Morris et al., 2010; McClain et al., 2011) similar to our findings just after AIE exposure at P57. They have found that adolescent binge alcohol exposure inhibits neurogenesis through alterations in NPC cell cycle kinetics, especially decreasing the proportion of NPCs in S-phase. Further, the 4 day binge model found reduced SOX2+IR did not persist following adolescent alcohol exposure (McClain et al., 2011) similar to our finding of SOX2+IR returning to control levels at P95, in adulthood. Overall, all studies agree adolescent ethanol exposure inhibits hippocampal neurogenesis through multiple mechanisms including increases in cell death. Recent studies have found that the AIE-induced persistent loss of neurogenesis that is not found following identical treatment in adults (Broadwater et al., 2014). The AIE studies presented here add maturational changes and new

TABLE 3 | Adolescent intermittent ethanol (AIE, 5 g/kg, i.g., 2 days on/2 days off) exposure did not impact the expression of BrdU+ (2 h after single injection), nestin+, β-2 microglobulin+ and activated caspase-3+IR expression in the SVZ of male rat brain at P57 and P95.

Age (day)	Group	BrdU + IR (2 h) (cell number × 1000/mm²)	Nestin + IR (cell number × 1000/mm²)	β-2 microglobulin + IR (cell number × 1000/mm²)	Activated caspase-3 + IR (cell number × 1000/mm²)
57	Control	1.90 ± 0.11	23.87 ± 1.12	2.81 ± 0.50	6.68 ± 0.41
	AIE	2.04 ± 0.13	22.24 ± 0.57	2.63 ± 0.27	6.36 ± 0.28
95	Control	1.95 ± 0.13	23.58 ± 0.72	4.01 ± 0.37	6.61 ± 0.38
	AIE	1.80 ± 0.16	23.33 ± 0.76	4.47 ± 0.034##	6.63 ± 0.33

$^{\#\#}p < 0.01$, compared to AIE group at P57.

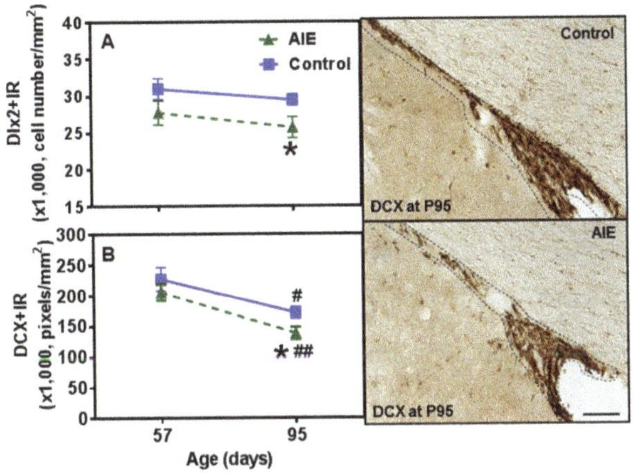

FIGURE 9 | Effects of AIE (5 g/kg, i.g., 2 days on/2 days off) exposure on Dlx2+ and DCX+IR expression in the SVZ of male rat brain at P57 and P95. Figure on the left: AIE remarkably decreased Dlx2+ (13%, **A**) and DCX+IR (20%, **B**) at P95 compared with control group. *$p < 0.05$ compared with control group. There was a significant maturational decline of DCX+IR (control: 26%; AIE: 33%) in control and AIE group. #$p < 0.05$, ##$p < 0.01$ compared with control or AIE group at P57, respectively. The data were expressed as the cell numbers of Dlx2+IR, and pixels of DCX+IR, each point is mean ± SEM per mm^2 ($n = 7{\sim}8$/group). Right panels: DCX+IR expression in the SVZ at P95 (Immunohistochemical staining, Bar scale = 100 μm).

progenitor stage specific markers (Lindsey and Tropepe, 2006; Kempermann et al., 2015). Assessment of NPC proliferation markers in hippocampal DG, e.g., Ki67+ and BrdU+IR at 2 h, indicates AIE exposure accelerate the maturational declines in NPC proliferation between P57, late adolescence, and young adulthood (P95). In contrast, early neuroprogenitor transcription factor markers of radial-glial and intermediate neuronal progenitors, e.g., SOX-2+ and Tbr2+IR, respectively, are decreased after AIE exposure (P57), but decline less during abstinent maturation to P95, consistent with AIE exposure insulting early progenitors that are maturing. Conditional null mutant Sox2 mice have reduced neurogenesis, stem/precursor cells and a smaller hippocampus in adulthood consistent with Sox2 and neurogenesis being required for normal hippocampal maturation (Favaro et al., 2009). Similarly, previous studies indicate Tbr2 is a transcription factor uniquely expressed in DG NPCs that regulates progenitor cell fate in adult DG that is lost as neurons mature (Hodge et al., 2008, 2012). Proxl is also a marker of the type-2 intermediate progenitors (Tbr2+ cells) in the DG (Urbán and Guillemot, 2014). AIE exposure resulted in the reduction of SOX2+, Tbr2+ and Proxl+IR expression in the DG at P57, suggesting that AIE-reduced radial glia and intermediate progenitor cells mainly happened after last ethanol exposure, but not on 41 days after abstinence in the hippocampal DG. Although AIE exposure causes an overall reduction in adult neurogenesis, the pools of SOX2+, Tbr2+ and Proxl+IR cells return to control levels in young adulthood (P95). Co-localized Tbr2+ and BrdU+ staining was reduced at P95 following AIE exposure consistent with fewer NPCs in S phase of cell cycle and a reduced rate of NPC proliferation and/or increased cell death. A reduced rate of progenitor proliferation is consistent with the reduced Ki67+ and BrdU+IR at 2 h, found after AIE exposure at P95. Further, we find AIE exposure increased activated caspase-3+IR cells at P57 that was further increased at P95. We also find increased activated caspase-3+IR at P57 correlates with decreased Ki67+IR in hippocampus DG consistent with increased cell death in early progenitors just after AIE exposure. In AIE exposed young adults at P95, activated caspase-3+IR cells only correlate with DCX+ cells suggesting increased cell death is an important mechanism contributing to the persistent loss of neurogenesis following AIE.

The mechanisms of persistent loss of neurogenesis following AIE exposure may be related to increased expression of proinflammatory cytokines and other innate immune signaling molecules. Previous studies have found that AIE exposure induces multiple proinflammatory cytokines, Toll-like receptors (TLRs) and RAGE, as well as HMGB1 an agonist at these immune receptors (Vetreno and Crews, 2012, 2014; Vetreno et al., 2013), that persists after AIE exposure and increases during maturation to young adulthood (Vetreno and Crews, 2012). Similarly, another study found that AIE exposure reduced adult hippocampal neurogenesis is associated with increases in adult hippocampal expression of the proinflammatory cytokines TNFα and MCP1 as well as the protease MMP9 and innate immune transcription factor NFκB (Vetreno and Crews, 2014). Further, this study found that treatment with lipopolysaccharide, a TLR4 agonist known to induce brain cytokines (Qin et al., 2007), reduces adult hippocampal neurogenesis (Vetreno and Crews, 2014). Another related finding is that AIE exposure reduces hippocampal BDNF expression (Sakharkar et al., 2016) suggesting loss of trophic support with increased neuroimmune gene expression after AIE exposure. β2M is a MHC1 protein that is expressed on monocytes and other cells as well as on brain microglia and neurons, where it is involved in synaptic stripping and is known to inhibit hippocampal neurogenesis (Smith et al., 2015; Yousef et al., 2015). In the current study, we found a marked increase in β2M+IR cells at P95, but not just after AIE exposure at P57, suggesting a progressive induction in expression of neuroimmune signaling β2M+IR cells. Proinflammatory cytokines (Fan and Pang, 2017) and TLRs (Rolls et al., 2007) can inhibit neurogenesis through increased progenitor death and/or increased differentiation to glia. Interestingly, β2M+IR expression similar to the receptor RAGE+IR (Vetreno and Crews, 2012; Vetreno et al., 2013) is not induced just after AIE treatment, but is triggered by AIE exposure and induced during maturation to young adulthood. Our study focused on adolescent maturation to adulthood and found increased β2M+IR expression and the greatest reductions in neurogenesis in young adulthood. Previous studies have reported that age-related increases in the DG β2M cause the age-related loss of neurogenesis during senescence (Smith et al., 2015; Yousef et al., 2015). Our findings are consistent with AIE-induced β2M+IR reflecting a progressive increase in neuroimmune signaling that reduces neurogenesis through increased cell death of hippocampal neuroprogenitors.

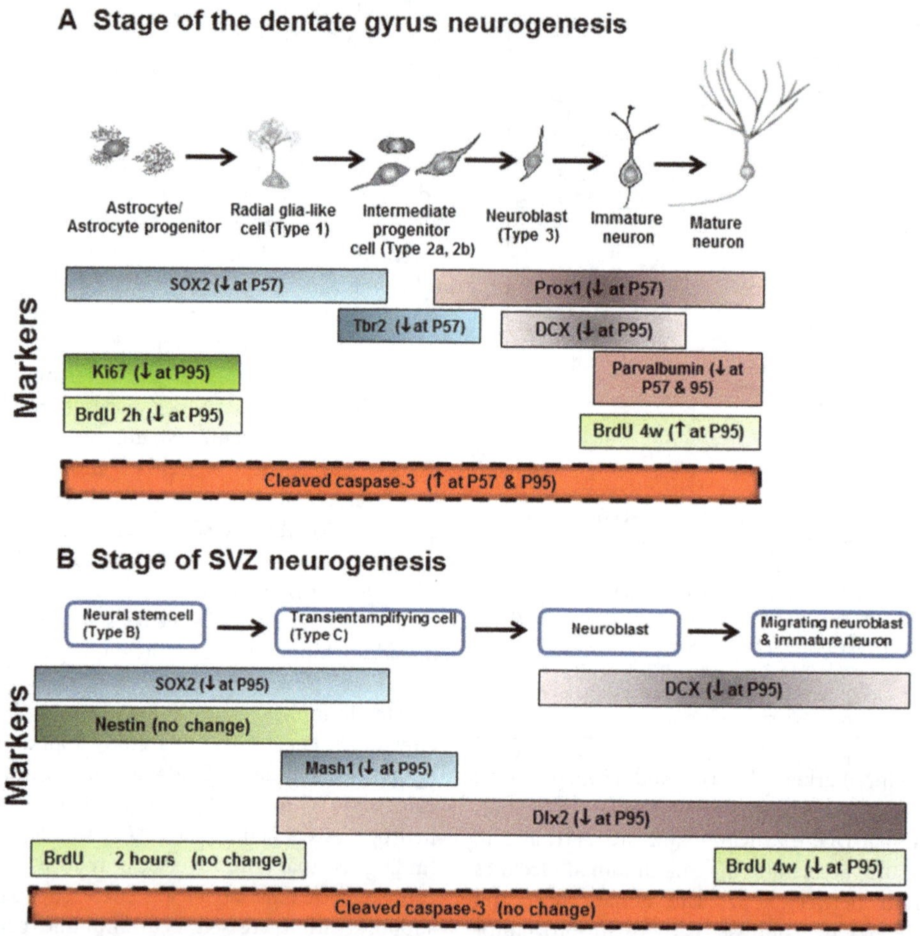

FIGURE 10 | Neurogenesis stages in the DG of the adult hippocampus and SVZ of lateral ventricle. **(A)** Schematic diagram representing the progression of neuronal development (Bonaguidi et al., 2012), and specific markers in the different developmental stages of the adult DG, such SOX2, Tbr2, Prox1, DCX and PV. Ki67 protein is present during all active phases of the cell cycle (G_1, S, G_2, and mitosis), but is absent from resting cells (G_0). Bromodeoxyuridine (BrdU), used in the detection of proliferating cells in living tissues as exogenous marker, is incorporated into the newly synthesized DNA of replicating cells (during the S phase of the cell cycle). For the proliferation study, animals were sacrificed 2 h after injecting BrdU with 300 mg/kg (i.p.). For the survival study, animals were sacrificed 4 weeks after injecting BrdU with 150 mg/kg (i.p.) for 14 days. **(B)** Schematic diagram representing the progression of neuronal development, and specific markers in the different developmental stages of the adult SVZ, such as SOX2, nestin, Mash1, DCX and Dlx2. ↓ at P57, decreased at postnatal day 57; ↓ at P95, decreased at postnatal day 95; ↑ at P57, increased at postnatal days 57; ↑ at P95, increased at postnatal days 95.

In the present study, we add new data on the impact of AIE on SVZ neurogenesis (**Figure 10**). SVZ NPCs are different from hippocampal NPCs (Kriegstein and Alvarez-Buylla, 2009; Ming and Song, 2011). In the adult mammalian brain, new neurons are generated in the SVZ and migrate through the white matter into the neocortex (Gould et al., 1999). Neurogenesis in adult SVZ is found along the walls of the lateral ventricles and has stages of adult SVZ neurogenesis that differ from DG (Ming and Song, 2005). Proliferating radial glia-like SOX2+ cells (type B cells), give rise to transient amplifying neuroblasts and immature Mash1+ neuroprogenitors (type C cells) that migrate through the rostral migratory stream (RMS). Hansson et al. (2010) in an adult rat 7 weeks chronic relapsing alcoholic model found that DCX+IR and SOX2+IR in the SVZ was reduced just after treatment and the reduced SVZ neurogenesis persisted for 21 days of abstinence. Other studies in adult mice have reported weeks of ethanol self-administration reduce SVZ BrdU+ cells (Campbell et al., 2014). We previously found that acute ethanol dose-dependently decreased cell proliferation in the SVZ of adolescent rats (Crews et al., 2006). A previous AIE exposure study in Sprague-Dawley rats that were sacrificed on P74, 26 days after the last ethanol exposure, found decreased hippocampal and SVZ neurogenesis with age, similar to that reported here, as well as the persistent loss in adulthood, although in SVZ the AIE reduction was not statistically significant at P74 (Broadwater et al., 2014), consistent with our finding of the AIE reduced SVZ neurogenesis increasing with age and being significant at P95. We studied AIE-treated rats 41 days after the last AIE exposure and found a significant, persistent loss of adult neurogenesis as indicated by decreased SOX2+, Mash1+, DCX+ and Dlx2+ cells in the SVZ. This is consistent with an emerging loss of SVZ neurogenesis during age-related maturation that requires time, e.g., at P95 we report here a significant loss of SVZ neurogenesis, but our studies reported here at P57 and Broadwater et al. (2014) at P74 found no change or a trend, respectively. Taken together, these studies suggest AIE exposure causes a progressive persistent change in the neurogenic niche of SVZ that weeks after AIE exposure ends reduces SOX2+ neural stem cells, Mash1+ progenitors, Dlx2+ neuroblasts and DCX+ immature neurons. These decreases in SVZ occur without an increase in activated caspase-3+ cells suggesting increased cell death is not a major contributor to the persistent loss of SVZ neurogenesis like it is in hippocampus DG. The AIE exposure induced loss of neurogenesis appears to be related to a progressive loss of SVZ neuroprogenitors. Mash1 is also known as achaete-scute homolog 1 (ASCL1) and is a transcription factor associated with stem cells neuronal differentiation commitment and Dlx2 is a neuroprogenitor-immature neuron transcription factor that are both decreased in young adults after AIE exposure consistent with a loss of early stem cells as well as differentiating progenitors. DCX marks immature neurons and BrdU (4 weeks) assesses neurogenesis. AIE exposure reduced both DCX+ and BrdU+IR (4 weeks) assessments indicating loss of neurogenesis. Thus, together these findings suggest AIE exposure leads to a persistent and growing loss of SVZ neuroprogenitors and neurogenesis.

Although our study did not investigate AIE-induced changes in behavior, loss of neurogenesis may contribute to AIE exposure induced behavior changes in adults. AIE exposure has been found to reduce adult cognitive flexibility and increase negative affect-anxiety (Crews et al., 2016). Loss of hippocampal neurogenesis has been proposed to reduce cognitive flexibility (Anacker and Hen, 2017) and to be associated with stress-induced depression-like behavior and the ability of anti-depressants to reverse depression. In addition, AIE-induced loss of neurogenesis has been found to correlate with loss of hippocampal volume (Ehlers et al., 2013b), a finding that mimics the reduced hippocampal volume found in human alcoholics and depressed individuals. Thus, the AIE induced loss of neurogenesis may contribute to cognitive and mood changes in adulthood that increase risks of adult psychopathology.

AUTHOR CONTRIBUTIONS

FTC and WL designed the study. WL performed the experiments and collected data. WL and FTC analyzed the data and wrote the manuscript. All authors read and approved the manuscript.

ACKNOWLEDGMENTS

We thank to the UNC-Bowles Center for Alcohol Studies for support. Authors would like to thank Ryan P. Vetreno for reviewing this manuscript.

REFERENCES

Abrous, D. N., Koehl, M., and Le Moal, M. (2005). Adult neurogenesis: from precursors to network and physiology. *Physiol. Rev.* 85, 523–569. doi: 10.1152/physrev.00055.2003

Anacker, C., and Hen, R. (2017). Adult hippocampal neurogenesis and cognitive flexibility—linking memory and mood. *Nat. Rev. Neurosci.* 18, 335–346. doi: 10.1038/nrn.2017.45

Bonaguidi, M. A., Song, J., Ming, G. L., and Song, H. (2012). A unifying hypothesis on mammalian neural stem cell properties in the adult hippocampus. *Curr. Opin. Neurobiol.* 22, 754–761. doi: 10.1016/j.conb.2012.03.013

Briones, T. L., and Woods, J. (2013). Chronic binge-like alcohol consumption in adolescence causes depression-like symptoms possibly mediated by the effects of BDNF on neurogenesis. *Neuroscience* 254, 324–334. doi: 10.1016/j.neuroscience.2013.09.031

Broadwater, M. A., Liu, W., Crews, F. T., and Spear, L. P. (2014). Persistent loss of hippocampal neurogenesis and increased cell death following adolescent, but not adult, chronic ethanol exposure. *Dev. Neurosci.* 36, 297–305. doi: 10.1159/000362874

Brown, J. P., Couillard-Despres, S., Cooper-Kuhn, C. M., Winkler, J., Aigner, L., and Kuhn, H. G. (2003). Transient expression of doublecortin during adult neurogenesis. *J. Comp. Neurol.* 467, 1–10. doi: 10.1002/cne.10874

Campbell, J. C., Stipcevic, T., Flores, R. E., Perry, C., and Kippin, T. E. (2014). Alcohol exposure inhibits adult neural stem cell proliferation. *Exp Brain Res.* 232, 2775–2784. doi: 10.1007/s00221-014-3958-1

Couillard-Despres, S., Winner, B., Schaubeck, S., Aigner, R., Vroemen, M., Weidner, N., et al. (2005). Doublecortin expression levels in adult brain reflect neurogenesis. *Eur. J. Neurosci.* 21, 1–14. doi: 10.1111/j.1460-9568.2004.03813.x

Crews, F. T., Mdzinarishvili, A., Kim, D., He, J., and Nixon, K. (2006). Neurogenesis in adolescent brain is potently inhibited by ethanol. *Neuroscience* 137, 437–445. doi: 10.1016/j.neuroscience.2005.08.090

Crews, F. T., Nixon, K., and Wilkie, M. E. (2004). Exercise reverses ethanol inhibition of neural stem cell proliferation. *Alcohol* 33, 63–71. doi: 10.1016/j.alcohol.2004.04.005

Crews, F. T., Vetreno, R. P., Broadwater, M. A., and Robinson, D. L. (2016). Adolescent alcohol exposure persistently impacts adult neurobiology and behavior. *Pharmacol. Rev.* 68, 1074–1109. doi: 10.1124/pr.115.012138

Dahl, R. E. (2004). Adolescent development and the regulation of behavior and emotion: introduction to part VIII. *Ann. N Y Acad. Sci.* 1021, 294–295. doi: 10.1196/annals.1308.034

Ehlers, C. L., Liu, W., Wills, D. N., and Crews, F. T. (2013a). Periadolescent ethanol vapor exposure persistently reduces measures of hippocampal neurogenesis that are associated with behavioral outcomes in adulthood. *Neuroscience* 244, 1–15. doi: 10.1016/j.neuroscience.2013.03.058

Ehlers, C. L., Oguz, I., Budin, F., Wills, D. N., and Crews, F. T. (2013b). Peri-adolescent ethanol vapor exposure produces reductions in hippocampal volume that are correlated with deficits in prepulse inhibition of the startle. *Alcohol. Clin. Exp. Res.* 37, 1466–1475. doi: 10.1111/acer.12125

Eriksson, P. S., Perfilieva, E., Björk-Eriksson, T., Alborn, A. M., Nordborg, C., Peterson, D. A., et al. (1998). Neurogenesis in the adult human hippocampus. *Nat. Med.* 4, 1313–1317. doi: 10.1038/3305

Ernst, A., Alkass, K., Bernard, S., Salehpour, M., Perl, S., Tisdale, J., et al. (2014). Neurogenesis in the striatum of the adult human brain. *Cell* 156, 1072–1083. doi: 10.1016/j.cell.2014.01.044

Fan, L. W., and Pang, Y. (2017). Dysregulation of neurogenesis by neuroinflammation: key differences in neurodevelopmental and neurological disorders. *Neural Regen. Res.* 12, 366–371. doi: 10.4103/1673-5374.202926

Favaro, R., Valotta, M., Ferri, A. L., Latorre, E., Mariani, J., Giachino, C., et al. (2009). Hippocampal development and neural stem cell maintenance require Sox2-dependent regulation of Shh. *Nat. Neurosci.* 12, 1248–1256. doi: 10.1038/nn.2397

Gould, E., Reeves, A. J., Graziano, M. S., and Gross, C. G. (1999). Neurogenesis in the neocortex of adult primates. *Science* 286, 548–552. doi: 10.1126/science.286.5439.548

Hansson, A. C., Nixon, K., Rimondini, R., Damadzic, R., Sommer, W. H., Eskay, R., et al. (2010). Long-term suppression of forebrain neurogenesis and loss of neuronal progenitor cells following prolonged alcohol dependence in rats. *Int. J. Neuropsychopharmacol.* 13, 583–593. doi: 10.1017/s1461145710000246

He, J., and Crews, F. T. (2007). Neurogenesis decreases during brain maturation from adolescence to adulthood. *Pharmacol. Biochem. Behav.* 86, 327–333. doi: 10.1016/j.pbb.2006.11.003

He, J., Nixon, K., Shetty, A. K., and Crews, F. T. (2005). Chronic alcohol exposure reduces hippocampal neurogenesis and dendritic growth of newborn neurons. *Eur. J. Neurosci.* 21, 2711–2720. doi: 10.1111/j.1460-9568.2005.04120.x

Herrera, D. G., Yague, A. G., Johnsen-Soriano, S., Bosch-Morell, F., Collado-Morente, L., Muriach, M., et al. (2003). Selective impairment of hippocampal neurogenesis by chronic alcoholism: protective effects of an antioxidant. *Proc. Natl. Acad. Sci. U S A* 100, 7919–7924. doi: 10.1073/pnas.1230907100

Hodge, R. D., and Hevner, R. F. (2011). Expression and actions of transcription factors in adult hippocampal neurogenesis. *Dev. Neurobiol.* 71, 680–689. doi: 10.1002/dneu.20882

Hodge, R. D., Kahoud, R. J., and Hevner, R. F. (2012). Transcriptional control of glutamatergic differentiation during adult neurogenesis. *Cell. Mol. Life Sci.* 69, 2125–2134. doi: 10.1007/s00018-011-0916-y

Hodge, R. D., Kowalczyk, T. D., Wolf, S. A., Encinas, J. M., Rippey, C., Enikolopov, G., et al. (2008). Intermediate progenitors in adult hippocampal neurogenesis: Tbr2 expression and coordinate regulation of neuronal output. *J. Neurosci.* 28, 3707–3717. doi: 10.1523/JNEUROSCI.4280-07.2008

Kempermann, G., Song, H., and Gage, F. H. (2015). Neurogenesis in the Adult Hippocampus. *Cold Spring Harb. Perspect. Biol.* 7:a018812. doi: 10.1101/cshperspect.a018812

Kempermann, G., Wiskott, L., and Gage, F. H. (2004). Functional significance of adult neurogenesis. *Curr. Opin. Neurobiol.* 14, 186–191. doi: 10.1016/j.conb.2004.03.001

Kriegstein, A., and Alvarez-Buylla, A. (2009). The glial nature of embryonic and adult neural stem cells. *Annu. Rev. Neurosci.* 32, 149–184. doi: 10.1146/annurev.neuro.051508.135600

Kuhn, H. G., Dickinson-Anson, H., and Gage, F. H. (1996). Neurogenesis in the dentate gyrus of the adult rat: age-related decrease of neuronal progenitor proliferation. *J. Neurosci.* 16, 2027–2033.

Lavado, A., Lagutin, O. V., Chow, L. M., Baker, S. J., and Oliver, G. (2010). Prox1 is required for granule cell maturation and intermediate progenitor maintenance during brain neurogenesis. *PLoS Biol.* 8:e1000460. doi: 10.1371/journal.pbio.1000460

Lavado, A., and Oliver, G. (2007). Prox1 expression patterns in the developing and adult murine brain. *Dev. Dyn.* 236, 518–524. doi: 10.1002/dvdy.21024

Lindsey, B. W., and Tropepe, V. (2006). A comparative framework for understanding the biological principles of adult neurogenesis. *Prog. Neurobiol.* 80, 281–307. doi: 10.1016/j.pneurobio.2006.11.007

Liu, W., and Crews, F. T. (2015). Adolescent intermittent ethanol exposure enhances ethanol activation of the nucleus accumbens while blunting the prefrontal cortex responses in adult rat. *Neuroscience* 293, 92–108. doi: 10.1016/j.neuroscience.2015.02.014

Lledo, P. M., Alonso, M., and Grubb, M. S. (2006). Adult neurogenesis and functional plasticity in neuronal circuits. *Nat. Rev. Neurosci.* 7, 179–193. doi: 10.1038/nrn1867

Mandyam, C. D., and Koob, G. F. (2012). The addicted brain craves new neurons: putative role for adult-born progenitors in promoting recovery. *Trends Neurosci.* 35, 250–260. doi: 10.1016/j.tins.2011.12.005

McClain, J. A., Hayes, D. M., Morris, S. A., and Nixon, K. (2011). Adolescent binge alcohol exposure alters hippocampal progenitor cell proliferation in rats: effects on cell cycle kinetics. *J. Comp. Neurol.* 519, 2697–2710. doi: 10.1002/cne.22647

Ming, G. L., and Song, H. (2011). Adult neurogenesis in the mammalian brain: significant answers and significant questions. *Neuron* 70, 687–702. doi: 10.1016/j.neuron.2011.05.001

Ming, G. L., and Song, H. (2005). Adult neurogenesis in the mammalian central nervous system. *Annu. Rev. Neurosci.* 28, 223–250. doi: 10.1146/annurev.neuro.28.051804.101459

Morris, S. A., Eaves, D. W., Smith, A. R., and Nixon, K. (2010). Alcohol inhibition of neurogenesis: a mechanism of hippocampal neurodegeneration in an adolescent alcohol abuse model. *Hippocampus* 20, 596–607. doi: 10.1002/hipo.20665

Nixon, K., and Crews, F. T. (2002). Binge ethanol exposure decreases neurogenesis in adult rat hippocampus. *J. Neurochem.* 83, 1087–1093. doi: 10.1046/j.1471-4159.2002.01214.x

Nixon, K., and Crews, F. T. (2004). Temporally specific burst in cell proliferation increases hippocampal neurogenesis in protracted abstinence from alcohol. *J. Neurosci.* 24, 9714–9722. doi: 10.1523/JNEUROSCI.3063-04.2004

Nixon, K., Kim, D. H., Potts, E. N., He, J., and Crews, F. T. (2008). Distinct cell proliferation events during abstinence after alcohol dependence: microglia proliferation precedes neurogenesis. *Neurobiol. Dis.* 31, 218–229. doi: 10.1016/j.nbd.2008.04.009

O'Malley, P. M., Johnston, L. D., and Bachman, J. G. (1998). Alcohol use among adolescents. *Alcohol. Health Res. World* 22, 85–93.

Paxinos, G., and Watson, C. (1997). *The Rat Brain in Stereotaxic Coordinates.* San Diego, CA: Academic Press.

Qin, L., Wu, X., Block, M. L., Liu, Y., Breese, G. R., Hong, J. S., et al. (2007). Systemic LPS causes chronic neuroinflammation and progressive neurodegeneration. *Glia* 55, 453–462. doi: 10.1002/glia.20467

Rao, M. S., and Shetty, A. K. (2004). Efficacy of doublecortin as a marker to analyse the absolute number and dendritic growth of newly generated neurons in the adult dentate gyrus. *Eur. J. Neurosci.* 19, 234–246. doi: 10.1111/j.0953-816x.2003.03123.x

Rolls, A., Shechter, R., London, A., Ziv, Y., Ronen, A., Levy, R., et al. (2007). Toll-like receptors modulate adult hippocampal neurogenesis. *Nat. Cell Biol.* 9, 1081–1088. doi: 10.1038/ncb1629

Sakharkar, A. J., Vetreno, R. P., Zhang, H., Kokare, D. M., Crews, F. T., and Pandey, S. C. (2016). A role for histone acetylation mechanisms in adolescent alcohol exposure-induced deficits in hippocampal brain-derived neurotrophic factor expression and neurogenesis markers in adulthood. *Brain Struct. Funct.* 221, 4691–4703. doi: 10.1007/s00429-016-1196-y

Smith, L. K., He, Y., Park, J. S., Bieri, G., Snethlage, C. E., Lin, K., et al. (2015). β2-microglobulin is a systemic pro-aging factor that impairs cognitive function and neurogenesis. *Nat. Med.* 21, 932–937. doi: 10.1038/nm.3898

Song, J., Olsen, R. H., Sun, J., Ming, G. L., and Song, H. (2016). Neuronal circuitry mechanisms regulating adult mammalian neurogenesis. *Cold Spring Harb. Perspect. Biol.* 8:a018937. doi: 10.1101/cshperspect.a018937

Spalding, K. L., Bergmann, O., Alkass, K., Bernard, S., Salehpour, M., Huttner, H. B., et al. (2013). Dynamics of hippocampal neurogenesis in adult humans. *Cell* 153, 1219–1227. doi: 10.1016/j.cell.2013.05.002

Spear, L. P. (2000). The adolescent brain and age-related behavioral manifestations. *Neurosci. Biobehav. Rev.* 24, 417–463. doi: 10.1016/s0149-7634(00)00014-2

Staples, M. C., and Mandyam, C. D. (2016). Thinking after drinking: impaired hippocampal-dependent cognition in human alcoholics and animal models of alcohol dependence. *Front. Psychiatry* 7:162. doi: 10.3389/fpsyt.2016.00162

Stevenson, J. R., Schroeder, J. P., Nixon, K., Besheer, J., Crews, F. T., and Hodge, C. W. (2009). Abstinence following alcohol drinking produces depression-like behavior and reduced hippocampal neurogenesis in mice. *Neuropsychopharmacology* 34, 1209–1222. doi: 10.1038/npp.2008.90

Urbán, N., and Guillemot, F. (2014). Neurogenesis in the embryonic and adult brain: same regulators, different roles. *Front. Cell. Neurosci.* 8:396. doi: 10.3389/fncel.2014.00396

Vetreno, R. P., and Crews, F. T. (2012). Adolescent binge drinking increases expression of the danger signal receptor agonist HMGB1 and Toll-like receptors in the adult prefrontal cortex. *Neuroscience* 226, 475–488. doi: 10.1016/j.neuroscience.2012.08.046

Vetreno, R. P., and Crews, F. T. (2014). Current hypotheses on the mechanisms of alcoholism. *Handb. Clin. Neurol.* 125, 477–497. doi: 10.1016/b978-0-444-62619-6.00027-6

Vetreno, R. P., and Crews, F. T. (2015). Binge ethanol exposure during adolescence leads to a persistent loss of neurogenesis in the dorsal and ventral hippocampus that is associated with impaired adult cognitive functioning. *Front. Neurosci.* 9:35. doi: 10.3389/fnins.2015.00035

Vetreno, R. P., Qin, L., and Crews, F. T. (2013). Increased receptor for advanced glycation end product expression in the human alcoholic prefrontal cortex is linked to adolescent drinking. *Neurobiol. Dis.* 59, 52–62. doi: 10.1016/j.nbd.2013.07.002

Wechsler, H., Dowdall, G. W., Davenport, A., and Castillo, S. (1995). Correlates of college student binge drinking. *Am. J. Public Health* 85, 921–926. doi: 10.2105/ajph.85.7.921

Yousef, H., Conboy, M. J., Morgenthaler, A., Schlesinger, C., Bugaj, L., Paliwal, P., et al. (2015). Systemic attenuation of the TGF-β pathway by a single drug simultaneously rejuvenates hippocampal neurogenesis and myogenesis in the same old mammal. *Oncotarget* 6, 11959–11978. doi: 10.18632/oncotarget.3851

15

Investigating the Role of Serotonin in Methamphetamine Psychosis: Unaltered Behavioral Effects of Chronic Methamphetamine in 5-HT1A Knockout Mice

*Emily J. Jaehne[1], Dzeneta Ameti[1], Tehani Paiva[1] and Maarten van den Buuse[1,2,3]**

[1] Department Psychology and Counselling, School of Psychology and Public Health, La Trobe University, Melbourne, VIC, Australia, [2] Department of Pharmacology, University of Melbourne, Melbourne, VIC, Australia, [3] The College of Public Health, Medical and Veterinary Sciences, James Cook University, Townsville, QLD, Australia

Edited by:
Jacqueline M. Barker,
Medical University of South Carolina,
USA

Reviewed by:
Eugene A. Kiyatkin,
National Institute on Drug Abuse,
USA
Jean-Philippe Guilloux,
Université Paris Sud UMRS-1178,
France

***Correspondence:**
Maarten van den Buuse
m.vandenbuuse@latrobe.edu.au

Methamphetamine (Meth) is a widely abused stimulant drug, but this abuse is associated with an increased risk of developing psychosis. In addition to its well-known action on brain dopamine, Meth also affects serotonergic (5-HT) neurons. The aim of this study was to investigate this role in mice, which lack one of the main serotonin receptors, the 5-HT_{1A} receptor, which has been implicated in both schizophrenia and Meth-induced psychosis. Male and female wild-type or 5-HT_{1A} knockout (KO) mice received daily treatment with increasing doses of methamphetamine from 6 to 9 weeks of age (1–4 mg/kg/day twice a day). At least 2 weeks after the last injection, the mice underwent a battery of behavioral tests focusing on psychosis-related behaviors, including Meth-induced hyperactivity, prepulse inhibition (PPI), social interaction, elevated plus maze (EPM), and Y-maze. Meth pretreatment resulted in significantly increased hyperlocomotion in response to an acute Meth challenge, but this effect was independent of genotype. Chronic Meth treatment resulted in decreased levels of anxiety in the EPM in both sexes, as well as increased startle responses in female mice only, again independent of genotype. 5-HT_{1A} KO mice showed an increased locomotor response to acute Meth in both sexes, as well as increased PPI and decreased startle responses in female mice only, independent of Meth pretreatment. In conclusion, the effects of chronic Meth appear unaffected by the absence of the 5-HT_{1A} receptor. These results do not support a role of the 5-HT_{1A} receptor in Meth-induced psychosis.

Keywords: methamphetamine, psychosis, serotonin, 5-HT_{1A} receptors, neuroplasticity

INTRODUCTION

Methamphetamine (Meth) use and availability has been increasing worldwide and is placing a huge burden on users, their relatives and friends, and society at large (1). One of the most severe consequences of Meth abuse in some users is the development of psychosis (2, 3), either acutely when the drug is active or as long-term symptoms, which may be similar to schizophrenia (2–4). Users may also develop other persistent psychiatric symptoms or impaired cognitive abilities following prolonged use of the drug (4, 5). However, the mechanisms involved in Meth psychosis, and its overlap with schizophrenia symptoms, remain unclear.

We have previously investigated the effects of chronic Meth on psychosis-like behavior in adulthood using a dosing schedule of escalating exposure during late adolescence/early adulthood. At least 2 weeks after the chronic treatment ended, the long-lasting effects of chronic Meth on a locomotor hyperactivity model of psychosis, as well as on cognition and other behaviors with relevance to psychiatric symptoms, were studied (6–8). Acute amphetamine- or Meth-induced locomotor hyperactivity is a widely used behavioral test in preclinical schizophrenia research, as it models the increase in dopamine signaling thought to contribute to psychosis (9). Sensitization of this dopaminergic signaling has been postulated to mimic developmental mechanisms in psychosis (10, 11). In our experiments, pretreatment with Meth led to sensitization to the acute effects of amphetamine in the hyperactivity model compared to control pretreatment (6), while Meth pretreatment reduced the effect of an acute injection of amphetamine on prepulse inhibition (PPI) of acoustic startle (PPI) (7). Further studies showed that the chronic dosing protocol altered social novelty behavior but not short-term memory in the Y-maze (8).

There is increasing evidence for a role of serotonin, as well as dopaminergic mechanisms, in schizophrenia. Postmortem studies have shown increased expression of 5-HT_{1A} receptors in the frontal cortex (12) but decreased binding in the amygdala in patients with schizophrenia (13). A polymorphism in the 5-HT_{1A} receptor was associated with schizophrenia psychopathology (14) and several atypical antipsychotic drugs have high affinity for serotonergic receptors, including the 5-HT_{1A} receptor (15–19). Extensive evidence suggests that 5-HT_{1A} receptor activation modulates dopamine activity and may enhance cognition in schizophrenia (15, 17, 20, 21). While much of the animal literature has focused on the role of 5-HT_{1A} in anxiety, where studies have shown 5-HT_{1A} knockout (KO) mice to have a robust anxiety phenotype behavior in the elevated plus maze (EPM) (22–25) and certain fear conditioning paradigms (26), more recent work has investigated its role in schizophrenia-related behaviors. For example, 5-HT_{1A} KO mice have an enhanced locomotor response to D-amphetamine compared to wild-type (WT) mice (27), an altered PPI response to methylenedioxymethamphetamine (28), and impaired cognition in the Morris Water maze (25, 29). The 5-HT_{1A} antagonist WAY100635 has also been shown to increase PPI in C57BL/6 mice (30).

These previous studies suggest a role for 5-HT_{1A} receptors in schizophrenia although it is less clear if this extends to Meth psychosis. While several studies have suggested a role for 5-HT_{1A} receptors in addiction to this drug (31), a role for this receptor in sensitization of Meth-induced hyperlocomotion is less clear (32). For example, the 5-HT_{1A} receptor antagonist, WAY100635, had no effect on amphetamine or Meth-induced hyperlocomotor activity (33, 34), while in contrast, the agonist, 8-OH-DPAT, was able to inhibit hyperlocomotion (33). 8-OH-DPAT and the 5-HT_{1A} receptor agonist, osemozotan, also prevented development and expression of amphetamine or Meth-induced behavioral sensitization (35, 36). However, the long-lasting effects of chronic Meth to induce psychosis-like behavior have not been studied in animals with genetically modified 5-HT_{1A} receptor levels. The current study was, therefore, designed to investigate the effect of 5-HT_{1A} receptor KO on the action of Meth to induce psychosis- and schizophrenia-related behaviors. We used the acute Meth-induced hyperactivity model of psychosis as well as a range of other relevant behavioral tests, including PPI for sensorimotor gating, social interaction as a model of some of the negative symptoms of schizophrenia, Y-maze and fear conditioning to assess cognitive changes, and EPM for anxiety. 5-HT_{1A} KO mice or WT controls were tested during adulthood after a 3-week binge protocol of Meth administration during late adolescence. As previous studies have shown sex differences in animal models of psychosis (37) as well as the effect of this Meth dosing protocol on some behaviors (7, 8), both male and female mice were included in this study.

MATERIALS AND METHODS

Animals

5-HT_{1A} receptor KO mice and their C57BL/6 WT control littermates (WT) (27) were derived from a breeding colony at the La Trobe Animal Research and Teaching Facility. Heterozygous mice were used as breeders to obtain WT and KO littermates for the current studies, while heterozygous offspring was not used. Genotypes were confirmed at weaning by Transnetyx Inc. (Cordova, TN, USA).

A total of 104 male and female mice were used for experiments ($n = 10$–16/group; **Table 1**). All mice were housed in groups of two to five during the experimental period in individually ventilated cages (Tecniplast, Buguggiate, Italy) with standard pellet food and water available *ad libitum*. Ambient temperature of housing and testing rooms was 21 ± 2°C and mice were housed under a 12-h light–dark cycle, lights on at 0700 hours, with all behavioral testing conducted between 0800 and 1600 hours.

Chronic Methamphetamine Treatment and Experimental Procedure

Mice were given either Meth or saline as a vehicle control for five consecutive days a week for a period of 3 weeks during

TABLE 1 | Number and mean weight of experimental groups.

Group	*n*	Body weight (g) at end of testing
Males		
WT-Saline	12	28.0 ± 0.7
WT-Meth	12	30.4 ± 0.6
5-HT_{1A} KO-Saline	12	28.8 ± 0.7
5-HT_{1A} KO-Meth	16	29.6 ± 0.5
Females		
WT-Saline	12	22.4 ± 0.3
WT-Meth	13	22.3 ± 0.3
5-HT_{1A} KO-Saline	16	22.5 ± 0.4
5-HT_{1A} KO-Meth	11	23.4 ± 0.4

Genotype: 5-HT_{1A} knockout (KO) or wild-type (WT).
Pretreatment: saline or methamphetamine (Meth).
Body weight: mean (±SEM).

adolescence, from the age of 6 to 9 weeks. Mice received 1 injection/day of 1 mg/kg during the first week, 2 injections/day of 2 mg/kg the second week, and 2 injections/day of 4 mg/kg the third week (6–8). This protocol was based on a binge-type Meth intake pattern seen in many abusers of the drug, including occasional interruptions of administration and a gradual increase of doses (38). The 2-week washout is required to be able to see the long-term effects of these chronic doses, which reflect increased effects in relapsed chronic users (38) as well as sensitization mechanisms similar to those postulated in psychosis development (10, 11). Meth and saline solutions were given intraperitoneally at a volume of 5 ml/kg. Meth was purchased from the National Measurement Institute (Pymble, NSW, Australia) and dissolved in 0.9% sterile saline.

Starting 2 weeks following the final injection, at 11 weeks of age, mice underwent a battery of behavioral tests over a period of 4 weeks, with less stressful tests performed first and more stressful tests, or tests involving acute drug challenge, performed at the end. Mice were given at least 2–3 days between behavioral tests. Tests were performed in the following order: Y-maze, social interaction, EPM, fear conditioning, PPI, and Meth-induced locomotor hyperactivity.

Behavioral Testing

Methamphetamine-Induced Locomotor Hyperactivity

Mice were placed into automated photocell arenas (Med Associates, Fairfax, VT, USA), 27 cm × 27 cm with walls 40 cm high, with a 16 × 16 array of photobeam sensors for detecting movement. Each time, they were first habituated in the arenas for 1 h, then were removed briefly and injected with the challenge drug, then placed back into the arena for a further 2 h (6, 27). During the first session, all mice received saline, followed by 1 mg/kg Meth in the second and 3 mg/kg Meth in the final session, with 3–4 days washout in between sessions. Distance traveled was automatically calculated in 5-min time bins.

PPI of Acoustic Startle

Prepulse inhibition was assessed as a measure of sensorimotor gating using automated SR-Lab startle chambers (San Diego Instruments, San Diego, CA, USA). Mice were placed in individual plexiglass cylinders (5 cm diameter) and the test session consisted of 104 stimulus trials as previously described (7, 27). PPI was quantified as the difference between stimulus responses during prepulse-pulse and pulse-alone trials and expressed as a percentage of pulse-alone responses. At 30 ms ISI, mice showed no effect of genotype or pretreatment, therefore, results analysis will focus on the 100 ms ISI.

Social Interaction

The test apparatus consists of a rectangular three chambered enclosure, 43 cm × 64 cm, with transparent walls 23 cm high. Two "stranger" enclosures, diameter 9 cm, height 10 cm, were placed in the two outer chambers. The test consisted of three phases, each 10 min in duration, which were conducted immediately after one another (8, 39). Stranger mice were adolescent 5-HT_{1A} heterozygous mice of the same sex as the test mouse. Interaction time was measured using Ethovision video tracking (Noldus, Wageningen, The Netherlands), with time spent in a "sniffing zone," 2.5 cm immediately surrounding stranger cages, defined as interaction.

Elevated Plus Maze

The EPM consisted of an elevated plus-shaped platform with two open and two closed arms, with a length of 40 cm and width of 5 cm, 50 cm above the ground, with a central square section between arms (40, 41). During the 5-min trial, time spent in open and closed arms and number of entries into arms were measured using Ethovision video tracking (Noldus). Mice that spend more time in the open arms are considered to have a lesser anxiety phenotype. The total number of arm entries was used as a control measure of locomotor activity.

Y-Maze

The Y-maze was a Y-shaped apparatus with three arms (start arm and two test arms), each 32 cm long and 10 cm wide with walls 15 cm high. The arms were at a 120° angle from each other. The test arms had different black and white symbols on either end wall. Behavior was tracked using Ethovision (Noldus), which measured time spent in, and number of entries to, each arm (42, 43). Sessions included a 10-min trial with access to only two arms followed 1 h later but a 5 min re-trial with access to all three arms. Time spent in the novel test arm compared to the other arms (familiar and start) during the retention phase was used as a measure of short-term spatial recognition memory.

Fear Conditioning

Fear memory was assessed using a 3-day fear conditioning protocol as previously used in mice (43, 44) using chambers equipped with footshock grid floors (Med Associates). Two different conditioning contexts were used, which differed in lux, scent, bedding, and structure due to a concave wall insert, and mice were pseudorandomly assigned to one context or the other. Freezing was defined as complete lack of any movement besides breathing and was measured in response to (1) the context where mice had previously been exposed to an unconditioned stimulus (scrambled foot-shocks of 1 s duration, 0.7 mA) or (2) a conditioned stimulus (30 s duration, 7,500 Hz, 70 dB) previously presented prior to the US, but in a new context.

Statistical Analysis

Data were expressed as the mean ± SEM and differences between groups were analyzed with analysis of variance (ANOVA), with repeated measures where appropriate, using IBM SPSS Statistics 23 (Armonk, New York, NY, USA). All data were first analyzed with genotype, Meth pretreatment and sex as between-group statistical factors. If significant interactions were seen, data were split and further analyzed by genotype, pretreatment, or sex as stated in the results. For locomotor activity analysis, repeated-measures factors were time and acute Meth treatment, while for social interaction and Y-maze analysis, repeated measures factors were stranger mouse interaction time and time spent in arms, respectively. Differences between groups were considered significant when $p < 0.05$.

RESULTS

Locomotor Activity

Analysis of locomotor activity following 1 and 3 mg/kg Meth compared to saline control showed a significant main effect of an acute Meth challenge [$F_{(2, 188)} = 273$, $p < 0.001$] and a treatment × pretreatment interaction [$F_{(2, 188)} = 73.3$, $p < 0.001$]. Data were, therefore, split and further ANOVAs were used to compare the effect of each dose of acute Meth with saline to further explore this relationship. Although females showed higher activity than males [$F_{(1, 94)} = 16.4$, $p < 0.001$], there were no significant interactions between sex and genotype, acute treatment or pretreatment, therefore, locomotor activity results for males and females were combined (**Figure 1**).

Following acute injection with 3 mg/kg Meth, all groups showed a significant main effect of treatment compared to saline injection [$F_{(1, 94)} = 307$, $p < 0.001$]. This effect was much greater in Meth-pretreated mice [treatment × pretreatment $F_{(1, 94)} = 87.3$, $p < 0.001$], indicating sensitization to a challenge dose of Meth following the binge dosing protocol used, and was also greater in 5-HT_{1A} KO mice than in WT controls [treatment × genotype $F_{(1, 94)} = 5.10$, $p = 0.026$]. There was, however, no treatment × pretreatment × genotype interaction, suggesting the genotype differences and Meth sensitization were independent of each other.

Acute injection with 1 mg/kg Meth showed similar results [treatment $F_{(1, 94)} = 24.9$, $p < 0.001$; treatment × pretreatment $F_{(1, 94)} = 18.0$, $p < 0.001$]; however, the effect of genotype in response to acute Meth failed to reach significance at this dose.

Prepulse Inhibition

Analysis of PPI at 100 ms ISI showed a significant genotype × sex interaction [$F_{(1, 104)} = 5.77$, $p = 0.018$]; therefore, data were further analyzed separately for male and female mice (**Figure 2A**). Female, but not male, 5-HT_{1A} KO mice showed significantly higher PPI than WT mice [main effect of genotype $F_{(1, 54)} = 9.08$, $p = 0.004$]. However, there was no effect of Meth pretreatment on PPI in any of the groups.

Analysis of startle response showed that male mice had significantly higher startle compared to females [$F_{(1, 104)} = 15.1$, $p < 0.001$] while there was also a significant main effect of genotype [$F_{(1, 104)} = 4.43$, $p = 0.038$] and a genotype × sex interaction [$F_{(1, 104)} = 4.52$, $p = 0.036$] suggesting a genotype effect, which was dependent on sex (**Figure 2B**). We, therefore, again further analyzed results separately for male and female mice. As with PPI, male mice showed no difference between groups, while in females, 5-HT_{1A} KO mice showed significantly lower startle than WT mice [main effect of genotype $F_{(1, 54)} = 17.6$, $p < 0.001$]. It was also shown that female Meth pretreated mice had significantly higher startle compared to controls [main effect of pretreatment $F_{(1, 54)} = 4.08$, $p = 0.048$]; however, there was no genotype × pretreatment effect, suggesting that these results were independent of each other.

Social Interaction

Analysis of total time spent interacting with the stranger mouse and empty cage showed a significant preference for the stranger mouse [$F_{(1, 78)} = 150$, $p < 0.001$], but there was no statistical interaction with genotype, pretreatment, or sex, indicating all groups showed similar sociability (**Figure 3A**).

In contrast, while analysis of the total time spent interacting with the familiar and novel stranger mice again showed a significant preference for the novel stranger [$F_{(1, 78)} = 51.6$, $p < 0.001$] and no statistical interaction with genotype or pretreatment, there was a significant interaction between stranger time and sex [$F_{(1, 78)} = 5.6$, $p = 0.021$; **Figure 3B**]. This suggests that there were no effects of genotype or Meth pretreatment on social novelty behavior, but that female mice show a decreased preference for the novel over the familiar stranger mouse.

Elevated Plus Maze

Analysis of time spent in the open arms of the EPM showed a significant main effect of Meth pretreatment [$F_{(1, 94)} = 8.17$, $p = 0.005$] reflecting that this pretreatment leads to increased time spent on the open arms of the EPM, suggesting decreased anxiety in these mice (**Figure 4A**). There was no significant main effect of genotype or sex; therefore, results have been presented for both sexes combined.

Total number of arm entries was analyzed as an indicator of activity on the plus maze (WT-Saline 42.2 ± 4.2, KO-Saline

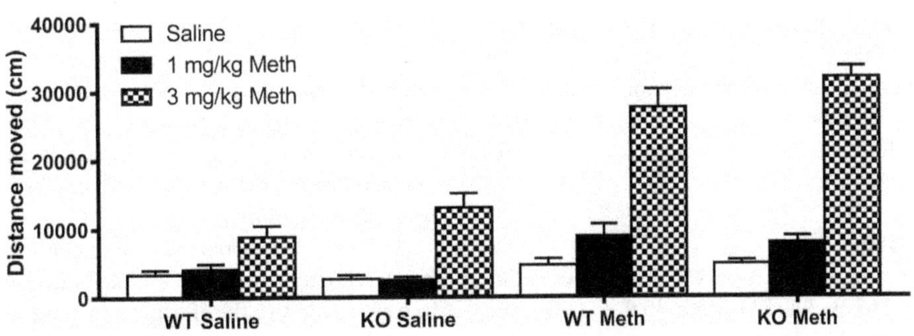

FIGURE 1 | Acute methamphetamine (Meth) induced hyperactivity following chronic Meth exposure. A low acute challenge dose of Meth (1 mg/kg) induced hyperactivity in mice previously pretreated with Meth. There was no genotype effect at this dose. A high acute challenge dose of Meth (3 mg/kg) induced hyperactivity to a significantly greater extent in Meth pretreated compared to saline pretreated mice. This dose also induced hyperactivity to a significantly greater extent in 5-HT_{1A} knockout (KO) mice compared to wild-type (WT) mice. Results are shown for males and females combined.

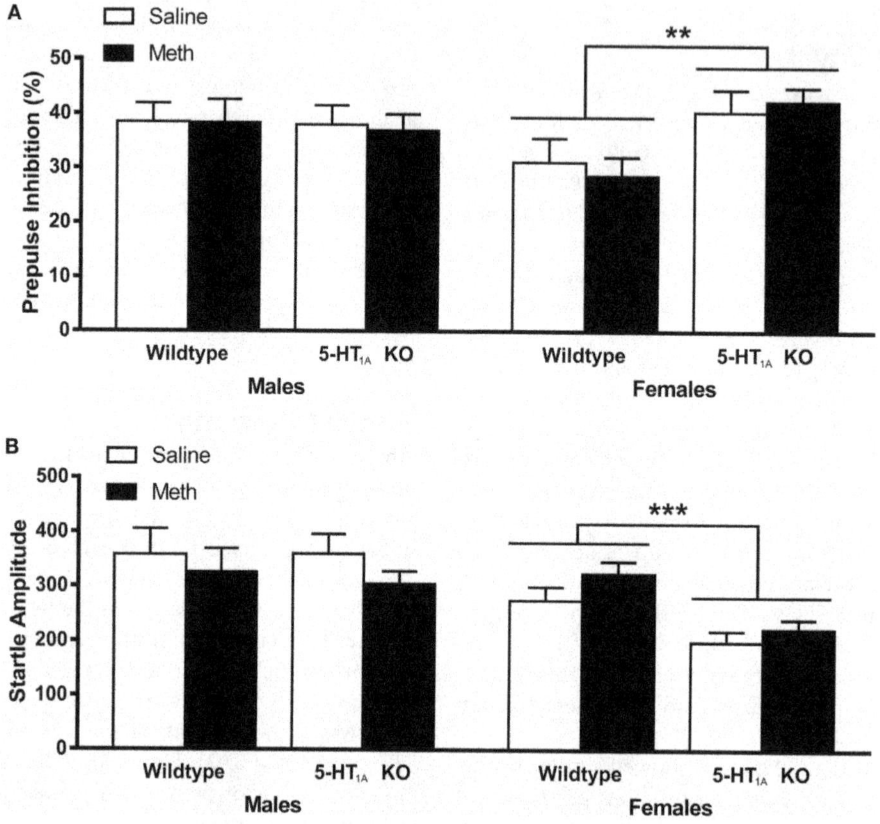

FIGURE 2 | (A) Average prepulse inhibition (PPI) across all four PP intensities was significantly higher in 5-HT$_{1A}$ knockout (KO) females compared to wild-type (WT) females. There was no difference in PPI between any groups in male mice. **(B)** Average startle responses across all four startle blocks were significantly lower in female 5-HT$_{1A}$ KO mice compared to WT, and higher in female Meth pretreated compared to saline pretreated mice. There was no difference in startle between any groups in male mice. ** signifies genotype effect $p < 0.01$, *** signifies $p < 0.001$.

45.1 ± 3.6, WT-Meth 46.5 ± 4.3, KO-Meth 47.0 ± 3.8). The results showed that there were no differences in activity between groups; therefore, overall activity did not have any effect on the different anxiety levels seen.

Y-Maze

Analysis of total time spent in each arm of the Y-maze showed a significant main effect of arms [$F_{(2, 184)} = 91.6$, $p < 0.001$], but no significant interaction of time in arms with genotype, pretreatment, or sex indicating all groups showed a similar preference for the novel arm and have intact short-term spatial memory (**Figure 4B**). There was no significant main effect of sex; therefore, results have been presented for both sexes combined.

Fear Conditioning

Analysis of context freezing (WT-Saline 42.3 ± 4.3, KO-Saline 45.6 ± 3.4, WT-Meth 44.7 ± 3.6, KO-Meth 40.9 ± 3.5%) and tone freezing (WT-Saline 43.5 ± 4.9, KO-Saline 55.5 ± 4.3, WT-Meth 49.0 ± 4.9, KO-Meth 48.1 ± 4.1) showed that there were no differences between the groups, suggesting that neither Meth pretreatment nor 5-HT$_{1A}$ genotype have any effect on fear memory.

DISCUSSION

This study showed that, while both the Meth binge dosing and 5-HT$_{1A}$ receptor KO genotype alter behavior in mice, 5-HT$_{1A}$ KO mice did not respond differently to chronic Meth pretreatment in any of the behaviors tested. Meth pretreatment resulted in a heightened response to acute Meth and decreased levels of anxiety in both sexes, as well as increased startle responses in female mice only, independent of genotype. However, 5-HT$_{1A}$ KO mice also showed an increased response to acute Meth in both sexes, as well as increased PPI and decreased startle response in female mice only, independent of Meth pretreatment. There were no effects on either short-term spatial memory in the Y-maze or conditioned fear memory induced by either Meth or 5-HT$_{1A}$ receptor KO genotype.

These studies were first able to confirm that chronic escalating Meth exposure during adolescence/young adulthood leads to sensitization to the effects of an acute challenge dose of Meth in adulthood, consistent with previous studies (6). We were also able to confirm that 5-HT$_{1A}$ KO mice have a greater response to acute Meth compared to WT consistent with their enhanced sensitivity seen following acute D-amphetamine previously (27). However, there was no statistical interaction between the

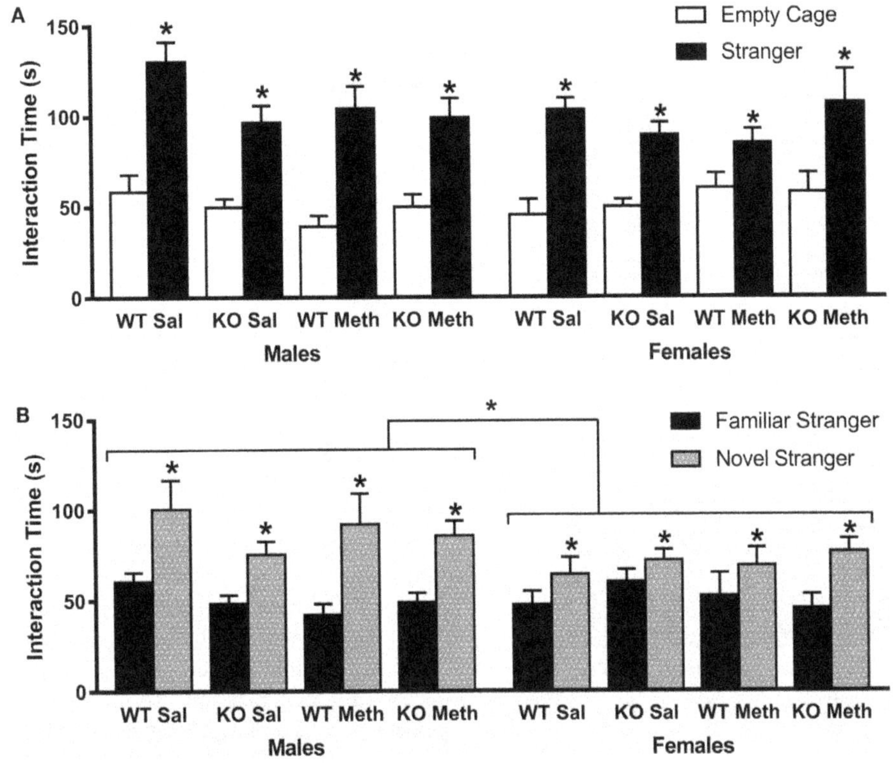

FIGURE 3 | Social behavior in the three-chamber task. (A) Sociability, as measured by preference to interact with a stranger mouse compared to an empty cage, was normal in all groups (indicated by * above stranger). **(B)** Social novelty preference, as measured by preference to interact with novel stranger mouse, was also normal in all groups (indicated by * above stranger), although female mice showed a lower preference compared to males. *$p < 0.05$.

two effects, as reflected by the observation that KO mice did not show an altered sensitivity to acute re-exposure to a single challenge dose of Meth compared to WT mice. These results suggest that the 5-HT_{1A} receptor is likely important in the acute action of Meth to induce hyperactivity but is not required for the development of sensitization induced by prior binge dosing of Meth. A previous study in the laboratory showed that the binding density of the dopamine transporter (DAT) and dopamine receptors D_1 and D_2 is only changed subtly in 5-HT_{1A} KO mice (27) and suggested that the interaction of 5-HT_{1A} receptors with dopamine release is at a more immediate functional level (45) rather that *via* more long-term changes in the expression of DAT or dopamine receptors.

Male mice showed no effect of genotype or Meth pretreatment on either PPI or startle response. Female 5-HT_{1A} KO mice, however, showed increased PPI and decreased startle responses compared to WT. The results are partly consistent with a previous study, which showed that administration of the 5-HT_{1A} antagonist, WAY100635, led to an increase in PPI in C57BL/6 mice (30); however, this was only done in male mice, which showed no changes in PPI between genotypes in the current study. While Meth pretreatment did not alter PPI in either sex, there was also a small but significant effect of Meth pretreatment to increase startle response in female mice; however, the effects of genotype and pretreatment were again independent of each other. Therefore, as with locomotor hyperactivity, Meth pretreatment had no specific effect in 5-HT_{1A} KO mice only. This is similar to previous studies using Meth pretreatment where no differences were seen in baseline PPI in either sex following binge Meth dosing (7).

There were no effects of Meth pretreatment or 5-HT_{1A} genotype on social behavior using the three-chamber sociability and social novelty preference tests. A previous study in the lab showed the same results for sociability, although suggested that Meth pretreatment decreased preference for social novelty to a lower level than saline pretreated mice in males only (8), while other studies have also shown impaired social behavior in animals previously exposed to Meth (46, 47).

5-HT_{1A} KO mice showed no signs of increased or decreased anxiety in the EPM, which is in contrast to other studies conducted in these mice, which have shown an anxious phenotype on the EPM and other tests of anxiety (22–26). Differences in experimental conditions such as conducting other behavioral tests prior to the elevated zero maze could contribute to the differences seen here compared to previous studies. Future studies should test for an anxiety phenotype in these mice prior to further behavioral testing to confirm presence of the phenotype. Importantly, however, Meth pretreatment led to increased time spent in the open arms of the plus maze, suggesting that these mice were less anxious than controls, but this effect was again

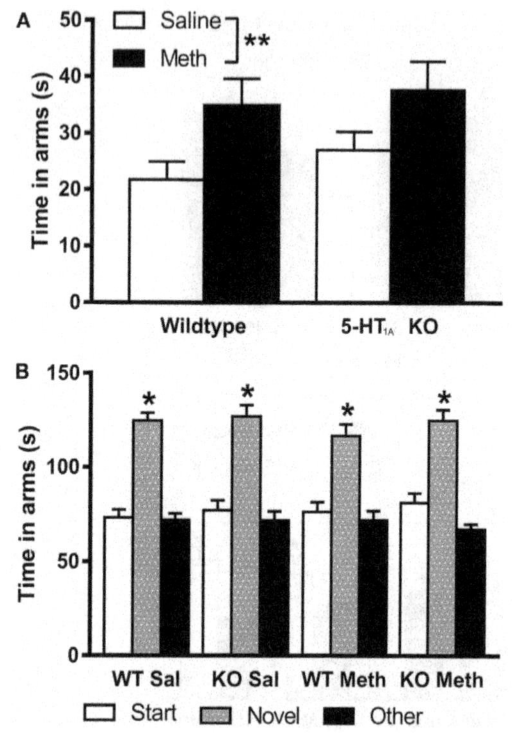

FIGURE 4 | (A) Time spent in the open arms of the elevated plus maze was higher in Meth pretreated mice compared to saline pretreated. **(B)** Short-term spatial memory, measured by preference to spend time in the novel arm of the Y-maze, was normal in all groups (indicated by * above novel arm). $^{*}p < 0.05$, $^{**}p < 0.01$. Results are shown for males and females combined.

independent of genotype. Previously, effects of chronic Meth pretreatment on anxiety have been variable. For example, a 10-day escalating dose protocol in mice induced no changes in anxiety measures in the EPM or light/dark box (48) while studies in rats showed increased anxiety or no change in the EPM depending on the age or extent of Meth exposure or time following exposure (49–51). These results suggest that dosing and testing protocol are very important for long-term effects of Meth on behavior.

A limitation of using 5-HT_{1A} KO mice is that the absence of these receptors during embryogenesis and development may influence the role of these receptors on behavior and the development of Meth sensitization. For example, changes in receptor density or function may change over time, and this could be altered by absence of the receptors during early development. Future studies could use conditional KO mice in which the receptor is deleted only in adulthood. Any differential role of presynaptic and postsynaptic 5-HT_{1A} receptors, which would both be absent in our KO mice, is also not addressed in this study. Previous research using 5-HT_{1A} agonists suggest that, while antagonists have no effect on behavioral sensitization (33, 34), the effects of the agonists may have been due to the activation of the presynaptic receptors preferentially over postsynaptic receptors (52). Studies show that both 8-OH-DPAT and osemozotan are able to prevent the development and expression of amphetamine or Meth-induced behavioral sensitization (35, 36), these effects were also reversed by the antagonist WAY100635, which has a greater affinity for presynaptic 5-HT_{1A} autoreceptors (53). Other limitations of this study are that the estrus cycle of female mice was not monitored, which could strengthen the results of any study using female animals, and the fact that we did not see an anxiety phenotype in the 5-HT_{1A} KO mice as discussed above.

While this study showed that there was no interaction between Meth pretreatment and the 5-HT_{1A} receptor in the protocols used, there is evidence that other 5-HT receptors may be involved in the long-term effects of Meth and Meth-induced sensitization. Repeated Meth administration failed to induce behavioral sensitization in 5-HT reuptake KO mice, but this was rescued by administration of a 5-HT_{1B} antagonist (54). Many different 5-HT receptor agonists and antagonists have been investigated for their role in behavioral sensitization induced by Meth. For example, the 5-HT_{1B} receptor antagonist, SB 216641, inhibited development but not expression of amphetamine-induced sensitization (55) while the 5-HT_2 receptor antagonist, ritanserin, inhibited the development, expression, and maintenance of Meth-induced behavioral sensitization (56, 57). Taken together, the current findings in 5-HT_{1A} receptor KO mice do not support a role of these receptors in Meth-induced psychosis, although this does not rule out a role of other serotonin receptors, which can be addressed in future studies with selected KO lines such as 5-HT_{1B} and 5-HT_2 receptor KO mice.

ETHICS STATEMENT

All experimentation was approved by the La Trobe University Animal Ethics Committee and was conducted in accordance with the Australian Code of Practice for the Care and Use of Animals for Scientific Purposes set out by the National Health and Medical Research Council of Australia.

AUTHOR CONTRIBUTIONS

MB designed the study. EJ, DA, and TP performed all behavioral testing and collected data. EJ performed analysis and wrote the manuscript with the help of MB who edited the final version. All authors contributed to and approved the final version of this manuscript.

ACKNOWLEDGMENTS

This study was supported by a Senior Research Fellowship (grant number 1041895) from the National Health and Medical Research Council of Australia. The authors would like to acknowledge and thank Camilla Hume for assistance with implementation and supervision of behavioral testing.

REFERENCES

1. United Nations. In: United Nations Office on Drugs and Crime, editor. *World Drug Report 2016*. Vienna (2016). Available from: http://www.unodc.org/wdr2016/
2. Callaghan RC, Cunningham JK, Allebeck P, Arenovich T, Sajeev G, Remington G, et al. Methamphetamine use and schizophrenia: a population-based cohort study in California. *Am J Psychiatry* (2012) 169(4):389–96. doi:10.1176/appi.ajp.2011.10070937
3. McKetin R, Hickey K, Devlin K, Lawrence K. The risk of psychotic symptoms associated with recreational methamphetamine use. *Drug Alcohol Rev* (2010) 29(4):358–63. doi:10.1111/j.1465-3362.2009.00160.x
4. Zweben JE, Cohen JB, Christian D, Galloway GP, Salinardi M, Parent D, et al. Psychiatric symptoms in methamphetamine users. *Am J Addict* (2004) 13(2):181–90. doi:10.1080/10550490490436055
5. Courtney KE, Ray LA. Methamphetamine: an update on epidemiology, pharmacology, clinical phenomenology, and treatment literature. *Drug Alcohol Depend* (2014) 143:11–21. doi:10.1016/j.drugalcdep.2014.08.003
6. Manning EE, Halberstadt AL, van den Buuse M. BDNF-deficient mice show reduced psychosis-related behaviors following chronic methamphetamine. *Int J Neuropsychopharmacol* (2016) 19(4):yv116. doi:10.1093/ijnp/pyv116
7. Manning EE, van den Buuse M. BDNF deficiency and young-adult methamphetamine induce sex-specific effects on prepulse inhibition regulation. *Front Cell Neurosci* (2013) 7:92. doi:10.3389/fncel.2013.00092
8. Manning EE, van den Buuse M. Altered social cognition in male BDNF heterozygous mice and following chronic methamphetamine exposure. *Behav Brain Res* (2016) 305:181–5. doi:10.1016/j.bbr.2016.03.014
9. van den Buuse M. Modeling the positive symptoms of schizophrenia in genetically modified mice: pharmacology and methodology aspects. *Schizophr Bull* (2010) 36(2):246–70. doi:10.1093/schbul/sbp132
10. Laruelle M. The role of endogenous sensitization in the pathophysiology of schizophrenia: implications from recent brain imaging studies. *Brain Res Brain Res Rev* (2000) 31(2–3):371–84. doi:10.1016/S0165-0173(99)00054-5
11. Weidenauer A, Bauer M, Sauerzopf U, Bartova L, Praschak-Rieder N, Sitte HH, et al. Making sense of: sensitization in schizophrenia. *Int J Neuropsychopharmacol* (2017) 20(1):1–10. doi:10.1093/ijnp/pyw081
12. Burnet PW, Eastwood SL, Harrison PJ. [^{3}H]WAY-100635 for 5-HT1A receptor autoradiography in human brain: a comparison with [^{3}H]8-OH-DPAT and demonstration of increased binding in the frontal cortex in schizophrenia. *Neurochem Int* (1997) 30(6):565–74. doi:10.1016/S0197-0186(96)00124-6
13. Yasuno F, Suhara T, Ichimiya T, Takano A, Ando T, Okubo Y. Decreased 5-HT1A receptor binding in amygdala of schizophrenia. *Biol Psychiatry* (2004) 55(5):439–44. doi:10.1016/j.biopsych.2003.11.016
14. Huang YY, Battistuzzi C, Oquendo MA, Harkavy-Friedman J, Greenhill L, Zalsman G, et al. Human 5-HT1A receptor C(-1019)G polymorphism and psychopathology. *Int J Neuropsychopharmacol* (2004) 7(4):441–51. doi:10.1017/s1461145704004663
15. De Deurwaerdere P, Di Giovanni G. Serotonergic modulation of the activity of mesencephalic dopaminergic systems: therapeutic implications. *Prog Neurobiol* (2017) 151:175–236. doi:10.1016/j.pneurobio.2016.03.004
16. Meltzer HY, Huang M. In vivo actions of atypical antipsychotic drug on serotonergic and dopaminergic systems. *Prog Brain Res* (2008) 172:177–97. doi:10.1016/s0079-6123(08)00909-6
17. Millan MJ. Improving the treatment of schizophrenia: focus on serotonin (5-HT)(1A) receptors. *J Pharmacol Exp Ther* (2000) 295(3):853–61.
18. Wood MD, Wren PB. Serotonin-dopamine interactions: implications for the design of novel therapeutic agents for psychiatric disorders. *Prog Brain Res* (2008) 172:213–30. doi:10.1016/s0079-6123(08)00911-4
19. Yadav PN, Abbas AI, Farrell MS, Setola V, Sciaky N, Huang XP, et al. The presynaptic component of the serotonergic system is required for clozapine's efficacy. *Neuropsychopharmacology* (2011) 36(3):638–51. doi:10.1038/npp.2010.195
20. Meltzer HY, Sumiyoshi T. Does stimulation of 5-HT(1A) receptors improve cognition in schizophrenia? *Behav Brain Res* (2008) 195(1):98–102. doi:10.1016/j.bbr.2008.05.016
21. Sumiyoshi T, Bubenikova-Valesova V, Horacek J, Bert B. Serotonin1A receptors in the pathophysiology of schizophrenia: development of novel cognition-enhancing therapeutics. *Adv Ther* (2008) 25(10):1037–56. doi:10.1007/s12325-008-0102-2
22. Heisler LK, Chu HM, Brennan TJ, Danao JA, Bajwa P, Parsons LH, et al. Elevated anxiety and antidepressant-like responses in serotonin 5-HT1A receptor mutant mice. *Proc Natl Acad Sci U S A* (1998) 95(25):15049–54. doi:10.1073/pnas.95.25.15049
23. Parks CL, Robinson PS, Sibille E, Shenk T, Toth M. Increased anxiety of mice lacking the serotonin1A receptor. *Proc Natl Acad Sci U S A* (1998) 95(18):10734–9. doi:10.1073/pnas.95.18.10734
24. Ramboz S, Oosting R, Amara DA, Kung HF, Blier P, Mendelsohn M, et al. Serotonin receptor 1A knockout: an animal model of anxiety-related disorder. *Proc Natl Acad Sci U S A* (1998) 95(24):14476–81. doi:10.1073/pnas.95.24.14476
25. Rogers J, Vo U, Buret LS, Pang TY, Meiklejohn H, Zeleznikow-Johnston A, et al. Dissociating the therapeutic effects of environmental enrichment and exercise in a mouse model of anxiety with cognitive impairment. *Transl Psychiatry* (2016) 6:e794. doi:10.1038/tp.2016.52
26. Klemenhagen KC, Gordon JA, David DJ, Hen R, Gross CT. Increased fear response to contextual cues in mice lacking the 5-HT1A receptor. *Neuropsychopharmacology* (2006) 31(1):101–11. doi:10.1038/sj.npp.1300774
27. van den Buuse M, Ruimschotel E, Martin S, Risbrough VB, Halberstadt AL. Enhanced effects of amphetamine but reduced effects of the hallucinogen, 5-MeO-DMT, on locomotor activity in 5-HT(1A) receptor knockout mice: implications for schizophrenia. *Neuropharmacology* (2011) 61(1–2):209–16. doi:10.1016/j.neuropharm.2011.04.001
28. van den Buuse M, Becker T, Kwek P, Martin S, Ruimschotel E, Risbrough V. Disruption of prepulse inhibition by 3,4-methylenedioxymethamphetamine (MDMA): comparison between male and female wild-type and 5-HT(1A) receptor knockout mice. *Int J Neuropsychopharmacol* (2011) 14(6):856–61. doi:10.1017/s1461145711000101
29. Wolff M, Costet P, Gross C, Hen R, Segu L, Buhot MC. Age-dependent effects of serotonin-1A receptor gene deletion in spatial learning abilities in mice. *Brain Res Mol Brain Res* (2004) 130(1–2):39–48. doi:10.1016/j.molbrainres.2004.07.012
30. van den Buuse M. Exploring the role of 5-HT1A receptors in the regulation of prepulse inhibition in mice: implications for cross-species comparisons. *ACS Chem Neurosci* (2013) 4(1):149–60. doi:10.1021/cn300118t
31. Müller CP, Carey RJ, Huston JP, De Souza Silva MA. Serotonin and psychostimulant addiction: focus on 5-HT1A-receptors. *Prog Neurobiol* (2007) 81(3):133–78. doi:10.1016/j.pneurobio.2007.01.001
32. Muller CP, Homberg JR. The role of serotonin in drug use and addiction. *Behav Brain Res* (2015) 277:146–92. doi:10.1016/j.bbr.2014.04.007
33. Przegalinski E, Filip M. Stimulation of serotonin (5-HT)1A receptors attenuates the locomotor, but not the discriminative, effects of amphetamine and cocaine in rats. *Behav Pharmacol* (1997) 8(8):699–706. doi:10.1097/00008877-199712000-00004
34. Steed E, Jones CA, McCreary AC. Serotonergic involvement in methamphetamine-induced locomotor activity: a detailed pharmacological study. *Behav Brain Res* (2011) 220(1):9–19. doi:10.1016/j.bbr.2011.01.026
35. Ago Y, Nakamura S, Uda M, Kajii Y, Abe M, Baba A, et al. Attenuation by the 5-HT1A receptor agonist osemozotan of the behavioral effects of single and repeated methamphetamine in mice. *Neuropharmacology* (2006) 51(4):914–22. doi:10.1016/j.neuropharm.2006.06.001
36. Przegaliński E, Siwanowicz J, Baran L, Filip M. Activation of serotonin (5-HT)1A receptors inhibits amphetamine sensitization in mice. *Life Sci* (2000) 66(11):1011–9. doi:10.1016/S0024-3205(99)00666-9
37. Hill RA. Sex differences in animal models of schizophrenia shed light on the underlying pathophysiology. *Neurosci Biobehav Rev* (2016) 67:41–56. doi:10.1016/j.neubiorev.2015.10.014
38. Segal DS, Kuczenski R, O'Neil ML, Melega WP, Cho AK. Escalating dose methamphetamine pretreatment alters the behavioral and neurochemical profiles associated with exposure to a high-dose methamphetamine binge. *Neuropsychopharmacology* (2003) 28(10):1730–40. doi:10.1038/sj.npp.1300247
39. Jaehne EJ, Klarić TS, Koblar SA, Baune BT, Lewis MD. Effects of Npas4 deficiency on anxiety, depression-like, cognition and sociability behaviour. *Behav Brain Res* (2015) 281:276–82. doi:10.1016/j.bbr.2014.12.044
40. Dawson GR, Tricklebank MD. Use of the elevated plus maze in the search for novel anxiolytic agents. *Trends Pharmacol Sci* (1995) 16(2):33–6. doi:10.1016/S0165-6147(00)88973-7

41. Wall PM, Messier C. Methodological and conceptual issues in the use of the elevated plus-maze as a psychological measurement instrument of animal anxiety-like behavior. *Neurosci Biobehav Rev* (2001) 25(3):275–86. doi:10.1016/S0149-7634(01)00013-6
42. Jaehne EJ, Baune BT. Effects of chemokine receptor signalling on cognition-like, emotion-like and sociability behaviours of CCR6 and CCR7 knockout mice. *Behav Brain Res* (2014) 261:31–9. doi:10.1016/j.bbr.2013.12.006
43. Notaras M, Hill R, Gogos JA, van den Buuse M. BDNF Val66Met genotype determines hippocampus-dependent behavior via sensitivity to glucocorticoid signaling. *Mol Psychiatry* (2016) 21(6):730–2. doi:10.1038/mp.2015.152
44. Chen ZY, Jing D, Bath KG, Ieraci A, Khan T, Siao CJ, et al. Genetic variant BDNF (Val66Met) polymorphism alters anxiety-related behavior. *Science* (2006) 314(5796):140–3. doi:10.1126/science.1129663
45. Fink KB, Gothert M. 5-HT receptor regulation of neurotransmitter release. *Pharmacol Rev* (2007) 59(4):360–417. doi:10.1124/pr.107.07103
46. Chiu HY, Chan MH, Lee MY, Chen ST, Zhan ZY, Chen HH. Long-lasting alterations in 5-HT2A receptor after a binge regimen of methamphetamine in mice. *Int J Neuropsychopharmacol* (2014) 17(10):1647–58. doi:10.1017/s1461145714000455
47. Strauss L, Brink CB, Möller M, Stein DJ, Harvey BH. Late-life effects of chronic methamphetamine exposure during puberty on behaviour and corticostriatal mono-amines in social isolation-reared rats. *Dev Neurosci* (2014) 36(1):18–28. doi:10.1159/000357495
48. Haidar M, Lam M, Chua BE, Smith CM, Gundlach AL. Sensitivity to chronic methamphetamine administration and withdrawal in mice with relaxin-3/RXFP3 deficiency. *Neurochem Res* (2016) 41(3):481–91. doi:10.1007/s11064-015-1621-2
49. Hruba L, Schutova B, Slamberova R. Sex differences in anxiety-like behavior and locomotor activity following prenatal and postnatal methamphetamine exposure in adult rats. *Physiol Behav* (2012) 105(2):364–70. doi:10.1016/j.physbeh.2011.08.016
50. Kitanaka N, Kitanaka J, Tatsuta T, Tanaka K, Watabe K, Nishiyama N, et al. Withdrawal from fixed-dose injection of methamphetamine decreases cerebral levels of 3-methoxy-4-hydroxyphenylglycol and induces the expression of anxiety-related behavior in mice. *Neurochem Res* (2010) 35(5):749–60. doi:10.1007/s11064-010-0132-4
51. Loxton D, Canales JJ. Long-term cognitive, emotional and neurogenic alterations induced by alcohol and methamphetamine exposure in adolescent rats. *Prog Neuropsychopharmacol Biol Psychiatry* (2017) 74:1–8. doi:10.1016/j.pnpbp.2016.11.003
52. Ago Y, Nakamura S, Baba A, Matsuda T. Neuropsychotoxicity of abused drugs: effects of serotonin receptor ligands on methamphetamine- and cocaine-induced behavioral sensitization in mice. *J Pharmacol Sci* (2008) 106(1):15–21. doi:10.1254/jphs.FM0070121
53. Ago Y, Koyama Y, Baba A, Matsuda T. Regulation by 5-HT1A receptors of the in vivo release of 5-HT and DA in mouse frontal cortex. *Neuropharmacology* (2003) 45(8):1050–6. doi:10.1016/S0028-3908(03)00304-6
54. Igari M, Shen HW, Hagino Y, Fukushima S, Kasahara Y, Lesch KP, et al. Attenuated methamphetamine-induced locomotor sensitization in serotonin transporter knockout mice is restored by serotonin 1B receptor antagonist treatment. *Behav Pharmacol* (2015) 26(1–2):167–79. doi:10.1097/fbp.0000000000000120
55. Przegalinski E, Siwanowicz J, Nowak E, Papla I, Filip M. Role of 5-HT(1B) receptors in the sensitization to amphetamine in mice. *Eur J Pharmacol* (2001) 422(1–3):91–9. doi:10.1016/S0014-2999(01)01079-2
56. Ago Y, Nakamura S, Kajita N, Uda M, Hashimoto H, Baba A, et al. Ritanserin reverses repeated methamphetamine-induced behavioral and neurochemical sensitization in mice. *Synapse* (2007) 61(9):757–63. doi:10.1002/syn.20421
57. Tanaka T, Ishigooka J, Watanabe S, Nagata E, Miura S. Partial inhibition of reverse tolerance by a high dose of ritanserin or low dose of haloperidol in methamphetamine-sensitized rat. *Nihon Shinkei Seishin Yakurigaku Zasshi* (1998) 18(1):1–7.

16

Age and Sex Interact to Mediate the Effects of Intermittent, High-Dose Ethanol Exposure on Behavioral Flexibility

Jacqueline M. Barker, Kathleen G. Bryant, Jennifer I. Osborne and L. J. Chandler**

Department of Neuroscience, Medical University of South Carolina, Charleston, SC, United States

Edited by:
Tod Edward Kippin,
University of California,
Santa Barbara, United States

Reviewed by:
Karen K. Szumlinski,
University of California,
Santa Barbara, United States
Scott Edwards,
LSU Health Sciences Center
New Orleans, United States

***Correspondence:**
Jacqueline M. Barker
barker.jacqui@gmail.com
L. J. Chandler
chandj@musc.edu

Human alcoholics have been shown to have impaired cognitive control over actions and increased reliance on habitual response strategies. While it is unclear in humans whether these differences predate ethanol exposure or result from chronic drinking, data from animal studies suggest that ethanol acts to promote the development of inflexible behaviors. Here, we investigated how intermittent exposure to high doses of ethanol impacts the ability to flexibly regulate behavior in a habit model. As adolescence, may represent a period of increased drug taking and developmental vulnerability that may impact adult behavior, we compared the effects of high-dose ethanol exposure during adolescence to exposure during adulthood in male and female rats. Our findings indicated that the effects of intermittent, high-dose ethanol exposure on habitual behavior is mediated by age and sex such that ethanol exposure during adolescence promoted the use of habitual response strategies in adult females, but not males, and that the opposite pattern emerged following intermittent, high-dose ethanol exposure in adult rats.

Keywords: adolescence, habit, behavioral flexibility, ethanol exposure, rat models, sex differences

INTRODUCTION

The development of alcohol use disorders is associated with a reduction in the ability to flexibly regulate behaviors. The ability to balance efficiency and flexibility in order to alter and adapt behavior is a critical function in changing environments. Shifting between cognitive regulation of behavior and inflexible stimulus-driven behavior can be modeled by the transition between goal-directed and habitual response strategies. When a new behavior is learned, it is typically performed in a goal-directed fashion. That is, behavior is performed in relationship to its outcome. After time and repeated performance, a transition to habitual response strategies may occur in which behavior is no longer mediated by its outcome.

Inflexible behavior is implicated in a number of neuropsychiatric illnesses characterized by deficits in cognitive control, such as addiction and obsessive compulsive disorder. Indeed, data from human neuroimaging studies revealed impairments in behavioral flexibility and an overreliance on habitual response strategies in abstinent alcoholics (Sjoerds et al., 2013). Though deficits in cognitive control are a hallmark of addictive disorders, it is unclear whether this phenotype is the result of chronic ethanol exposure in humans, or rather is a risk factor predating the development of alcohol use disorders. Evidence from animal models has suggested that innate individual differences in cue reactivity and incentive motivation can predict subsequent differences in drug self-administration (Flagel et al., 2009; Saunders and Robinson, 2013) as well as the development of inflexible behaviors (Barker et al., 2012, 2014). In addition, sex differences in the propensity to develop habits have been reported such that while female rodents develop sucrose-seeking habits more quickly than males (Quinn et al., 2007), male rodents show more rapid development of habitual ethanol seeking (Barker et al., 2010). It is possible that sex differences in habit formation relate to differences in motivation to consume ethanol or differences in ethanol reinforcement. While sex differences in ethanol consumption have been observed, females generally self-administer ethanol at higher rates than males (e.g., Barker et al., 2010). It is alternatively possible that sub-chronic ethanol exposure differentially impacts loss of cognitive control over actions in males versus females. Indeed, while a growing body of literature indicates that ethanol exposure itself may act to promote the development of inflexible behaviors, including habits (Corbit et al., 2012), the bulk of this research has been performed in males.

In humans, the onset of drinking behavior during adolescence is highly predictive of subsequent development of alcohol use disorders, and as such, adolescence may mark a period of unique vulnerability to the effects of alcohol on cognitive control. Adolescence is characterized by increased risk-taking (Laviola et al., 2003) and goal-seeking behavior (Doremus-Fitzwater and Spear, 2016), and adolescent males are resistant to the development of habitual ethanol seeking (Serlin and Torregrossa, 2014). Binge-like ethanol exposure during adolescence has been shown to have long-lasting effects on behavior, including impairments in fear learning and extinction (Broadwater and Spear, 2013) and in set-shifting (Gass et al., 2014). These findings suggest that the impact of ethanol exposure on the development of habitual reward seeking may not only be sex-specific, but may also depend upon the developmental age when exposure occurs. Here, we investigated how intermittent, high-dose ethanol exposure during either adolescence or adulthood impacted the development of habitual reward seeking in male and female rats.

MATERIALS AND METHODS

Animals

Male and female Long Evans rats (Harlan Labs) were delivered to the Medical University of South Carolina animal facility at either postnatal day (PND) 22 (adolescent ethanol exposure) or 60 (adult ethanol exposure). Rats were housed on a reverse light cycle with 12 h light:12 h dark. All behavioral procedures occurred during the dark cycle. Adolescent rats were housed with litter-mates of the same sex, and adult rats were pair housed unless separation was required because of injury or fighting. All procedures were conducted with approval of the Medical University of South Carolina Institutional Animal Care and Use Committee.

Intermittent Ethanol Exposure Procedure

Adolescent and adult rats assigned to undergo ethanol exposure were subjected to five cycles of ethanol exposure via vapor inhalation (**Figure 1A**). Control rats were moved to the chamber exposure room each day but did not undergo vapor inhalation of ethanol. Each cycle of ethanol exposure consisted of two consecutive episodes of exposure, with each exposure lasting 14 h in the vapor chambers (**Figure 1B**). Vapor chamber exposure began 3 h prior to the onset of the light cycle, and rats are removed from vapor chambers 1 h prior to the onset of the dark cycle at which time intoxication ratings and tail-vein blood samples are obtained. Adolescent ethanol exposure spanned the period from early to mid- adolescence (PND 28–44) and involved exposure to ethanol vapor on PND 28 and 29 (Cycle I), 31 and 32 (Cycle II), 35 and 36 (Cycle III), 38 and 39 (Cycle IV), and 42 and 43 (Cycle V). Following ethanol exposure, rats were returned to the colony where they were maintained on *ad libitum* food and water until at least PND 80. To investigate the effects of intermittent, high-dose ethanol exposure during adulthood, exposure began at PND 70 and rats were exposed to ethanol vapor on PND 70 and 71 (Cycle I), 73 and 74 (Cycle II), 77 and 78 (Cycle III), 80 and 81 (Cycle IV), and 84 and 85 (Cycle V). Rats that underwent intermittent, high-dose ethanol exposure in adulthood were maintained on *ad libitum* food and water for 36 days prior to any behavioral testing in order to match the time between adolescent ethanol exposure and assessment of the development of habitual reward seeking in adulthood. Tail vein blood was collected on a subset of ethanol vapor exposure sessions for both adolescent and adult-exposed animals in order to measure blood ethanol concentration (BEC), and the level of intoxication was determined at the end of each vapor chamber exposure using a previously described 5-point behavioral intoxication rating scale (Nixon and Crews, 2002; Gass et al., 2014) as follows: 1 = not intoxicated (no apparent signs of intoxication); 2 = low intoxication (slight motor impairment); 3 = moderate intoxication (obvious motor impairment, but able to walk); 4 = high intoxication (loss of righting reflex for >30 s, dragging of abdomen when walking, severe motor impairment, maintains eye blink reflex); 5 = extreme intoxication (loss of righting reflex, loss of eye blink reflex, may be unconscious, or difficult to arouse). We targeted intoxication ratings between 2 and 3 (low to moderate intoxication levels; **Figures 2C,D**). Targeted BECs between 250 and 350 mg/dL and low to moderate intoxication ratings were chosen to model ethanol consumption patterns in young adults drinkers. Recent reports suggest that in natural environments (i.e., at a bar) adolescent and young adults achieve estimated blood alcohol concentrations within this range (Treloar et al., 2017). Intoxication ratings have been shown previously to correlate with BEC, and indeed our findings revealed that intoxication ratings in both adolescent and adult ethanol exposed animals significantly correlated with BECs (**Figures 2E,F**). Since obtaining tail vein blood from

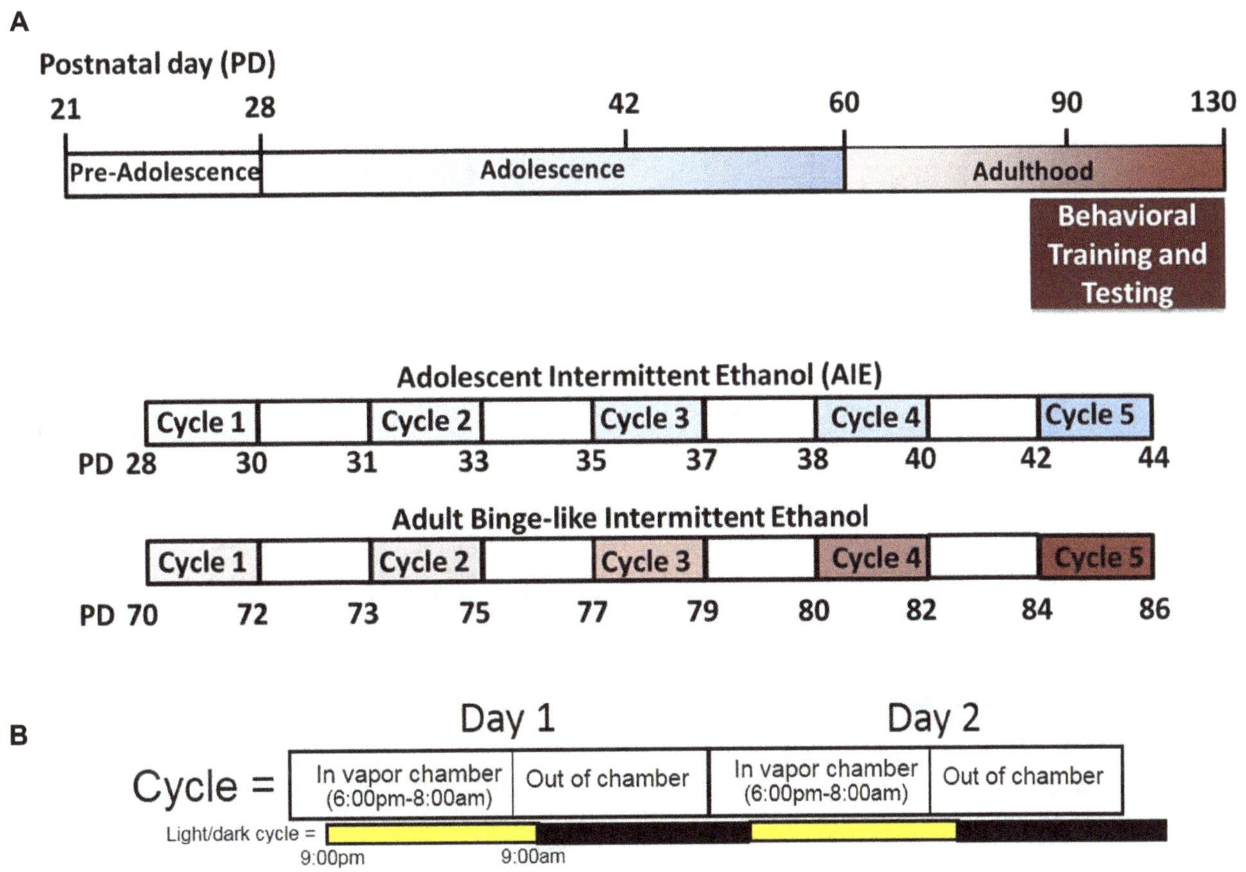

FIGURE 1 | Experimental design and time-line. **(A)** Male and female rats were exposed to intermittent ethanol exposure during either adolescence (blue) or adulthood (red). All rats underwent five cycles of exposure to ethanol. For adolescent ethanol exposed rats, exposure occurred between PND 28–44 and testing occurred after PND 80. For adult exposed rats, exposure occurred between PND 70–86 and testing occurred after PND 120. **(B)** Each cycle of ethanol exposure consisted of two 14-h exposures that began 3 h prior to the start of the light cycle and ended 1 h prior to the start of the dark cycle.

unintoxicated rats is a much more stressful procedure than it is with intoxicated rats, blood was not obtained from control rats so as not to introduce this stress as an experimental confound.

Behavioral Training and Testing

After at least 36 days from the last cycle of ethanol exposure, rats were food restricted to approximately 90% of their free feeding weights and then trained to self-administer 10% sucrose via two levers in a standard rat operant chamber from Med-Associates (St. Albans, VT, United States). Operant chambers were housed within a sound-attenuating box. Each chamber was equipped with a 28 V house light and had two retractable levers on the left and right panels of the right wall. A magazine was located at the bottom of the middle panel on the right side of the wall. Sucrose was delivered to a well in the magazine via a syringe pump housed within the sound attenuating chamber but outside of the operant box. A fan provided background noise and ventilation. No additional tones or cues were presented.

Each day, rats had a 30-min training session during which each lever was presented separately. Each lever was only available for 15 min and the order of lever availability was alternated daily. A press on either lever was initially reinforced on a fixed ratio 1 (FR1) schedule in which each lever press resulted in a single delivery of sucrose. After stable responding ($\geq$ to 3 consecutive days) of at least 30 presses per lever, reinforcement schedules were transitioned to either an action-promoting random ratio (RR) 5 or a habit-promoting random interval (RI) 30 schedule (Adams and Dickinson, 1981; Gremel and Costa, 2013). The use of these schedules enabled within-subjects assessment of response strategy under conditions where either goal-directed actions (RR schedule) or habitual response strategies were expected (RI schedule). On the RR5 schedule, the number of lever presses controlled reinforcer delivery. On average, the fifth response was reinforced, but the program software randomly generated the actual response requirement. On the RI30 schedule, the first lever pressed after a randomly determined interval (averaging 30 s) had elapsed was reinforced. Unlike the RR schedule, reinforcer delivery on the RI schedule was not related to the number of lever presses. The response schedule assigned to each lever was consistent across training for each animal (i.e., left lever was always the

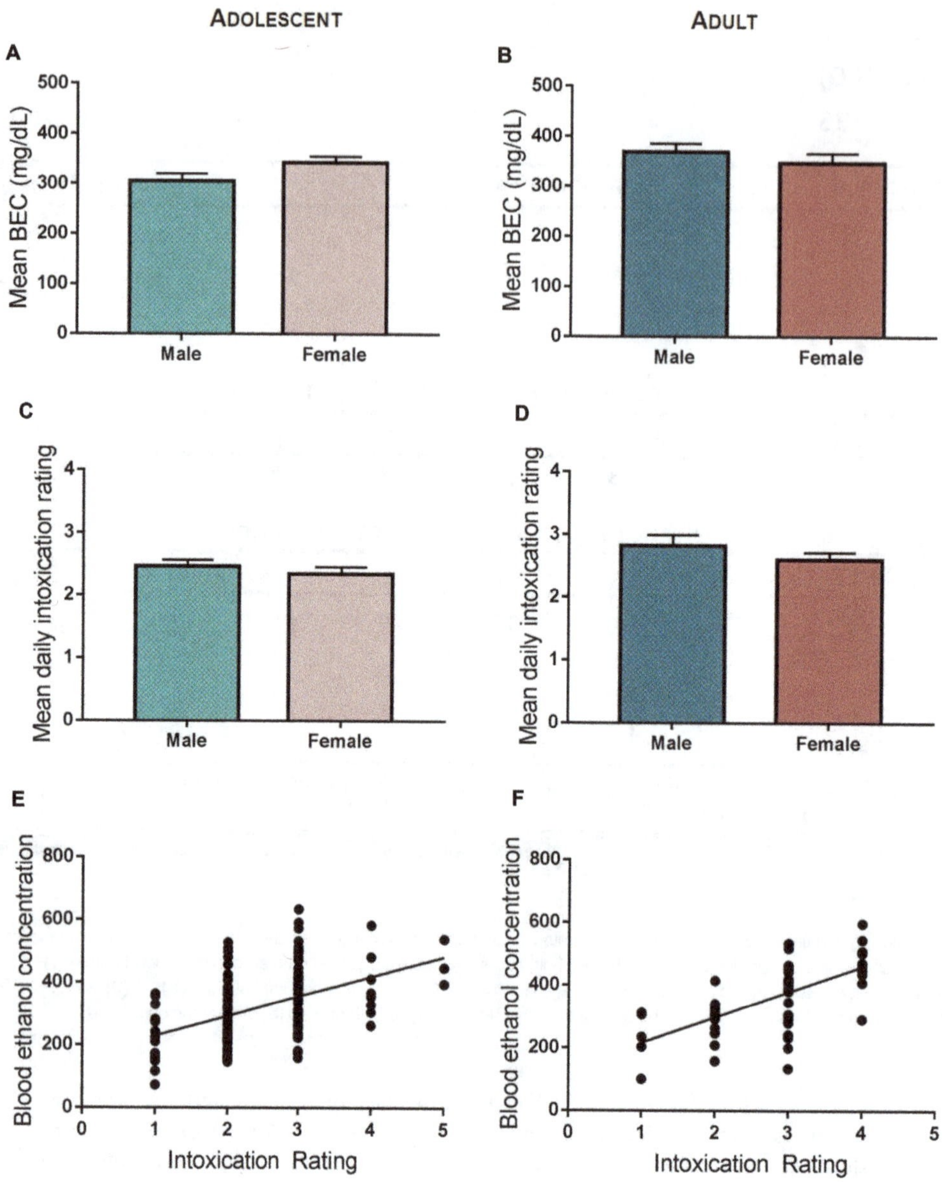

FIGURE 2 | Ethanol vapor exposure. Mean intoxication ratings were comparable for adolescent **(A)** and adult **(B)** ethanol exposed rats and did not differ between male and female rats. Male and female rats had similar blood ethanol levels during adolescent **(C)** or adult **(D)** ethanol vapor exposure. BECs and intoxication ratings were significantly correlated in both adolescent exposed **(E)** and adult exposed rats **(F)**.

'interval' lever and right lever was always the 'ratio' lever). After two sessions on the RR5/RI30 schedules, these were transitioned to RR10 and RI60 schedules for an additional eight sessions.

Following eight sessions on the RR10/RI60 schedule, response strategy was assessed using a specific satiety outcome devaluation procedure. Because habits are by definition insensitive to changes in outcome value, devaluation procedures enable the determination of whether rats are relying on habitual response strategies in which responding is unaffected by devaluation, or are using goal-directed strategies in which reward seeking behavior is reduced following devaluation. Rats underwent both a 'non-devalued' and 'devalued' testing procedure for the RR and RI levers. During the 'devalued' condition, rats received access to a 10% sucrose bottle for 1 h prior to a 10 min test session in a novel cage. During these test sessions, conditions were identical to training except that they were performed in extinction in which lever presses did not result in reinforcer delivery. Following this test session, rats were again provided 1-h access to a 10% sucrose bottle to confirm devaluation. In the 'non-devalued' condition, rats received 1-h access to home cage chow prior to testing. Between all devaluation tests, rats had 1 additional training session on the RR10/RI60 schedule and the order of testing was counterbalanced.

Statistical Analyses

Analysis was performed in SPSS using repeated measures ANOVA and *t*-tests as appropriate. *Post hoc t*-test comparisons were Bonferroni corrected.

RESULTS

Intoxication Ratings

Comparison of daily intoxication ratings with BEC values across groups revealed no difference between male and females, or between adult and adolescent rats. Data were collapsed across exposure cycles for analysis. Neither mean BECs nor intoxication ratings significantly differed between males and females in adolescent rats ($t = 0.1828$, $p > 0.5$; $t = 0.755$, $p > 0.4$; **Figures 2A,C**) or in adult rats ($t = 0.876$, $p > 0.3$; $t = 1.084$, $p > 0.2$, respectively; **Figures 2B,D**). Intoxication ratings and BECs were positively correlated on days that BEC's were taken, indicating that intoxication ratings reliably reflect BEC (adolescent ethanol exposure, Pearson's correlation, $r^2 = 0.208$, $p < 0.001$; adult ethanol exposure, Pearson's correlation, $r^2 = 0.407$; $p < 0.001$; **Figures 2E,F**).

Acquisition of Sucrose Seeking

Adolescent Ethanol Exposure

A rmANOVA on total lever presses across acquisition indicated main effects of reinforcement schedule [$F(1,37) = 26.233$, $p < 0.001$] and day of training [$F(12,444) = 50.527$, $p < 0.001$]. In addition, significant interactions between schedule, day of training, and sex were observed [$F(12, 444) = 2.427$, $p < 0.01$], as well as schedule x day x ethanol exposure [$F(12,444) = 3.104, p < 0.001$]. Follow-up rmANOVA indicated that in male rats, reinforcement schedule, ethanol exposure, and day of training interact to moderate responding [$F(12,228) = 2.656, p < 0.01$]. *Post hoc* comparisons further indicated that in air control males, responding on the RR vs RI levers was significantly different on days 3, 10, 11, 12, and 13 of training (*p*-values < 0.05; **Figure 3A**). In contrast, in ethanol exposed rats, responding differed on RR and RI levers only on day 2 and 12 of training (*p*-values < 0.05). In females, ethanol exposure did not impact responding during acquisition [main effect $p > 0.2$, no significant interactions], but a schedule by day interaction was present [$F(12, 216) = 5.070, p < 0.001$]. Follow-up comparisons indicated differences in responses on the RI vs RR lever on days 11, 12, and 13 for female rats ($p < 0.05$; **Figure 3B**).

Adult Ethanol Exposure

A rmANOVA on total lever presses across acquisition indicated a main effect of schedule on responding [$F(1,26) = 4.723$, $p < 0.05$] and a main effect of day of training [$F(12,312) = 17.437$, $p < 0.001$], consistent with an increase in responding across training. In addition, a significant day x sex interaction was observed [$F(12, 312) = 2.843, p < 0.01$] as well as a reinforcement schedule x day of training interaction [$F(12,312) = 3.102$, $p < 0.001$]. No significant main effect of ethanol exposure was observed [$F(1,26) = 0.243$, $p > 0.6$], and no significant ethanol exposure interactions were observed with any other measures (*p*-values > 0.4). In male rats, no main effect of schedule [$F(1,12) = 0.505$, $p > 0.4$] or schedule × day interaction were observed [$F(12,180) = 0.605$, $p > 0.8$] indicating comparable levels of responding on the RR and RI schedules. However, a main effect of day was observed [$F(12,180) = 5.529$, $p < 0.001$] consistent with increased responding across training (**Figure 3C**). In female rats, in addition to a significant effect of day [$F(12,156) = 12.724$, $p < 0.001$], a significant schedule × day interaction was observed [$F(12,156) = 3.4$, $p < 0.001$], indicating that response rates were distinct on RI and RR schedules. While a main effect of schedule [$F(1,156) = 4.591$, $p = 0.05$] is consistent with a higher response rate on the RR schedule than the RI schedule, post-hoc comparisons did not indicate significant differences in responding on the RR versus RI schedule on individual days of training (**Figure 3D**).

Adolescent Ethanol Exposure Promoted Used of Habitual Response Strategies in Females

For adult rats exposed to alcohol during adolescence, a rmANOVA of response rates during the outcome devaluation test indicated a reinforcement schedule × devaluation × ethanol exposure interaction [$F(1,41) = 5.621$, $p < 0.05$] as well as a significant schedule × devaluation interaction [$F(1,41) = 9.791$, $p < 0.01$]. Main effects of reinforcement schedule [$F(1,41) = 11.947$, $p < 0.01$] and devaluation [$F(1,41) = 27.303$, $p < 0.001$] were also observed. Follow-up comparisons indicated that in males, no main effect of ethanol exposure [$F(1,21) = 0.035, p > 0.8$] or interactions with ethanol exposure were observed (*p*-values > 0.2). A significant schedule × devaluation was observed [$F(1,21) = 7.928, p < 0.01$], as well as main effects of schedule [$F(1,21) = 8.407$, $p < 0.01$] and devaluation [$F(1,21) = 15.417, p < 0.001$]. *Post hoc* analyses indicated no difference between response rates on the RI lever during valued versus devalued conditions ($p > 0.3$), consistent with habitual behavior. In contrast, response rates on the RR lever were lower during the devalued test than the valued test ($p < 0.01$; **Figure 4A**), consistent with goal-directed behavior. In female rats, a schedule × devaluation × ethanol exposure interaction was indicated by rmANOVA [$F(1,20) = 4.709$, $p < 0.05$], as well as a devaluation × ethanol exposure interaction [$F(1,20) = 2.37, p < 0.05$). In addition, a significant main effect of devaluation was observed [$F(1,20) = 12.013$, $p < 0.01$]. Subsequent comparisons indicated that adolescent air exposed female rats exhibited habitual responding on the RI lever and did not change response rates when the outcome was devalued ($p > 0.4$). In contrast, air exposed females exhibited goal-directed reward seeking on the RR lever and lower response rates on the RR lever ($p < 0.05$). Female rats that had been subjected to intermittent, high-dose ethanol exposure during adolescence, however, showed habitual behavior on both the RR and RI levers ($p > 0.8$ and $p > 0.1$, respectively), consistent with increased reliance on habitual

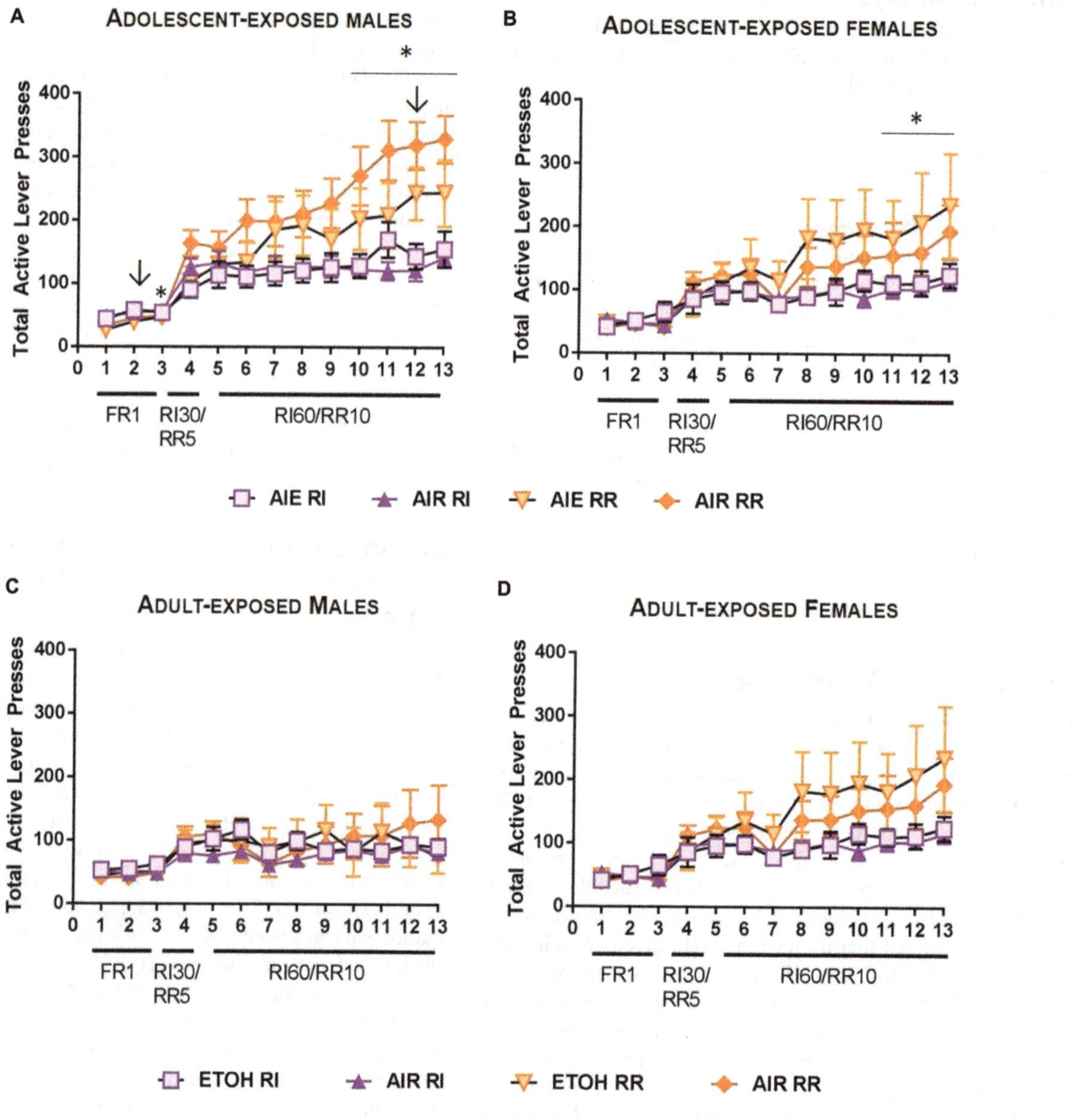

FIGURE 3 | Acquisition of sucrose seeking in rats exposed to ethanol. **(A)** In adult male rats that had been subject to adolescent intermittent ethanol (AIE), responding on the RR lever was significantly higher than responding on the RI lever on days 2 and 12 (arrows). In control (AIR) male rats, responding was significantly higher on the RR lever on days 3, and 10–13. **(B)** In adult female rats that had been subject to AIE, no differences in response rates were observed between AIE and AIR exposed rats. Responding was significantly higher on the RR lever than the RI lever on the final 3 days or RI60/RR10 responding for both groups. **(C)** In male rats subjected to intermittent ethanol (ETOH) exposure in adulthood, no differences in responding between ethanol-exposed and control rats were observed, nor did adult ethanol exposure alter response rates on the RR and RI levers. **(D)** In female rats exposed to ethanol in adulthood, no significant differences in responding on RR versus RI levers were observed. ↓$p < 0.05$; *$p < 0.05$.

response strategies in female rats following adolescent ethanol exposure (**Figure 4B**).

Adult Ethanol Exposure Promoted the Use of Habitual Response Strategies in Males

For rats exposed to ethanol during adulthood, a rmANOVA of response rates during the outcome devaluation tests indicated a four-way interaction between schedule × sex × ethanol exposure × devaluation [$F(1,26) = 4.276$, $p < 0.05$], as well as a main effect of schedule [$F(1,26) = 13.378$, $p < 0.01$], a schedule × sex interaction [$F(1,26) = 9.216$, $p < 0.01$] and a devaluation × schedule interaction [$F(1,26) = 4.725$, $p < 0.05$]. No main effect of devaluation was present [$F(1,26) = 1.78$, $p = 0.194$] or main effect of ethanol exposure [$F(1,26) = 1.172$, $p = 0.289$]. There was however, a main effect of sex on response rates [$F(1,26) = 7.566$, $p < 0.05$].

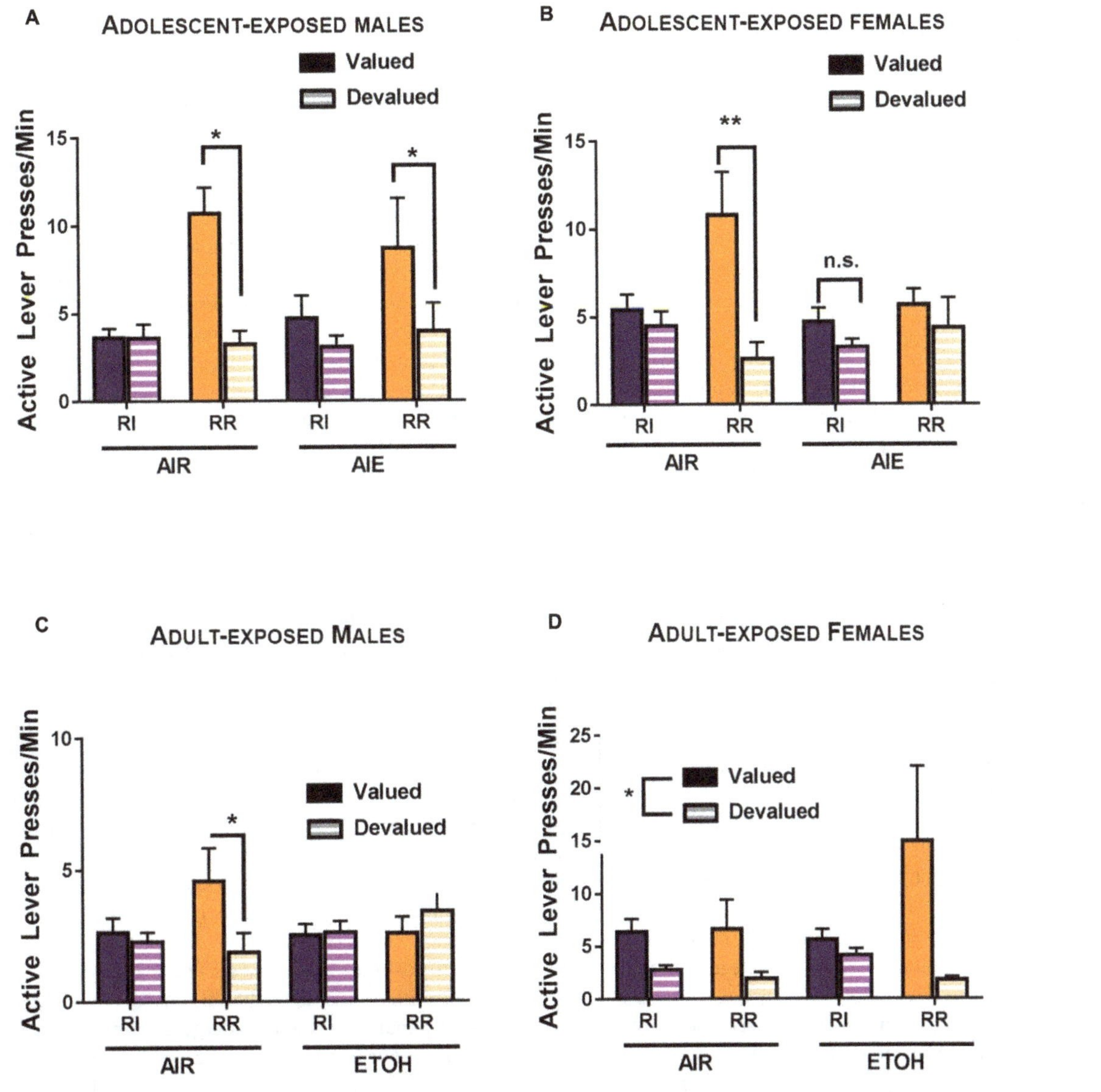

FIGURE 4 | Response strategy selection in an outcome devaluation test in adult rats following ethanol exposure. **(A)** In adult male rats, responding on the RI habit-promoting lever was habitual in both air control and AIE exposed groups, as evidenced by a lack of reduction in response rate when the outcome was devalued by specific satiety. In contrast, responding on the RR lever was goal-directed (sensitive to outcome devaluation) in male rats in both the control (AIR) and ethanol exposed groups. **(B)** AIR exposed female rats showed similar patterns of responding to males. In control female rats, responding on the RI schedule was habitual (i.e., was insensitive to outcome devaluation), while responding on the RR lever was goal-directed and sensitive to outcome devaluation. In contrast, AIE exposed females showed habitual response strategies on both the RI lever and the RR lever; responding on both the RR and RI levers was insensitive to outcome devaluation. **(C)** Air exposed male rats were insensitive to outcome devaluation on the RI lever, consistent with habitual behavior, but were sensitive to outcome devaluation on the RR lever, indicative of goal-directed actions. In contrast, adult ETOH exposed males were insensitive to outcome devaluation on both levers, indicative of habitual response strategies during responding in both action- and habit-promoting conditions. **(D)** In female rats, a main effect of devaluation was present, indicating lower response rates during devaluation in all conditions. This was not mediated by schedule or adult ethanol exposure. *$p < 0.05$.

To deconstruct significant interactions, rmANOVAs were performed separately on response rates for male and female rats. In male rats, this analysis revealed a significant interaction of schedule × devaluation × ethanol exposure [$F(1,14) = 7.349$, $p < 0.05$] and a schedule × ethanol interaction [$F(1,14) = 5.847$, $p < 0.05$]. *Post hoc* analysis indicated no significant effect of devaluation on responding on the RI schedule for ethanol exposed ($p > 0.8$) or air exposed males ($p > 0.4$). In contrast, air exposed control males showed lower rates of responding on the devalued lever in the RR schedule ($p < 0.5$) (**Figure 4C**), indicative of goal-directed behavior. In adult ethanol exposed males, however, response rates did not differ between the valued and devalued conditions on the RR schedule ($p > 0.2$), indicative of habitual responding on the 'action-promoting' lever.

In female rats, rmANOVA indicated a main effect of devaluation [$F(1,12) = 10.295, p < 0.01$), and a non-significant trend toward a devaluation x schedule interaction [$F(1,12) = 3.299, p = 0.09$) (**Figure 4D**), suggesting that ethanol exposure in adult females did not impact response strategy selection.

DISCUSSION

Our findings indicate that age and sex interact to determine the effects of intermittent, high-dose ethanol exposure on habitual behavior. In particular, we found that intermittent ethanol exposure during adolescence promoted the reliance on habitual response strategies in female rats, while response strategy was not impacted in males. In contrast, exposure to ethanol in adulthood using an identical exposure paradigm was associated with facilitation of habit formation in males but not females. These findings suggest that while intermittent high-dose ethanol exposure altered the ability to flexibly regulate behavior, the effect is dependent upon the age of ethanol exposure as well as sex.

In the adult exposure paradigm, air exposed control males exhibited habitual reward seeking when responding on an interval (habit promoting) schedule, but retained sensitivity to outcome devaluation on a ratio (action promoting) schedule. In males that were exposed to ethanol during adulthood, however, outcome devaluation had no impact on responding on either the RI or the RR schedule, indicating a greater propensity toward habitual response strategies. Female rats showed no effect of adult ethanol exposure on response strategy selection. Given previous reports that adult males develop ethanol seeking habits more rapidly than sucrose seeking habits (Dickinson et al., 2002), and that males form ethanol seeking habits more quickly than females (Barker et al., 2010), these data suggest that in adults, intermittent ethanol exposure may act to promote habitual response strategies in males but not females.

As with investigation of the consequences of adolescent ethanol exposure in females, there is a paucity of data describing sex differences in the impact of intermittent ethanol exposure in adult animals. Current findings suggest that males and females may be differentially sensitive to the both the aversive and rewarding effects of ethanol exposure. For example, while both adult males and females exhibit increases in anxiety following a bout of intoxication, this effect is exaggerated in adult males (Varlinskaya and Spear, 2004). This study also observed protracted elevation in BECs in adult males as compared to adult females, and that this effect was absent in adolescents (Varlinskaya and Spear, 2004). Together with additional literature demonstrating more rapid recovery from early withdrawal in females than in males (Devaud and Chadda, 2001), these findings suggest that adult males may be differentially sensitive to repeated bouts of intoxication and withdrawal than females. Consistent with these sex differences, male rats show persistent elevations in corticosterone following ethanol withdrawal, while corticosterone levels return to baseline in females (Alele and Devaud, 2006). Because chronic corticosterone itself can facilitate reliance on habitual response strategies in males (Gourley et al., 2012; Swanson et al., 2013), it is possible that repeated ethanol intoxication and withdrawal in adult males facilitates habitual behavior via its effects on the glucocorticoid system.

Interestingly, adolescent ethanol exposed male rats did not differ in response strategy selection compared to air exposed controls when tested in adulthood. Both ethanol-exposed and air control males showed habitual response strategies on the interval schedule and goal-directed actions when responding on the ratio schedule. Adolescent males have been shown to be resistant to habitual ethanol seeking relative to adult males (Serlin and Torregrossa, 2014), which is consistent with increased goal-oriented behavior in adolescent males (Doremus-Fitzwater and Spear, 2016). This suggests that ethanol exposure may not act on neurocircuitry to facilitate habit formation and expression in adolescent males in the same way it does in adults (Dickinson et al., 2002; Barker et al., 2010; Corbit et al., 2012). While a number of groups have identified protracted adolescent-like phenotypes following binge-like and intermittent ethanol exposure, our findings were not consistent with this in regard to response strategy selection. We observed that adult males were capable of habit formation following adolescent ethanol exposure – i.e., male rats showed habitual responding under habit-promoting conditions - and thus did not exhibit an adolescent-like resistance to habit formation.

In contrast to our observations in male rats, adolescent ethanol-exposed female rats demonstrated facilitated habitual reward seeking in adulthood. The precise timing of ethanol exposure during adolescence has been shown to have distinct effects on adult behavior (Spear, 2015). In particular, ethanol exposure in early adolescence that encompasses the onset of puberty may have greater effects on adult behavior than ethanol exposure restricted to later adolescence (Spear, 2015). It is possible that the sex differences we observed result from differences in pubertal onset – females mature more rapidly than males and undergo puberty earlier than male rats. Because our ethanol vapor procedure is restricted to early- to mid- adolescence (i.e., is ended at PND 44), this period encompasses the pubertal maturation period of female rats, but may not cover the entire pubertal period of male rats. The timing of drug alcohol exposure relative to puberty may mediate the effect of exposure on neuronal maturation. For example, the effects of amphetamine withdrawal on dopamine receptor expression in the medial prefrontal cortex (mPFC) was dependent upon the timing of drug exposure such that reductions in dopamine D1 receptors in mPFC occurred only in animals exposed to amphetamine prior to pubertal onset (Kang et al., 2016). Recent studies from our lab also suggest that intermittent ethanol exposure during this time period of development in males resulted in profound changes in dopamine neurotransmission in the prelimbic cortex, including reductions in both D1 receptor expression and expression of COMT, which together with the norepinephrine transporter, is the primary mediator of the extracellular levels of dopamine in the PFC (Trantham-Davidson et al., 2017). It is important to note that to date,investigation of dopamine system alterations following intermittent ethanol exposure in this model is largely limited tomales, and the effects of adolescent ethanol exposure on mPFC dopamine neurotransmission in females is poorly understood. Prefrontal dopamine signaling regulates behavioral flexibility and cognitive control in a number of different tasks including impairments in the ability to detect change in reward value (Winter et al., 2009) and set shifting (Floresco et al., 2006). It has also previously been reported that mPFC dopamine signaling can acutely and bidirectionally regulate habitual reward seeking (Barker et al., 2013). Importantly, changes in dopamine signaling following intermittent ethanol exposure are long lasting. Though findings on the role of PFC dopamine signaling specifically are lacking, chronic changes in dopamine following chronic cocaine (Halbout et al., 2016) or amphetamine (Nelson and Killcross, 2006) are known to promote reliance on habit-like response strategies that are PFC-dependent (Nelson and Killcross, 2013).

In addition to changes in prefrontal dopamine signaling, intermittent ethanol exposure during adolescence has been shown to disrupt GABAergic neurotransmission in the PFC in both male and female adult rats (Centanni et al., 2017; Trantham-Davidson et al., 2017), including impairments in tonic $GABA_A$ currents (Centanni et al., 2017). Normal maturation of the mPFC GABA system has been shown to be required for appropriate goal-directed behaviors in adulthood (Butkovich et al., 2015), suggesting that alterations in $GABA_A$ signaling following adolescent alcohol exposure could contribute to the alterations in response strategy selection in adulthood observed in the present study. However, the absence of sex differences in tonic GABA current in the Centanni et al. (1999) study suggests that dysregulation of GABAergic transmission in the PFC following adolescent ethanol exposure is unlikely to explain the increased reliance on habitual response strategies in female rats. Interestingly, sex-specific effects of adult ethanol exposure on $GABA_A$ receptor subunit expression have been reported (Devaud et al., 1999). Female ethanol withdrawn rats show inceased sensitivity to neuroactive steroids thought to act at.

SUMMARY AND IMPLICATIONS

The ability to toggle between actions and habits is critical to maximize behavioral efficiency. Our findings indicate that intermittent, high-dose ethanol exposure impacts the ability to flexibly regulate behavior in a sex- and age- dependent manner. We observed that high-dose ethanol exposure during adolescence promoted reliance on habitual response strategy in adult female but not male rats. In contrast, this same intermittent, high-dose ethanol exposure paradigm in adults facilitated the use of habits in male but not female rats. Together, these findings point to a need for an increased understanding of sex differences in the impact of drugs and alcohol on the neurocircuits that mediate cognitive control and behavioral flexibility, and how restricted access to drugs and alcohol may have long-lasting effects on the plasticity and function of these circuits.

AUTHOR CONTRIBUTIONS

JB, JO, KB performed the experiments. JB and LC designed the experiments and wrote the manuscript.

ACKNOWLEDGMENTS

We thank the members of the Chandler lab for their assistance with ethanol vapor exposure procedures. This work was supported by NIH grants AA023141 and AA024499 (JB) and AA010761 (LC).

REFERENCES

Adams, C., and Dickinson, A. (1981). "Actions and habits: variations in associative representations during instrumental learning," in *Information Processing in Animals: Memory Mechanisms*, eds N. E. Spear and R. R. Miller (Hillsdale, NJ: Erlbaum).

Alele, P. E., and Devaud, L. L. (2006). Sex differences in steroid modulation of ethanol withdrawal in male and female rats. *J. Pharmacol. Exp. Ther.* 320, 427–436. doi: 10.1124/jpet.106.107896

Barker, J. M., Torregrossa, M. M., Arnold, A. P., and Taylor, J. R. (2010). Dissociation of genetic and hormonal influences on sex differences in alcoholism-related behaviors. *J. Neurosci.* 30, 9140–9144. doi: 10.1523/JNEUROSCI.0548-10.2010

Barker, J. M., Torregrossa, M. M., and Taylor, J. R. (2012). Low prefrontal PSA-NCAM confers risk for alcoholism-related behavior. *Nat. Neurosci.* 15, 1356–1358. doi: 10.1038/nn.3194

Barker, J. M., Torregrossa, M. M., and Taylor, J. R. (2013). Bidirectional modulation of infralimbic dopamine D1 and D2 receptor activity regulates flexible reward seeking. *Front. Neurosci.* 7:126. doi: 10.3389/fnins.2013.00126

Barker, J. M., Zhang, H., Villafane, J. J., Wang, T. L., Torregrossa, M. M., and Taylor, J. R. (2014). Epigenetic and pharmacological regulation of 5HT3 receptors controls compulsive ethanol seeking in mice. *Eur. J. Neurosci.* 39, 999–1008. doi: 10.1111/ejn.12477

Broadwater, M., and Spear, L. P. (2013). Consequences of ethanol exposure on cued and contextual fear conditioning and extinction differ depending on timing of exposure during adolescence or adulthood. *Behav. Brain Res.* 256, 10–19. doi: 10.1016/j.bbr.2013.08.013

Butkovich, L. M., DePoy, L. M., Allen, A. G., Shapiro, L. P., Swanson, A. M., and Gourley, S. L. (2015). Adolescent-onset GABAA α1 silencing regulates reward-related decision making. *Eur. J. Neurosci.* 42, 2114–2121. doi: 10.1111/ejn.12995

Centanni, S. W., Burnett, E. J., Trantham-Davidson, H., and Chandler, L. J. (2017). Loss of δ-GABA A receptor-mediated tonic currents in the adult prelimbic cortex following adolescent alcohol exposure. *Addict. Biol.* 22, 616–628. doi: 10.1111/adb.12353

Corbit, L. H., Nie, H., and Janak, P. H. (2012). Habitual alcohol seeking: time course and the contribution of subregions of the dorsal striatum. *Biol. Psychiatry* 72, 389–395. doi: 10.1016/j.biopsych.2012.02.024

Devaud, L. L., and Chadda, R. (2001). Sex differences in rats in the development of and recovery from ethanol dependence assessed by changes in seizure susceptibility. *Alcohol. Clin. Exp. Res.* 25, 1689–1696. doi: 10.1111/j.1530-0277.2001.tb02176.x

Devaud, L. L., Matthews, D. B., and Morrow, A. L. (1999). Gender impacts behavioral and neurochemical adaptations in ethanol-dependent rats. *Pharmacol. Biochem. Behav.* 64, 841–849. doi: 10.1016/S0091-3057(99)00164-1

Dickinson, A., Wood, N., and Smith, J. W. (2002). Alcohol seeking by rats: action or habit? *Q. J. Exp. Psychol. B* 55, 331–348. doi: 10.1080/02724990244 00016

Doremus-Fitzwater, T. L., and Spear, L. P. (2016). Reward-centricity and attenuated aversions: an adolescent phenotype emerging from studies in laboratory animals. *Neurosci. Biobehav. Rev.* 70, 121–134. doi: 10.1016/j.neubiorev.2016. 08.015

Flagel, S. B., Akil, H., and Robinson, T. E. (2009). Neuropharmacology individual differences in the attribution of incentive salience to reward-related cues: implications for addiction. *Neuropharmacology* 56, 139–148. doi: 10.1016/j. neuropharm.2008.06.027

Floresco, S. B., Magyar, O., Ghods-Sharifi, S., Vexelman, C., and Tse, M. T. L. (2006). Multiple dopamine receptor subtypes in the medial prefrontal cortex of the rat regulate set-shifting. *Neuropsychopharmacology* 31, 297–309. doi: 10.1038/sj.npp.1300825

Gass, J. T., Glen, W. B., McGonigal, J. T., Trantham-Davidson, H., Lopez, M. F., Randall, P. K., et al. (2014). Adolescent alcohol exposure reduces behavioral flexibility, promotes disinhibition, and increases resistance to extinction of ethanol self-administration in adulthood. *Neuropsychopharmacology* 39, 2570–2583. doi: 10.1038/npp.2014.109

Gourley, S. L., Swanson, A. M., Jacobs, A. M., Howell, J. L., Mo, M., Dileone, R. J., et al. (2012). Action control is mediated by prefrontal BDNF and glucocorticoid receptor binding. *Proc. Natl. Acad. Sci. U.S.A.* 109, 20714–20719. doi: 10.1073/ pnas.1208342109

Gremel, C. M., and Costa, R. M. (2013). Orbitofrontal and striatal circuits dynamically encode the shift between goal-directed and habitual actions. *Nat. Commun.* 4:2264. doi: 10.1038/ncomms3264

Halbout, B., Liu, A. T., and Ostlund, S. B. (2016). A closer look at the effects of repeated cocaine exposure on adaptive decision-making under conditions that promote goal-directed control. *Front. Psychiatry* 7:44. doi: 10.3389/fpsyt.2016. 00044

Kang, S., Wu, M. M., Galvez, R., and Gulley, J. M. (2016). Timing of amphetamine exposure in relation to puberty onset determines its effects on anhedonia, exploratory behavior, and dopamine D1 receptor expression in young adulthood. *Neuroscience* 339, 72–84. doi: 10.1016/j.neuroscience.2016. 09.044

Laviola, G., Macrì, S., Morley-Fletcher, S., and Adriani, W. (2003). Risk-taking behavior in adolescent mice: psychobiological determinants and early epigenetic influence. *Neurosci. Biobehav. Rev.* 27, 19–31. doi: 10.1016/S0149-7634(03)00006-X

Nelson, A., and Killcross, S. (2006). Amphetamine exposure enhances habit formation. *J. Neurosci.* 26, 3805–3812. doi: 10.1523/JNEUROSCI.4305-05.2006

Nelson, A. J. D., and Killcross, S. (2013). Accelerated habit formation following amphetamine exposure is reversed by D1, but enhanced by D2, receptor antagonists. *Front. Neurosci.* 7:76. doi: 10.3389/fnins.2013. 00076

Nixon, K., and Crews, F. T. (2002). Binge ethanol exposure decreases neurogenesis in adult rat hippocampus. *J. Neurochem.* 83, 1087–1093. doi: 10.1046/j.1471-4159.2002.01214.x

Quinn, J. J., Hitchcott, P. K., Umeda, E. A., Arnold, A. P., and Taylor, J. R. (2007). Sex chromosome complement regulates habit formation. *Nat. Neurosci.* 10, 1398–1400. doi: 10.1038/nn1994

Saunders, B. T., and Robinson, T. E. (2013). Individual variation in resisting temptation: implications for addiction. *Neurosci. Biobehav. Rev.* 37(9 Pt A), 1955–1975. doi: 10.1016/j.neubiorev.2013.02.008

Serlin, H., and Torregrossa, M. M. (2014). Adolescent rats are resistant to forming ethanol seeking habits. *Dev. Cogn. Neurosci.* 16, 183–190. doi: 10.1016/j.dcn. 2014.12.002

Sjoerds, Z., de Wit, S., van den Brink, W., Robbins, T. W., Beekman, A. T. F., Penninx, B. W. J. H., et al. (2013). Behavioral and neuroimaging evidence for overreliance on habit learning in alcohol-dependent patients. *Transl. Psychiatry* 3, e337. doi: 10.1038/tp.2013.107

Spear, L. P. (2015). Adolescent alcohol exposure: are there separable vulnerable periods within adolescence? *Physiol. Behav.* 148, 122–130. doi: 10.1016/j. physbeh.2015.01.027

Swanson, A. M., Shapiro, L. P., Whyte, A. J., and Gourley, S. L. (2013). Glucocorticoid receptor regulation of action selection and prefrontal cortical dendritic spines. *Commun. Integr. Biol.* 6:e26068. doi: 10.4161/cib.26068

Trantham-Davidson, H., Centanni, S. W., Garr, S. C., New, N. N., Mulholland, P. J., Gass, J. T., et al. (2017). Binge-like alcohol exposure during adolescence disrupts dopaminergic neurotransmission in the adult prelimbic cortex. *Neuropsychopharmacology* 42, 1024–1036. doi: 10.1038/npp.2016.190

Treloar, H., Celio, M. A., Lisman, S. A., Miranda, R., and Spear, L. P. (2017). Subjective alcohol responses in a cross-sectional, field-based study of adolescents and young adults: effects of age, drinking level, and dependence/consequences. *Drug Alcohol Depend.* 170, 156–163. doi: 10.1016/ j.drugalcdep.2016.11.009

Varlinskaya, E. I., and Spear, L. P. (2004). Acute ethanol withdrawal (hangover) and social behavior in adolescent and adult male and female Sprague-Dawley rats. *Alcohol Clin. Exp. Res.* 28, 40–50. doi: 10.1097/01.ALC.0000108655.51087.DF

Winter, S., Dieckmann, M., and Schwabe, K. (2009). Dopamine in the prefrontal cortex regulates rats behavioral flexibility to changing reward value. *Behav. Brain Res.* 198, 206–213. doi: 10.1016/j.bbr.2008.10.040

17

Adolescent Executive Dysfunction in Daily Life: Relationships to Risks, Brain Structure and Substance Use

Duncan B. Clark[1], Tammy Chung[1], Christopher S. Martin[1], Brant P. Hasler[1], Douglas H. Fitzgerald[1], Beatriz Luna[1], Sandra A. Brown[2], Susan F. Tapert[2], Ty Brumback[2], Kevin Cummins[2], Adolf Pfefferbaum[3,4], Edith V. Sullivan[4], Kilian M. Pohl[3], Ian M. Colrain[3], Fiona C. Baker[3], Michael D. De Bellis[5], Kate B. Nooner[6] and Bonnie J. Nagel[7]*

[1] Department of Psychiatry, University of Pittsburgh, Pittsburgh, PA, United States, [2] Department of Psychology and Psychiatry, University of California, San Diego, La Jolla, CA, United States, [3] Center for Health Sciences, SRI International, Menlo Park, CA, United States, [4] Department of Psychiatry and Behavioral Sciences, School of Medicine, Stanford University, Palo Alto, CA, United States, [5] Department of Psychiatry, Duke University, Durham, NC, United States, [6] Department of Psychology, University of North Carolina Wilmington, Wilmington, NC, United States, [7] Department of Psychiatry, Oregon Health and Science University, Portland, OR, United States

Edited by:
Shannon Leigh Gourley,
Emory University School of Medicine,
United States

Reviewed by:
Frauke Nees,
Zentralinstitut für Seelische Gesundheit, Germany
Christos Frantzidis,
Aristotle University of Thessaloniki, Greece

***Correspondence:**
Duncan B. Clark
clarkdb@upmc.edu

During adolescence, problems reflecting cognitive, behavioral and affective dysregulation, such as inattention and emotional dyscontrol, have been observed to be associated with substance use disorder (SUD) risks and outcomes. Prior studies have typically been with small samples, and have typically not included comprehensive measurement of executive dysfunction domains. The relationships of executive dysfunction in daily life with performance based testing of cognitive skills and structural brain characteristics, thought to be the basis for executive functioning, have not been definitively determined. The aims of this study were to determine the relationships between executive dysfunction in daily life, measured by the Behavior Rating Inventory of Executive Function (BRIEF), cognitive skills and structural brain characteristics, and SUD risks, including a global SUD risk indicator, sleep quality, and risky alcohol and cannabis use. In addition to bivariate relationships, multivariate models were tested. The subjects ($n = 817$; ages 12 through 21) were participants in the National Consortium on Alcohol and Neurodevelopment in Adolescence (NCANDA) study. The results indicated that executive dysfunction was significantly related to SUD risks, poor sleep quality, risky alcohol use and cannabis use, and was not significantly related to cognitive skills or structural brain characteristics. In multivariate models, the relationship between poor sleep quality and risky substance use was mediated by executive dysfunction. While these cross-sectional relationships need to be further examined in longitudinal analyses, the results suggest that poor sleep quality and executive dysfunction may be viable preventive intervention targets to reduce adolescent substance use.

Keywords: adolescents, executive functioning, neurocognitive testing, neuroimaging, alcohol

INTRODUCTION

Executive functioning is a broad construct comprised of behavioral competencies and cognitive skills, including attention, inhibition, mental flexibility, working memory, self-monitoring, planning, and emotional control (Chan et al., 2008). These self-control capabilities and higher order cognitive skills support the optimization of responding to environmental and personal challenges so as to maximize reward opportunities and achieve long-term goals (Best and Miller, 2010; Diamond and Lee, 2011). Problems in executive functioning in daily life (i.e., executive dysfunction) and cognitive skills assessed by performance-based testing may, in fact, reflect different constructs.

Characteristics reflecting executive dysfunction has been found to be associated with substance use disorder (SUD) risks and outcomes (Clark and Winters, 2002; Tarter et al., 2003; Clark et al., 2008). Pertinent indicators include dysregulation in cognitive (e.g., attention deficits), behavioral (e.g., impulsivity), and affective (e.g., affective lability) domains (Clark and Winters, 2002; Vanyukov et al., 2009; Clark et al., 2012). Most studies on these relationships have not explicitly and comprehensively measured executive dysfunction dimensions, however, leaving remaining questions on the extent to which SUD risks and outcomes may relate to specific dimensions or global executive dysfunction indicators.

Several studies have examined executive dysfunction in relationship to SUD risks and outcomes using a comprehensive multidimensional executive dysfunction measure, the Behavior Rating Inventory of Executive Function (BRIEF-SR: Gioia et al., 2002a,b; Roth et al., 2015). Expressly developed to measure eight executive dysfunction dimensions, the BRIEF has been demonstrated to be a valid and practical tool in school and clinical settings as well as in research (Egeland and Fallmyr, 2010; Roth et al., 2015). The BRIEF has been utilized in adolescent research to study executive dysfunction in relationship to SUD risks and outcomes, including disruptive behavior disorders (Wang et al., 2012; Long et al., 2015), sleep problems (Anderson et al., 2009; Caruso et al., 2014), academic achievement (Langberg et al., 2013; Samuels et al., 2016), performance-based cognitive tests (Shimoni et al., 2012; Long et al., 2015), brain structure and function (Clark et al., 2012; Ziegler et al., 2013; Zhai et al., 2015), and substance use (Clark et al., 2012). While comprehensively measuring executive dysfunction dimensions, most of these prior studies have had small sample sizes. Compared with prior studies, the present study includes a broader array of assessment domains with a considerably larger sample.

Among adolescents, poor sleep has been found to be associated with difficulties that may reflect executive dysfunction, such as inattention and depression (Millman, 2005). Limited research has specifically addressed the relationship between sleep quality and expressly measured executive dysfunction among adolescents. In 236 healthy adolescents (age 13–16 years: Anderson et al., 2009), increased sleepiness was significantly associated with more problems on dimensions including Working Memory, Task Planning, Orderliness, and Task Completion (i.e., BRIEF Metacognition) and not associated with Inhibitory Control, Flexibility, Emotional Control and Monitoring (i.e., BRIEF Behavioral Regulation). Sleep problems and circadian misalignment have been found to predict adolescent alcohol and other substance use (Hasler and Clark, 2013; Hasler et al., 2014, 2016, 2017). A study with a larger sample is needed to determine whether the relationships observed between executive dysfunction and poor sleep (Anderson et al., 2009) can be confirmed. Since poor sleep may influence executive dysfunction and executive dysfunction may, in turn, influence substance use, an examination of the relationships among these characteristics may suggest mechanisms, preventive intervention targets, and directions for future research.

The construct of executive functioning refers to behaviors in daily life as well as specific cognitive skills. A hypothesis about executive functioning in daily life is that variations in specific cognitive skills reflect the capabilities needed for effective functioning (Willcutt et al., 2005). To the extent that variations in objectively assessed cognitive skills correlate with executive dysfunction, such testing may be useful in depicting a mechanism for functional deficits. Relevant constructs assessed by performance-based cognitive testing include attention (e.g., Continuous Performance Test: Kurtz et al., 2001) and working memory (e.g., N-Back Test: Ragland et al., 2002). Several studies with small adolescent samples have noted, however, that performance-based cognitive tests and executive dysfunction ratings have little or no correspondence (Mahone et al., 2009; Cyders and Coskunpinar, 2012; Boschloo et al., 2014; Long et al., 2015; see Toplak et al., 2013 for review), with some exceptions (e.g., BRIEF and Working Memory by cognitive testing: Faridi et al., 2015). These studies suggest that cognitive testing of these constructs may not be particularly informative in understanding executive dysfunction in daily life. The present study examined these relationships in a large sample.

Executive dysfunction may reflect delays or deficits in neuromaturation. To the extent that variations in structural brain characteristics are found to correlate with executive dysfunction, such findings would support a hypothesis that specific observable brain characteristics reflect the neurobiological foundation for executive functioning. Prefrontal cortex (PFC) development has been hypothesized to be the neurobiological foundation for maturing executive functioning during adolescence, with the interaction of PFC with other functionally specialized brain regions critical for integrative executive functions (Spear, 2000). During adolescence, the maturation of executive cognitive skills occurs in parallel with increasing organization or integrity of white matter tracts projecting to PFC (Klingberg et al., 1999; Chambers et al., 2003; Takahashi et al., 2004; Lenroot and Giedd, 2006; Ashtari et al., 2007; Paus, 2010). The frontoparietal network (Fassbender et al., 2006), including tracts such as the superior longitudinal fasciculus (SLF) that connect the frontal and parietal cortex. The delay or disruption in the maturation of white matter integrity has been implicated as a neurobiological substrate for executive dysfunction (Lipton et al., 2009; Skranes et al., 2009; Clark et al., 2012). A few studies with adolescents have examined executive dysfunction, measured by BRIEF, in relationship to structural brain characteristics. Among 35 adolescents with SUD and 20 controls, worse executive dysfunction was significantly correlated with less PFC and parietal white matter integrity by diffusion tensor imaging fractional anisotropy (FA: Clark et al., 2012). Among 35 children and adolescents (Mahone et al., 2009), problems indicated on the BRIEF Working Memory scale were significantly correlated with smaller frontal gray matter volume, but not with temporal, parietal or occipital gray matter volume. In the NIH MRI study (Faridi et al., 2015), BRIEF Inhibitory Control was not significantly correlated with cortical gray thickness, while BRIEF Working Memory and Emotional

Control showed greater cortical thickness associated with fewer problems only in the parahippocampal gyri. These studies do not clearly establish consistent relationships between adolescent executive dysfunction and structural brain characteristics, and the present larger study will clarify these relationships.

To the extent that executive dysfunction is found to correlate with the early development of risky substance use patterns, such findings would support the hypothesis that deficits in self-control reflected in executive dysfunction may contribute to SUD. In a few adolescent samples, executive dysfunction, indicated by BRIEF, have been found to be associated with substance involvement. BRIEF Global Composite (GEC) has been found to be significantly different among adolescents with SUD ($n = 35$) and control adolescents ($n = 20$), with 29% of the SUD group showing scores considered to indicate clinical problems (i.e., ≥70; Clark et al., 2012). In this sample, BRIEF GEC mediated the relationship between disruption of frontoparietal white matter integrity and cannabis symptoms. More everyday executive functioning problems indicated by BRIEF scores have also been observed in young adults with substance use (Hadjiefthyvoulou et al., 2012). More extensive study of these relationships is needed, particularly the examination of the relationship between executive dysfunction and the adolescent onset of risky substance use patterns.

This study examined these relationships at the initial assessment among subjects in National Consortium on Alcohol and Neurodevelopment in Adolescents (NCANDA), providing the opportunity to examine executive dysfunction in a relatively large, representative sample with a broad array of hypothetically related psychosocial, neurocognitive and brain measures. The aims of this study were to determine the relationships between executive dysfunction in daily life, measured by the Behavior Rating Inventory of Executive Function (BRIEF), cognitive skills and structural brain characteristics, and SUD risks, including a global SUD risk indicator, sleep quality, and risky alcohol and cannabis use. In addition to bivariate relationships, multivariate models were tested.

METHODS

Participants

NCANDA participants were 831 youth ranging in age from 12 to 21 years. NCANDA examines adolescent neurodevelopmental risks for and outcomes of alcohol use in a large, multisite, accelerated longitudinal design (see Brown et al., 2015 for additional details). NCANDA subjects were recruited from five sites: Duke University, University of Pittsburgh, Oregon Health and Science University, University of California, San Diego, and SRI International. For this analysis, 10 subjects were missing BRIEF, and 4 were excluded for invalid results (see below). The demographic characteristics were as follows: age: mean: 16.2 years, s.d. 2.5, range: 12.0–21.9; female: $n = 417$, male: $n = 400$; race: white: $n = 586$ (71.7%), African American: 95 (11.6%), Asian: $n = 62$ (7.6%); Native American: $n = 3$ (<1%); Pacific Islander: $n = 4$ (<1%); multiple: $n = 67$ (8.2%); ethnicity: Hispanic: $n = 96$ (11.8%), non-Hispanic: $n = 721$ (88.2%). These race and ethnicity proportions are similar to the U.S. population (Brown et al., 2015). Most subjects ($n = 692$, 83%) had little or no alcohol use history, and a subsample ($n = 139$, 17%) had a history of risky alcohol use based on exceeding established alcohol use thresholds (National Institute on Alcohol Abuse and Alcoholism, 2011). Youth at increased risk for problematic alcohol use, based on one or more risk factors including early alcohol use, family SUD history, disruptive behavior disorder symptoms, or two or more anxiety or depression symptoms, comprised approximately 50% of the sample. The institutional review board at each site approved the study. Adult participants consented to participate, and minors provided assent with parental or legal guardian consent.

Design

NCANDA uses an accelerated longitudinal design (Duncan et al., 1996, 2006), sampling subjects from a broad age span with subsequent follow-up assessments to characterize development across an expansive period. At the initial assessment, youth completed a comprehensive assessment of substance use, psychiatric symptoms and diagnoses, personality factors, and functioning in major life domains (Brown et al., 2015); a neurocognitive battery (Sullivan et al., 2016), and a neuroimaging assessment with structural and diffusion tensor imaging (Pfefferbaum et al., 2016; Pohl et al., 2016). One parent of each youth also completed an assessment. These analyses utilized the initial assessment data.

Measures

BRIEF

Behavior Rating Inventory of Executive Function-Self-Report Version (BRIEF-SR: Baron, 2000; Gioia et al., 2002a,b; Guy et al., 2004; Roth et al., 2015): The BRIEF-SR is an 80-item adolescent self-report behavior rating scale of purposeful, goal-directed, problem-solving behavior. For each item, the subject is asked: "Over the past 6 months, how often has each of the following behaviors been a problem?" The response choices are "Often" (3 points), "Sometimes" (2 points) and "Never" (1 point). The instrument yields a summary score, the Global Executive Composite (GEC), two composite indices, and eight scales: (1) The ***Inhibitory Control*** scale (13 items) assesses inhibitory control and impulsivity (e.g., *"I have problems waiting my turn," "I don't think of consequences before acting," "I get out of control more than my friends"*). (2) The ***Flexibility*** scale (10 items), including behavioral and cognitive characteristics, assesses the ability to make transitions and flexibly solve problems (e.g., *"I have trouble changing from one activity to another"*). (3) The ***Emotional Control*** scale (10 items) assesses the ability to modulate emotional responses in response to situational demands (e.g., *"I overreact to small problems," "I get upset easily"*). (4) The ***Monitoring*** scale (5 items) assesses self-awareness of interpersonal strengths and weaknesses (e.g., *"I don't know when my actions bother others"*). (5) The ***Working Memory*** scale (12 items) assesses holding information in mind for the purpose of completing a task (e.g., *"I forget instructions easily," "I have trouble with jobs or tasks that have more than one step"*). (6) The Task ***Planning*** scale (Plan: 13 items) assesses planning steps to complete a task and the anticipation of future consequences (e.g.,

"I don't plan ahead for school assignments," "I don't think ahead about possible problems" "I have trouble carrying out the things that are needed to reach a goal, such as saving money for special needs, studying to get good grades, etc."). (7) The ***Organization*** scale (Organize: 7 items) assesses the ability to keep work and school materials organized (e.g., *"My backpack/schoolbag is disorganized"*). (8) The ***Task Completion*** assesses the ability to complete school or work in a timely fashion by 10 items (e.g., *"I have difficulty finishing a task on my own"*). The ***Behavioral Regulation Index (BRI)*** combines Inhibit, Shift, Emotional Control, and Monitor scales (internal consistency: 0.96). The ***Metacognition Index (MCI)*** is comprised of Initiate, Working Memory, Plan and Organize, Task Monitor, and Organization of Materials subscales (internal consistency: 0.72). In addition, validity scales include the ***Inconsistency*** scale, which determines whether the subject responded in a consistent manner by comparing 10 pairs of similar items, and the ***Negativity*** scale (10 items), which determines whether the subject responds to selected items in an unusually negative manner. Raw scores are converted to age indexed t-scores, with higher scores indicating more problems. Subjects with missing ($n = 10$) or invalid ($n = 4$) BRIEF scores were excluded from all analyses.

Risk Factors for Alcohol Use Disorder (AUD)

The NCANDA sample (Brown et al., 2015) was configured to include approximately 50% of the sample at higher risk for problematic alcohol use based on screening evidence for one of the following: (1) early alcohol use (i.e., first standard drink before age 15 years old); (2) a family history of alcohol or other substance problems; (3) endorsement of one or more conduct disorder or antisocial personality disorder symptoms or t score ≥ 60 on the externalizing score of the Achenbach system of Empirically Based Assessments (ASEBA: Achenbach and Rescorla, 2001a,b); (4) endorsement of two or more internalizing symptoms or $t \geq 60$ on ASEBA internalizing. ***Risk Density*** was calculated as the sum of the presence (1) or absence (0) of each of these characteristics (range: 0–4).

Subjective Sleep Quality

The Pittsburgh Sleep Quality Index (PSQI: Buysse et al., 1989) has been shown to be comprised of two factors, sleep efficiency and perceived sleep quality (Mollayeva et al., 2016). The PSQI has been validated in adolescent samples (de la Vega et al., 2015) and has been commonly used in adolescent research (e.g., Noone et al., 2014). The perceived sleep quality factor includes a subjective sleep quality item which correlates highly with the factor score and loads more strongly on this factor than do other items (Mollayeva et al., 2016). The subjective sleep quality item asks "During the past month, how would you rate your sleep quality overall?" with response options "very good," "fairly good," "fairly bad," and "very bad."

Performance Based Cognitive Tests

The NCANDA performance based cognitive testing protocol was designed to assess functional domains relevant for alcohol involvement risks and outcomes (see Sullivan et al., 2016 for details). The NCANDA cognitive and motor battery assessed eight domains: general ability, attention, abstraction, emotion, working memory, balance, and motor speed (Sullivan et al., 2016, 2017). Most of these domains were assessed with computer-administered WebCNP tests (Gur et al., 2010). For examining cognitive skills that may be pertinent to executive dysfunction here, the domains of attention, emotion and working memory are particularly pertinent, and the examination of general ability may provide information on the global effects of problems in this arena. The functional domains and tests included here were: (1) Attention: Continuous Performance Test (Kurtz et al., 2001); (2) Emotion: Emotion Recognition Test (Gur et al., 2002), Measured Emotion Differentiation (Fossati, 2012); (3) Working Memory: Short Fractal N-Back Test (Ragland et al., 2002); and (4) General Ability: Vocabulary Test (Lee et al., 2014), WRAT-4 Math Calculations and Word Reading (Wilkinson and Robertson, 2006). These computer administered WebCNP tests were used to generate domain specific accuracy and speed (response time) z scores. In prior analyses, older age was associated with better scores on attention, emotion, and general ability (Sullivan et al., 2016), so age was used as a covariate in these analyses.

MRI Acquisition and Analysis

The NCANDA neuroimaging battery includes structural indices (Pfefferbaum et al., 2016) and diffusion tensor imaging (DTI: Pohl et al., 2016), and more detailed descriptions of the protocols may be found in those publications. Briefly, T1-weighted, 3D images were collected in the sagittal plane on systems from two manufacturers: 3T General Electric (GE) Discovery MR750 at three sites and 3T Siemens TIM TRIO scanners at two sites. The GE sites used an Array Spatial Sensitivity Encoding Technique (ASSET) for parallel and accelerated imaging with an 8-channel head coil and acquired an Inversion Recovery-Spoiled Gradient Recalled (IR-SPGR) echo sequence. The Siemens sites used a 12-channel head coil and parallel imaging and temporal acceleration with iPAT and acquired an MPRAGE sequence. Each site scanned the ADNI phantom on each day that participants were scanned. Analysis proceeded via the NCANDA NeuroInformatics Platform (Rohlfing et al., 2014) and involved skull stripping applied to the extracted maps. The SRI24 atlas-based analysis pipeline was used to identify intracranial volume (ICV), supratentorial volume (svol), and pons, corpus callosum, subcortical white matter (including the centrum semiovale), and lateral ventricular volumes. FreeSurfer (Dale et al., 1999) was used on skull-stripped data to create bilateral surface area, volume, and thickness of frontal, temporal, parietal, occipital, cingulate cortices derived from the Desikan-Killiany regions-of-interest (ROI) scheme (Desikan et al., 2006) plus the insular cortex. Volume was expressed in cc, surface area in cm^2, and thickness in mm. All ROIs were adjusted for linear scaling factors from the ADNI phantom (Clarkson et al., 2009). To acquire Diffusion-Weighted Images (DWI, a.k.a. diffusion tensor imaging or DTI), GE and Siemens sites applied a 2D Axial Spin Echo, Echo-Planar protocol, as well as a reverse phase acquisition of the 2D Axial Spin Echo-Planar protocol for B0-field inhomogeneity spatial distortion correction. To achieve common anatomical coordinates across subjects, each subject's fractional anisotropy (FA) data set was registered to the FA channel of the SRI24 atlas. Cortical volume and thickness were smaller with increasing age, and cortical volumes greater in males than females (Pfefferbaum et al., 2016). For DTI indices, increasing age was associated with higher FA and lower diffusivity measures (Pohl et al., 2016). Consequently, statistical analyses on structural brain characteristics in the present study were controlled for age and sex.

Substance Use

Past and recent alcohol and other substance use were determined by the Customary Drinking and Drug Use Record (CDDR: Brown et al., 1998). The measure includes items on alcohol and marijuana use, including use frequency in the past year, and the maximum number of drinks in a drinking episode during the past year. At **Risk Alcohol Use:** Alcohol use frequency in the past year has been found to useful for identifying use patterns associated with alcohol use disorder (AUD) among adolescents (e.g., Chung et al., 2012; Clark et al., 2016). The National Institute on Alcohol Abuse and Alcoholism (NIAAA) Alcohol Screening and Brief Intervention for Youth: A Practitioner's Guide (NIAAA Youth Guide) recommends age specific stratified past year alcohol use frequency thresholds to define low, moderate and high risk for AUD. Moderate Risk is defined at age 12–15 as: $\geq$1 days; ages 16–17: $\geq$3 days; ages 18: $\geq$12 days. High Risk is defined at age 12–15 as: $\geq$3 days; age 16: $\geq$12 days; age 17: $\geq$24 days; age 18: $\geq$52 days. Subjects below these thresholds were classified as Low Risk. **Binge Alcohol Use:** While the traditional definition of a drinking binge has typically been applied across development, binge definitions appropriate for younger adolescents have been developed to account for smaller body size among youth (Donovan, 2009). Using the "lifetime greatest number of drinks" response, age-specific binge thresholds were calculated as follows: ages 9 to 13 years: $\geq$3 drinks; 14 or 15 years: $\geq$4 for males, $\geq$3 for females; 16 or 17 years: $\geq$5 for males, $\geq$3 for females.

Statistical Analyses

Overall NCANDA data management has been described (Rohlfing et al., 2014). (NCANDA Data releases used in these analyses: 000001_V1; 00010_V3; 00011; 00012_V2.) The analyses presented to test hypotheses were by analysis of variance (ANOVA) for categorical variables or Pearson correlations for continuous variables. Covariates for all analyses were age, sex and SES. A sequential procedure (Ludbrook, 1998) was used to reduce Type 1 error or family wise error rate, first testing the global hypothesis represented by the BRIEF Global Composite (i.e., GEC), followed by tests examining the BRIEF indices and scales with Šidák corrections (Šidák, 1967; Ludbrook, 1998). For analyses examining BRIEF composite, indices and scales, BRIEF GEC was examined first ($p < 0.05$) and, where the relationship between GEC and the dependent measure were significant, relationships with Behavioral Regulation Index (BRI) and Metacognition Index (MCI), then the eight scales, were interpreted. Corrections for multiple tests were implemented as follows: Behavioral Regulation Index or BRI and Metacognition Index or MCI: $\alpha = 0.05$ for 2 tests: $p < 0.025$; 8 scales: $\alpha = 0.05$ for 8 tests: $p < 0.0064$). To reduce type 1 error in sets of analyses examining correlations between multiple continuous variables (i.e., cognitive test scores and brain structure variables) and BRIEF GEC, the Šidák procedure was applied, in which the overall number of comparisons was taken into consideration to determine the significance threshold (Cognitive skill domains, with scores for accuracy and speed: $\alpha = 0.05/2$ or $p < 0.025$; MR Structural Gray Indices: $\alpha = 0.05/18$ or $p < 0.0028$; DTI: $\alpha = 0.05/32$ or $p < 0.0016$). For variables with significant relationships with BRIEF GEC, multivariate models were constructed to test mediation hypotheses (Baron and Kenny, 1986).

RESULTS

BRIEF Description

For subjects with valid BRIEF data ($n = 817$), mean scale t-scores ranged from 43.5 ± 8.6 (BRIEF Inhibitory Control) to 46.1 ± 9.9 (BRIEF Task Completion), with composite t-scores also in this range (BRI: 43.6 ± 9.4; MCI: 44.6 ± 10.6; GEC: 43.9 ± 10.4).

Demographic Characteristics

BRIEF composite scores did not significantly differ by gender (e.g., GEC: F: 44.0 ± 11.1; M: 43.8 ± 9.6; $t = 0.2$, d.f. 815, $p = 0.8$). BRIEF GEC was not significantly correlated with age ($r = 0.06$, $n = 817$, $p = 0.10$). BRIEF GEC was significantly correlated with SES ($r = -0.15$, $n = 731$, $p < 0.001$). Race (White: $n = 586$, 43.7 ± 10.1; African American: $n = 95$, 43.3 ± 11.7; Asian: $n = 62$, 43.9 ± 8.9; Other: $n = 67$, 46.6 ± 12.0) was not significantly associated with BRIEF GEC ($F = 1.7$, d.f. 3,806, $p = 0.16$). Ethnicity (Non-Hispanic: $n = 721$, 43.2 ± 11.9; Hispanic: 49.1 ± 11.9) was significantly associated with BRIEF GEC ($F = 28.4$, 1,815, $p < 0.001$). To a substantial extent, this relationship was accounted for by SES (multivariate model: $n = 725$; SES: $F = 13.1$, $p < 0.001$; Race: $F = 1.6$, $p = 0.6$; Ethnicity: $F = 4.9$, $p = 0.03$).

NCANDA Risk Density

Risk Density (**Table 1**) was determined by summing the number of risks present (range: 0–4; 0: $n = 381$, 46.6%; 1: 276, 33.8%; 2: 119, 14.6%; 3: 37, 4.5%; 4: 4, 0.5%). Due to few participants with 4 risk characteristics, participants with 3 or 4 risk factors were combined for analyses. Risk Density was significantly associated with BRIEF GEC, with higher Risk Density associated with greater dysfunction (**Table 1**; **Figure 1**). All BRIEF indices and scales were similarly significantly related to Risk Density. Abnormal BRIEF GEC scores ($\geq$70), present in 2% of the sample, were associated with Risks (0 Risks, 0%; 1 risk, 2%, 2 risks, 4%, 3 or 4 Risks, 20%: Likelihood Ratio $\chi^2 = 68.0$, d.f. = 3, $p < 0.001$). Risk Density was significantly associated with At Risk Alcohol Use ($F = 40.5$, $p < 0.001$), Binge Alcohol Episodes ($F = 7.4$, $p < 0.01$), and Marijuana Use ($F = 10.3$, $p < 0.01$) (**Table 8**).

Sleep Quality

Sleep Quality was significantly associated with BRIEF GEC, with poorer slep quality associated with greater dysfunction (**Table 2**; **Figure 2**). All BRIEF indices and scales were similarly significantly related to Sleep Quality. Sleep Quality was significantly associated with At Risk Alcohol Use ($F = 5.6$,

TABLE 1 | BRIEF global composite, indexes and scales by NCANDA risk density categories.

	0	1	2	3–4	*F*
	n = 381	*n* = 276	*n* = 119	*n* = 41	
Inhibitory control	40.8 ± 7.2	44.5 ± 8.2	46.9 ± 9.0	54.0 ±12.0	37.3[c]
Flexibility	42.7 ± 9.3	46.9 ± 10.1	51.1 ± 12.4	55.4 ± 11.1	28.9[c]
Emotional control	42.4 ± 7.3	46.2 ± 8.5	50.9 ± 10.6	53.3 ± 11.5	36.6[c]
Monitoring	42.5 ± 7.6	45.3 ± 8.6	50.2 ± 9.2	54.1 ± 10.1	33.5[c]
Behavioral regulation	40.1 ± 7.7	44.7 ± 8.7	49.5 ± 10.2	55.0 ± 11.0	51.3[b]
Working memory	41.9 ± 8.4	46.9 ± 10.0	50.1 ± 10.8	56.9 ± 12.0	40.0[c]
Task plan	41.9 ± 8.7	46.7 ± 9.9	50.6 ± 1.5	56.7 ± 10.8	39.9[c]
Orderly	43.0 ± 8.7	46.9 ± 9.5	49.2 ± 10.0	54.4 ± 11.2	24.4[c]
Completion	42.3 ± 7.3	47.5 ± 9.8	51.4 ± 11.0	57.9 ± 12.7	47.6[c]
Metacognition	40.9 ± 8.5	46.6 ±10.2	50.4 ± 11.2	57.7 ± 11.9	50.1[b]
Global composite	39.9 ± 8.2	45.0 ± 9.6	50.0 ± 10.9	56.5 ± 11.7	55.8[a]

d.f. 3, 724; covariates: sex, age, SES.
[a]*$p < 0.05$ for test of GEC.*
[b]*$p < 0.025$ for 2 tests of Indexes.*
[c]*$p < 0.0064$ for 8 tests of Scales.*

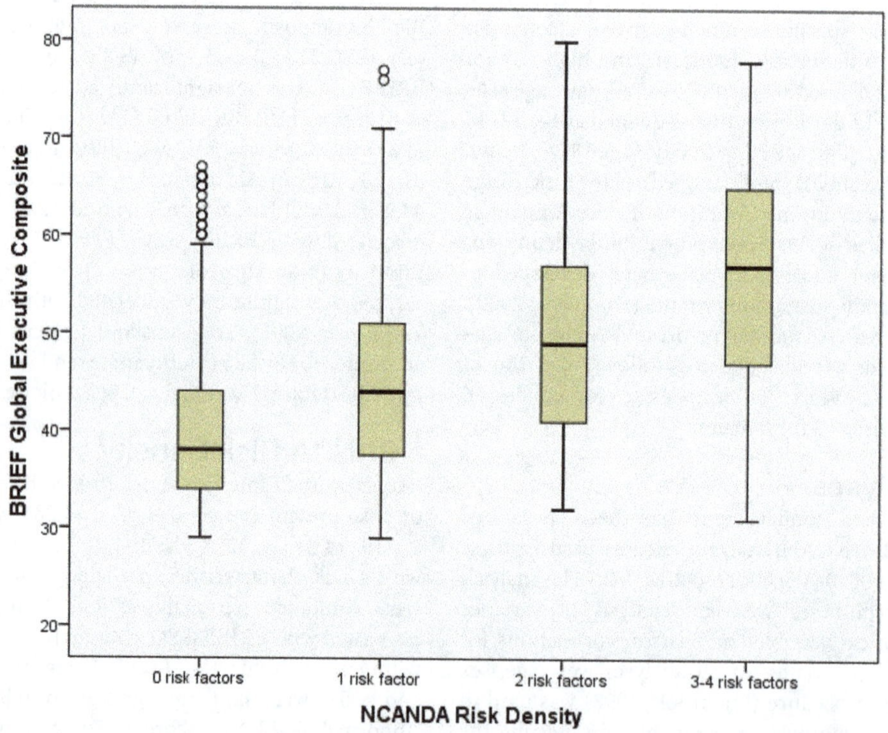

FIGURE 1 | Box plot of BRIEF global composite by NCANDA risk density categories. The figure shows box plots for NCANDA Risk Density categories. The box plot represents the interquartile range (IQR), with the shaded box representing the second and third quartiles and center demarcations indicating the median. The whiskers represent the maximum and minimum values up to 1.5 × IQR, and the circles represent values beyond 1.5 × IQR.

$p < 0.05$), Binge Alcohol Episodes ($F = 3.9$, $p < 0.05$), and Marijuana Use ($F = 5.8$, $p < 0.05$) (**Table 8**).

Cognitive Skill Domain Scores

Cognitive Skill Domain Scores were not significantly correlated with BRIEF GEC (**Table 3**). Note that, while a correction for two tests per domain (i.e., accuracy and speed) was thought applicable, a less stringent threshold of $p < 0.05$ did not change the interpretation of the results. Since there may be some interest in the observed correlations for specific variable pairs (e.g., Working Memory by BRIEF scale by Cognitive Skill Domain), the full table of analyses is presented.

TABLE 2 | BRIEF global composite, indexes and scales by sleep quality categories.

	Very good	Fairly good	Fairly bad	Very bad	*F*
	$n = 218$	$n = 430$	$n = 71$	$n = 12$	
Inhibitory control	41.0 ± 7.1	44.0 ± 8.7	48.3 ± 10.7	47.2 ± 9.8	14.5[c]
Flexibility	42.7 ± 9.6	46.5 ± 10.7	51.5 ± 10.6	53.8 ± 15.4	15.4[c]
Emotional control	42.9 ± 8.1	46.2 ± 9.3	48.2 ± 9.5	49.5 ± 9.8	9.6[c]
Monitoring	42.3 ± 7.7	45.9 ± 8.9	48.6 ± 9.3	48.5 13.2	12.8[c]
Behavioral regulation	40.4 ± 8.2	44.4 ± 9.4	48.9 ± 10.3	49.7 ± 11.8	18.7[b]
Working memory	42.0 ± 9.3	46.0 ± 9.8	52.3 ± 11.9	54.9 ± 11.9	24.2[c]
Task plan	41.3 ± 9.3	46.0 ± 9.8	53.3 ± 11.9	53.5 ± 11.3	28.5[c]
Orderly	42.2 ± 7.9	46.5 ± 9.7	50.6 ± 11.3	55.4 ± 9.6	20.4[c]
Task completion	42.9 ± 8.3	46.2 ± 9.6	54.4 ± 11.8	54.3 ± 12.5	27.1[c]
Metacognition	40.9 ± 9.2	45.5 ± 10.0	53.3 ± 12.2	55.3 ± 12.6	31.8[b]
Global composite	39.9 ± 9.0	44.7 ± 10.3	51.4 ± 11.8	52.9 ± 12.4	28.3[a]

d.f. 2, 723; covariates: sex, age, SES.
[a] *$p < 0.05$ for test of BRIEF GEC.*
[b] *$p < 0.025$ for 2 tests of Indexes.*
[c] *$p < 0.0064$ for 8 tests of Scales.*

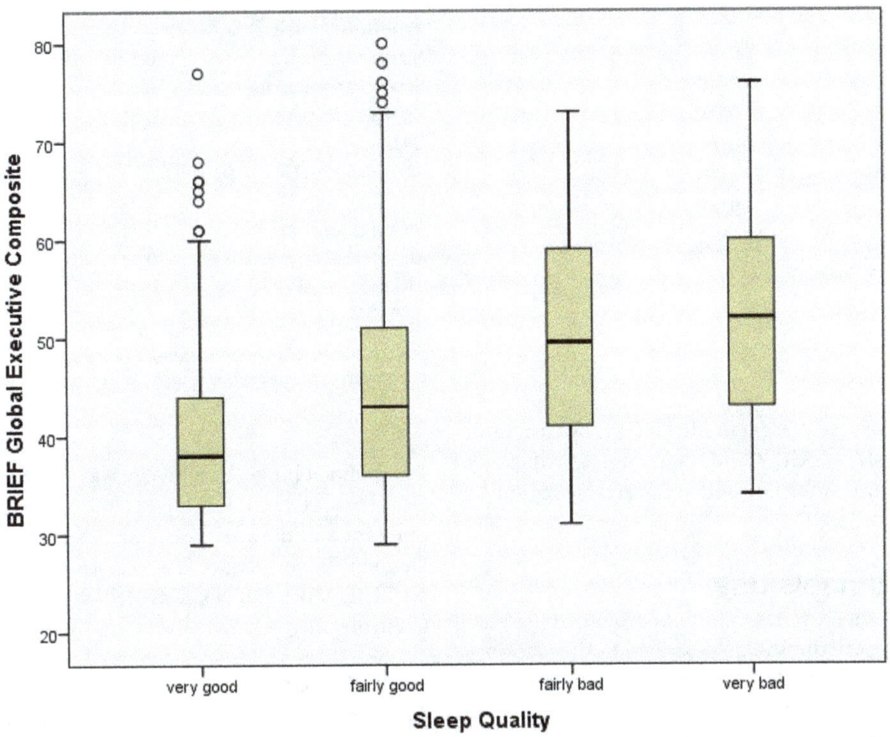

FIGURE 2 | Box plot of BRIEF global executive composite by sleep quality categories. The figure shows box plots for Sleep Quality categories. The box plot represents the interquartile range (IQR), with the shaded box representing the second and third quartiles and center demarcations indicating the median. The whiskers represent the maximum and minimum values up to 1.5 × IQR, and the circles represent values beyond 1.5 × IQR.

Cortical Structure

Using a correction for multiple comparisons for tests across the BRIEF GEC by structural variables matrix (i.e., 18 tests), BRIEF GEC was not significantly correlated with gray matter volume, cortical thickness or cortical surface area in frontal temporal, parietal, occipital, cingulate, or insula regions (**Table 4**).

TABLE 3 | BRIEF global composite, indexes and scales by cognitive skill domain scores.

	Attention		Emotion recognition		Working memory		General ability	
	a	s	a	s	a	s	a	s
Inhibitory control	−0.08	−0.01	−0.01	0.13	0.01	0.00	−0.04	0.08
Flexibility	−0.02	−0.04	−0.02	0.03	0.02	−0.02	−0.01	0.02
Emotional control	−0.03	−0.01	0.03	0.05	0.04	0.02	−0.04	0.01
Monitoring	−0.03	−0.05	−0.03	0.07	−0.02	−0.02	−0.04	0.04
Behavioral regulation	−0.05	−0.03	−0.01	0.08	0.02	0.00	−0.04	0.04
Working memory	−0.05	−0.03	0.03	0.06	0.00	0.00	−0.04	0.04
Task planning	−0.04	−0.03	0.04	0.09	0.04	−0.02	0.01	0.07
Organization	0.01	−0.03	0.06	0.06	0.03	−0.02	0.01	0.07
Task completion	−0.05	−0.06	0.01	0.05	0.00	−0.05	−0.13	−0.02
Metacognition	−0.04	−0.03	0.04	0.07	0.02	−0.03	−0.04	0.05
Global composite	−0.05	−0.03	0.02	0.08	0.02	−0.01	−0.04	0.05

A, accuracy; s, speed; Pearson correlations [r]; d.f. 707; covariates: sex, age, SES.
With corrections for multiple comparisons, none of the above statistical test reached statistical significance.

TABLE 4 | BRIEF global composite by MR structural gray segment volume, thickness and surface area.

	Volume	Thickness	Surface area
Frontal	−0.01	−0.04	0.02
Temporal	0.02	0.00	0.04
Parietal	0.01	0.00	0.03
Occipital	−0.02	−0.01	0.00
Cingulate	0.00	−0.02	0.02
Insula	−0.03	−0.05	−0.01

Pearson correlations [r]; d.f. 707; covariates: sex, age, SES.
With corrections for multiple comparisons, none of the above statistical test reached statistical significance.

TABLE 5 | BRIEF global composite by DTI indices for fasciculi and tracts.

	FA	MD	L1	LT
FASCICULI				
Superior longitudinal	−0.07	0.08	0.03	0.04
Superior frontal-occipital	−0.07	0.00	−0.06	0.02
Sagittal stratum	0.01	0.01	0.04	−0.02
Uncinate	−0.09	0.08	0.00	0.08
LIMBIC TRACTS				
Fornix	0.01	0.01	0.02	0.00
Striatia terminalis	0.01	0.06	0.09	−0.01
Anterior middle cingulum	−0.03	0.11	0.09	0.03
Inferior cingulum	0.01	0.00	0.01	−0.01

FA, fractional anisotrophy; MD, mean diffusivity; L1, axial diffusivity; LT, radial diffusivity. Pearson correlations [r]; d.f. 703; covariates: sex, age, SES. With corrections for multiple comparisons, none of the above statistical test reached statistical significance.

DTI

Using a correction across the presented BRIEF GEC by structural variables (i.e., 32 tests), BRIEF GEC was not significantly correlated with DTI indices for fasciculi and tracts by region or DTI variable (**Table 5**).

Alcohol and Cannabis Use

At Risk Alcohol Use Category was determined by the past year alcohol use days frequency thresholds described in the National Institute on Alcohol Abuse and Alcoholism Youth Guide (2011). Overall (**Table 6**), 83% ($n = 676$) were Low Risk, 12% ($n = 95$) were Moderate Risk, and 5% ($n = 41$) were High Risk. At Risk Alcohol Use Category was significantly related to BRIEF GEC ($F = 7.0$, d.f. 2,723, $p = 0.001$), with higher risk associated with more problems. At Risk Alcohol Use Category was significantly associated with BRIEF BRI and MCI, and scales including Inhibitory Control, Emotional Control, and Task Planning.

Age Defined Binge Alcohol Use

Past year age defined binge alcohol use (**Table 7**) was present in 129 subjects (15.9%). Including sex, age and SES as covariates, Age Defined Binge Alcohol Use was significantly related to BRIEF GEC ($F = 11.1$, d.f. 1,721, $p = 0.001$), with the presence of at least one binge in the past year associated with more problems. Age Defined Binge Alcohol Use was associated with more problems on BRIEF BRI and MCI, as well as on the including Inhibitory Control scale.

Cannabis Use

Past year cannabis use was present in 123 subjects (**Table 7**: 15.2%). Cannabis Use was significantly related to BRIEF GEC ($F = 9.1$, d.f. 1,720, $p = 0.003$), with the presence of cannabis use in the past year associated with more problems. Cannabis Use was associated with more problems on BRIEF BRI and MCI, as well as scales including Inhibitory Control, Emotional Control, and Task Planning.

Multivariate Models

For variables shown to be significantly related to BRIEF GEC (i.e., NCANDA Risk Density and Sleep Quality), multivariate

TABLE 6 | At Risk Alcohol Use Frequency x BRIEF scales.

	Low risk	Moderate risk	High risk	*F*
	n = 616	*n* = 82	*n* = 31	
Inhibitory control	43.1 ± 8.4	46.3 ± 10.7	47.3 ± 9.0	8.1[c]
Flexibility	45.7 ± 10.8	48.0 ± 11.4	48.1 ± 11.7	2.3
Emotional control	45.1 ± 9.1	48.9 ± 9.2	47.1 ± 10.6	7.3[c]
Monitoring	44.8 ± 8.8	47.3 ± 10.0	47.6 ± 8.8	3.7
Behavioral regulation	43.3 ± 9.5	47.1 ± 10.5	46.7 ± 10.3	7.4[b]
Working memory	45.1 ± 10.3	48.6 ± 11.7	48.5 ± 9.4	5.4
Task plan	45.0 ± 10.4	47.9 ± 11.0	51.8 ± 11.0	8.0[c]
Orderly	45.5 ± 9.8	47.5 ± 10.1	48.9 ± 9.0	2.4
Task completion	45.7 ± 10.0	49.2 ± 11.0	48.1 ± 11.4	3.9
Metacognition	44.5 ± 10.7	48.0 ± 11.6	49.3 ± 10.5	5.9[b]
Global composite	43.5 ± 10.5	47.5 ± 11.2	48.1 ± 10.6	7.0[a]

d.f. 2, 723; covariates: sex, age, SES.
[a]*$p < 0.05$ for test of BRIEF GEC.*
[b]*$p < 0.025$ for 2 tests of Indices.*
[c]*$p < 0.0064$ for 8 tests of Scales.*

models were tested (**Table 8**). NCANDA Risk Density was significantly related to Past Year At Risk Alcohol Use Frequency, Age Defined Binge Alcohol Use and Cannabis Use (i.e., substance use). In multivariate models including BRIEF GEC, the relationship between Risk Density and substance use variables diminished but remained significant, suggesting that mediation was not demonstrated. Sleep Quality was significantly related to substance use variables. In multivariate models including BRIEF GEC, the relationship between Sleep Quality and substance use variables was not statistically significant, suggesting mediation. In a model with NCANDA Risk Density, Sleep Quality and BRIEF GEC, the relationship between NCANDA Risk Density and substance use remained significance while Sleep Quality was not significantly related to substance use.

DISCUSSION

In NCANDA, BRIEF (Guy et al., 2004) was utilized as an ecologically valid complement to performance based cognitive testing to measure executive functioning constructs. While BRIEF scores were noted to be, on average, somewhat lower than might be expected from the scale construction samples, subsequent studies have similarly noted that normative samples have mean calculated *t*-scores similar to the NCANDA sample (Roth et al., 2015). BRIEF scores were not related to age, sex, or race, and showed a significant relationship with SES. Prior studies have shown relationships between SES and executive functioning, with attributions of this correlation interpreted as related to parent education and other home and family environment characteristics (Hackman et al., 2015).

As expected, higher BRIEF scores were systematically correlated with NCANDA Risk Density. Previous studies have indicated that characteristics related to executive functioning are associated with SUD risk indicators, including externalizing characteristics (Familiar et al., 2015; Long et al., 2015), internalizing characteristics (Clark et al., 1997), family SUD history (Tapert and Brown, 2000), and the early adolescent onset of alcohol use (Tarter et al., 2003). However, the multivariate models indicated that the inclusion of BRIEF was accompanied by only a modest reduction in the relationship between NCANDA Risk Density and substance use, suggesting that the mediation hypothesis was not supported. These analyses of cross-sectionally collected data were not ideal for determining directional influences, and subsequent NCANDA analyses will be able to further examine the extent to which the relationship between risk factors and later substance use may be mediated by executive dysfunction.

Poor sleep quality was significantly and consistently correlated with all executive dysfunction dimensions. While prior research has suggested that sleep problems are associated with executive dysfunction in daily life, the robust correlations observed here indicates a more extensive relationship than has been previously reported. Since prior research utilizing BRIEF in relationship to sleep has involved smaller samples, the present finding may benefit from greater statistical power. The multivariate models indicated that the inclusion of BRIEF was accompanied by a reduction in the relationship between Sleep Quality and substance use, indicating that the mediation hypothesis was supported. Since the present findings are based on cross-sectional data, however, analyses informed by changes in these relationships over time will be undertaken in the course of the NCANDA study. In addition, polysomnography being examined in an NCANDA subset will complement subjective sleep assessments (Baker et al., 2016). Sleep difficulties have been shown to predict problematic alcohol use (Hasler and Clark, 2013; Hasler et al., 2014), and subsequent NCANDA analyses will be able to examine the extent to which executive dysfunction mediates this relationship over the course of adolescent development.

The self-report of executive dysfunction in daily life assessed by BRIEF were not significantly correlated with performance based cognitive test results. While one might expect there to be some correspondence between these indicators, our results are consistent with several prior studies. A recent review of 20 studies (Toplak et al., 2013) on the relationship between self-report and performance-based executive functioning assessments found that, of 286 relevant correlations, only 68 (24%) were statistically significant, and the median correlation was only 0.19. The authors concluded that these approaches generally assess different underlying constructs. The results here were consistent with these observations. Broadly conceived, performance-based cognitive tests and BRIEF scores assess executive functioning dimensions. However, our results, consistent with prior studies (Toplak et al., 2013), indicate that executive dysfunction in daily life, measured by BRIEF, and performance based cognitive testing measure distinct constructs.

BRIEF Global Composite scores were not significantly correlated with cortical structure or DTI indicators. These findings were consistent with some prior observations (e.g., Faridi et al., 2015). The current study had a substantially larger and more representative sample than some other pertinent prior studies with positive findings (Mahone et al., 2009;

TABLE 7 | Past year age defined binge and marijuana use × BRIEF scales.

	Age defined binges			Marijuana use		
	No $n = 626$	Yes $n = 100$	F	No $n = 621$	Yes $n = 104$	F
Inhibitory control	43.2 ± 8.6	46.1 ± 9.6	11.1[c]	43.1 ± 8.5	46.5 ± 9.9	12.2[c]
Flexibility	45.7 ± 10.7	48.0 ± 11.4	4.4	45.6 ± 10.6	48.3 ± 11.5	4.9
Emotional control	45.3 ± 9.5	46.9 ± 9.5	3.4	45.1 ± 9.1	48.1 ± 9.3	8.4[c]
Monitoring	44.8 ± 8.8	47.3 ± 9.8	6.5	44.8 ± 8.8	47.4 ± 9.3	5.5
Behavioral regulation	43.4 ± 9.4	46.3 ± 9.9	8.7[b]	43.2 ± 9.4	47.0 ± 10.2	11.0[b]
Working memory	45.3 ± 10.5	47.4 ± 9.5	4.4	45.1 ± 10.4	48.0 ± 10.1	5.3
Task plan	45.1 ± 10.4	48.1 ± 10.7	5.5	45.0 ± 10.5	48.6 ± 10.1	7.5[c]
Orderly	45.4 ± 9.7	48.1 ± 9.6	3.7	45.3 ± 9.8	48.2 ± 9.3	4.5
Task completion	45.8 ± 9.8	48.2 ± 11.1	3.7	45.8 ± 10.0	48.3 ± 10.4	2.7
Metacognition	44.7 ± 10.6	47.6 ± 10.8	5.6[b]	44.6 ± 10.7	48.8 ± 10.3	6.2[b]
Global composite	43.6 ± 10.4	46.8 ± 10.6	7.4[a]	43.5 ± 10.4	47.4 ± 10.5	9.1[a]

Binge: d.f. 1, 721; covariates: sex, age, SES; Marijuana: d.f. 1, 720.
[a]*$p < 0.05$ for test of Composite.*
[b]*$p < 0.025$ for 2 tests of Indexes.*
[c]*$p < 0.0064$ for 8 tests of Scales.*

TABLE 8 | Contributions to ANOVA models of substance use outcomes.

	At Risk Alcohol		Binge alcohol		Cannabis use	
Tested covariates	F	(R^2)	F	(R^2)	F	(R^2)
BRIEF alone	13.7***	(0.070)	7.4**	(0.126)	10.3**	(0.141)
Risk alone	40.5 ***	(0.102)	14.1***	(0.134)	28.6***	(0.162)
Risk with BRIEF	27.6***	(0.103)	8.2**	(0.134)	19.1***	(0.162)
BRIEF with risk	1.3		1.5		1.1	
Sleep alone	5.6*	(0.059)	3.9*	(0.122)	5.8*	(0.136)
Sleep with BRIEF	1.6	(0.070)	1.4	(0.126)	2.1	(0.143)
BRIEF with sleep	9.7**		4.8*		6.6**	
BRIEF with risk and sleep	0.7	(0.103)	0.8	(0.135)	0.4	(0.163)
Risk with BRIEF and sleep	27.0***		7.8**		18.5***	
Sleep with BRIEF and risk	1.0		1.1		1.6	

*Adjusted R^2 for the model; F-statistic with d.f. 1, 701; covariates: sex, age, SES; *$p < 0.05$, **$p < 0.01$, ***$p < 0.001$; BRIEF, BRIEF Global Composite; Risk, NCANDA Risk Density; Sleep, Sleep Quality; At Risk Alcohol, At Risk Alcohol Frequency (Past Year); Binge Alcohol, Age Defined Binge Alcohol Use (Past Year); Marijuana Use, Marijuana Use (Past Year).*

Clark et al., 2012). Alternative statistical approaches, such as latent variable modeling, may provide additional insights. For example, among 286 healthy children and adolescents, a latent variable modeling approach revealed a systematic pattern of relationships between cortical networks and BRIEF scores (Ziegler et al., 2013). The examination of network based brain activation patterns, using techniques such as resting state MRI, may show relationships between functional brain development and executive functioning difficulties (Fair et al., 2009; Casey et al., 2016). The neurobiological foundations of executive dysfunction may be more reflected in functional MRI indicators of activation during tasks that require cognitive and behavioral skills in this arena. For example, among 59 young adolescents (ages 12–15), BRIEF cognitive flexibility was associated with orbitofrontal cortex activation during a behavioral inhibition task (Zhai et al., 2015).

Consistent with prior studies (Clark et al., 2012; Hadjiefthyvoulou et al., 2012), BRIEF scores were associated with indicators of risky substance use, including a frequency of alcohol use indicating risk for AUD, age defined binge drinking, and marijuana use. Difficulties with executive functioning and risky substance use may reflect both preexisting psychological dysregulation and substance use resulting in disruption of executive functioning (Clark et al., 2012). While the cross-sectional structure of these NCANDA data from the initial assessment do not support interpretations on the direction of the observed associations, multivariate models were presented that may suggest directions for future studies. The age range in this study was broad, a feature which limits the size of subsamples representing each adolescent stage. For this examination of the initial assessment data, the sample was insufficient to subgroup subjects by age. When data collection for NCANDA has been completed, the acquisition of additional follow-up data in this accelerated longitudinal design and the application of statistical modeling techniques developed for such studies will support the examination of changes in these relationships over the course of adolescence. In addition, analyses with the longitudinal data will clarify the extent to which alternative hypotheses are reflected in observed relationships. While this sample size is larger than many other similar studies, the recruitment strategy and sample characteristics were designed to optimally provide data for later analyses taking advantage of the accelerated longitudinal design, and were not ideal for some of the analyses presented here.

In summary, these analyses found significant and systematic relationships between executive dysfunction in daily life and SUD risk indicators, including a composite risk indicator (i.e., NCANDA Risk Density), poor sleep quality, and risky alcohol and marijuana use. In addition, the study contributed to the available literature on the relationship between BRIEF scores and performance based cognitive testing, indicating that these methods assess complimentary but distinct constructs. Everyday executive functioning was not systematically related to cortical structure or white matter integrity by DTI. With the on-going collection and analysis of additional follow-up assessments with the measures described here, and the examination of functional brain characteristics and other variables, NCANDA will provide insights on the relationships among difficulties with everyday executive functioning, performance-based cognitive testing of skills reflecting executive functions, structural and functional brain development, and alcohol and other substance use effects on these neurodevelopmental trajectories.

These results suggest that executive dysfunction in daily life is not accounted for by deficits in the cognitive skills measured in the NCANDA protocol. This observation has clinical implications, in that the results here imply that such testing may not provide the expected insights into the origins of executive dysfunction. Also, executive dysfunction was not accounted for by cortical structural or DTI characteristics. While some support has been presented that cognitive tests relate to some related mental disorders (e.g., ADHD: Willcutt et al., 2005), these results are consistent with other negative studies in suggesting that cognitive testing and MRI studies may not provide clinical insights explaining executive dysfunction with typical adolescents.

Consistent with several prior studies (Hasler and Clark, 2013; Hasler et al., 2014, 2016, 2017), poor sleep quality was related to both executive dysfunction and risky substance use. These findings suggest interventions to improve sleep may benefit executive functioning as well as risky substance use. Individually applicable clinical interventions to improve sleep quality have demonstrated effectiveness in adolescents (Gradisar et al., 2014). On a more general level, early school times may be detrimental to sleep quality, later sleep times warrant consideration (Hasler et al., 2014; Minges and Redeker, 2016).

Interventions to improve executive functioning, in addition to having inherent value, may also be be a viable preventive intervention target. Interventions that improve inhibitory control in childhood, for example, hold promise for preventing SUD in adolescence (Riggs and Greenberg, 2009; Diamond and Lee, 2011).

ETHICS STATEMENT

This study was carried out in accordance with the recommendations of Human Subjects Institutional Review Boards as noted below with written informed consent from all subjects. Institutional review boards approved the study for each site. University of California, San Diego (UCSD) Human Subjects Institutional Review Boards approved the study at each site: University of California, San Diego; Oregon Health & Science University; SRI International; Duke University; University of Pittsburgh. The protocol was approved by these committees. All subjects gave written informed consent in accordance with the Declaration of Helsinki. For participants under 18 years old, a parent provided written informed consent and the under 18 participant provided assent. Participants 18 years old or older provided written informed consent.

AUTHOR CONTRIBUTIONS

All authors (DC, TC, CM, BH, DF, BL, SB, ST, TB, KC, AP, ES, KP, IC, FB, MD, KN, and BN) were involved in study conception, data collection, and manuscript editing.

REFERENCES

Achenbach, T. M., and Rescorla, L. A. (2001a). *Manual for the ASEBA School-Age Forms and Profiles*. Burlington, VT: University of Vermont, Research Center for Children, Youth, and Families.

Achenbach, T. M., and Rescorla, L. A. (2001b). *Manual for the ASEBA Adult Forms and Profiles*. Burlington, VT: University of Vermont, Research Center for Children, Youth, and Families.

Anderson, B., Storfer-Isser, A., Taylor, H. G., Rosen, C. L., and Redline, S. (2009). Associations of executive function with sleepiness and sleep duration in adolescents. *Pediatrics* 123, e701–e707. doi: 10.1542/peds.2008-1182

Ashtari, M., Cervellione, K. L., Hasan, K. M., Wu, J., McIlree, C., Kester, H., et al. (2007). White matter development during late adolescence in healthy males: a cross-sectional diffusion tensor imaging study. *Neuroimage* 35, 501–510. doi: 10.1016/j.neuroimage.2006.10.047

Baker, F. C., Willoughby, A. R., de Zambotti, M., Franzen, P. L., Prouty, D., Javitz, H., et al. (2016). Age-related differences in sleep architecture and electroencephalogram in adolescents in the NCANDA sample. *Sleep* 39, 1429–1439. doi: 10.5665/sleep.5978

Baron, I. S. (2000). Behavior Rating Inventory of Executive Function. *Child Neuropsychol.* 6, 235–238. doi: 10.1076/chin.6.3.235.3152

Baron, R. M., and Kenny, D. A. (1986). The moderator-mediator variable distinction in social psychology research: conceptual, strategic, and statistical considerations. *J. Pers. Soc. Psychol.* 51, 1173–1182.

Best, J. R., and Miller, P. H. (2010). A developmental perspective on executive function. *Child Dev.* 81, 1641–1660. doi: 10.1111/j.1467-8624.2010.01499.x

Boschloo, A., Krabbendam, L., Aben, A., de Groot, R., and Jolles, J (2014). Sorting test, tower test, and BRIEF-SR do not predict school performance of healthy adolescents in preuniversity education. *Front. Psychol.* 5:287. doi: 10.3389/fpsyg.2014.00287

Brown, S. A., Brumback, T., Tomlinson, K., Cummins, K., Thompson, W. K., Nagel, B. J., et al. (2015). The National Consortium on Alcohol and Neurodevelopment in Adolescence (NCANDA): a multi-site study of adolescent development and substance use. *J. Stud. Alcohol Drugs* 76, 895–908. doi: 10.15288/jsad.2015.76.895

Brown, S. A., Myers, M. G., Lippke, L., Tapert, S. F., Stewart, D. G., and Vik, P. W. (1998). Psychometric evaluation of the customary drinking and drug use record (CDDR): a measure of adolescent alcohol and drug involvement. *J. Stud. Alcohol* 59, 427–438.

Buysse, D., Reynolds, C., Monk, T., Berman, S., and Kupfer, D (1989). The pittsburgh sleep quality index: a new instrument for psychiatric practice and research. *Psychiatry Res.* 28, 193–213

Caruso, N. C., Radovanovic, B., Kennedy, J. D., Couper, J., Kohler, M., Kavanagh, P. S., et al. (2014). Sleep, executive functioning and behavior in children and adolescents with type 1 diabetes. *Sleep Med.* 15, 1490–1499. doi: 10.1016/j.sleep.2014.08.011

Casey, B. J., Galvan, A., and Somerville, L. H. (2016). Beyond simple models of adolescence to an integrated circuit-based account: a commentary. *Dev. Cogn. Neurosci.* 17, 128–130. doi: 10.1016/j.dcn.2015.12.006

Chambers, R. A., Taylor, J. R., and Potenza, M. N. (2003). Developmental neurocircuitry of motivation in adolescence: a critical period of addiction vulnerability. *Am. J. Psychiatry* 160, 1041–1052. doi: 10.1176/appi.ajp.160.6.1041

Chan, R. C. K., Shum, D., Toulopoulou, T., and Chen, E. Y. H. (2008). Assessment of executive functions: review of instruments and identification of critical issues. *Arch. Clin. Neuropsychol.* 23, 201–216. doi: 10.1016/j.acn.2007.08.010

Chung, T., Smith, G. T., Donovan, J. E., Windle, M., Faden, V. B., Chen, C. M., et al. (2012). Drinking frequency as a brief screen for adolescent alcohol problems. *Pediatrics* 129, 1–8. doi: 10.1542/peds.2011-1828

Clark, D. B., Chung, T., Thatcher, D. L., Pajtek, S., and Long, E. C. (2012). Psychological dysregulation, white matter disorganization and substance use disorders in adolescence. *Addiction* 107, 206–214. doi: 10.1111/j.1360-0443.2011.03566.x

Clark, D. B., Martin, C. S., Chung, T., Gordon, A. J., Fiorentino, L., Tootell, M., et al. (2016). Screening for underage drinking and DSM-5 alcohol use disorder in rural primary care practice. *J. Pediatr.* 173, 214–220. doi: 10.1016/j.jpeds.2016.02.047

Clark, D. B., Pollock, N. A., Bromberger, J. T., Bukstein, O. G., Mezzich, A. C., and Donovan, J. E. (1997). Gender and comorbid psychopathology in adolescents with alcohol use disorders. *J. Am. Acad. Child Adolesc. Psychiatry* 36, 1195–1203.

Clark, D. B., Thatcher, D. L., and Tapert, S. (2008). Alcohol, psychological dysregulation and adolescent brain development. *Alcohol. Clin. Exp. Res.* 32, 375–385. doi: 10.1111/j.1530-0277.2007.00601.x

Clark, D. B., and Winters, K. C. (2002). Measuring risks and outcomes in substance use disorders prevention research. *J. Consult. Clin. Psychol.* 70, 1207–1223. doi: 10.1037/0022-006X.70.6.1207

Clarkson, M. J., Ourselin, S., Nielsen, C., Leung, K. K., Barnes, J., Whitwell, J. L., et al. (2009). Comparison of phantom and registration scaling corrections using the ADNI cohort. *Neuroimage* 47, 1506–1513. doi: 10.1016/j.neuroimage.2009.05.045

Cyders, M. A., and Coskunpinar, A (2012). The relationship between self-report and lab task conceptualizations of impulsivity. *J. Res. Pers.* 46, 121–124. doi: 10.1016/j.jrp.2011.11.005

Dale, A. M., Fischl, B., and Sereno, M. I. (1999). cortical surface-based analysis. I. segmentations and surface reconstruction. *Neuroimage* 9, 179–194.

de la Vega, R., Tome-Pires, C., Sole, E., Racine, M., Castarlenas, E., Jensen, M. P., et al. (2015). The Pittsburgh sleep quality index: validity and factor structure in young people. *Psychol. Assess.* 27, e22–e27. doi: 10.1037/pas0000128

Desikan, R. S., Segonne, F., Fischl, B., Quinn, B. T., Dickerson, B. C., Blacker, D., et al. (2006). An automated labeling system for subdividing the human cerebral cortex on MRI scans into gyral based regions of interest. *Neuroimage* 31, 968–980. doi: 10.1016/j.neuroimage.2006.01.021

Diamond, A., and Lee, K (2011). Interventions shown to aid executive function development in children 4 to 12 years old. *Science* 333, 959–964. doi: 10.1126/science.1204529

Donovan, J. E. (2009). estimated blood alcohol concentrations for child and adolescent drinking and their implications for screening instruments. *Pediatrics* 123, e975–e981. doi: 10.1542/peds.2008-0027

Duncan, S. C., Duncan, T. E., and Hops, H. (1996). Analysis of longitudinal data within accelerated longitudinal designs. *Psychol. Methods* 1, 236–248. doi: 10.1037/1082-989X.1.3.236

Duncan, S. C., Duncan, T. E., and Strycker, LA (2006). Alcohol use from ages 9 to 16: a cohort-sequential latent growth model. *Drug Alcohol Depend.* 81, 71–81. doi: 10.1016/j.drugalcdep.2005.06.001

Egeland, J., and Fallmyr, O. (2010). Confirmatory factor analysis of the Behavior Rating Inventory of Executive Function (BRIEF): support for a distinction between emotional and behavioral regulation. *Child Neuropsychol.* 164, 326–337. doi: 10.1080/09297041003601462

Fair, D. A., Cohen, A. L., Power, J. D., Dosenbach, N. U., Church, J. A., Miezin, F, et al. (2009). Functional brain networks develop from "local to distributed" organization. *PLoS Comput. Biol.* 5, 1–14. doi: 10.1371/journal.pcbi.1000381

Familiar, I., Ruisenor-Escudero, H., Giordani, B., Bangirana, P., Nakasujja, N., Opoka, R., et al. (2015). Use of the Behavior Rating Inventory of Executive Function and child behavior checklist in Ugandan children with HIV or a history of severe malaria. *J. Dev. Behav. Pediatr.* 36, 277–284. doi: 10.1097/DBP.0000000000000149

Faridi, N., Karama, S., Burgaleta, M., White, M. T., Evans, A. C., Fonov, V., et al. (2015). Neuroanatomical correlates of behavioral rating versus performance measures of working memory in typically developing children and adolescents. *Neuropsychology* 29, 82–91. doi: 10.1037/neu0000079

Fassbender, C., Simoes-Franklin, C., Murphy, K., Hester, R., Meaney, J., Robertson, I. H., et al. (2006). The role of a right fronto-parietal network in cognitive control - common activations for "cues-to-attend" and response inhibition. *J. Psychophysiol.* 20, 286–296. doi: 10.1027/0269-8803.20.4.286

Fossati, P. (2012). Neural correlates of emotion processing: from emotional to social brain. *Eur. Neuropsychopharmacol.* 22, 487–491. doi: 10.1016/j.euroneuro.2012.07.008

Gioia, G. A., Isquith, P. K., Guy, S. C., and Kenworthy, L. (2002a). *Behavior Rating Inventory of Executive Function (BRIEF).* Lutz, FL: Psychological Assessment Resources.

Gioia, G. A., Isquith, P. K., Retzlaff, P. D., and Espy, K. A. (2002b). Confirmatory factor analysis of the Behavior Rating Inventory of Executive Function (BRIEF) in a clinical sample. *Child Neuropsychol.* 8, 249–257. doi: 10.1076/chin.8.4.249.13513

Gradisar, M., Smits, M. G., and Bjorvatn, B (2014). Assessment and treatment of delayed sleep phase disorder in adolescents: recent innovations and cautions. *Sleep Med. Clin.* 9, 199–210. doi: 10.1016/j.jsmc.2014.02.005

Gur, R. C., Richard, J., Hughett, P., Calkins, M. E., Macy, L., Bilker, W. B., et al. (2010). A cognitive neuroscience-based computerized battery for efficient measurement of individual differences: standardization and initial construct validation. *J. Neurosci. Methods* 187, 254–262. doi: 10.1016/j.jneumeth.2009.11.017

Gur, R. C., Sara, R., Hagendoorn, M., Marom, O., Hughett, P., Macy, L., et al. (2002). A method for obtaining 3-dimensional facial expressions and its standardization for use in neurocognitive studies. *J. Neurosci. Methods* 15, 137–143. doi: 10.1016/S0165-0270(02)00006-7

Guy, S. C., Isquith, P. K., and Gioia, G. A. (2004). *Behavior Rating Inventory of Executive Function – Self-Report Version.* Lutz, FL: Psychological Assessment Resources.

Hackman, D. A., Gallop, R., Evans, G. W., and Farah, M. J. (2015). Socioeconomic status and executive function: developmental trajectories and mediation. *Dev. Sci.* 18, 686–702. doi: 10.1111/desc.12246

Hadjiefthyvoulou, F., Fisk, J. E., Montgomery, C., and Bridges, N. (2012). Self-reports of executive dysfunction in current ecstasy/polydrug users. *Cogn. Behav. Neurol.* 25, 128–138. doi: 10.1097/WNN.0b013e318261459c

Hasler, B., and Clark, D. B. (2013). Circadian misalignment, reward-related brain function, and adolescent alcohol involvement. *Alcohol. Clin. Exp. Res.* 37, 558–565. doi: 10.1111/acer.12003

Hasler, B. P., Franzen, P., de Zambotti, M., Prouty, D., Brown, S., Tapert, S., et al. (2017). Eveningness and later sleep timing are associated with greater risk for alcohol and marijuana use in adolescence: initial findings from the NCANDA study. *Alcohol. Clin. Exp. Res.* 41, 1154–1165. doi: 10.1111/acer.13401

Hasler, B. P., Kirisci, L., and Clark, D. B. (2016). Restless sleep and variable sleep timing during late childhood accelerate the onset of alcohol and drug involvement. *J. Stud. Alcohol Drugs* 77, 649–655. doi: 10.15288/jsad.2016.77.649

Hasler, B. P., Martin, C. S., Wood, D. S., Rosario, B., and Clark, D. B. (2014). A longitudinal study of insomnia and other sleep complaints in adolescents with and without alcohol use disorders. *Alcohol. Clin. Exp. Res.* 38, 2225–2233. doi: 10.1111/acer.12474

Klingberg, T., Vaidya, C. J., Gabrieli, J. D., Moseley, M. E., and Hedehus, M. (1999). Myelination and organization of the frontal white matter in children: a diffusion tensor MRI study. *Neuroreport* 10, 2817–2921. doi: 10.1097/00001756-199909090-00022

Kurtz, M. M., Ragland, J. D., Bilker, W., Gur, R. C., and Gur, R. E. (2001). Comparison of the continuous performance test with and without working memory demands in healthy controls and patients with schizophrenia. *Schizophr. Res.* 48, 307–316. doi: 10.1016/S0920-9964(00)00060-8

Langberg, J. M., Dvorsky, M. R., and Evans, S. W. (2013). What specific facets of executive function are associated with academic functioning in youth with attention-deficit/hyperactivity disorder? *J. Abnorm. Child Psychol.* 41, 1145–1159. doi: 10.1007/s10802-013-9750-z

Lee, N. R., Raznahan, A., Wallance, G. L., Alexander-Bloch, A., Clasen, L. S., Lerch, J. P., et al. (2014). anatomical coupling among distributed cortical regions in youth varies as a function of individual differences in vocabulary abilities. *Hum. Brain Mapp.* 35, 1885–1895. doi: 10.1002/hbm.22299

Lenroot, R. K., and Giedd, J. N. (2006). Brain development in children and adolescents: insights from anatomical magnetic resonance imaging. *Neurosci. Biobehav. Rev.* 30, 718–729. doi: 10.1016/j.neubiorev.2006.06.001

Lipton, M. L., Gulko, E., Zimmerman, M. E., Friedman, B. W., Kim, M., Gellella, E., et al. (2009). Diffusion-tensor imaging implicates prefrontal axonal injury in executive function impairment following very mild traumatic brain injury. *Radiology* 252, 816–824. doi: 10.1148/radiol.2523081584

Long, E., Luna, B., Verhulst, B., and Clark, D. B. (2015). Disruptive behavior disorders and indicators of disinhibition in adolescents: the BRIEF-SR, anti-saccade task, and D-KEFS color-word interference test. *J. Adolesc.* 44, 182–190. doi: 10.1016/j.adolescence.2015.07.003

Ludbrook, J. (1998). Multiple comparison procedures updated. *Clin. Exp. Pharmacol. Physiol.* 25, 1032–1037. doi: 10.1111/j.1440-1681.1998.tb02179.x

Mahone, E. M., Martin, R., Kates, W. R., Hay, T., and Horska, A. (2009). Neuroimaging correlates of parent ratings of working memory in typically developing children. *J. Int. Neuropsychol. Soc.* 15, 31–41. doi: 10.1017/S1355617708090164

Millman, R. P. (2005). Excessive sleepiness in adolescents and young adults: causes, consequences, and treatment strategies. *Pediatrics* 115, 1774–1786. doi: 10.1542/peds.2005-0772

Minges, K. E., and Redeker, N. S. (2016). Delayed school start times and adolescent sleep: a systematic review of the experimental evidence. *Sleep Med. Rev.* 28, 82–91. doi: 10.1016/j.smrv.2015.06.002

Mollayeva, T., Thurairajah, P., Burton, K., Mollayeva, S., Shapiro, C. M., and Colantonio, A. (2016). The Pittsburgh Sleep Quality Index as a screening tool for sleep dysfunction in clinical and non-clinical samples: a systematic review and meta-analysis. *Sleep Med. Rev.* 25, 52–73. doi: 10.1016/j.smrv.2015.01.009

National Institute on Alcohol Abuse and Alcoholism (2011). *Alcohol Screening and Brief Intervention for Youth: A Practitioner's Guide. NIH Publications 11-7805.* Bethesda, MD: National Institute on Alcohol Abuse and Alcoholism.

Noone, D. M., Willis, T. A., Cox, J., Harkness, F., Ogilvie, J., Forbes, E., et al. (2014). Catastrophizing and poor sleep quality in early adolescent females. *Behav. Sleep Med.* 12, 41–52. doi: 10.1080/15402002.2013.764528

Paus, T (2010). Growth of white matter in the adolescent brain: myelin or axon? *Brain Cogn.* 72, 26–35. doi: 10.1016/j.bandc.2009.06.002

Pfefferbaum, A., Rohlfing, T., Pohl, K. M., Lane, B., Chu, W., Kwon, D., et al. (2016). Adolescent development of cortical and white matter structure in the NCANDA sample: role of sex, ethnicity, puberty, and alcohol drinking. *Cereb. Cortex* 26, 4101–4121. doi: 10.1093/cercor/bhv205

Pohl, K. M., Sullivan, E. V., Rohlfing, T., Chu, W., Kwon, D., Nichols, B. N., et al. (2016). Harmonizing DTI measurements across scanners to examine the development of white matter microstructure in 803 adolescents of the NCANDA study. *Neuroimage* 130, 194–213. doi: 10.1016/j.neuroimage.2016.01.061

Ragland, J. D., Turetsky, B. I., Gur, R. C., Gunning-Dixon, F., Turner, T., Schroeder, L., et al. (2002). Working memory for complex figures: an fMRI comparison of letter and fractal n-back tasks. *Neuropsychology* 16, 370–379. doi: 10.1037/0894-4105.16.3.370

Riggs, N. R., and Greenberg, M. T. (2009). Neurocognition as a moderator and mediator in adolescent substance misuse prevention. *Am. J. Drug Alcohol Abuse* 35, 209–213. doi: 10.1080/00952990903005940

Rohlfing, T., Cummins, K., Henthorn, T., Chu, W., and Nichols, B. N. (2014). N-CANDA data integration: anatomy of an asynchronous infrastructure for multi-site, multi-instrument longitudinal data capture. *J. Am. Med. Inform. Assoc.* 21, 758–762. doi: 10.1136/amiajnl-2013-002367

Roth, R. M., Erdodi, L. A., McColloch, L. J., and Isquith, P. K. (2015). Much ado about norming: the Behavior Rating Inventory of Executive Function. *Child Neuropsychol.* 21, 225–233. doi: 10.1080/09297049.2014.897318

Samuels, W. E., Tournaki, N., Blackman, S., and Zilinski, C (2016). Executive functioning predicts academic achievement in middle school: a four-year longitudinal study. *J. Educ. Res.* 109, 478–490. doi: 10.1080/00220671.2014.979913

Šidák, Z. K. (1967). Rectangular confidence regions for the means of multivariate normal distributions. *J. Am. Stat. Assoc.* 62, 626–633. doi: 10.1080/01621459.1967.10482935

Shimoni, M., Engel-Yeger, B., and Tirosh, E. (2012). Executive dysfunctions among boys with attention deficit hyperactivity disorder (ADHD): performance-based test and parents report. *Res. Dev. Disabil.* 33, 858–865. doi: 10.1016/j.ridd.2011.12.014

Skranes, J., Lohaugen, G. C., Martinussen, M., Indredavik, M. S., Dale, A. M., Haraldseth, O., et al. (2009). White matter abnormalities and executive function in children with very low birth weight. *Neuroreport* 20, 263–266. doi: 10.1097/WNR.0b013e32832027fe

Spear, L. P. (2000). The adolescent brain and age-related behavioral manifestations. *Neurosci. Biobehav. Rev.* 24, 417–463. doi: 10.1016/S0149-7634(00)00014-2

Sullivan, E., Brumback, T., Tapert, S., Fama, R., Prouty, D., Brown, S. A., et al. (2016). Cognitive, emotion control, and motor baseline performance of adolescents in the NCANDA study: contributions from alcohol consumption, age, puberty, sex, ethnicity, and family history of addiction. *Neuropsychol.* 30, 449–473. doi: 10.1037/neu0000259

Sullivan, E., Brumback, T., Tapert, S., Prouty, D., Fama, R., Brown, S., et al. (2017). Effects of prior testing lasting a full year in NCANDA adolescents: contributions from age, sex, socioeconomic status, ethnicity, site, family history of alcohol or drug abuse, and baseline performance. *Develop. Cogn. Neurosci.* 24, 72–83. doi: 10.1016/j.dcn.2017.01.003

Takahashi, T., Murata, T., Omori, M., Kosaka, H., Takahashi, K., Yonekura, Y., et al. (2004). Quantitative evaluation of age-related white matter microstructural changes on MRI by multifractal analysis. *J. Neurol. Sci.* 225, 33–37. doi: 10.1016/j.jns.2004.06.016

Tapert, S. F., and Brown, S. A. (2000). Substance dependence, family history of alcohol dependence and neuropsychological functioning in adolescence. *Addiction* 95, 1043–1053. doi: 10.1046/j.1360-0443.2000.95710436.x

Tarter, R. E., Kirisci, L., Mezzich, A., Cornelius, J., Pajer, K., Vanyukov, M., et al. (2003). Neurobehavioral disinhibition in childhood predicts early age onset substance use disorder.*Am. J. Psychiatry* 160, 1078–1085. doi: 10.1176/appi.ajp.160.6.1078

Toplak, M. E., West, R. F., and Stanovich, K. E. (2013). Practitioner review: do performance-based measures and ratings of executive function assess the same construct? *J. Child Psychol. Psychiatry* 54, 131–143. doi: 10.1111/jcpp.12001

Vanyukov, M., Kirisci, L., Tarter, R. E., Ridenour, T. A., Reynolds, M. D., Maher, B., et al. (2009). Measurement of the risk for substance use disorders: phenotypic and genetic analysis of an index of common liability. *Behav. Genet.* 39, 233–244. doi: 10.1007/s10519-009-9269-9

Wang, Y., Horst, K. K., Kronenberger, W. G., Hummer, T. A., Mosier, K. M., Kalnin, A. J., et al. (2012). White matter abnormalities associated with disruptive behavior disorder in adolescents with and without attention-deficit./hyperactivity disorder. *Psychiatry Res. Neuroimag.* 202, 245–251. doi: 10.1016/j.pscychresns.2012.01.005

Wilkinson, G. S., and Robertson, G. J. (2006). *WRAT 4: Wide Range Achievement Test: Professional Manual.* Lutz, FL: Psychological Assessment Resources, Incorporated.

Willcutt, E. G., Doyle, A. E., Nigg, J. T., Faraone, S. V., and Pennington, B. F. (2005). Validity of the executive function theory of attention-deficit/hyperactivity disorder: a meta-analytic review. *Biol. Psychiatry* 57, 1336–1346. doi: 10.1016/j.biopsych.2005.02.006

Zhai, Z., Pajtek, S., Luna, B., Geier, C., Ridenour, T., and Clark, D. B. (2015). Reward modulated response inhibition, cognitive shifting, and the orbital frontal cortex in early adolescence. *J. Res. Adolesc.* 24, 753–764. doi: 10.1111/jora.12168

Ziegler, G., Dahnke, R., Winkler, A. D., and Gaser, C. (2013). Partial least squares correlation of multivariate cognitive abilities and local brain structure in children and adolescents. *Neuroimage* 82, 284–294. doi: 10.1016/j.neuroimage.2013.05.088

18

Effects of Intermittent Alcohol Exposure on Emotion and Cognition: A Potential Role for the Endogenous Cannabinoid System and Neuroinflammation

Laura Sanchez-Marin [†], Francisco J. Pavon [†], Juan Decara, Juan Suarez, Ana Gavito, Estela Castilla-Ortega, Fernando Rodriguez de Fonseca * and Antonia Serrano *

Unidad de Gestion Clinica de Salud Mental, Instituto de Investigacion Biomedica de Malaga, Hospital Regional Universitario de Malaga, Universidad de Malaga, Malaga, Spain

Edited by:
Mary M. Torregrossa,
University of Pittsburgh, USA

Reviewed by:
Tommy Pattij,
VU University Medical Center,
Netherlands
Consuelo Guerri,
Centro de Investigación Príncipe
Felipe, Spain

***Correspondence:**
Fernando Rodriguez de Fonseca
fernando.rodriguez@ibima.eu
Antonia Serrano
antonia.serrano@ibima.eu

[†] These authors have contributed equally to this work.

Intermittent alcohol exposure is a common pattern of adolescent alcohol use that can lead to binge drinking episodes. Alcohol use is known to modulate the endocannabinoid system (ECS), which is involved in neuronal communication, neuroplasticity, neuroinflammation and behavior. Adolescent male Wistar rats were exposed to 4-week intermittent alcohol intoxication (3 g/kg injections for 4 days/week) or saline ($N = 12$ per group). After alcohol deprivation, adult rats were assessed for emotionality and cognition and the gene expression of the ECS and other factors related to behavior and neuroinflammation was examined in the brain. Alcohol-exposed rats exhibited anxiogenic-like responses and impaired recognition memory but no motor alterations. There were brain region-dependent changes in the mRNA levels of the ECS and molecular signals compared with control rats. Thus, overall, alcohol-exposed rats expressed higher mRNA levels of endocannabinoid synthetic enzymes (N-acyl-phosphatidylethanolamine phospholipase D and diacylglycerol lipases) in the medial-prefrontal cortex (mPFC) but lower mRNA levels in the amygdala. Furthermore, we observed lower mRNA levels of receptors CB_1 CB_2 and peroxisome proliferator-activated receptor-α in the striatum. Regarding neuropeptide signaling, alcohol-exposed rats displayed lower mRNA levels of the neuropeptide Y signaling, particularly NPY receptor-2, in the amygdala and hippocampus and higher mRNA levels of corticotropin-releasing factor in the hippocampus. Additionally, we observed changes of several neuroinflammation-related factors. Whereas, the mRNA levels of toll-like receptor-4, tumor necrosis factor-α, cyclooxygenase-2 and glial fibrillary acidic protein were significantly increased in the mPFC, the mRNA levels of cyclooxygenase-2 and glial fibrillary acidic protein were decreased in the striatum and hippocampus. However, nuclear factor-κβ mRNA levels were lower in the mPFC and striatum and allograft inflammatory factor-1 levels were differentially expressed in the amygdala and hippocampus. In conclusion, rats exposed to adolescent intermittent alcohol displayed anxiety-like behavior and cognitive deficits in adulthood and these alterations were accompanied by brain region-dependent changes in the gene expression of the ECS and other signals associated with neuroinflammation and behavior. An intermittent adolescent alcohol exposure has behavioral and molecular consequences in the adult brain, which might be linked to higher vulnerability to addictive behaviors and psychopathologies.

Keywords: rats, intermittent alcohol, adolescence, endocannabinoid system, neuroinflammation, anxiety, brain, recognition memory

INTRODUCTION

Alcohol is the most widely used recreational drug, and its consumption is increasing in young people and adolescents. A common pattern of alcohol intake among adolescents is the intermittent alcohol exposure, which can lead eventually to heavy episodic drinking. Thus, adolescent binge drinking is a major public health concern and it is associated with long-term health consequences, including mental problems (e.g., anxiety, mood and personality disorders) and substance use disorders, primarily alcoholism (Oesterle et al., 2004; Dawson et al., 2008; Read et al., 2008). Further, the potential role of alcohol use as a risk factor for adult psychiatric disorders cannot be discarded.

The molecular actions of alcohol on the brain are complex, and involve several mechanisms and signaling systems and some of these actions occur in both the adult and the adolescent brain. Brain maturation mainly happens during adolescence, when numerous plastic and dynamic processes are happening, and the vulnerability of the developing brain to the toxic effects of alcohol is higher. Therefore, early alcohol exposure can produce alterations in the brain structure and function, resulting in behavioral and cognitive deficits (Nagel et al., 2005; Zeigler et al., 2005; Guerri et al., 2009). These long-term harmful effects of alcohol exposure on behavior have also been confirmed in animal models (e.g., learning dysfunctions in adolescent rats exposed to repeated alcohol continue into adulthood) (Crews et al., 2000; Pascual et al., 2007).

Alcohol and other drugs of abuse induce changes in the Central Nervous System (CNS) that can lead to pathological behaviors related to addiction. In fact, the transition to alcoholism involves changes in the reinforcing and rewarding effects of alcohol use, a dysregulation of synaptic plasticity and the development of maladaptive stress responses (Kalivas and O'Brien, 2008; Koob, 2008). A variety of signals and neurotransmitters (e.g., dopamine, serotonin, glutamate, GABA, opioids, endocannabinoids...) in the CNS are implicated in the pathophysiology and development of alcoholism which play a prominent role in mediating behavioral and pharmacological effects of alcohol (Koob et al., 1998).

Over the past years, numerous studies have demonstrated the involvement of the endogenous cannabinoid system (ECS) in the behavioral and pharmacological effects of alcohol (Serrano and Parsons, 2011). The ECS includes endogenous ligands, cannabinoid receptors and the enzymatic machinery for the synthesis and inactivation of endocannabinoids. The main endocannabinoids are arachidonoylethanolamide (AEA) and 2-arachidonoylglycerol (2-AG), which bind to cannabinoid receptors to exert their effects. The cannabinoid receptors are G protein-coupled receptors and two types have been characterized and cloned, CB_1 and CB_2 (Howlett et al., 1990; Munro et al., 1993). Regarding the metabolic pathways for endocannabinoids, there are very complex enzymatic cascades for synthesis and inactivation that are crucial in regulating their levels. The primary pathway for AEA synthesis is mediated by a specific phospholipase D (NAPE-PLD) (Okamoto et al., 2004), while the synthetic pathway for 2-AG is mainly mediated by two sn-1-selective diacylglycerol lipases (DAGL-α and DAGL-β) (Bisogno et al., 2003). Finally, the inactivation of endocannabinoids is mediated by cellular reuptake and subsequent intracellular hydrolysis and both fatty acid amide hydrolase (FAAH) and monoacylglycerol lipase (MAGL) have been identified as enzymes primarily responsible for the degradation of AEA and 2-AG, respectively (Cravatt et al., 1996; Dinh et al., 2002).

The ECS has been widely studied in recent years due to its anti-inflammatory and homeostatic properties, which is of interest because alcohol abuse is associated with the induction of neuroinflammatory and neurodegenerative processes. In this regard, binge-like alcohol exposure increases the nuclear factor-*kappa* β (NF-κβ)-DNA binding activity, up-regulates the expression of cyclooxygenase-2 (COX-2), causes microglia activation (Knapp and Crews, 1999; Obernier et al., 2002a; Crews et al., 2006) and induces brain injury in the cortex and hippocampus associated with cognitive deficits (Crews et al., 2000; Obernier et al., 2002b; Tajuddin et al., 2014; Antón et al., 2016). However, it is important to consider that all the mentioned effects of alcohol use depend on several factors, including age of the subject, amount of alcohol consumed, duration and pattern of alcohol consumption (Kovacs and Messingham, 2002; Goral et al., 2008).

Long-term effects of alcohol exposure in animal models have revealed clear deleterious impact on emotional and cognitive processing, as well as on underlying inflammatory responses triggered by the unique ability of alcohol to direct activate natural immunity through toll-like receptor-4 (TLR4) (Fernandez-Lizarbe et al., 2009; Pascual et al., 2011). In fact, recent studies have reported the role of TLR4 in behavioral and cognitive dysfunctions using models of intermittent alcohol exposure in adolescence (Montesinos et al., 2015, 2016).

In this context, the present study aimed to characterize the impact of an adolescent intermittent alcohol exposure in emotional behaviors (open field and elevated-plus maze), cognitive responses (novel object recognition memory) and gene expression of primary signaling systems related to neuroinflammation, anxiety and stress in adult rats. The medial prefrontal cortex, amygdala, striatum and hippocampus were selected for gene expression analysis since they play a predominant role in alcohol-related behaviors and neuroadaptations.

MATERIALS AND METHODS

Animals and Ethical Statement

Twenty-four male Wistar rats (Charles River Laboratories, Barcelona, Spain) weighing 100–125 g on postnatal day (pnd) 24 were housed individually in a humidity and temperature-controlled vivarium on a 12 h light/dark cycle (lights off at 19:00 h). Rats were allowed to acclimatize to the new environment for 7 days before any experimental procedure was performed (pnd 31). Water and rat chow pellets were available *ad libitum*.

This study was carried out in accordance with the European Directive 2010/63/EU for the protection of animals used for scientific purposes and Spanish regulations (Real Decreto 53/2013 and 178/2004, Ley 32/2007 and 9/2003 and Decreto 320/2010) for the care and use of laboratory animals. The protocol was approved by the Ethic and research Committee at the Universidad de Malaga. All efforts were made to minimize animal suffering and social isolation, as well as to reduce the number of animals used.

Experimental Design

As shown in **Figure 1**, adolescent rats (pnd 31) were randomly assigned to the experimental alcohol group following 4 weeks of intermittent alcohol exposure ($n = 12$) or control group ($n = 12$).

Intermittent Alcohol Procedure

An intraperitoneal (i.p.) administration of ethanol solution was used as intermittent intoxication during 4 weeks. Rats were injected weekly with 3 g/kg of ethanol (20% in saline, w/v) for 4 consecutive days followed by 3 days of alcohol deprivation. After the adolescent alcohol exposure, rats were left undisturbed in their home-cages before performing behavioral tests to evaluate locomotor activity, cognitive responses and anxiety-like behaviors. Following a schedule similar to the alcohol group, control animals received an injection of saline and they were also individually maintained in their home-cages for controlling the effects of social isolation on behavioral experiments and biochemical determinations previously reported in adolescence (Skelly et al., 2015).

Determination of Blood Ethanol Concentration

Rats were tail-bled 1 h after the last alcohol exposure. Blood was collected into a microtube containing anticoagulant (4 μl heparin; 1000 USP units/ml) and centrifuged at 2000 × g for 10 min. Serum was extracted and assayed for ethanol concentration (BEC) using the alcohol oxidase method with an AM1 Alcohol Analyzer (Analox Instrument, London, UK).

Behavioral Studies

Behavioral tests were conducted by trained observers who were unaware of the experimental conditions.

Open Field Test

Motor and anxiety-like behaviors were studied in an opaque open field (100 × 100 × 40 cm) divided into 16 squares with two zones; the center (4 squares) and periphery (12 squares) of the field. The open field was illuminated using a ceiling halogen lamp that was regulated to yield 350 lux at the center of the field. On the experimental day, the animals were placed in the center and the locomotor activity and time spent in the center and periphery were scored for 15 min. The number of crossings (expressed as number lines/squares crossed) and the percent of time spent in the center (time spent in the center/total time × 100) were calculated.

This task was also used as habituation session for the novel object recognition test.

Novel Object Recognition Test

The novel object recognition procedure consists of habituation, familiarization, and test phases. Familiarization phase was conducted 24 h after the habituation phase. During the familiarization phase, animals were placed in the test field and allowed to explore for 3 min two identical objects. Then, animals were returned to their home-cage for 1 h. Test phase was conducted by placing rats for 3 min in the test field with 2 different objects, one was familiar and the other one was novel. Objects were made in plastic but different in shape, size and color. Between each test, the relative position of both objects were counterbalanced and permuted.

The time spent in exploring these objects were recorded in both phases. The exploration time was defined as the time that animals spent in licking, sniffing or touching each object, but it was not considered the time spent in standing or sitting on or leaning against each object (expressed in seconds). The novel object preference was determined using the discrimination ratio (expressed as the difference in time exploring the novel and the familiar objects/total exploration time).

Elevated Plus-Maze

The elevated plus-maze was made of opaque plastic and was composed of 2 oppositely positioned open arms (45 × 10 cm), 2 oppositely positioned closed arms of the same size and 50-cm-high walls. The arms were connected by a central and neutral area (10 × 10 cm). The entire apparatus was elevated 75 cm above a white floor and exposed to dim illumination (70 lux). At the beginning, rats were placed in the center of the maze, facing an open arm, and were allowed to freely explore the maze for 5 min. The number of entries (an arm entry was defined as all four paws in the arm zone) and the time spent in each arm were scored using a video monitor. The number of entries into the closed arms (expressed as number of entries into the closed arms) and the percent of time spent in the exposed arm (time spent in the open arms/total time × 100) were calculated.

Sample Collection

Two weeks after the last alcohol exposure (pnd 70), rats were anesthetized with sodium pentobarbital (50 mg/kg, i.p.) and brain samples were collected. The brains were quickly removed, immediately frozen on dry ice and stored at −80°C,

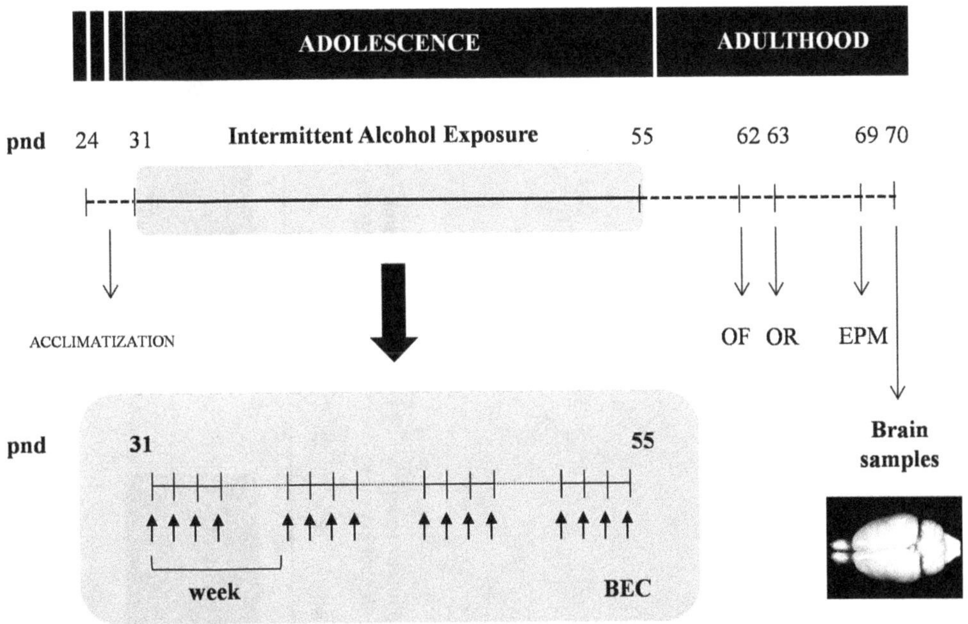

FIGURE 1 | Experimental design of the study. Rats were exposed to an intermittent alcohol exposure for 4 weeks (from pnd 31 to 55). During this period, rats were randomly assigned to alcohol (repeated i.p. administration) or control (saline) group. Blood ethanol concentrations (BEC) were determined 60 min after the last alcohol exposure. The analyzes of behavior on the open field (OF), novel object recognition (OR) and elevated plus-maze (EPM) were carried out in the different groups at 1 and 2 weeks after the alcohol exposure. All animals were sacrificed 2 weeks after the last alcohol exposure and brain samples were collected.

until determination of the gene expression of proteins using quantitative real-time reverse transcription polymerase chain reaction (RT-qPCR).

Dissection of the Brain

The frozen brains were placed in acrylic rat brain matrices, and 2-mm thick slices were obtained using brain matrix razor blades. The medial prefrontal cortex (mPFC), striatum (accumbens, caudate, and putamen nucleus), entire amygdala and dorsal and ventral hippocampus were dissected out bilaterally and collected using a scalpel (mPFC and hippocampus) and a sample corer (striatum and amygdala). The localization of the brain regions was performed using a rat brain atlas and considering the bregma point as zero coordinate in the rostral-caudal coordinates: mPFC, +3.0 mm to +5.0 mm from bregma; striatum, +1.0 mm to −1.0 mm from bregma; amygdala, −1.0 mm to −3.0 mm from bregma; and hippocampus, −3.0 mm to −5.0 mm from bregma (Paxinos and Watson, 1998).

RNA Isolation and RT-qPCR Analysis

Total RNA was extracted from brain samples using Trizol Reagent (Gibco BRL Life Technologies, Baltimore, MD, USA) and the concentrations were quantified using a spectrophotometer to ensure ratios of absorbance at 260 to 280 nm of 1.8–2.0. The reverse transcription was performed using the Transcriptor Reverse Transcriptase kit and random hexamer primers (Transcriptor RT; Roche Diagnostic, Mannheim, Germany). The RT-qPCR was performed using an ABI PRISM® 7300 Real-Time PCR System (Applied Biosystems, Foster City, CA, USA) and the FAM dye label format for the TaqMan Gene Expression Assays (Applied Biosystems). The absolute values from each sample were normalized relative to the housekeeping β-actin gene (*Actb*). The relative quantification was calculated using the $\Delta\Delta$Ct method and normalized to the control group. Primers for the RT-qPCR were obtained based on the Applied Biosystems genome database of rat mRNA references (http://bioinfo.appliedbiosystems.com/genome-database/gene-expression.html) (**Table 1**).

Statistical Analysis

All the data in the graphs are expressed as the means ± SEM. The statistical analysis was performed using GraphPad Prism version 5.04 (GraphPad Software, San Diego, CA, USA) and the normal distribution of data was evaluated by D'Agostino-Pearson omnibus test. Student's *t*-test and Welch's *t*-test for unequal variances were conducted to compare continuous variables between the two experimental groups (Control and Alcohol). Two-way analysis of variance (ANOVA) was conducted in the Novel Object Recognition Test using alcohol exposure (control and alcohol) and type of object (familiar and novel) as factors and using Bonferroni as *post hoc* test. Benjamini–Hochberg false discovery rate (FDR) approach was used for multiple comparisons (Benjamini et al., 2001) of the mRNA expression analysis. The statistics (*t*-statistic and *F*-statistic) and degrees of freedom were indicated in the description of results. The significance level was established at 0.05 and a *p*-value of less than 0.05 was considered statistically significant. Additionally,

TABLE 1 | Primers references for TaqMan® Gene Expression Assays.

Gene symbol	Assay ID	GenBank accession number	Amplicon length
Actb	Rn00667869_m1	NM_031144.3	91
Cnr1	Rn02758689_s1	NM_012784.4	92
Cnr2	Rn01637601_m1	NM_020543.4	68
Dagla	Rn01454304_m1	NM_001005886.1	67
Daglb	Rn01453771_m1	NM_001107120.1	98
Faah	Rn00577086_m1	NM_024132.3	63
Mgll	Rn00593297_m1	NM_138502.2	78
Napepld	Rn01786262_m1	NM_199381.1	71
Ppara	Rn00566193_m1	NM_013196.1	98
Crh	Rn01462137_m1	NM_031019.1	112
Crhr1	Rn00578611_m1	XM_006247542.2	58
Crhr2	Rn00575617_m1	NM_022714.1	82
Npy	Rn00561681_m1	NM_012614.2	63
Npy1r	Rn02769337_s1	NM_001113357.1	98
Npy2r	Rn00576733_s1	NM_023968.1	65
Npy5r	Rn02089867_s1	NM_012869.1	107
Aif1	Rn00574125_g1	NM_017196.3	126
Gfap	Rn01253033_m1	NM_017009.2	75
Ptgs2	Rn01483830_g1	NM_017232.3	69
Rela	Rn01502266_m1	NM_199267.2	67
Tlr4	Rn00569848_m1	NM_019178.1	127
Tnf	Rn99999017_m1	NM_012675.3	108

FDR adjusted significance levels were indicated for the multiple comparisons in each case.

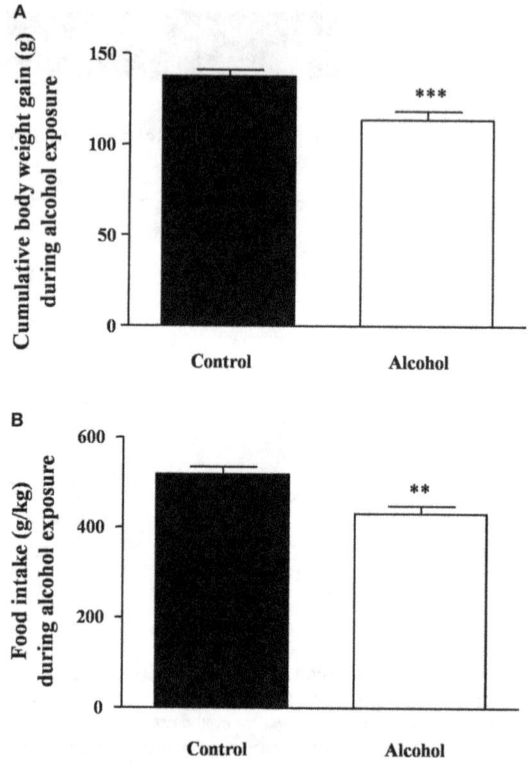

FIGURE 2 | Body weight gain and food intake during intermittent alcohol exposure in adolescent rats. Cumulative body weight gain **(A)** and food intake **(B)** after 4 weeks of alcohol exposure. Bars represent the mean ± SEM (8–12 animals per group). Data were analyzed by Student's *t*-test (Welch's correction). $^{**}p < 0.01$ and $^{***}p < 0.001$ denote significant differences compared with the control group.

RESULTS

In the present study, we examined adult rats exposed to intermittent alcohol exposures during adolescence. We assessed anxiety-like and cognitive behaviors as well as the mRNA expression of numerous enzymes and receptors involved in the ECS and other mediators linked to behavior, neuroinflammation and plasticity.

Body Weight Gain and Food Intake during Adolescent Intermittent Alcohol Exposure

As shown in **Figure 2A**, during the period of alcohol exposure, there was a significant decrease in body weight gain in the alcohol group compared with the control group [$t_{(22)} = 4.00, p < 0.001$]. Similarly, the averages of food intake during these 4 weeks were also significantly different [$t_{(22)} = 3.68, p = 0.001$] (**Figure 2B**).

After the last alcohol exposure, the BEC in the alcohol group reached an average of 201 ± 6 mg/dl.

Effects of Intermittent Alcohol Exposure on Locomotion and Anxiety-Like Behaviors

We next explored whether alcohol exposure during adolescence induced locomotor or emotional alterations.

One week after the last adolescent alcohol exposure, we measured spontaneous locomotor and exploratory activity using the open field test in rats. We observed no significant differences in the number of crossings between both groups (**Figure 3A**). Additionally, we measured anxiety-like behavior by time spent in the center area of the field (**Figure 3B**) and we detected a significant decrease in the time spent in the center area in the alcohol group compared with the control group [$t_{(14)} = 4.19$, $p < 0.001$].

The rats were also tested on the elevated plus-maze under novelty conditions 2 weeks after alcohol exposure. Regarding the locomotor activity in the elevated plus-maze, we found no differences in the number of entries in the closed arms between groups (**Figure 3C**). In this maze, we measured anxiety-like behavior by the time spent in the open arms and significant differences were found. As shown in **Figure 3D**, there was a significant decrease in the time of open arm exploration in the alcohol group compared with the control group [$t_{(14)} = 4.65$, $p < 0.001$].

Effects of Intermittent Alcohol Exposure on Novel Object Recognition

One week after adolescent alcohol exposure, the recognition memory was measured using the novel object recognition task. During the familiarization phase, none of the groups displayed any preference for the objects but the statistical analysis revealed

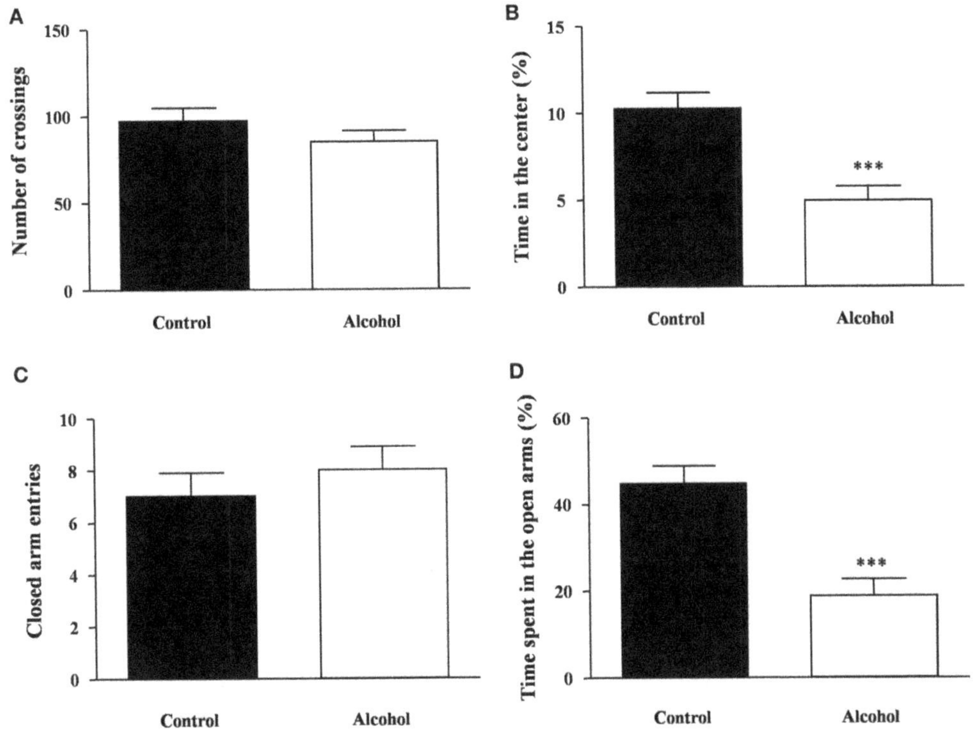

FIGURE 3 | Locomotion and anxiety-like behavior in adult rats exposed to intermittent adolescent alcohol. Number of crossings **(A)** and time spent in the center of the field **(B)** were evaluated in the open field test 1 week after the last alcohol exposure (pnd 62). Closed arm entries **(C)** and time spent exploring the open arms **(D)** were evaluated in the elevated plus-maze 2 weeks after the last alcohol exposure (pnd 69). Bars represent the mean ± SEM (8–12 animals per group). Data were analyzed by Student's *t*-test (Welch's correction). $^{***}p < 0.001$ denotes significant differences compared with the control group.

significant differences on the total exploration time (**Figure 4A**). Thus, the alcohol group spent less time to explore both objects than the control group [$t_{(21)} = 4.73, p < 0.001$].

One hour later, the test session was repeated using a novel object. A two-way ANOVA revealed a main effect of alcohol exposure on the exploration time [$F_{(1, 42)} = 12.76, p < 0.001$] but also an interaction between alcohol exposure and type of object [$F_{(1, 42)} = 14.40$, $p < 0.001$]. As shown in **Figure 4B**, the *post hoc* comparison indicated that the control group had a higher preference for the novel object relative to the familiar object ($p < 0.05$), whereas the alcohol group displayed a lower preference for the novel object ($p < 0.05$). Additionally, there was a significant decrease in the preference of the novel object in the alcohol group compared with the control group ($p < 0.001$).

Consequently, the alcohol group exhibited a negative discrimination ratio that indicated an impaired recognition memory [$t_{(21)} = 5.83, p < 0.001$] (**Figure 4C**).

Effects of Intermittent Alcohol Exposure on the Gene Expression of Endocannabinoid System

We examined the effect of adolescent alcohol exposure on the gene expression encoding relevant enzymes and receptors involved in endocannabinoid signaling [receptors: CB_1 (*Cnr1*), CB_2 (*Cnr2*) and peroxisome proliferator-activated receptor-α (PPAR-α) (*Ppara*); synthesis enzymes: NAPE-PLD (*Napepld*), DAGL-α (*Dagla*) and DAGL-β (*Daglb*); degradation enzymes: FAAH (*Faah*) and MAGL (*Mgll*)] following 2 weeks after the last exposure.

Medial Prefrontal Cortex

In the mPFC (**Figure 5A**), the observed effects were mostly activatory. The mRNA expression of *Ppara* [$t_{(7)} = 4.96$, $p = 0.002$]; the synthesis enzymes *Napepld* [$t_{(14)} = 6.12$, $p < 0.001$], *Dagla* [$t_{(7)} = 12.47, p < 0.001$] and *Daglb* [$t_{(7)} = 9.47$, $p < 0.001$]; and *Faah* [$t_{(14)} = 2.53, p = 0.024$] were significantly increased in the alcohol group relative to the control group before adjustment for multiple comparisons. The FDR adjusted significance level ($q = 0.031$) indicated that all differences in the mRNA levels were still significant.

Striatum

Conversely, the adolescent exposure during adolescence produced only inhibitory effects, as shown in **Figure 5B**. Thus, rats exposed to alcohol displayed a significant decrease in the striatal mRNA expression of the receptors: *Cnr1* [$t_{(7)} = 6.66$, $p < 0.001$], *Cnr2* [$t_{(7)} = 2.94, p = 0.022$] and *Ppara* [$t_{(8)} = 14.55$, $p < 0.001$] compared with the control group. However, the FDR adjusted significance level ($q = 0.013$) showed a significant decrease in the expression of *Cnr1* and *Ppara*.

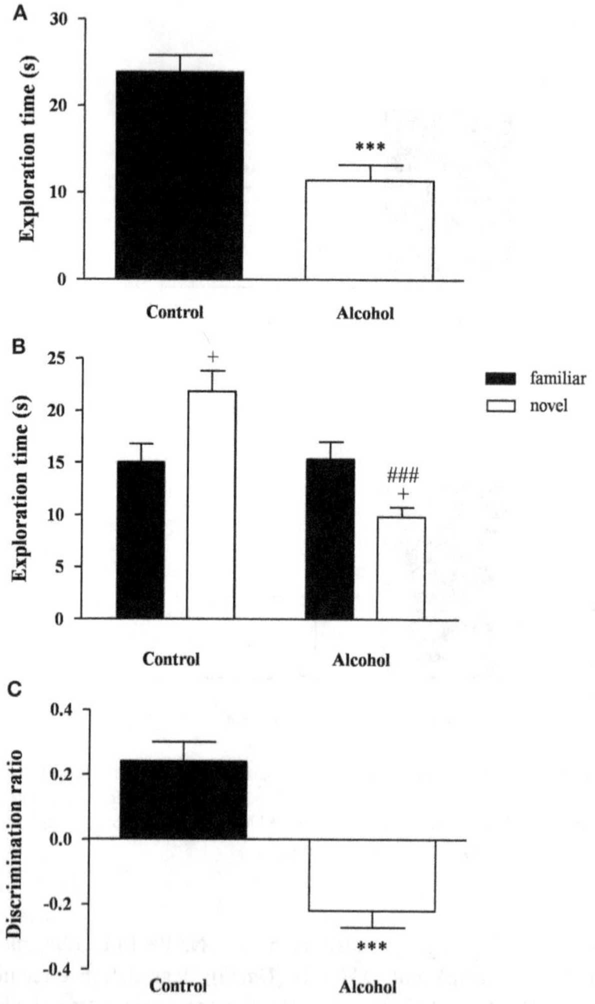

FIGURE 4 | Recognition memory in adult rats exposed to intermittent adolescent alcohol. Exploration time **(A)** during the familiarization phase, exploration time for both familiar and novel object **(B)** during the test phase and discrimination ration **(C)** of the novel object. Bars represent the mean ± SEM (8–12 animals per group). Data were analyzed by Student's *t*-test (Welch's correction) and two-way ANOVA. $^{***}p < 0.001$ denotes significant differences compared with the control group. $^{+}p < 0.05$ denotes significant differences compared with time exploring the familiar object; and $^{\#\#\#}p < 0.001$ denotes significant differences compared with time exploring the novel object in the control group.

Amygdala

Similar to the striatum, we found again inhibitory effects in the amygdala (**Figure 5C**). The mRNA levels of *Cnr1* [$t_{(14)} = 4.12$, $p = 0.001$], *Napepld* [$t_{(9)} = 2.69$, $p = 0.025$] and *Dagla* [$t_{(14)} = 3.44$, $p = 0.004$] were significantly decreased in the alcohol group relative to the control group before adjustment for multiple comparisons. The subsequent correction ($q = 0.013$) revealed significant differences in the expression of *Cnr1* and *Dagla* but not in *Napepld*.

Hippocampus

In the hippocampus (**Figure 5D**), the alcohol group displayed a significant decrease in the mRNA levels of *Cnr2* [$t_{(7)} = 3.96$, $p = 0.006$] and a significant increase in both *Dagla* [$t_{(14)} = 2.81$, $p = 0.014$] and *Mgll* [$t_{(9)} = 3.02$, $p = 0.015$] relative to the control group. Consistently, the FDR adjusted significance level ($q = 0.019$) revealed that these differences in the mRNA expression were still significant.

Table S1 summarizes the adjustment for multiple comparisons of the mRNA expression of the ECS in each brain region.

Effects of Intermittent Alcohol Exposure during Adolescence on the Gene Expression of Neuropeptides Linked to Anxiety and Stress

We also evaluated the effect of alcohol exposure during adolescence on the gene expression of neuropeptides linked to anxiety/stress responses and their receptors [neuropeptides: corticotropin-releasing factor (CRF) (*Crh*) and neuropeptides Y (NPY) (*Npy*); and receptors: CRF1R (*Crhr1*), CRF2R (*Crhr2*), NPY1R (*Npy1r*), NPY2R (*Npy2r*) and NPY5R (*Npy5r*)]. Determinations were conducted in the amygdala and hippocampus, two main regions belonging to the circuit that modulates emotional responses.

Amygdala

As shown in **Figure 6A**, the statistical analysis indicated no differences in the mRNA expression of *Crh* and its receptors but there were significant decreases in the expression of *Npy* [$t_{(9)} = 2.40$, $p = 0.040$] and *Npy2r* [$t_{(14)} = 3.07$, $p = 0.007$] in the alcohol group compared with the control group. However, the FDR adjusted significance level ($q = 0.007$) only remained significant differences between groups for *Npy2r*.

Hippocampus

In the hippocampus (**Figure 6B**), repeated *t*-tests showed significant differences in the mRNA levels of *Crh*, *Npy*, *Npy2r*, and *Npy5r* between groups. Thus, the alcohol group displayed higher *Crh* mRNA expression [$t_{(14)} = 3.76$, $p = 0.002$] and lower mRNA expression of *Npy* [$t_{(14)} = 2.22$, $p = 0.043$], *Npy2r* [$t_{(14)} = 6.60$, $p < 0.001$] and *Npy5r* [$t_{(14)} = 2.46$, $p = 0.027$] than the control group. After adjusting for multiple comparisons ($q = 0.014$) in the hippocampus, the significant differences were only observed in *Crh* and *Npy2r*.

Table S2 summarizes the adjustment for multiple comparisons of the mRNA expression of neuropeptides and receptors in the amygdala and hippocampus.

Effects of Intermittent Alcohol Exposure during Adolescence on the Gene Expression of Neuroinflammatory Factors

Finally, we examined the effect of alcohol exposure during adolescence on the gene expression of relevant inflammatory-related markers [pro-inflammatory mediators: tumor necrosis factor-α (TNF-α) (*Tnf*), TLR4 (*Tlr4*), COX-2 (*Ptgs2*) and NF-κβ (*Rela*); and glia-activating factors: glial fibrillary acidic protein (GFAP) (*Gfap*) and allograft inflammatory factor-1 or microglia response factor (MRF-1) (*Aif1*)] following 2 weeks after the last alcohol exposure.

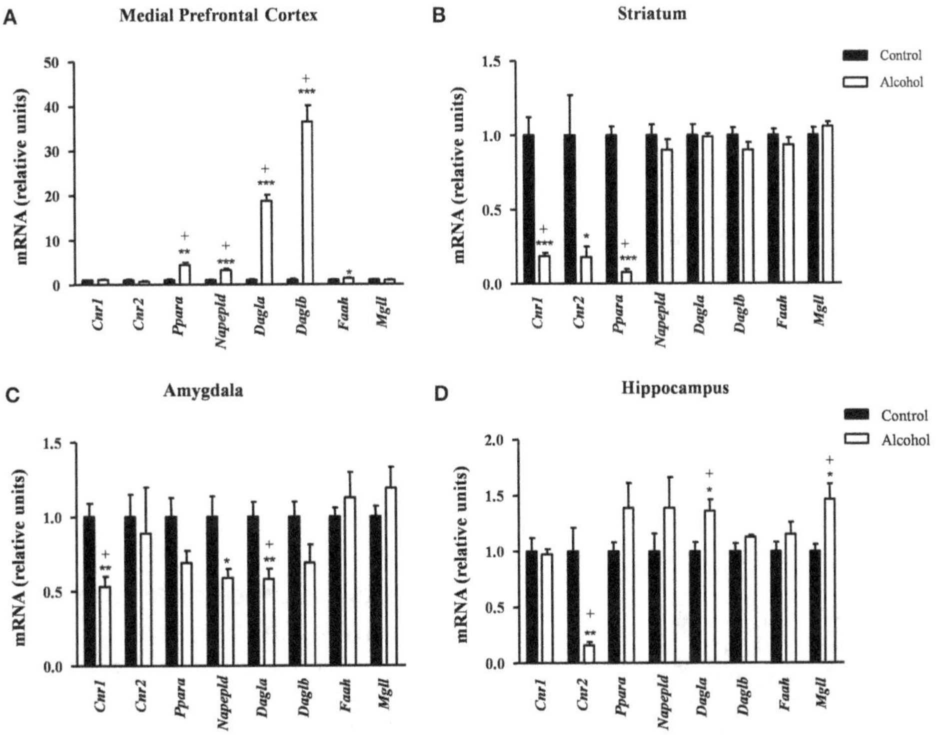

FIGURE 5 | Relative mRNA expression of endocannabinoid signaling-related genes in different brain regions of adult rats exposed to intermittent adolescent alcohol. Relative mRNA expression of *Cnr1*, *Cnr2*, *Ppara*, *Napepld*, *Dagla*, *Daglb*, *Faah* and *Mgll* in the medial prefrontal cortex **(A)**, striatum **(B)**, amygdala **(C)**, and hippocampus **(D)**. Bars represent the mean ± SEM (8 animals per group). Data were analyzed by Student's *t*-test (Welch's correction) and Benjamini-Holchberg false discovery rate procedure for multiple comparisons. *$p < 0.05$, **$p < 0.01$ and ***$p < 0.001$ denote significant differences compared with the control group. (+) denotes significant differences compared with the control group after adjustment for multiple comparisons in each brain region.

Medial Prefrontal Cortex

In the mPFC (**Figure 7A**), the mRNA levels of *Tnf* [$t_{(9)} = 3.55$, $p = 0.006$], *Tlr4* [$t_{(14)} = 12.50$, $p < 0.001$], *Ptgs2* [$t_{(14)} = 2.67$, $p = 0.018$] and *Gfap* [$t_{(7)} = 9.08$, $p < 0.001$] were significantly increased in the alcohol group in comparison with the control group. By contrast, the mRNA expression of *Rela* was significantly decreased in the alcohol group [$t_{(14)} = 4.17$, $p < 0.001$]. The adjustment for multiple comparisons ($q = 0.042$) confirmed all the significant differences found after repeated *t*-tests.

Striatum

In the striatum (**Figure 7B**), the statistical analysis showed a significant decrease in the mRNA levels of *Ptgs2* [$t_{(14)} = 4.34, p < 0.001$], *Rela* [$t_{(9)} = 5.91, p < 0.001$], *Gfap* [$t_{(14)} = 2.48, p = 0.027$] and *Aif1* [$t_{(7)} = 2.51, p = 0.041$] in the alcohol group compared with the control group. However, the FDR adjusted significance level ($q = 0.018$) remained significant differences only in the expression of *Ptgs2* and *Rela*.

Amygdala

As shown in **Figure 7C**, the alcohol group only displayed lower *Aif1* mRNA levels compared with the control group [$t_{(8)} = 3.45$, $p = 0.008$] and this difference was still observed after the correction for multiple comparisons ($q = 0.008$).

Hippocampus

Regarding the hippocampus (**Figure 7D**), the statistical analysis indicated that the alcohol group displayed lower mRNA levels of *Ptgs2* [$t_{(14)} = 2.72, p = 0.017$] and *Gfap* [$t_{(14)} = 2.74, p = 0.016$] and higher *Aif1* mRNA levels [$t_{(8)} = 2.84, p = 0.022$] compared with the control group. The adjustment for multiple comparisons ($q = 0.025$) confirmed the significance of all differences found using repeated *t*-tests.

Table S3 summarizes the adjustment for multiple comparisons of the mRNA expression of neuroinflammation-related factors in each brain region.

DISCUSSION

The present study in adult rats investigated the effects of intermittent alcohol intoxication on emotional behavior, cognition and the relative mRNA expression of genes from the endocannabinoid system (ECS), neuropeptides regulating anxiety- and alcohol-related behavior and mediators of neuroinflammation and plasticity. We must keep in mind that the social isolation of the animals in their home-cages throughout the experiments can affect the basal values in emotional behaviors (e.g., isolation induces anxiety-like behaviors and impairs fear extinction) and the

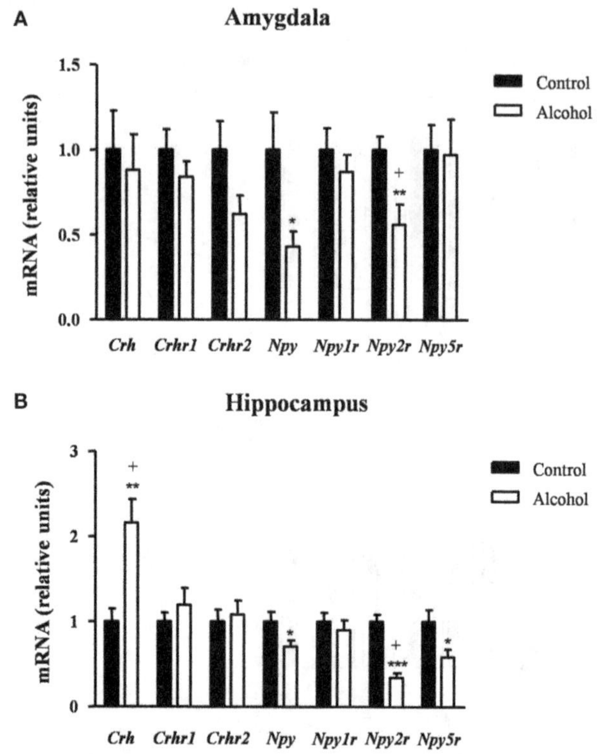

FIGURE 6 | Relative mRNA expression of markers of anxiety in different brain regions of adult rats exposed to intermittent adolescent alcohol. Relative mRNA expression of *Crh, Crhr1, Crhr2, Npy, Npy1r, Npy2r,* and *Npy5r* in the amygdala **(A)** and hippocampus **(B)**. Bars represent the mean ± SEM (8 animals per group). Data were analyzed by Student's *t*-test (Welch's correction) and Benjamini-Holchberg false discovery rate procedure for multiple comparisons. $^{*}p < 0.05$, $^{**}p < 0.01$ and $^{***}p < 0.001$ denote significant differences compared with the control group. (+) denotes significant differences compared with the control group after adjustment for multiple comparisons in each brain region.

expression of signaling systems in the brain (Skelly et al., 2015).

Intermittent Alcohol Intoxication

As expected, the alcohol group showed elevated ethanol levels in the blood. These BECs were about 200 mg/dl and they are comparable to the concentrations reported in other studies conducted in adolescent Wistar rats using a model of binge-like drinking with i.p. injections of 3 g/kg, which reported 150–180 mg/dl 1 h postinjection (Przybycien-Szymanska et al., 2010, 2012). Although our procedure raised plasma alcohol levels in a binge-like manner [binge drinking is indeed defined as heavy episodic drinking within a BEC of 80 mg/dl or higher (NIAAA, 2004)], the alcohol administration was injected and it is possible that our model would yield higher alcohol doses than animals would consume voluntarily as it is expected in a binge drinking pattern (Spanagel, 2000). However, both patterns of excessive alcohol consumption are characterized by high BECs, and this can be critical in the effects of adolescent alcohol on behavior and expression of signaling systems in the brain.

During the alcohol exposure, we monitored the feeding behavior of adolescent rats by measuring body weight and food intake. Thus, the alcohol group displayed a lower body weight gain accompanied by a reduction in food intake during the alcohol exposure. These observations agree with previous studies reporting a significant decrease in body weight after i.p. administration of ethanol (Luz et al., 1996; Iwaniec and Turner, 2013). In fact, Lauing and colleagues reported decreased weight gain after modeling binge drinking using i.p. alcohol administration delivered on 2 consecutive days followed by 5 days of abstinence (Lauing et al., 2008). Several factors such as local inflammation and pain related to repeated injections, repeated acute ethanol intoxications with subsequent physical discomfort... could participate in this negative energy balance. However, there are studies reporting no differences in the final body weight after an intermittent binge-drinking exposure (Przybycien-Szymanska et al., 2010) although the total duration of this protocol was only 8 days.

Effects on Emotional Behaviors and Cognitive Responses

After the alcohol exposure, locomotor activity, anxiety-like behavior and cognitive responses were assessed using a behavioral test battery consisting of the open field, elevated plus maze and novel object recognition task.

One week after the last alcohol session, we observed no differences in locomotor activity in the open field but there was an anxiogenic-like response to the test in the alcohol group compared with the control group, which could be related to the effects of alcohol deprivation on emotional behavior. These results are consistent with previous studies in rodents exposed to repeated binge-drinking during adolescence, which reported long-term anxiety disorders (Gilpin et al., 2012; Montesinos et al., 2016). One week later, the same rats were assessed in the elevated plus-maze and the anxiogenic-like behavior was also detected in the alcohol group. Ethanol withdrawal in rodents is associated with a negative affective state, including an enhanced anxiety-like behavior. Following a period of abstinence, rats spent significantly less time in the open arms of the elevated-plus maze than control animals (File et al., 1993; Moy et al., 1997; Wilson et al., 1998; Pandey et al., 2003). This behavioral profile can persist for as long as 28 days (Rasmussen et al., 2001). In our animals, the elevated anxiety in the alcohol group persisted unchanged for at least 2 weeks following the last alcohol exposure, suggesting enduring changes on emotionality.

A novel object recognition task was used to detect the existence of cognitive impairments because this paradigm relies on the innate preference that rodents display for exploring novel rather than familiar objects (Ennaceur and Delacour, 1988). To perform the task, we used a 1 h delay interval between the familiarization and novelty phases to consolidate a short-term memory that depends on the integrity of the hippocampal formation (García-Moreno et al., 2002). The results showed that rats exposed to alcohol displayed a decreased preference for the novel object over the familiar object but similar exploration time of the familiar object. This attracted our attention, because this

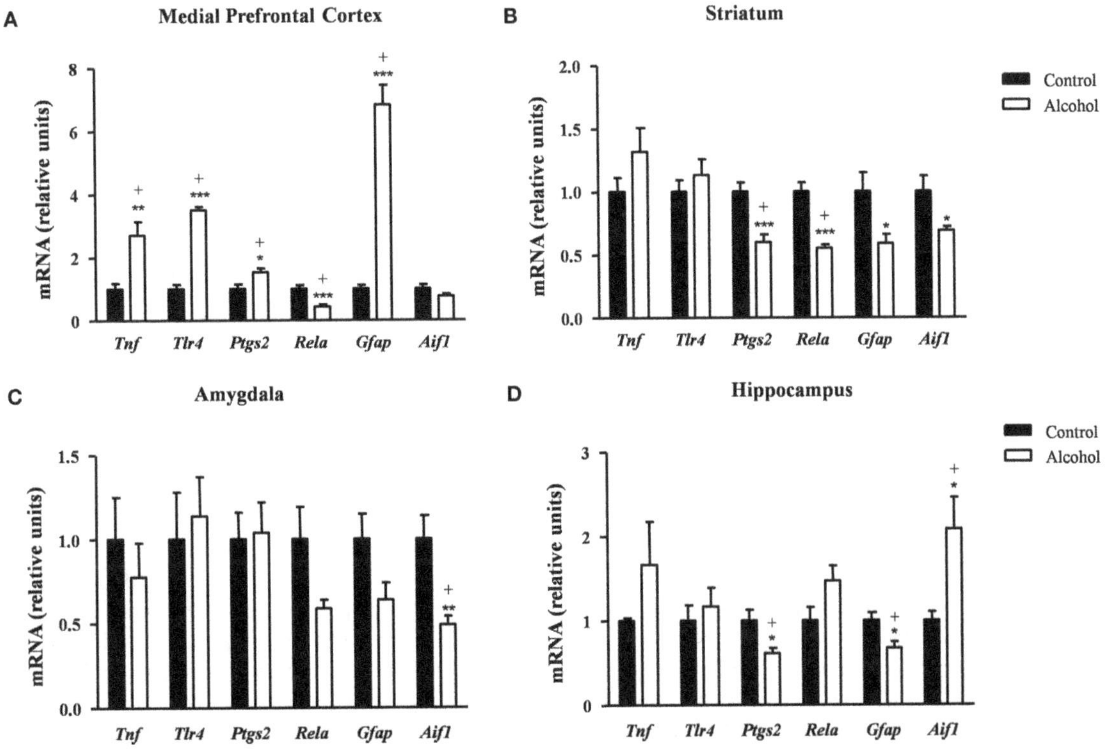

FIGURE 7 | Relative mRNA expression of neuroinflammatory factors in different brain regions of adult rats exposed to intermittent adolescent alcohol. Relative mRNA expression of *Tnf, Tlr4, Ptgs2, Rela, Gfap* and *Aif1* mRNA in the medial prefrontal cortex **(A)**, striatum **(B)**, amygdala **(C)**, and hippocampus **(D)**. Bars represent the mean ± SEM (8 animals per group). Data were analyzed by Student's *t*-test (Welch's correction) and Benjamini–Holchberg false discovery rate procedure for multiple comparisons. $^*p < 0.05$, $^{**}p < 0.01$ and $^{***}p < 0.001$ denote significant differences compared with the control group. (+) denotes significant differences compared with the control group after adjustment for multiple comparisons in each brain region.

less exploration time of the novel object was not associated with a locomotor impairment in this task, which was in agreement with the open field observations. In fact, the alcohol group displayed less exploration time during the familiarization phase when both identical objects were considered novel. Thus, the reduced preference for the novel object exhibited by the rats exposed to alcohol might be associated with the development of neophobia-induced anxiety and cognitive deficit, which is thought to prevent exploratory behavior (Myhrer, 1988).

Effects on Endocannabinoid System Components

The brain is undergoing extensive maturation during adolescence. Similarly, the ECS is also undergoing maturational changes and some alteration of these processes of maturation can produces long-term alterations, including deficits in emotional behavior and cognition.

Several lines of evidence indicate that alcohol leads to neuroadaptations in endocannabinoid signaling mechanisms (Basavarajappa and Hungund, 1999; Basavarajappa et al., 2003). The present results showed that rats exposed to adolescent alcohol displayed alterations in the expression of endocannabinoid enzymes and receptors that appear to be reliant on the brain region, which is consistent with previous studies reporting regionally distinct effects on brain endocannabinoid levels after alcohol exposure (González et al., 2002, 2004; Rubio et al., 2007).

The mPFC is a key region for multiple cognitive functions, including executive function or anxiety. In addition, the ECS is involved in the regulation of emotional behaviors in this brain region (Rubino et al., 2008; McLaughlin et al., 2014; Morena et al., 2016). Thus, the negative impact of the alcohol to the adolescent mPFC may be associated to the observed alterations in cognition and behavior. We found that rats exposed to adolescent alcohol had a strong increase in the mRNA expression of *Napepld* and *Dagl* in this region. These observations suggest that the ECS is activated in response to the negative affective state associated to alcohol withdrawal. Additionally, the alcohol group displayed an increase in the mRNA expression of *Faah* and the receptor *Ppara*. It has been described that localized infusion of the FAAH inhibitor URB597 into the mPFC increases ethanol consumption by rats (Hansson et al., 2007). Also, a recent study has reported that pretreatment with an inhibitor of FAAH prevents against oxidative stress caused by binge ethanol consumption in the mPFC of adolescent rats (Pelição et al., 2016). Furthermore, PPAR-α is involved in the actions of other N-acylethanolamines with no endocannabinoid activity (e.g., oleoylethanolamide and palmitoylethanolamide) that have been reported to exhibit neuroprotective effects (Fu et al., 2003; Scuderi et al., 2012).

Collectively these findings suggest a strengthening of the ECS that may reflect a homeostatic mechanism to prevent the neurotoxic effects induced by alcohol with a relevant role of other non-cannabinoid congeners in the alcohol exposure.

The ECS is an important modulator of neuroplasticity in the striatum. Overall, we observed that alcohol-exposed rats displayed a decreased mRNA expression of *Cnr1* and *Ppara*, as well as a decreasing trend in *Cnr2*. These results agree with preclinical studies that indicate a decrease in *Cnr1* mRNA levels after alcohol exposure in mice (Vinod et al., 2006) and rats (Adermark et al., 2011). Regarding the *Cnr2* mRNA levels, it is known that alcohol consumption alters the *Cnr2* expression in the brain and that an increased ethanol preference is associated with a reduced *Cnr2* expression in the striatum (Onaivi et al., 2008).

The amygdala is a crucial subcortical area that integrates reward, emotions, and conditioned learning. Previous studies have demonstrated drug-induced alterations in amygdalar endocannabinoid function (Orio et al., 2009; Kamprath et al., 2011; Schmidt et al., 2011). In the present study, we observed a decreasing trend in the receptors and synthesis enzymes but not in the degradative enzymes. Consistently, we have reported that chronic alcohol treatment alters the expression of different cannabinoid signaling-related genes in the amygdala (Serrano et al., 2012).

The hippocampus is a brain region involved in learning which cooperates with the amygdala to modulate emotion and belongs to the reward circuit. Numerous studies have shown that alcohol exposure alters hippocampal function (for review see Kutlu and Gould, 2016). Regarding the expression of the endocannabinoid signaling in the hippocampus, we found a dramatic decrease in the expression of *Cnr2*. In the hippocampus, such cannabinoid receptor is involved in the modulation of excitatory synapses (García-Gutiérrez et al., 2013; Kim and Li, 2015). A recent study has demonstrated a role of the hippocampal CB_2 to modulate cognitive functions in mice (Li and Kim, 2016). Thus, the effects on *Cnr2* mRNA expression in our alcohol-exposed rats may be associated to the adverse effects of alcohol on synaptic plasticity (basically long-term potentiation and long-term depression processes) and the consequent defects in learning and memory (Lovinger and Roberto, 2013).

Effects on Neuropeptides Linked to Emotional Behaviors

As mentioned above, the presence of anxiety is one of the most consistent features of alcohol withdrawal. Since the amygdala and hippocampus are key brain regions in the modulation of emotional behaviors and the ECS is also involved in the regulation of emotionality (Hill and Gorzalka, 2009), the present findings suggest that the differential changes observed in the ECS after adolescent alcohol exposure may be associated with different responses to anxiety. In this regard, to get a better understanding of the potential mechanisms underlying the anxiety effects that were observed, we analyzed the CRF and NPY signals in these regions. Furthermore, both neuropeptides are clearly involved in alcohol-related behaviors and binge alcohol drinking (Pleil et al., 2015).

Interestingly, we found an increase in the hippocampal expression of *Crh* mRNA in the alcohol group with no changes in the CRF receptors. In line with this, previous studies have associated CRF with binge drinking and alcohol dependence (Lowery et al., 2010; Gilpin et al., 2012; Pleil et al., 2015).

Regarding the NPY signal, in both brain areas the alcohol group displayed a down-regulation of this system with a strong decrease in the mRNA levels of *Npy2r* that may be associated with the anxiogenic-like behavior observed in this group. These findings are in agreement with a recent study showing that a decrease in the expression of receptors for NPY are associated with an increase in the anxiety-like behavior in adolescent rats exposed to repeated binge-like alcohol drinking (McClintick et al., 2016).

Effects on Neuroinflammatory Signals

Since alcohol increases neuroinflammation through its ability of activating natural immunity, we evaluated the gene expression of factors involved in pro-inflammatory signaling pathways but also factors associated with plasticity and neurodevelopment.

The data indicate a region-specific susceptibility to the alcohol regulation of the mRNA expression of these factors, being these alterations more prominent in the mPFC. In line with this, binge drinking has been reported to produce alcohol-induced inflammatory PFC damage and this can be accompanied by reduced executive functions and compulsive behavior (Crews et al., 2000). Thus, we observed that adult rats exposed to adolescent alcohol displayed an overall increase in the mRNA expression of the neuroinflammation-related factors *Tlr4, Tnf* and *Ptgs2* in the mPFC. Several evidence indicates that alcohol induces the TLR4 signaling in the PFC (Vetreno and Crews, 2012; Pascual et al., 2014), triggering the induction of a cascade of pro-inflammatory mediators that affect, among others, cognitive impairments and anxiety-like behaviors associated with the alcohol abuse (Montesinos et al., 2015; Pascual et al., 2015).

TLR4 receptors are mediators of alcohol-induced inflammatory damage in the adolescent and adult brain (Alfonso-Loeches et al., 2010). In fact, Crews and colleagues have reported an increased *Tlr4* expression in the brain of alcoholics as well as in mice treated chronically with ethanol (Crews et al., 2013). In addition to TLR4, there was an up-regulation of *Tnf* and *Ptgs2* mRNA levels in alcohol-exposed rats, which is consistent with previous studies reporting that ethanol binge drinking is associated with increased cortical levels of TNF-α and COX-2 (Knapp and Crews, 1999; Antón et al., 2016). By contrast, the gene expression of various pro-inflammatory mediators were down-regulated (e.g., COX-2 mRNA levels were decreased in the striatum and hippocampus and NF-κβ mRNA levels were decreased in the mPFC and striatum), which appears to be incongruent with literature since alcohol exposure activates COX-2 and NF-κβ by triggering cytokine and chemokine release and neuroinflammation. In the mPFC, the decreased gene expression of *Rela* may be associated with the up-regulation of *Ppara* receptor observed in this brain region because it has been described that the activation of this nuclear receptor inhibits *Rela* (Stahel et al., 2008). Nevertheless, we have to keep in mind that changes in gene expression are often not concordant with protein expression (Vogel and Marcotte, 2012).

In addition to these factors and receptors, the inflammatory response is associated with astrocytes activation (Ransohoff and Brown, 2012). In fact, previous studies have demonstrated that *Gfap* levels are affected by alcohol exposure (Miguel-Hidalgo et al., 2006; Udomuksorn et al., 2011). Consistently, the gene expression of GFAP and MRF-1 were found up-regulated in the mPFC and hippocampus. Similar to COX-2 and NF-κβ, the gene expression of both astrocyte marker *Gfap* and microglial marker *Aif1* were also down-regulated in other brain regions (hippocampus and amygdala, respectively) and this was only reported in human alcoholic brain in conjunction with astrocytic loss (Lewohl et al., 2005).

Summary

In summary, adult rats exposed to intermittent alcohol exposure during adolescence displayed anxiety-like behaviors and cognitive deficits related to recognition memory. Furthermore, the mRNA expression of some components of signaling systems involved in behavior, neuroinflammation and plasticity were found altered in these animals, with brain region-dependent changes.

Although adult rats exposed to adolescent alcohol had no alterations in locomotor activity, they exhibited a strong anxiogenic-like behavior. In addition to the anxiety-like response, we observed a clear cognitive deficit with a reduced preference for the novelty. These behavioral and cognitive effects in adulthood were accompanied by molecular changes in the brain.

Alterations in the mRNA expression of genes of the ECS appear to be reliant on the brain region. However, we observed an overall decreasing trend in the mRNA expression of the cannabinoid receptors in the alcohol group. This down-regulation can be associated to the adverse effects of alcohol on synaptic plasticity with cognitive consequences in adulthood such as deficits in learning and memory.

Whereas, the ECS is also associated with emotionality, neuropeptides such as CRF and NPY are clearly involved in alcohol-related behaviors and binge alcohol drinking. Thus, we observed changes in both signals that were linked to anxiogenic-like behaviors, in particular a decrease in the NPY signaling expression.

Regarding neuroinflammatory-related factors, our data indicated a brain region-specific susceptibility in the adult rats exposed to intermittent alcohol. These alterations were more prominent in the mPFC with an up-regulation of the mRNA levels of *Tlr4, Tnf, Ptgs2,* and *Gfap* and a decrease of *Rela*. The activation of PPAR-α inhibits NF-κβ and the mRNA expression of *Ppara* was increased in the mPFC, a key region for multiple cognitive functions. Interestingly, *Ppara* is involved in the anti-inflammatory and neuroprotective actions of endocannabinoid congeners. In contrast to the mPFC, the mRNA expression of *Ptgs2* and *Gfap* were down-regulated in the rest of brain regions.

Limitations and Perspectives

We are aware of the limitations of our study, mainly because of the exploratory nature of the present investigation and the necessity of performing future studies that include female subjects and alcohol exposure during adulthood. Furthermore, the protein expression and function of signaling systems and factors involved in behavior, neuroinflammation and neuroplasticity will open new lines of research using pharmacological and genetic approaches to characterize the association and regulation of these systems with emotional behavior and cognition in the context of adolescent alcohol and its long-term consequences.

The existence of sex differences in the response to alcohol and other drugs has been extensively reported (Becker and Koob, 2016) but we have conducted our experiments only in male rats for clarity. Studies using female rats will reveal whether the estrous cycle and gonadal hormones influence the behavioral and molecular alterations that we have observed here.

Although our data indicate changes in the mRNA expression of signaling systems in the brain and alterations in both emotional and cognitive responses of adult rats exposed to adolescent alcohol, we cannot link these molecular and behavioral effects exclusively to an alcohol exposure during adolescence because we have no rats exposed to alcohol during adulthood for comparison. Consequently, the specificity of the effects associated with intermittent alcohol exposure on these biological substrates will have to be elucidated.

Finally, additional studies will have to resolve the lack of the protein expression of these enzymes, factors and receptors because changes in gene expression level are frequently not reflected at the protein level. In fact, post-transcriptional, translational and degradation regulation must also be taken into account in the determination of protein concentrations because contribute at least as much as transcriptional itself (Vogel and Marcotte, 2012). Also, functional assays will be required to elucidate the role of these signaling systems in the appearance of emotional behaviors and addictive behaviors related to an adolescent alcohol exposure.

AUTHOR CONTRIBUTIONS

All authors had full access to all data in the study and take responsibility for the integrity of the data and the accuracy of the data analyzes. Study concept and design: FR, AS. Acquisition of data: LS, FP, JD, JS, AG, EC. Analysis and interpretation of data: FP, FR, AS. Drafting of the manuscript: FR, AS. Critical revision of the manuscript for important intellectual content, obtained funding and study supervision: FP, FR, AS.

REFERENCES

Adermark, L., Jonsson, S., Ericson, M., and Söderpalm, B. (2011). Intermittent ethanol consumption depresses endocannabinoid-signaling in the dorsolateral striatum of rat. *Neuropharmacology* 61, 1160–1165. doi: 10.1016/j.neuropharm.2011.01.014

Alfonso-Loeches, S., Pascual-Lucas, M., Blanco, A. M., Sanchez-Vera, I., and Guerri, C. (2010). Pivotal role of TLR4 receptors in alcohol-induced neuroinflammation and brain damage. *J. Neurosci.* 30, 8285–8295. doi: 10.1523/JNEUROSCI.0976-10.2010

Antón, M., Alén, F., Gómez de Heras, R., Serrano, A., Pavón, F. J., Leza, J. C. et al. (2016). Oleoylethanolamide prevents neuroimmune HMGB1/TLR4/NF-kB danger signaling in rat frontal cortex and depressive-like behavior induced by ethanol binge administration. *Addict. Biol.* doi: 10.1111/adb.12365. [Epub ahead of print].

Basavarajappa, B. S., and Hungund, B. L. (1999). Chronic ethanol increases the cannabinoid receptor agonist anandamide and its precursor N-arachidonoylphosphatidylethanolamine in SK-N-SH cells. *J. Neurochem.* 72, 522–528. doi: 10.1046/j.1471-4159.1999.0720522.x

Basavarajappa, B. S., Saito, M., Cooper, T. B., and Hungund, B. L. (2003). Chronic ethanol inhibits the anandamide transport and increases extracellular anandamide levels in cerebellar granule neurons. *Eur. J. Pharmacol.* 466, 73–83. doi: 10.1016/S0014-2999(03)01557-7

Becker, J. B., and Koob, G. F. (2016). Sex Differences in animal models: focus on addiction. *Pharmacol. Rev.* 68, 242–263. doi: 10.1124/pr.115.011163

Benjamini, Y., Drai, D., Elmer, G., Kafkafi, N., and Golani, I. (2001). Controlling the false discovery rate in behavior genetics research. *Behav. Brain Res.* 125, 279–284. doi: 10.1016/S0166-4328(01)00297-2

Bisogno, T., Howell, F., Williams, G., Minassi, A., Cascio, M. G., Ligresti, A., et al. (2003). Cloning of the first sn1-DAG lipases points to the spatial and temporal regulation of endocannabinoid signaling in the brain. *J. Cell Biol.* 163, 463–468. doi: 10.1083/jcb.200305129

Cravatt, B. F., Giang, D. K., Mayfield, S. P., Boger, D. L., Lerner, R. A., and Gilula, N. B. (1996). Molecular characterization of an enzyme that degrades neuromodulatory fatty-acid amides. *Nature* 384, 83–87. doi: 10.1038/384083a0

Crews, F., Nixon, K., Kim, D., Joseph, J., Shukitt-Hale, B., Qin, L., et al. (2006). BHT blocks NF-*k*B activation and ethanol-induced brain damage. *Alcohol. Clin. Exp. Res.* 30, 1938–1949. doi: 10.1111/j.1530-0277.2006.00239.x

Crews, F. T., Braun, C. J., Hoplight, B., Switzer, R. C. III, and Knapp, D. J. (2000). Binge ethanol consumption causes differential brain damage in young adolescent rats compared with adult rats. *Alcohol. Clin. Exp. Res.* 24, 1712–1723. doi: 10.1111/j.1530-0277.2000.tb01973.x

Crews, F. T., Qin, L., Sheedy, D., Vetreno, R. P., and Zou, J. (2013). High mobility group box 1/Toll-like receptor danger signaling increases brain neuroimmune activation in alcohol dependence. *Biol. Psychiatry* 73, 602–612. doi: 10.1016/j.biopsych.2012.09.030

Dawson, D. A., Goldstein, R. B., Chou, S. P., Ruan, W. J., and Grant, B. F. (2008). Age at first drink and the first incidence of adult-onset DSM-IV alcohol use disorders. *Alcohol. Clin. Exp. Res.* 32, 2149–2160. doi: 10.1111/j.1530-0277.2008.00806.x

Dinh, T. P., Carpenter, D., Leslie, F. M., Freund, T. F., Katona, I., Sensi, S. L., et al. (2002). Brain monoglyceride lipase participating in endocannabinoid inactivation. *Proc. Natl. Acad. Sci. U.S.A.* 99, 10819–10824. doi: 10.1073/pnas.152334899

Ennaceur, A., and Delacour, J. (1988). A new one-trial test for neurobiological studies of memory in rats. 1: behavioral data. *Behav. Brain Res.* 31, 47–59. doi: 10.1016/0166-4328(88)90157-X

Fernandez-Lizarbe, S., Pascual, M., and Guerri, C. (2009). Critical role of TLR4 response in the activation of microglia induced by ethanol. *J. Immunol.* 183, 4733–4744. doi: 10.4049/jimmunol.0803590

File, S. E., Andrews, N., and Al-Farhan, M. (1993). Anxiogenic responses of rats on withdrawal from chronic ethanol treatment: effects of tianeptine. *Alcohol. Alcohol.* 28, 281–286.

Fu, J., Gaetani, S., Oveisi, F., Lo Verme, J., Serrano, A., Rodriguez De Fonseca, F., et al. (2003). Oleylethanolamide regulates feeding and body weight through activation of the nuclear receptor PPAR-alpha. *Nature* 425, 90–93. doi: 10.1038/nature01921

García-Gutiérrez, M. S., Ortega-Alvaro, A., Busquets-Garcia, A., Perez-Ortiz, J. M., Caltana, L., Ricatti, M. J., et al. (2013). Synaptic plasticity alterations associated with memory impairment induced by deletion of CB2 cannabinoid receptors. *Neuropharmacology* 73, 388–396. doi: 10.1016/j.neuropharm.2013.05.034

García-Moreno, L. M., Conejo, N. M., Capilla, A., Garcia-Sanchez, O., Senderek, K., and Arias, J. L. (2002). Chronic ethanol intake and object recognition in young and adult rats. *Prog. Neuropsychopharmacol. Biol. Psychiatry* 26, 831–837. doi: 10.1016/S0278-5846(01)00327-X

Gilpin, N. W., Karanikas, C. A., and Richardson, H. N. (2012). Adolescent binge drinking leads to changes in alcohol drinking, anxiety, and amygdalar corticotropin releasing factor cells in adulthood in male rats. *PLoS ONE* 7:e31466. doi: 10.1371/journal.pone.0031466

González, S., Cascio, M. G., Fernandez-Ruiz, J., Fezza, F., Di Marzo, V., and Ramos, J. A. (2002). Changes in endocannabinoid contents in the brain of rats chronically exposed to nicotine, ethanol or cocaine. *Brain Res.* 954, 73–81. doi: 10.1016/S0006-8993(02)03344-9

González, S., Valenti, M., De Miguel, R., Fezza, F., Fernandez-Ruiz, J., Di Marzo, V., et al. (2004). Changes in endocannabinoid contents in reward-related brain regions of alcohol-exposed rats, and their possible relevance to alcohol relapse. *Br. J. Pharmacol.* 143, 455–464. doi: 10.1038/sj.bjp.0705963

Goral, J., Karavitis, J., and Kovacs, E. J. (2008). Exposure-dependent effects of ethanol on the innate immune system. *Alcohol* 42, 237–247. doi: 10.1016/j.alcohol.2008.02.003

Guerri, C., Bazinet, A., and Riley, E. P. (2009). Foetal alcohol spectrum disorders and alterations in brain and behaviour. *Alcohol Alcohol.* 44, 108–114. doi: 10.1093/alcalc/agn105

Hansson, A. C., Bermudez-Silva, F. J., Malinen, H., Hyytia, P., Sanchez-Vera, I., Rimondini, R., et al. (2007). Genetic impairment of frontocortical endocannabinoid degradation and high alcohol preference. *Neuropsychopharmacology* 32, 117–126. doi: 10.1038/sj.npp.1301034

Hill, M. N., and Gorzalka, B. B. (2009). The endocannabinoid system and the treatment of mood and anxiety disorders. *CNS Neurol. Disord. Drug Targets* 8, 451–458. doi: 10.2174/187152709789824624

Howlett, A. C., Bidaut-Russell, M., Devane, W. A., Melvin, L. S., Johnson, M. R., and Herkenham, M. (1990). The cannabinoid receptor: biochemical, anatomical and behavioral characterization. *Trends Neurosci.* 13, 420–423. doi: 10.1016/0166-2236(90)90124-S

Iwaniec, U. T., and Turner, R. T. (2013). Intraperitoneal injection of ethanol results in drastic changes in bone metabolism not observed when ethanol is administered by oral gavage. *Alcohol. Clin. Exp. Res.* 37, 1271–1277. doi: 10.1111/acer.12105

Kalivas, P. W., and O'Brien, C. (2008). Drug addiction as a pathology of staged neuroplasticity. *Neuropsychopharmacology* 33, 166–180. doi: 10.1038/sj.npp.1301564

Kamprath, K., Romo-Parra, H., Haring, M., Gaburro, S., Doengi, M., Lutz, B., et al. (2011). Short-term adaptation of conditioned fear responses through endocannabinoid signaling in the central amygdala. *Neuropsychopharmacology* 36, 652–663. doi: 10.1038/npp.2010.196

Kim, J., and Li, Y. (2015). Chronic activation of CB2 cannabinoid receptors in the hippocampus increases excitatory synaptic transmission. *J. Physiol.* 593, 871–886. doi: 10.1113/jphysiol.2014.286633

Knapp, D. J., and Crews, F. T. (1999). Induction of cyclooxygenase-2 in brain during acute and chronic ethanol treatment and ethanol withdrawal. *Alcohol. Clin. Exp. Res.* 23, 633–643. doi: 10.1111/j.1530-0277.1999.tb04165.x

Koob, G. F. (2008). A role for brain stress systems in addiction. *Neuron* 59, 11–34. doi: 10.1016/j.neuron.2008.06.012

Koob, G. F., Roberts, A. J., Schulteis, G., Parsons, L. H., Heyser, C. J., Hyytia, P., et al. (1998). Neurocircuitry targets in ethanol reward and dependence. *Alcohol. Clin. Exp. Res.* 22, 3–9. doi: 10.1111/j.1530-0277.1998.tb03611.x

Kovacs, E. J., and Messingham, K. A. (2002). Influence of alcohol and gender on immune response. *Alcohol Res. Health* 26, 257–263.

Kutlu, M. G., and Gould, T. J. (2016). Effects of drugs of abuse on hippocampal plasticity and hippocampus-dependent learning and memory: contributions to development and maintenance of addiction. *Learn. Mem.* 23, 515–533. doi: 10.1101/lm.042192.116

Lauing, K., Himes, R., Rachwalski, M., Strotman, P., and Callaci, J. J. (2008). Binge alcohol treatment of adolescent rats followed by alcohol abstinence is associated with site-specific differences in bone loss and incomplete recovery of bone mass and strength. *Alcohol* 42, 649–656. doi: 10.1016/j.alcohol.2008.08.005

Lewohl, J. M., Wixey, J., Harper, C. G., and Dodd, P. R. (2005). Expression of MBP, PLP, MAG, CNP, and GFAP in the human alcoholic brain. *Alcohol. Clin. Exp. Res.* 29, 1698–1705. doi: 10.1097/01.alc.0000179406.98868.59

Li, Y., and Kim, J. (2016). CB2 cannabinoid receptor knockout in mice impairs contextual long-term memory and enhances spatial working memory. *Neural Plast.* 2016:9817089. doi: 10.1155/2016/9817089

Lovinger, D. M., and Roberto, M. (2013). Synaptic effects induced by alcohol. *Curr. Top. Behav. Neurosci.* 13, 31–86. doi: 10.1007/978-3-642-28720-6_143

Lowery, E. G., Spanos, M., Navarro, M., Lyons, A. M., Hodge, C. W., and Thiele, T. E. (2010). CRF-1 antagonist and CRF-2 agonist decrease binge-like ethanol drinking in C57BL/6J mice independent of the HPA axis. *Neuropsychopharmacology* 35, 1241–1252. doi: 10.1038/npp.2009.209

Luz, J., Griggio, M. A., Plapler, H., De-Meo-Bancher, M., and Carvalho-Kosmiskas, J. V. (1996). Effects of ethanol on energy balance of rats and the inappropriateness of intraperitoneal injection. *Alcohol* 13, 575–580. doi: 10.1016/S0741-8329(96)00070-5

McClintick, J. N., McBride, W. J., Bell, R. L., Ding, Z. M., Liu, Y., Xuei, X., et al. (2016). Gene expression changes in glutamate and GABA-A receptors, neuropeptides, ion channels, and cholesterol synthesis in the periaqueductal gray following binge-like alcohol drinking by adolescent alcohol-preferring (P) rats. *Alcohol. Clin. Exp. Res.* 40, 955–968. doi: 10.1111/acer.13056

McLaughlin, R. J., Hill, M. N., and Gorzalka, B. B. (2014). A critical role for prefrontocortical endocannabinoid signaling in the regulation of stress and emotional behavior. *Neurosci. Biobehav. Rev.* 42, 116–131. doi: 10.1016/j.neubiorev.2014.02.006

Miguel-Hidalgo, J. J., Overholser, J. C., Meltzer, H. Y., Stockmeier, C. A., and Rajkowska, G. (2006). Reduced glial and neuronal packing density in the orbitofrontal cortex in alcohol dependence and its relationship with suicide and duration of alcohol dependence. *Alcohol. Clin. Exp. Res.* 30, 1845–1855. doi: 10.1111/j.1530-0277.2006.00221.x

Montesinos, J., Pascual, M., Pla, A., Maldonado, C., Rodriguez-Arias, M., Minarro, J., et al. (2015). TLR4 elimination prevents synaptic and myelin alterations and long-term cognitive dysfunctions in adolescent mice with intermittent ethanol treatment. *Brain Behav. Immun.* 45, 233–244. doi: 10.1016/j.bbi.2014.11.015

Montesinos, J., Pascual, M., Rodriguez-Arias, M., Minarro, J., and Guerri, C. (2016). Involvement of TLR4 in the long-term epigenetic changes, rewarding and anxiety effects induced by intermittent ethanol treatment in adolescence. *Brain Behav. Immun.* 53, 159–171. doi: 10.1016/j.bbi.2015.12.006

Morena, M., Patel, S., Bains, J. S., and Hill, M. N. (2016). Neurobiological interactions between stress and the endocannabinoid system. *Neuropsychopharmacology* 41, 80–102. doi: 10.1038/npp.2015.166

Moy, S. S., Knapp, D. J., Criswell, H. E., and Breese, G. R. (1997). Flumazenil blockade of anxiety following ethanol withdrawal in rats. *Psychopharmacology (Berl).* 131, 354–360. doi: 10.1007/s002130050303

Munro, S., Thomas, K. L., and Abu-Shaar, M. (1993). Molecular characterization of a peripheral receptor for cannabinoids. *Nature* 365, 61–65. doi: 10.1038/365061a0

Myhrer, T. (1988). Exploratory behavior and reaction to novelty in rats with hippocampal perforant path systems disrupted. *Behav. Neurosci.* 102, 356–362. doi: 10.1037/0735-7044.102.3.356

Nagel, B. J., Schweinsburg, A. D., Phan, V., and Tapert, S. F. (2005). Reduced hippocampal volume among adolescents with alcohol use disorders without psychiatric comorbidity. *Psychiatry Res.* 139, 181–190. doi: 10.1016/j.pscychresns.2005.05.008

NIAAA (2004). *NIAAA Council Approves Definition of Binge Drinking.* Bethesda: National Institutes of Health NIAAA Newsletter.

Obernier, J. A., Bouldin, T. W., and Crews, F. T. (2002a). Binge ethanol exposure in adult rats causes necrotic cell death. *Alcohol. Clin. Exp. Res.* 26, 547–557. doi: 10.1111/j.1530-0277.2002.tb02573.x

Obernier, J. A., White, A. M., Swartzwelder, H. S., and Crews, F. T. (2002b). Cognitive deficits and CNS damage after a 4-day binge ethanol exposure in rats. *Pharmacol. Biochem. Behav.* 72, 521–532. doi: 10.1016/S0091-3057(02)00715-3

Oesterle, S., Hill, K. G., Hawkins, J. D., Guo, J., Catalano, R. F., and Abbott, R. D. (2004). Adolescent heavy episodic drinking trajectories and health in young adulthood. *J. Stud. Alcohol.* 65, 204–212. doi: 10.15288/jsa.2004.65.204

Okamoto, Y., Morishita, J., Tsuboi, K., Tonai, T., and Ueda, N. (2004). Molecular characterization of a phospholipase D generating anandamide and its congeners. *J. Biol. Chem.* 279, 5298–5305. doi: 10.1074/jbc.M306642200

Onaivi, E. S., Ishiguro, H., Gong, J. P., Patel, S., Meozzi, P. A., Myers, L., et al. (2008). Functional expression of brain neuronal CB2 cannabinoid receptors are involved in the effects of drugs of abuse and in depression. *Ann. N.Y Acad. Sci.* 1139, 434–449. doi: 10.1196/annals.1432.036

Orio, L., Edwards, S., George, O., Parsons, L. H., and Koob, G. F. (2009). A role for the endocannabinoid system in the increased motivation for cocaine in extended-access conditions. *J. Neurosci.* 29, 4846–4857. doi: 10.1523/JNEUROSCI.0563-09.2009

Pandey, S. C., Roy, A., and Zhang, H. (2003). The decreased phosphorylation of cyclic adenosine monophosphate (cAMP) response element binding (CREB) protein in the central amygdala acts as a molecular substrate for anxiety related to ethanol withdrawal in rats. *Alcohol. Clin. Exp. Res.* 27, 396–409. doi: 10.1097/01.ALC.0000056616.81971.49

Pascual, M., Balino, P., Alfonso-Loeches, S., Aragon, C. M., and Guerri, C. (2011). Impact of TLR4 on behavioral and cognitive dysfunctions associated with alcohol-induced neuroinflammatory damage. *Brain Behav Immun.* 25(Suppl. 1), S80–S91. doi: 10.1016/j.bbi.2011.02.012

Pascual, M., Balino, P., Aragon, C. M., and Guerri, C. (2015). Cytokines and chemokines as biomarkers of ethanol-induced neuroinflammation and anxiety-related behavior: role of TLR4 and TLR2. *Neuropharmacology* 89, 352–359. doi: 10.1016/j.neuropharm.2014.10.014

Pascual, M., Blanco, A. M., Cauli, O., Minarro, J., and Guerri, C. (2007). Intermittent ethanol exposure induces inflammatory brain damage and causes long-term behavioural alterations in adolescent rats. *Eur. J. Neurosci.* 25, 541–550. doi: 10.1111/j.1460-9568.2006.05298.x

Pascual, M., Pla, A., Minarro, J., and Guerri, C. (2014). Neuroimmune activation and myelin changes in adolescent rats exposed to high-dose alcohol and associated cognitive dysfunction: a review with reference to human adolescent drinking. *Alcohol. Alcohol.* 49, 187–192. doi: 10.1093/alcalc/agt164

Paxinos, G., and Watson, C. (1998). *The Rat Brain in Stereotaxic Coordinates.* New York, NY: Academic Press; Spiral Bound.

Pelição, R., Santos, M. C., Freitas-Lima, L. C., Meyrelles, S. S., Vasquez, E. C., Nakamura-Palacios, E. M., et al. (2016). URB597 inhibits oxidative stress induced by alcohol binging in the prefrontal cortex of adolescent rats. *Neurosci. Lett.* 624, 17–22. doi: 10.1016/j.neulet.2016.04.068

Pleil, K. E., Rinker, J. A., Lowery-Gionta, E. G., Mazzone, C. M., McCall, N. M., Kendra, A. M., et al. (2015). NPY signaling inhibits extended amygdala CRF neurons to suppress binge alcohol drinking. *Nat. Neurosci.* 18, 545–552. doi: 10.1038/nn.3972

Przybycien-Szymanska, M. M., Gillespie, R. A., and Pak, T. R. (2012). 17beta-Estradiol is required for the sexually dimorphic effects of repeated binge-pattern alcohol exposure on the HPA axis during adolescence. *PLoS ONE* 7:e32263. doi: 10.1371/journal.pone.0032263

Przybycien-Szymanska, M. M., Rao, Y. S., and Pak, T. R. (2010). Binge-pattern alcohol exposure during puberty induces sexually dimorphic changes in genes regulating the HPA axis. *Am. J. Physiol. Endocrinol. Metab.* 298, E320–E328. doi: 10.1152/ajpendo.00615.2009

Ransohoff, R. M., and Brown, M. A. (2012). Innate immunity in the central nervous system. *J. Clin. Invest.* 122, 1164–1171. doi: 10.1172/JCI58644

Rasmussen, D. D., Mitton, D. R., Green, J., and Puchalski, S. (2001). Chronic daily ethanol and withdrawal: 2. Behavioral changes during prolonged abstinence. *Alcohol. Clin. Exp. Res.* 25, 999–1005. doi: 10.1111/j.1530-0277.2001.tb02308.x

Read, J. P., Beattie, M., Chamberlain, R., and Merrill, J. E. (2008). Beyond the "Binge" threshold: heavy drinking patterns and their association with alcohol involvement indices in college students. *Addict. Behav.* 33, 225–234. doi: 10.1016/j.addbeh.2007.09.001

Rubino, T., Realini, N., Castiglioni, C., Guidali, C., Vigano, D., Marras, E., et al. (2008). Role in anxiety behavior of the endocannabinoid system in the prefrontal cortex. *Cereb. Cortex* 18, 1292–1301. doi: 10.1093/cercor/bhm161

Rubio, M., Mchugh, D., Fernandez-Ruiz, J., Bradshaw, H., and Walker, J. M. (2007). Short-term exposure to alcohol in rats affects brain levels of anandamide, other N-acylethanolamines and 2-arachidonoyl-glycerol. *Neurosci. Lett.* 421, 270–274. doi: 10.1016/j.neulet.2007.05.052

Schmidt, K., Krishnan, B., Xia, Y., Sun, A., Orozco-Cabal, L., Pollandt, S., et al. (2011). Cocaine withdrawal reduces group I mGluR-mediated long-term potentiation via decreased GABAergic transmission in the amygdala. *Eur. J. Neurosci.* 34, 177–189. doi: 10.1111/j.1460-9568.2011.07769.x

Scuderi, C., Valenza, M., Stecca, C., Esposito, G., Carratu, M. R., and Steardo, L. (2012). Palmitoylethanolamide exerts neuroprotective effects in mixed neuroglial cultures and organotypic hippocampal slices via peroxisome proliferator-activated receptor-alpha. *J. Neuroinflammation* 9:49. doi: 10.1186/1742-2094-9-49

Serrano, A., and Parsons, L. H. (2011). Endocannabinoid influence in drug reinforcement, dependence and addiction-related behaviors. *Pharmacol. Ther.* 132, 215–241. doi: 10.1016/j.pharmthera.2011.06.005

Serrano, A., Rivera, P., Pavon, F. J., Decara, J., Suárez, J., Rodriguez de Fonseca, F., et al. (2012). Differential effects of single versus repeated alcohol withdrawal on the expression of endocannabinoid system-related genes in the rat amygdala. *Alcohol Clin. Exp. Res.* 36, 984–894. doi: 10.1111/j.1530-0277.2011.01686.x

Skelly, M. J., Chappell, A. E., Carter, E., and Weiner, J. L. (2015). Adolescent social isolation increases anxiety-like behavior and ethanol intake and impairs fear extinction in adulthood: possible role of disrupted noradrenergic signaling. *Neuropharmacology* 97, 149–159. doi: 10.1016/j.neuropharm.2015.05.025

Spanagel, R. (2000). Recent animal models of alcoholism. *Alcohol Res. Health* 24, 124–131.

Stahel, P. F., Smith, W. R., Bruchis, J., and Rabb, C. H. (2008). Peroxisome proliferator-activated receptors: "key" regulators of neuroinflammation after traumatic brain injury. *PPAR Res.* 2008:538141. doi: 10.1155/2008/538141

Tajuddin, N., Moon, K. H., Marshall, S. A., Nixon, K., Neafsey, E. J., Kim, H. Y., et al. (2014). Neuroinflammation and neurodegeneration in adult rat brain from binge ethanol exposure: abrogation by docosahexaenoic acid. *PLoS ONE* 9:e101223. doi: 10.1371/journal.pone.0101223

Udomuksorn, W., Mukem, S., Kumarnsit, E., Vongvatcharanon, S., and Vongvatcharanon, U. (2011). Effects of alcohol administration during adulthood on parvalbumin and glial fibrillary acidic protein immunoreactivity in the rat cerebral cortex. *Acta Histochem.* 113, 283–289. doi: 10.1016/j.acthis.2009.11.001

Vetreno, R. P., and Crews, F. T. (2012). Adolescent binge drinking increases expression of the danger signal receptor agonist HMGB1 and Toll-like receptors in the adult prefrontal cortex. *Neuroscience* 226, 475–488. doi: 10.1016/j.neuroscience.2012.08.046

Vinod, K. Y., Yalamanchili, R., Xie, S., Cooper, T. B., and Hungund, B. L. (2006). Effect of chronic ethanol exposure and its withdrawal on the endocannabinoid system. *Neurochem. Int.* 49, 619–625. doi: 10.1016/j.neuint.2006.05.002

Vogel, C., and Marcotte, E. M. (2012). Insights into the regulation of protein abundance from proteomic and transcriptomic analyses. *Nat. Rev. Genet.* 13, 227–232. doi: 10.1038/nrg3185

Wilson, J., Watson, W. P., and Little, H. J. (1998). CCK(B) antagonists protect against anxiety-related behaviour produced by ethanol withdrawal, measured using the elevated plus maze. *Psychopharmacology* 137, 120–131. doi: 10.1007/s002130050601

Zeigler, D. W., Wang, C. C., Yoast, R. A., Dickinson, B. D., Mccaffree, M. A., Robinowitz, C. B., et al. (2005). The neurocognitive effects of alcohol on adolescents and college students. *Prev. Med.* 40, 23–32. doi: 10.1016/j.ypmed.2004.04.044

19

Ex-Drug Users' and Health Professionals' Perspectives About School-Based Drug Use Prevention Programs

Teuku Tahlil[1*] *and Aiyub Aiyub*[2]

[1] *Department of Community Health Nursing, Nursing Faculty, Universitas Syiah Kuala, Banda Aceh, Indonesia,* [2] *Department of Psychiatry, Nursing Faculty, Universitas Syiah Kuala, Banda Aceh, Indonesia*

Edited by:
Michal Grivna,
United Arab Emirates University,
United Arab Emirates

Reviewed by:
Nualnong Wongtongkam,
James Cook University, Australia
Masoud Mohammadnezhad,
Fiji National University, Fiji

***Correspondence:**
Teuku Tahlil
ttahlil@unsyiah.ac.id

Adolescents have become a prime target for drug dealers in various countries around the world, including in Indonesia. To reduce the high number of drug users amongst adolescents, effective drug prevention programs should be developed and implemented. The present study aimed to identify effective school-based drug prevention programs for adolescents from the perspectives of former drug users and health professionals. This qualitative research used Focus Group Discussions (FGDs) to collect the data. The study participants consisted of eight Ex-Drug Users (EDUs) and eight Health Professionals (HPs) from health educational institutions and health service settings that were selected through purposive sampling. Data analysis was performed using the qualitative content analysis. Five themes were identified from both EDUs and HPs, including the negative effects of drugs, the socialization of drug abuse, the rehabilitation of drug addicts, the partner collaboration, and the obstacles in preventing drug use. All participants agreed that the drug prevention programs such as school-based drug prevention programs are necessary in order to minimize the adverse effects of drug use. While EDUs tended to focus on the social and psychological effects of drugs, the HPs were more inclined toward the risks of diseases, social impacts, and economic problems of the drugs as the reasons for program importance. In terms of the intervention programs, both EDUs and HPs proposed conducting socialization through the use of active methods and agreed that rehabilitation as an effective way for addict students. Also, both groups of participants agreed on the significance of internal and external support, as well as coordination and collaboration to produce an effective and quality program. While the EDUs cited external factors as the main obstacle to the success of program implementation, the HPs mentioned internal factors of the users. School-based drug prevention programs are an important and potentially effective strategy to reduce the use and the effects of drug use among adolescents. The support of various relevant stakeholders is needed to further increase the effectiveness of the programs and eliminate possible barriers to the implementation of the intervention programs.

Keywords: drug abuse, students, prevention program, healthcare professional, ex-drug users, qualitative study, Indonesia

INTRODUCTION

Adolescents are at a transitional period in which they try to search for identity and to engage in numerous high-risk behaviors. Adolescents tend to seek pleasure and to be aggressive and moral free; thus, they often encounter conflict psychologically and socially with their families, peer groups, and social environment (1, 2). Psychological and social distress often triggers the occurrence of unhealthy behaviors such as smoking, consuming alcohol, and using drugs (3).

Drugs are dangerous substances. The use of drugs will interfere with the formation and distribution of neurotransmitters and hormone secretion, affecting the growth of the brain area, and nerve circuits (4, 5). Moreover, the use of drugs in adolescents can cause various adverse effects such as low thinking, low academic achievement, high-risk sexual behaviors, increased criminal behaviors, poor interpersonal and social relationships, and increased risk of morbidity and mortality (6, 7).

Despite the harmful effects, drug abuse has become a common problem faced by many countries in the world, including in Indonesia. A survey of the European Monitoring Center for Drugs and Drug Addiction (8) showed that cannabis users in Europe reached 23.5 million people, cocaine 3.5 million people, and opioid 13.5 million people. In Indonesia, the National Narcotics Board (9) reported that the prevalence of drug use in 2017 reached 2.9% for regular users and 9.1% for experimental users, both of which equaled to 1 million (regular users) and 1.8 million (experimental users) of Indonesians. Additionally, the users who had been addicted reached 500,000 people (10). In terms of age, the highest prevalence was at age under 30 years (3%), while in terms of gender, the prevalence of men was greater than women of 12% compared to 4.6% (experimental users) and of 3.7% against 1.7% (regular users), respectively. From the educational background, drug abuse was mostly done by those with low education (9).

Drug abuse among adolescents has been increasingly worrying in Indonesia. Kusumawardhani et al. (11) reported that around 2.5% of 10,736 junior and senior high school students in their survey had used drugs. About 1.1% of the surveyed children started using drugs at the age of seven or younger, and 1.7% consumed drugs from one to more than twenty times during their lifetime (11).

Adolescents are at a critical period for the onset of drug abuse (12). The risk of drug abuse begins to emerge since a child separates from parents and starts entering school. The greatest risk is when an adolescent enters high school. In this period, the adolescent's social condition changes considerably because he/she will face many challenges from social, psychological, and educational aspects. At the age of 15–18 years, adolescents begin to get the trust of parents to regulate themselves, and therefore, they are free to do social activities with peer groups outside their homes (13). This situation will then become the beginning of drug abuse attempts.

Allowing adolescents to be exposed to drugs is similar to letting young people become physically, socially, mentally, and spiritually weak. Drug prevention efforts need to start early, such as between 11 and 12 years (14). During this period, adolescents begin to be exposed to drugs, and usually start using drugs while they are in high school. Therefore, all stakeholders should be fully involved in an effort to eradicate the distribution and use of drugs. Drug prevention is not only the responsibility of the school, but the involvement of all parties, both internal and external, so that a good and drug-free environment can be established. Motivated by this issue, this study was conducted to explore various ideas in a participatory manner from relevant stakeholders. The study was a preliminary research that attempted to identify an effective school-based drug prevention program appropriate for adolescents.

METHODS

Study Design

This qualitative study used Focus Group Discussions (FGDs) to explore the perspectives of Ex-Drug Users (EDUs) and Health Professionals (HPs) about an effective and appropriate drug prevention program for adolescents in schools. Two FGDs were conducted, included one group of EDUs and one group of HPs. Each FGDs comprised of eight participants.

Study Participants

Two groups of participants were recruited as samples, namely [1] eight EDUs who have worked as addiction consultants at one of the Provincial National Narcotics Boards, and; [2] eight HPs, comprising health educators (25%), health workers in hospitals (50%) and community health centers (25%) from two districts/cities in Indonesia. The participants were selected by using the purposive sampling technique, taking into account that the selected participants had sufficient knowledge and capacity to provide information in accordance with the objectives of the study. The inclusion criteria of EDUs were: [1] adult participants (20–58 years), [2] have totally quit using drug, [3] have experienced to use rehabilitation unit for recovery, and [4] have experienced as counselor in drug rehabilitation unit. For the HPs, inclusion criteria included: [1] aged between 20 and 60 years, [2] worked as a health worker (services provider or educator), and, [3] have never used drug.

Data Collection

Data for this qualitative study were obtained through two FGDs (one for EDUs and one for HPs). Semi-structured open ended interview questions related to the implementation of school-based drug prevention programs for adolescents were asked to the participants during each FGDs, including the significance of the program, the appropriate format of the program, the parties needed to be involved in the program, and the use of religious elements in the program. Each FGDs was carried out separately lasting about 60–90 min and recorded using a Voice Recorder. All FGDs were led by the research team and took place at the appointed time and location, as agreed between the research team and participants. The audio recorded of FGDs were transcribed for unit analysis.

TABLE 1 | Characteristics of participants.

Characteristics		Group (f,%)	
		Health professionals	Ex-drug users
Sex			
	Male	3 (37.50)	8 (100.00)
	Female	5 (62.50)	0 (0)
Age			
	25–30	0 (0)	3 (37.50)
	31–35	1 (12.50)	3 (37.50)
	36–40	2 (25.00)	1 (12.50)
	41–45	4 (50.00)	1 (12.50)
	46–50	1 (12.50)	0 (0)
Marital status			
	Married	7 (87.50)	6 (75.00)
	Not married	1 (12.50)	2 (25.00)
Education			
	Senior high school	0 (0.00)	7 (87.50)
	Diploma III	1 (12.50)	1 (12.50)
	Bachelor/Diploma IV/Profession	4 (50.00)	0 (0)
	Master/Specialist–1	2 (25.00)	0 (0)
	Doctorate/ Specialist–2	1 (12.50)	0 (0)

Data Analysis

The data were analyzed by using the qualitative content analysis. The analysis process began by identifying the meaning units of the interview transcripts. The identified meaning units were then inferred in the form of condensed meaning units. Afterwards, the textual and the latent meanings were also identified to determine the themes and the categories relevant with the purpose of the study (15).

RESULTS

Characteristics of Participants

The characteristics of participants involved in this study are shown in **Table 1**. Most study participants were male (68.75%), aged over 35 years (56.25%), married (81.25%), and had above Diploma education (56.25%).

Participants' Perception on School-Based Drug Use Prevention Programs

The perceptions of HPs and EDUs on school-based drug use prevention programs are summarized in **Table 2**. Overall there is no difference in perspective between EDUs and HPs on the implementation of school-based drug abuse prevention programs. There are five main themes suggested, namely (1) The negative effects of drugs, (2) Drug abuse socialization programs, (3) Rehabilitation of addicts, (4) Cooperation partners, and (5) Obstacles to the implementation of drug prevention programs.

The Negative Effects of Drugs Use

There was a slight difference in perspective between EDUs and HPs on the theme of the negative effects of drugs. The EDUs consider the social and psychological effects of drug users is lack of empathy. One EDU stated as follow:

> *"Teenage drug users like to look for fun and don't really care about others."*

In addition, the EDUs also stated that drug users were difficult to regulate, liked to lie, often committed crimes, making them often legally troubled, as stated by the participants as follows:

> *"The signs of drug users include stealing, cheating, lying, and being unruly and stubborn"*
> *"Teenage drug users often commit crimes to buy drugs"*
> *"... often violate the law."*

On the other hand, the HPs considered that social, disease, and economic problems as the negative aspects of drugs. The social problems experienced by drug users included decreased academic achievement and disruption of relationships with family and society. The HPs participants' remarks are shown below:

> *"The impact of the use of drugs on adolescents is that [drugs] can disturb the harmonious relationships with parents"*
> *"The behaviors of teenage drug users are very disruptive to the community environment."*

Drug Abuse Socialization Programs

The HPs said that socialization media, models, and material should be highly noted. Socialization should guarantee that the students are not so lured that they want to try drugs, as described by the HPs participants below:

> *"Socialization can be done through presentations, videos and role play so it can be more interesting"*
> *"Socialization in schools must ensure that the students do not want to try to the drugs."*

According to the EDUs, socialization should be tailored to the target groups, the media, the models, and the material. Their responses are stated in the following:

> *"Socialization material needs to be appropriate to the target groups"*
> *"Socialization material should not be too vulgar because that can stimulate the teenagers to try the drugs"*
> "Consisting of...*early detection...* and. *the dangers of drugs for health and social affairs."*

In regard with the time of socialization, the EDUs perceived that socialization should begin from when the students enter junior high school, in which the socialization contains actual, real, and worry-free information.

Rehabilitation of Addicts

In addition to drug prevention socialization, the EDUs and HPs also consider the medical and social rehabilitation program for the addicts are especially important. Both EDUs and HPs agreed that an outpatient and inpatient rehabilitation model, specifically designated for children/adolescents, need to be provided so that

TABLE 2 | Perceptions of ex-drug users and health professionals on the implementation of school based drug prevention programs.

Participants	Themes	Categories	Sub-Categories
Ex-drug users	Negative effects of drugs	Social problems	Users are less empathetic and unruly, commit crime & violate laws.
		Psychological problems	Mind disorders, low concentration, emotional disturbances, and messy lifestyles
	Socialization of drug prevention programs	Media Outreach	Social media, films & posters
		Target groups	Early life and from the beginning of entering school
		Socialization models	Intra and Extracurricular
		Socialization material	Early detection, the dangers of drugs, materials must be in accordance with the target groups, and information conveyed is real and actual and not too vulgar
	Rehabilitation	Rehabilitation models	Outpatient and inpatient rehabilitation specifically for children, and not combined with adults
	Cooperation partners	Internal	Teachers, peer groups, and parents
		External	BNN, Offices of Education and Health, and universities
	Barriers to program implementation	Government support	Financial and legal
		Social support	Stigma and discrimination
Health professionals	Negative effects of drugs	Social problems	Decrease academic achievement and damage social relations (family & community)
		Diseases	Neurological disease, HIV/AIDS and tuberculosis
		Economy	Economic need to obtain substances increases
	Socialization of drug prevention programs	Media outreach	Videos, socio-dramas and advertisements
		Socialization models	Intra and Extracurricular
		Socialization material	Early detection, the dangers of drugs, prohibition of drugs in religion, and information conveyed is not too vulgar
	Rehabilitation	Rehabilitation models	Outpatient and inpatient rehabilitation specifically for children, and not combined with adults
	Cooperation partners	Internal	Students, teachers, and family
		External	Health workers in Puskesmas, hospitals (general & mental), pesantren (Islamic Boarding School) and BNN
	Barriers to program implementation	Government support	Rules and law enforcement
		Users	Low medications awareness, relapse, and substance use suggestions
		Social support	Stigma and discrimination

rehabilitation will not cause any negative psychological effects on the children. The participants' statements are shown below:

> *"To date, we still do not have a rehabilitation unit specifically for children"* [EDUs].
> *"...combining rehabilitation of children with adults can cause psychological pressure for the children."* [HPs].

The participants also expected that outpatient rehabilitation ensure that addict students can undergo rehabilitation without having their educational process interrupted. The following are one of the EDU participant's responses:

> *"If students are identified as drug addicts, they should not be expelled. They can undergo outpatient rehabilitation managed by the national narcotic board."*

Cooperation Partners

In order to ensure the success of drug prevention programs, the participants pointed out the need for coordination and cooperation among related stakeholders. The EDUs and HPs agreed that peer groups, teachers and parents, being important internal parties, should be involved. Their responses are stated below:

> *"Schools play an important role in an effort to prevent drug abuse and the role of teachers is very important..."* [HPs].
> *"... teachers can become addiction counselors...."* [EDUs].
> *"In addition to teachers, peer groups need to be trained so that they can disseminate the prevention of drug abuse."* [HPs].

There was a different view among the participants on the issue of the external parties. The EDUs perceived that the Indonesia National Narcotics Agency, the Departments of Health and

Education, as well as higher educational institutions should be involved, as stated in the following:

> *"Cooperation across sectors, such as the Office of Education, National Narcotic Agency, academics and schools are very important".*

The HPS, on the other side, mentioned that it is necessary to involve the National Narcotics Agency, the center of health services (e.g., community health centers, general and mental hospitals) and the religious elements (Muslim scholars and Islamic boarding schools) in the programs, as stated below:

> *"Mental hospital has addiction counselors..."* so *"...[they] can be professional trainers..."*
>
> *"Our people have a strong belief in religious leaders; therefore, their involvement is seen as very important."*

Programs Obstacles

In relation with the obstacles that might be encountered in the implementation of the drug abuse prevention programs, the EDUs considered the government and social support as the obstacles, whereas the HPs added the users as a constraint, in addition to government and social support. Some of their statements are as follows:

> *"Families are not open when asked about their children, and some families say their children have migrated even though they are being rehabilitated...* "and *"Suggestion for using drugs is very high, so the relapse cases are also quite high."*
>
> *"...many important programs previously existed had to stop due to lack of funding."*

DISCUSSIONS

The study aimed to identify effective interventions for school-based drug use prevention programs from the perspectives of EDUs and HPs. When both EDUs and HPs were asked about the importance of drug use prevention programs in schools, the EDUs conveyed that drugs have caused detrimental effects on the growth and development of adolescence period. They had lack of empathy, been difficult to regulate, been highly emotional, and liked to violate and commit crimes, making them often face legal problems during their addiction period of their adolescence. As a result, their lives fell apart and had no future. In addition, the HPs remarked that teenage drug addicts have been often alone and had no harmonious relationships with their families and social environments. The situation happened because these addicts needed a lot of money to buy drugs, and so they often committed theft and other types of crimes. Also, many teenage addicts suffered from chronic illnesses and dropped out of school due to delinquency and inability to adapt academically.

Researchers have investigated potential effects of drug abuse on adolescents. Previous studies (16, 17) have linked drug abuse with school students' low quality of life in mental, psychological, physical, and social dimensions; low of academic performance, absenteeism, school drop-out, getting involve in a crime, low of self-esteem, pleasure seeking, lack of communication skills, and lack of safe recreational space.

Given the magnitude of the destructive effects of drugs, it is crucial to develop effective and quality prevention programs. It is acknowledged (18) that the most essential aspects in improving the quality of a prevention strategy framework are accountability, capacity, and effectiveness. To achieve these, this study attempted to develop a drug prevention model by exploring stakeholder ideas and opinions (EDUs and HPs), and in doing so their participation could be beneficial to produce quality, effective, and acceptable prevention programs.

The FGD results have shown that there are two major themes suggested by the participants for drug abuse prevention programs, including information dissemination of anti-drugs as a preventative measure and rehabilitation of drug addicts as treatment for drug users. Education is the main prevention strategy against drug abuse (19). Dissemination of information about drugs is carried out to increase the target group's knowledge in recognizing substances that are often abused, the consequences of the use of the substances, and to promote anti-drug use attitudes (20).

The results of the FGD further revealed that the EDUs wanted the anti-drug socialization material to be adjusted to the target group (adolescents). In a similar vein, Edalati and Conrod (21) conclude that the drug prevention program material should be designed by taking into consideration the cultural values, the developmental needs, and the attitudes of the target group so that the material will be more effective and relevant to the personality of the target group members. The EDUs also suggested that early detection and the dangers of drugs need to be included in the materials, along with real and actual information. The information should not frighten the target group, but still provide the facts of drugs in real life. The HPs were also in favor of putting early detection and the dangers of drugs in the material. In addition, the HPs considered that a religious perspective on substance abuse needs to be conveyed to increase adolescent beliefs about the dangers of drugs. In terms of the way information is delivered, both EDUs and HPs agreed that the information should not have vulgar content in order to prevent teenagers to try the drugs. One way to disseminate information properly is, according to the HPs, through a field trip to a rehabilitation unit to see the real impact of drug abuse.

Regarding the methods of socialization, the EDUs and HPs also agreed that the use of models, media and material should be adapted to the target group (adolescents). However, the EDUs advocated the use of social media, films, and posters in anti-drug socialization, while the HPs recommended the use of videos, social drama, field trips (rehabilitation units and mental hospitals) and advertisements as the media for disseminating anti-drug information. Buller et al. (22) have written about drug prevention campaigns using mass media and social media for the past 15 years. They assert that the selection of media (broadcasting media, print media, online media, social media, and mobile media) and media content need to be adjusted to the target of the disseminated information. Some media content that can be chosen, according to Botvin and Griffin (20), in the dissemination of information on drug abuse are didactic instruction, discussion, audio/video presentations, displays of substances, posters, pamphlets, and school assembly programs. Further, according to the EDUs, field trips can also provide experience about the dangers of drug abuse, and so these can be considered an effective method for preventing drug abuse behavior among adolescents.

There are three issues targeted by the drug use prevention programs in schools, namely: [1] demand reduction (by giving students skills to say "no to drug"), [2] supply reduction (by crating and developing relevant policies), and [3] reduce the adverse consequences (by treating and referring students with substances abuse to appropriate counseling and treatment (23). The effectiveness of drug use prevention programs in schools are very dependent on the models of anti-drug socialization in schools. In the FGDs, both EDUs and HPs wanted the intra and extracurricular activities to be integrated in the socialization. Both also agreed to insert drug-related material in existing school subjects rather than adding a new subject. The participants stated that drug-related material may be integrated in civics, religion, biology, and physical education. In addition to the intra-curricular model, drug socialization can also be inserted in extracurricular activities such as scouting and school health units.

In the literature review written by Edalati and Conrod (21) of several intervention tests using Randomized Controlled Trials (RCTs) in adolescents and adults, it was found that brief group based intervention sessions (psycho-education, motivational enhancement therapy, and cognitive behavioral therapy) given to high-risk students during school hours were quite successful in reducing the range of drug use to 50% with the effects lasting for up to 3 years. Sloboda and Ringwalt (23) pinpoint that the impacts expected from the dissemination of information about drug use prevention in schools include creating a safe (physical and emotional) and inclusive school environment, promoting positive relationships, and instilling anti-drug norms and behaviors.

Aside of drug use prevention, drug use treatment, and rehabilitation are also the concerns of the participants in the FGDs. When asked about what to do with children who experience drug dependence, the EDUs and HPs agreed that treatment and rehabilitation are important for adolescents who have already been dependent. In the Indonesian Law and Narcotics (24), the Indonesian government incurs severe penalties (maximum death penalty) for drug dealers; however, drug users or addicts, as the victims, are given the opportunity to undergo treatment and rehabilitation programs outside prison (10). Considering the importance of treatment and rehabilitation for drug users (especially adolescents), the EDUs and HPs viewed that a special rehabilitation for adolescents is necessary. The EDUs claimed it is very harmful to combine youth with adults in a rehabilitation unit as this can cause discomfort and stress for the youth. The EDUs also said that outpatient rehabilitation units are better for adolescents whose dependency levels are still low and because inpatient rehabilitation will disrupt their educational process at school. However, in Indonesia, the availability of treatment and rehabilitation units is not yet balanced with drug addicts. In addition, the use of treatment and rehabilitation is also still low. It is therefore necessary to add and improve the quality of treatment and rehabilitation unit services to meet the needs of drug users addiction (10).

Drug abuse prevention programs cannot only be conducted by schools. Thus, the EDUs and HPs suggested the involvement of all stakeholders, both internal and external, to the programs. Both groups agreed that teachers, peer groups, and parents need to be involved as the internal stakeholders in the strategy to prevent drug abuse. There are three parties that need to be involved in the process of preventing and overcoming the victims of drug abuse, such as teachers and parents (internal parties) and health services (external) (21). The involvement of teachers and school counselors as the internal parties is highly required. Some previous studies found that the efforts made by teachers and school counselors were as effective as prevention efforts done by trained clinicians. In addition, the EDUs and HPs also noted the involvement of the National Narcotics Board, the education and health departments, and Islamic boarding schools.

During FGDs, the obstacles to implementing drug use prevention were also discussed. In this case, both groups of participants stated that the government support was not yet optimal. The EDUs further claimed that many prevention and rehabilitation programs had to be canceled due to the lack of funds. Moreover, the legal issue concerned was the lack of legal rules that could ensnare drug dealers. The Indonesian Criminal Code does not specifically regulate drug offenses (25). However, many regulations regarding drug offenses are regulated through the Narcotics Law (No. 35/2009) (24). The opportunity given by the Narcotics Law regarding rehabilitation opportunities for drug addicts is often used by law enforcers to conduct transactions with captured users/dealers. This situation occurs because the standard definition between users and dealers is not yet clear, allowing rise to legal loopholes. In addition to involving the legal rules, the HPs also highlighted the low level of law enforcement in Indonesia, causing the circulation of drug has yet to overcome.

Other than the government support, public support for drug users is also still low. Both EDUs and HPs believed that stigma and discrimination against drug users was still very high within the Indonesian society. Stigma has been very high in society (26). Families cannot trust drug users and health care workers provide poor care to the users. This has an effect on the low help-seeking behavior of drug users, leading to low participation in treatment and rehabilitation. Sabarinah (10) found that the rate of drug users utilizing treatment and rehabilitation (TR) in Indonesia was about 15%. While this figure was not merely affected by the stigma, the number and quality of services from TR were indeed a problem.

The main limitation of the current study is the findings were merely based on data obtained from FGDs with EDUs and HPs. The findings may not represent the need of adolescents. Thus, further studies which include students and other relevant stakeholders are required to further explore the most appropriate and effective school-based drug use prevention programs for adolescents.

CONCLUSION AND SUGGESTIONS

Drug prevention programs among junior high school students are considered highly significant in order to prevent the adverse effects of drug abuse. The results showed that in addition to the prevention program, treatment, and rehabilitation should also be carried out to cure addict students. In the process of treatment and rehabilitation, the aspects of education and psychology should always be considered. Therefore, special rehabilitation of children and adolescents is needed to minimize their psychological stress compared to when treated together with adults. In addition, outpatient rehabilitation units should also be developed so that the addict students can undergo treatment and rehabilitation without having to leave school.

Drug prevention programs are not only the responsibility of schools, and thus, internal and external coordination and cooperation are necessary to produce an effective and quality program. Support from various relevant stakeholders will also be needed to help improve the effectiveness of drug abuse prevention programs.

ETHICS STATEMENT

The studies involving human participants were reviewed and approved by Research Ethics Committee of the Nursing Faculty of Universitas Syiah Kuala, Banda Aceh, Indonesia. The patients/participants provided their written informed consent to participate in this study.

AUTHOR CONTRIBUTIONS

TT wrote a proposal for funding, led the study design and data collection, and assisted in data analysis and writing of the manuscript. AA assisted in data collection, analyzed the data, and wrote the manuscript.

INFORMED CONSENT

Information about the study was delivered orally and in writing to all study participants. All participants provided their written consent for their involvement in this study.

FUNDING

This study was funded by the Director of Research and Community Services (DRPM), the Ministry of Research, Technology and Higher Education RI [Grant No. 215/SP2H/LT/DRPM/2019].

REFERENCES

1. Townsed MC. *Psychiatric Mental Health Nursing: Concepts of Care in Evidence-Based Practice, 6th Edn.* Philadelphia, PA: F.A. Davis Company (2015).
2. Videbeck SL. *Psychiatric Mental Health Nursing, 5th Edn.* New York, NY: Lippincott Williams and Wilkins.
3. Das JK, Salam RA, Arshad A, Finkelstein Y, Bhutta ZA. Interventions for adolescent substance abuse: an overview of systematic reviews. *J Adolescent Health.* (2016) 59:S61–75. doi: 10.1016/j.jadohealth.2016.06.021
4. Guerri C, Pascual M. Impact of neuroimmune activation induced by alcohol or drug abuse on adolescent brain development. *Int J Dev Neurosci.* (2019) 77:89–98. doi: 10.1016/j.ijdevneu.2018.11.006
5. Vakonaki E, Tzatzarakis M, Tsiminikaki K, Nathena D, Fragkiadaki P, Kalliantasi K, Tsatsakis A. Effect of chronic and heavy drug abuse on biological aging. *World Acad Sci J.* (2019) 2019:67–73. doi: 10.3892/wasj.2019.7
6. Carney T, Myers BJ, Louw J, Okwundu CI. Brief school-based interventions and behavioural outcomes for substance-using adolescents. *Cochrane Database Syst Rev.* (2016) 2016:Cd008969. doi: 10.1002/14651858.CD008969.pub3
7. Welsh JW, Hou SS, Shentu Y, Le Cook B. Assessing the association between the strength of state policies on school drug prevention and substance use disorders. *Subst Use Misuse.* (2019) 54:811–7. doi: 10.1080/10826084.2018.1544644
8. European Monitoring Centre for Drugs and Drug Addiction. *Prevalence of Drug Use.* (2017). Retrieved from: http://www.emcdda.europa.eu/data/stats2017/gps
9. Indonesia National Narcotic Board. *(Badan Narkotika Nasional RI) Survey Nasional Penyalahgunaan Narkoba di 34 Povinsi Tahun 2017.* Jakarta: Pusat Penelitian Data dan Informasi Badan Narkotika Nasional (2017).
10. Sabarinah. Use of drug treatment and rehabilitation services in indonesia: findings of the 2014 National Narcotic Survey. *Asia Pac J Public Health.* (2019) 31:548–58. doi: 10.1177/1010539519872343
11. Kusumawardani N, Rachmalina WY, Anwar A, Handayani K, Mubasyiroh R. *Perilaku Berisiko Kesehatan Pada Pelajar SMP Dan SMA Di Indonesia.* Jakarta: Puslitbang Upaya Kesehatan Masyarakat Kemenkes RI (2015).
12. Winters K, Botzet A, Stinchfield R, Gonzales-Castaneda R, Finch A, Piehler T, Hemze A. *Adolescent Substance Abuse Treatment: A Review of Evidence-Based Research: Evidence-Based Approaches to Prevention and Treatment.* Cham: Springer International Publishing (2018). p. 141–71. doi: 10.1007/978-3-319-90611-9_5
13. National Institute on Drug Abuse. *Preventing Drug Abuse Among Children and Adolescents. A Research-Based Guide for Parents, Educators and Community Leaders,* 2nd Edn. Bethesda, MD: National Institute on Drug Abuse (2003).
14. Chie QT, Tam CL, Bonn G, Wong CP, Dang HM, Khairuddin R. Drug abuse, relapse, and prevention education in malaysia: perspective of university students through a mixed methods approach. *Front. Psychiatr.* (2015) 6:65. doi: 10.3389/fpsyt.2015.00065
15. Graneheim UH, Lundman B. Qualitative content analysis in nursing research: concepts, procedures and measures to achieve trustworthiness. *Nurse Educ Today.* (2004) 24:105–12. doi: 10.1016/j.nedt.2003.10.001
16. Fadaei M, Farokhzadian J, Miri S, Goojani R. Promoting drug abuse preventive behaviors in adolescent students based on the health belief model. *Int J Adolesc Med Health.* (2020) 1–8. doi: 10.1515/ijamh-2019-0170
17. Momtazi S, Rawson R. Substance abuse among Iranian high school students. *Curr Opin Psychiatr.* (2010) 23:221–6. doi: 10.1097/YCO.0b013e328338630d
18. Substance Abuse and Mental Health Services Administration. *Focus on Prevention.* Rockville, MD: Center for Substance Abuse Prevention, Substance Abuse and Mental Health Services Administration (2017).
19. Lanfredi M, Macis A, Ferrari C, Rillosi L, Ughi EC, Fanetti A, Rossi R. Effects of education and social contact on mental health-related stigma among high-school students. *Psychiatr Res.* (2019) 281:112581. doi: 10.1016/j.psychres.2019.112581

20. Botvin G, Griffin K. Chapter 3: Drug Abuse Prevention Curricula in Schools. In: Z. Sloboda and WJ. Bukoski, edItors. *Handbook of Drug Abuse Prevention.* Springer (2006). p. 45–74. doi: 10.1007/0-387-35408-5_3
21. Edalati H, Conrod PJ. A review of personality-targeted interventions for prevention of substance misuse and related harm in community samples of adolescents. *Front Psychiatr.* (2018). 9:770. doi: 10.3389/fpsyt.2018.00770
22. Buller DB, Walkosz BJ, Gill Woodall W. Use of Media and Social Media in the Prevention of Substance Use. In: Z. Sloboda, H. Petras, E. Robertson, R. Hingson, editors. *Prevention of Substance Use.* Cham: Springer International Publishing (2019). p. 319–34. doi: 10.1007/978-3-030-00627-3_20
23. Sloboda Z, Ringwalt CL. The school: a setting for evidence-based prevention interventions and policies. In: Z. Sloboda, H. Petras, E. Robertson, R Hingson, editors. *Prevention of Substance Use.* Cham: Springer International Publishing (2019). p. 147–63. doi: 10.1007/978-3-030-00627-3_9
24. Setyowati I. Sanctions policy in the Indonesian Act. No. 35 of 2009 on narcotics. *J Pembaharuan Hukum.* (2018) 5:55. doi: 10.26532/jph.v5i1.3022
25. Nicholson P, Lindsey T. *Drugs Law and Legal Practice in Southeast.* Asia: Bloomsbury (2016).
26. Benz MB, Palm Reed K, Bishop LS. Stigma and help-seeking: the interplay of substance use and gender and sexual minority identity. *Addict Behav.* (2019) 97:63–9. doi: 10.1016/j.addbeh.2019.05.023

20

Chronic Nicotine Exposure Initiated in Adolescence and Unpaired to Behavioral Context Fails to Enhance Sweetened Ethanol Seeking

Aric C. Madayag[1,2†], Kyle S. Czarnecki[1†], Lynde M. Wangler[1] and Donita L. Robinson[1,3]*

[1]Bowles Center for Alcohol Studies, University of North Carolina, Chapel Hill, NC, United States, [2]Department of Pharmacology, University of North Carolina, Chapel Hill, NC, United States, [3]Department of Psychiatry, University of North Carolina, Chapel Hill, NC, United States

Edited by:
Jacqueline M. Barker,
Medical University of South Carolina,
United States

Reviewed by:
Sheketha R. Hauser,
Indiana University School of Medicine, United States
Jee Hyun Kim,
Florey Institute of Neuroscience and Mental Health, Australia
Jean-Marie N. Maddux,
Lake Forest College, United States

***Correspondence:**
Donita L. Robinson
dlr@unc.edu

†These authors have contributed equally to this work.

Nicotine use in adolescence is pervasive in the United States and, according to the Gateway Hypothesis, may lead to progression towards other addictive substances. Given the prevalence of nicotine and ethanol comorbidity, it is difficult to ascertain if nicotine is a gateway drug for ethanol. Our study investigated the relationship between adolescent exposure to nicotine and whether this exposure alters subsequent alcohol seeking behavior. We hypothesized that rats exposed to nicotine beginning in adolescence would exhibit greater alcohol seeking behavior than non-exposed siblings. To test our hypothesis, beginning at P28, female rats were initially exposed to once daily nicotine (0.4 mg/kg, SC) or saline for 5 days. Following these five initial injections, animals were trained to nose-poke for sucrose reinforcement (10%, w/v), gradually increasing to sweetened ethanol (10% sucrose; 10% ethanol, w/v) on an FR5 reinforcement schedule. Nicotine injections were administered after the behavioral sessions to minimize acute effects of nicotine on operant self-administration. We measured the effects of nicotine exposure on the following aspects of ethanol seeking: self-administration, naltrexone (NTX)-induced decreases, habit-directed behavior, motivation, extinction and reinstatement. Nicotine exposure did not alter self-administration or the effectiveness of NTX to reduce alcohol seeking. Nicotine exposure blocked habit-directed ethanol seeking. Finally, nicotine did not alter extinction learning or cue-induced reinstatement to sweetened ethanol seeking. Our findings suggest that nicotine exposure outside the behavioral context does not escalate ethanol seeking. Further, the Gateway Hypothesis likely applies to scenarios in which nicotine is either self-administered or physiologically active during the behavioral session.

Keywords: alcohol use disorder, adolescent, addiction, cigarette smoking, tobacco

INTRODUCTION

Conventional cigarette use among youth is in steady decline; however, novel modes of consumption have arisen and are more readily available, potentially leading to increased levels of nicotine exposure. In 2016, according to the National Institutes of Health "Monitoring the Future Survey 2016", the percent of youth using conventional cigarettes in the past month among 8th, 10th and 12th grades was 2.6%, 4.9% and 10.5% respectively. Conversely, e-cigarette use encompassed 6.2%,

11.0% and 12.5% at the same grade level. These statistics argue that consumption of nicotine by conventional tobacco sources, e-cigarettes, or smokeless tobacco may pose a health threat to the future of the youth in the United States. In turn, alcohol use among adolescents is widespread, with over 35% of youth grades 8–12 in the United States reporting regular consumption and approximately 15% reporting heavy drinking or binge-drinking episodes (Bachman, 2002). Binge-level alcohol consumption is associated with elevated risk for numerous adverse outcomes including drug abuse susceptibility (Brown et al., 2000). Despite the prevalence of nicotine and ethanol use during adolescence, and their comorbidity, it is unknown if the two substances interact directly or through long-term physiological mechanisms to elicit a synergistic behavioral response. With apparent ease of access to nicotine and ethanol, the aim of this study was to determine if adolescents that are exposed to nicotine are also more susceptible to escalate ethanol seeking.

Preclinical studies suggest that adolescent animals are prone to nicotine and alcohol use. Compared to adults, adolescent rodents exhibit a higher preference for nicotine (Torres et al., 2009; Nesil et al., 2011) and higher rewarding effects of nicotine (Shram and Lê, 2010), though lower operant responding for nicotine (Shram et al., 2008; Schassburger et al., 2016). In turn, adolescent rodents show greater propensity to self-administer ethanol (Tambour et al., 2008; Walker and Ehlers, 2009; Doherty and Gonzales, 2015; Serlin and Torregrossa, 2015) and a higher preference for ethanol over water control (Truxell et al., 2007; Melendez, 2011). These findings collectively suggest adolescents are more prone to substance use and potential abuse, which could render them susceptible to addiction in adulthood. The Common Liability Hypothesis (Palmer et al., 2012) posits that underlying genetic or environmental predispositions are the important factors leading to addiction, and the developmental preference for addictive drugs during adolescence may fall into a "predisposition," albeit developmentally limited. Alternatively, the Gateway Hypothesis (Kandel et al., 1992; Degenhardt et al., 2010) theorizes that drug exposure "primes" the brain in such a way as to promote later addiction to a variety of drugs. Discerning the respective contributions of drug exposure, genetic, and environmental factors has proved to be difficult in human studies due to the inability to manipulate such variables ethically.

Nicotine has been suggested as a potent gateway drug (Kandel and Kandel, 2014). Specifically, animal studies found that nicotine produces molecular, physiological and behavioral changes to render higher susceptibility to later cocaine use (Levine et al., 2011). However, it is not clear whether nicotine use during adolescence—when many people initiate drug use—is associated with more profound "gateway" effects towards ethanol. Studies indicate that animals will escalate ethanol self-administration when it is co-administered with nicotine (Lárraga et al., 2017), suggesting that nicotine exposure escalates ethanol seeking. In Pavlovian-based tasks, when given concurrently with the initiation of a conditioned approach session where ethanol is the unconditioned stimulus, nicotine enhances approach behavior, though not when administered repeatedly in days leading up to the beginning of behavior sessions (Maddux and Chaudhri, 2017). Moreover, we and others have observed that nicotine is sufficient to elevate conditioned responding to cues predicting sucrose or water reward (Olausson et al., 2004a,b; Stringfield et al., 2017), suggesting non-specific elevation of conditioned responding. It is unknown if exposure to nicotine *prior to* ethanol self-administration sessions can lead to such an escalation of ethanol seeking, as would be indicated by the Gateway Hypothesis for nicotine (Kandel and Kandel, 2014).

Consistent with the Gateway Hypothesis for nicotine, we hypothesized that exposure to nicotine in adolescence would increase the rewarding and motivational properties of ethanol. To test this, we exposed adolescent female rats to daily nicotine injections and tested operant responding for sweetened ethanol under multiple conditions to ascertain ethanol seeking, habit-directed behavior, motivation for ethanol and extinction-reinstatement. Nicotine exposure continued through the operant training and testing. Notably, operant sessions and nicotine administration were separated in time so that any changes in behavior between groups would be due to nicotine exposure and associated neuroplasticity rather than acute effects.

MATERIALS AND METHODS

Subjects

Eighteen Sprague-Dawley female rats were bred at the University of North Carolina at Chapel Hill and maintained under a 12:12 h light:dark cycle, lights on from 07:00 to 19:00. Animals were weaned into pair-housed cages on postnatal day (P) 21 with *ad libitum* access to water and standard chow except when indicated. All experimental procedures were performed during the light cycle between 09:00 and 12:00. This study was carried out in accordance with the recommendations of University of North Carolina Division of Laboratory Animal Medicine. The protocol was approved by the Institutional Animal Care and Use Committee of the University of North Carolina. The dataset consisted of four litters grouped into three behavior cohorts. The following is a breakdown of experimental group distribution: cohort 1, 4 saline and 4 nicotine; cohort 2, 2 saline and 4 nicotine; cohort 3, 2 saline and 2 nicotine. Every animal performed the entirety of behavior experiments.

Drugs

Nicotine hydrogen tartrate (Sigma Aldrich, St. Louis, MO, USA) was dissolved in 0.9% saline and pH adjusted to 7.0 ± 0.2 via NaOH solution. Nicotine was administered via subcutaneous injection at 0.4 mg/kg, calculated using the free base form (Palmatier et al., 2013; Stringfield et al., 2017). Ethanol (95% Decon Labs, King of Prussia, PA, USA) was diluted to concentrations of up to 10% (w/v) in 10% sucrose as previously described (Shnitko and Robinson, 2015). Naltrexone (NTX) HCl (Sigma Aldrich) was dissolved in sterile saline. All injections delivered 1 ml/kg volume.

Operant Acquisition and Maintenance

The experimental timeline is outlined in **Table 1**. Rats were administered saline or nicotine, with cage-mates assigned the

TABLE 1 | Experimental timeline.

Age range at start of epoch	Experimental epoch	
P28	Daily nicotine injections for 5 days	
P33	**Operant training**	
	Sessions 1–3:	*FR1, 10S (water restricted)*
	Session 4:	*FR1, 10S*[a]
	Sessions 5, 6:	*FR1, 10S/2.5E*
	Sessions 7, 8:	*FR1, 10S/5E*
	Session 9:	*FR1, 10S/10E*
	Sessions 10:	*FR3, 10S/10E*
	Sessions 11–21:	*FR5, 10S/10E*
P57–P61	Naltrexone dose-response sessions	
	Maintenance sessions, FR5, 10S/10E	
P76–P90	Satiety-specific devaluation session	
	Maintenance sessions, FR5, 10S/10E	
P84–P95	Progressive ratio session	
P85–P96	12 extinction sessions	
P97–P108	Reinstatement session	

[a]*4/18 rats did not undergo this session (2 saline and 2 nicotine rats).*

same treatment to minimize differences in behavior within a cage after drug exposure. Starting P28, animals received daily saline or nicotine injections for five consecutive days prior to the first behavior session. Behavioral experiments were performed in 12.0″ × 9.5″ × 8.25″ operant chambers (Med Associates, Inc., St. Albans, VT, USA). Beam break detectors were used to measure a nosepoke response. A cue light was located above the reward delivery well to indicate the availability to retrieve the reward. Animals underwent one session per day for 6–7 days per week. To avoid acute effects of nicotine on operant behavior (Chaudhri et al., 2005), nicotine or saline injections were made 2 h after each training session.

To encourage acquisition of operant responding for reward, on P34 animals were water restricted the day prior and concurrently with the three initial days of nosepoke training; one nosepoke resulted in concurrent delivery of a cue light and a tone for 3.5 s, 100 μL of reward solution, and a 20 s time out. Nosepoke training consisted of 100 μL of 10% sucrose reward (10S) on an FR1 schedule of reinforcement; each session lasted 2–3 h, immediately followed by home cage access to water for 1 h. After the third session, animals returned to *ad libitum* water access in their home cages for the duration of the study. Next, each phase of training took place during 20–30 min sessions as described in **Table 1** (reinforcement schedule-reward): FR1-10S; FR1-10S/2.5E (10% sucrose, 2.5% ethanol, both w/v); FR1-10S/5E; FR1-10S/10E; FR3-10S/10E. The age of first exposure to ethanol (10% sucrose, 2.5% ethanol) was P37–38. Following this schedule, animals were maintained on 30-min sessions of an FR5 schedule of reinforcement with 10S/10E reward. Prior to experimental manipulations below, each animal underwent 11 maintenance sessions on FR5-10S/10E. Note that sweetened alcohol was used to promote rapid acquisition of ethanol seeking during the short period of rodent adolescence (approximately P28–P42).

Naltrexone

Each animal received 0, 0.3, 1 and 3 mg/kg (SC) NTX 30 min prior to a standard FR5-10S/10E self-administration session. The doses were counterbalanced such that every animal received every dose, but also equal numbers of rats from each group received the same dose order. Animals underwent two maintenance self-administration sessions between NTX sessions to allow wash-out of the prior NTX dose and to re-establish baseline behavior.

Satiety Specific Devaluation

Next we assessed habitual vs. goal-directed reward seeking with the satiety specific devaluation as previously described (Hay et al., 2013; Shillinglaw et al., 2014), except in the present study we used a between-subjects approach. After the last NTX session, over 3 days leading up to the devaluation session, animal pairs were separated in their home cage by a plastic divider and allowed to drink water from inserted water bottles freely for 60 min prior to standard maintenance sessions; this habituated the rats to the separation and bottle placement. On the test day, animals were separated and allowed to freely drink either 2% maltodextrin solution (control) or 10S/10E solution (devaluation) in a between-subjects design in the 60 min prior to behavioral session. The devaluation test session consisted of a 10-min operant session during which nosepokes were recorded but cue and reward reinforcements were absent.

Progressive Ratio

Following devaluation, animals underwent 4 days of maintenance self-administration sessions to re-establish baseline behavior. Animals were then assessed for motivation for sweetened ethanol with a progressive ratio schedule of reinforcement as previously described (Walker and Koob, 2007). Animals were placed in the operant conditioning boxes and the number of responses required for reinforcement increased according to the schedule of 1, 1, 2, 2, 3, 3, 4, 4, 5, 5, 7, 7, 9, 9, 11, 11, 13, 13, 15, 15, 18, 18, 21, 21, 24, 24, etc. The session ended after an animal failed to respond for 30 min with a maximum session of 3 h. Nosepokes and "breakpoint" was recorded. The "breakpoint" was the last level of required responding achieved by an animal prior to the end of the session.

Extinction and Reinstatement

Following the progressive ratio session, with no maintenance sessions between, animals underwent 12 30-min extinction sessions in which they were placed in the operant boxes and nosepokes were recorded but cues and rewards were not delivered. After the last extinction session, animals underwent a 30-min extinction-reinstatement session that began as an extinction session, where cues and reward reinforcements were not delivered. Ten minutes into the session, a single cue delivery consisting of cue light and tone for 3.5 s was delivered. Thereafter, the conditioned (cue) reinforcements were delivered on an

FR5 schedule but no reward was delivered, similar to previous studies (Bienkowski et al., 2000; Hay et al., 2013).

Statistical Analysis

All figures were generated using GraphPad Prism software (GraphPad Software, La Jolla, CA, USA). Statistical analyses were performed using Statistica Software (Statistica, Tulsa, OK, USA). Most experiments were analyzed using two-way ANOVA with session, time bin, or dose as repeated measures and exposure history (saline or nicotine) as the between-subjects factor. Satiety-induced reward devaluation analysis was performed as a two-way ANOVA with no repeated measure. Bonferroni corrected t-tests were performed for *post hoc* analyses as appropriate. Progressive ratio analyses were performed as independent sample t-tests.

RESULTS

Acquisition and Maintenance of Self-Administration of Sweetened Ethanol

We first measured if nicotine exposure beginning during adolescence altered acquisition of operant self-administration of sweetened ethanol. The first four sessions were variable as the rats learned the operant response under water restriction and then were removed from water restriction. Thus, we compared the six sessions in which ethanol was gradually added to the sucrose solution. Nicotine injections 2 h after each behavioral session did not alter acquisition of sweetened ethanol self-administration (**Table 2**). A two-way repeated measures ANOVA yielded a main effect of session ($F_{(1,5)} = 7.35$, $p < 0.001$), but no significant effect of exposure ($F_{(1,5)} = 1.37$, $p = 0.26$) or session by exposure interaction ($F_{(1,5)} = 1.56$, $p = 0.18$). Collapsed across exposure group, *post hoc* analysis revealed that animals made significantly more nosepokes in the second session on FR1-10S/2.5E than in the first session on that schedule, and that animals made significantly fewer nosepokes in the session on FR1-10S10E than in the previous three sessions (Bonferroni t-test, $p < 0.05$).

We next measured whether saline and nicotine groups differed in their maintenance of operant behavior. Saline- and nicotine-exposed animals exhibited similar levels of self-administration as measured by nosepokes and sweetened ethanol consumed (**Figure 1**). A two-way ANOVA for nosepokes per session revealed a main effect of session ($F_{(10,160)} = 5.53$, $p < 0.0001$), no main effect of exposure ($F_{(1,16)} = 0.13$, $p = 0.72$) and no significant session by exposure interaction ($F_{(10,160)} = 0.66$, $p = 0.76$). Collapsed across exposure group, *post hoc* analysis showed significant increase in nosepokes in sessions 7 through 10 compared to the first session (Bonferroni t-test, $p < 0.05$). Similarly, a two-way ANOVA for ethanol consumed per session yielded a significant main effect of session ($F_{(10,160)} = 3.18$, $p < 0.001$), but no main effect of exposure ($F_{(1,16)} = 0.04$, $p = 0.85$), and no significant session-by-exposure interaction ($F_{(10,160)} = 0.91$, $p = 0.53$). Specifically, rats self-administered an average of 0.6–1.2 g/kg ethanol in a session. We also compared body weight during these sessions (data not shown), and detected the expected effect of session (weight gain over days; ($F_{(10,160)} = 156.3$, $p < 0.001$), but no significant effect of exposure ($F_{(1,16)} = 0.25$, $p = 0.62$) or interaction ($F_{(10,160)} = 0.19$, $p = 0.99$). Thus, exposure to nicotine starting in adolescence but administered after the operant sessions had no impact on self-administration of sweetened ethanol.

TABLE 2 | Acquisition of operant self-administration, after water restriction.

Session	Saline	Nicotine
FR1, 10S/2.5E	131.9 ± 23.7	82.3 ± 16.7
FR1 10S/2.5E[a]	155.6 ± 14.2	135.3 ± 12.7
FR1, 10S/5E	151.1 ± 18.5	112.8 ± 13.0
FR1, 10S/5E	146.3 ± 20.8	135.4 ± 14.9
FR1, 10S/10E[b]	78.5 ± 11.1	85.2 ± 10.4
FR3, 10S/10E	115.4 ± 21.8	116.2 ± 12.5

Data shown as mean nosepokes ± SEM. [a]Collapsed across exposure group, higher than the previous session. [b]Collapsed across exposure group, lower than the previous three sessions.

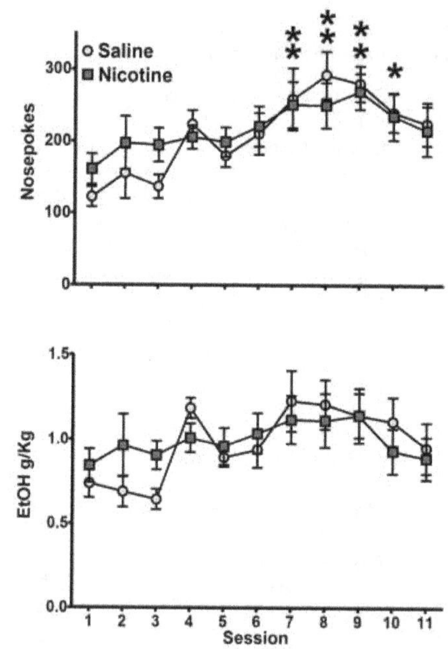

FIGURE 1 | Animals exposed to saline and nicotine self-administered sweetened ethanol similarly. Both nosepokes (Top) and consumption (Bottom) were not significantly different between exposure groups (Bonferroni *post hoc* t-test, collapsed across drug exposure groups: *$p < 0.05$, **$p < 0.01$ compared to first session; N = 8 saline, 10 nicotine).

Naltrexone Effects on Sweetened Ethanol Seeking

To determine if adolescent nicotine exposure affects the ability of NTX to alter ethanol seeking in animals, we administered a dose range of NTX that has been shown to differentially decrease ethanol vs. sucrose self-administration (Czachowski and Delory, 2009; Hay et al., 2013), using a within-subject design (**Figure 2**). A two-way ANOVA on nosepokes revealed a significant main effect of NTX ($F_{(3,48)} = 8.03$, $p < 0.001$), but no main effect

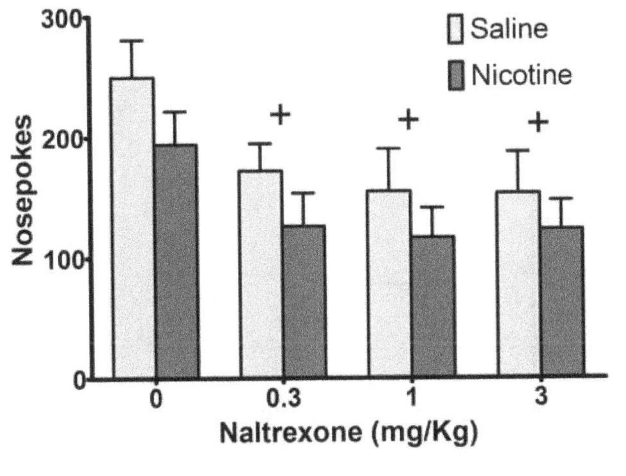

FIGURE 2 | Naltrexone (NTX) reduced operant behavior similarly in saline- and nicotine-exposed rats. While all doses of NTX decreased operant responding, no significant differences in responding were observed between groups (Bonferroni *post hoc t*-test, collapsed across drug exposure groups: $^+p < 0.01$ compared to vehicle; $N = 8$ saline, 10 nicotine).

of adolescent drug exposure history ($F_{(1,16)} = 1.81$, $p = 0.20$) and no significant dose-by-exposure interaction ($F_{(3,48)} = 0.15$, $p = 0.93$). *Post hoc* analysis collapsed across drug exposure history indicated significant decreases in sweetened ethanol seeking for all NTX doses compared to control ($p < 0.01$). Therefore, while NTX reduced sweetened ethanol self-administration, exposure to nicotine did not alter NTX's effects on ethanol seeking.

Satiety-Specific Reward Devaluation

Repeated exposure to nicotine can induce habitual nicotine seeking (Clemens et al., 2014). However, it is unknown if this inflexible behavior is generalizable to rewards other than nicotine. Thus, we used satiety-specific reward devaluation to determine if exposure to nicotine also renders an animal more susceptible to habitual behavior. Animals received *ad libitum* access to either 10S/10E or 2% maltodextrin control solution for 60 min prior to a 10 min extinction session (**Figure 3**). Saline-exposed animals did not alter reward seeking after 10S/10E devaluation compared to rats receiving the 2% maltodextrin control, indicating habitual reward seeking. In contrast, nicotine-exposed rats decreased operant responding following reward devaluation compared to rats under non-devalued conditions. A two-way ANOVA for nosepokes revealed no significant main effect of consumed solution ($F_{(1,14)} = 2.70$, $p = 0.12$), and no significant main effect of drug exposure ($F_{(1,14)} = 1.14$, $p = 0.30$), but a significant solution-by-exposure interaction ($F_{(1,14)} = 12.83$, $p < 0.01$). *Post hoc* analysis resulted in significant decrease in responding after 10S/10E devaluation compared to maltodextrin only in the nicotine-exposed rats ($p < 0.01$). This difference in reward seeking was not due to differences in liquid consumption during the 60-min access period, as there was no significant difference in volume of solution consumed prior to behavioral testing between exposure groups. A two-way ANOVA of liquid consumed

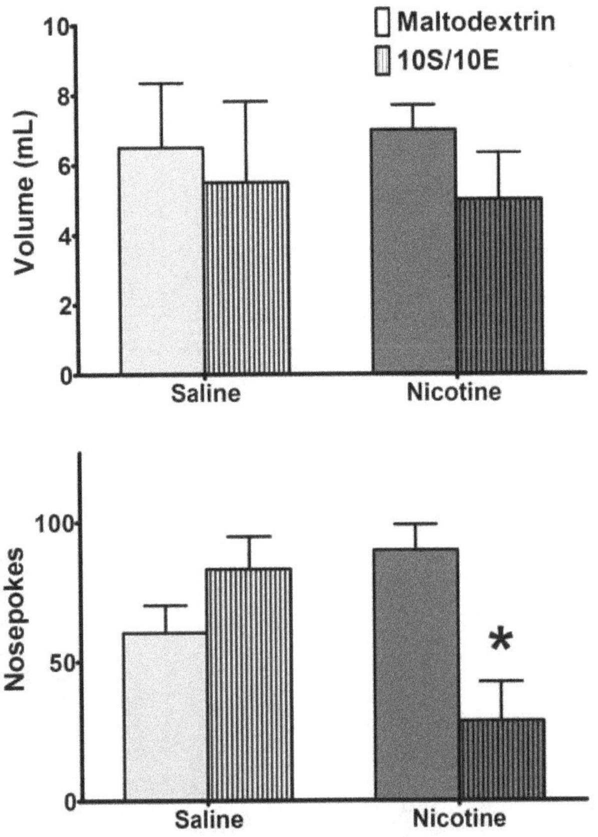

FIGURE 3 | Animals exhibited sustained habitual behavior following reward devaluation except when exposed to nicotine. (Top) Saline and nicotine animals consumed similar volumes of maltodextrin (solid bars) and sweetened ethanol (patterned bars) prior to behavioral measurement. (Bottom) Compared to maltodextrin, a control for consumed volume, pre-exposure to sweetened ethanol altered reward seeking only in nicotine exposed rats (Bonferroni *post hoc t*-test: $^*p < 0.01$ compared to maltodextrin access nicotine group; $N = 4$ Maltodextrin-Saline, 4 10S/10E-Saline, 5 Maltodextrin-Nicotine, 5 10S/10E-Nicotine).

prior to behavioral testing revealed no significant main effects of solution ($F_{(1,14)} = 0.92$, $p = 0.35$) and drug exposure ($F_{(1,14)} < 0.0001$, $p \approx 1.00$), nor a significant solution-by-exposure interaction ($F_{(1,14)} = 0.10$, $p = 0.75$). Though nicotine was expected to induce habitual behavior, nicotine exposed animals were more responsive to reward devaluation, and therefore resistant to habit formation towards sweetened ethanol in this experiment.

Progressive Ratio

Nicotine can enhance motivation for cue-reward pairing (Chaudhri et al., 2006, 2007). To test whether exposure to nicotine in adolescence alters motivation for sweetened ethanol, we recorded nosepokes and the breakpoint in a progressive ratio session (**Figures 4A,B**). Independent samples *t*-tests indicated that nicotine had no effect on nosepokes ($t_{(16)} = 0.49$, $p = 0.63$) or breakpoint ($t_{(16)} = 0.37$, $p = 0.72$). Thus, chronic nicotine exposure had no impact on motivation for sweetened ethanol.

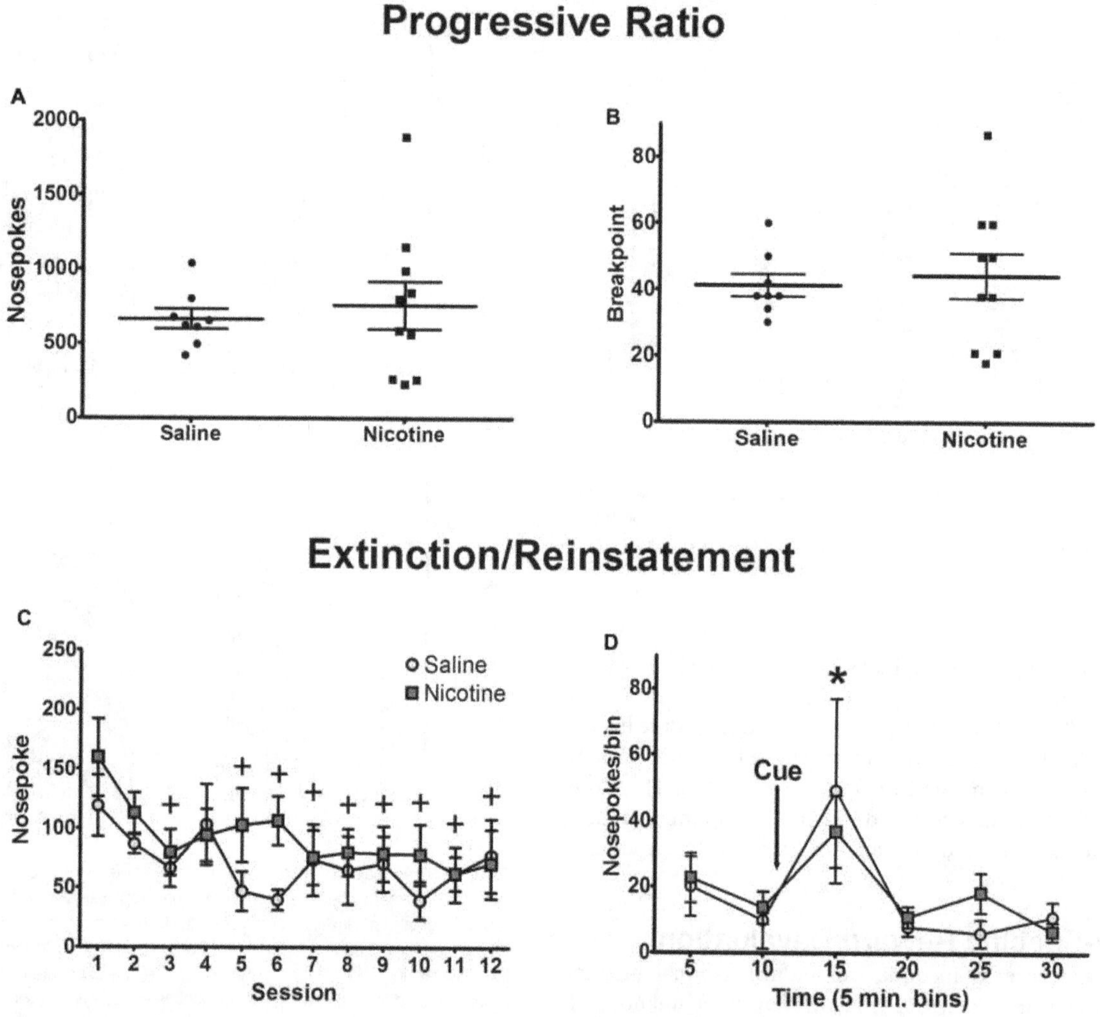

FIGURE 4 | Exposure to nicotine did not affect behavior during progressive ratio, extinction and reinstatement sessions. Motivation towards sweetened ethanol as measured by progressive ratio testing did not differ between exposure groups, indicated by **(A)** total nosepokes and **(B)** behavioral breakpoint. Individual rat data points are presented, with the mean ± SEM overlaid. **(C)** Behavioral responding decreased across 12 extinction sessions similarly between exposure groups. **(D)** Cue-induced reinstatement of operant responding was not different between groups (Bonferroni *post hoc t*-test, collapsed across drug exposure groups: $^{+}p < 0.01$ compared to session 1; $^{*}p < 0.05$ compared to 10, 20, 25 and 30 min bins; $N = 8$ saline, 10 nicotine).

Extinction and Reinstatement of Operant Behavior

Extinction learning was measured over 12 sessions. No significant difference in decreased reward seeking was observed between saline and nicotine exposed animals (**Figure 4C**). A two-way ANOVA of nosepokes resulted in a main effect of session ($F_{(11,176)} = 4.33, p < 0.0001$), but no main effect of drug exposure ($F_{(1,16)} = 0.59, p = 0.45$), and no significant session-by-exposure interaction ($F_{(11,176)} = 1.38, p = 0.18$). Nosepokes decreased significantly in the last eight sessions of extinction as indicated by *post hoc* analysis collapsed across drug exposure groups ($p < 0.01$).

As exposure to nicotine during adolescence has been shown to increase responding for conditioned reinforcers when compared to saline-exposed animals (Quick et al., 2014), we measured reinstatement of reward seeking after exposure to reward-associated cues. Reinstatement of operant responding for the cues previously associated with sweetened ethanol was measured in a single extinction-reinstatement session. Presentation of the cue (light and tone) 10 min into the session resulted in a significant increase in responding, but no significant difference was found between saline- and nicotine-exposed animals (**Figure 4D**). A two-way ANOVA of nosepokes across 5-min bins revealed a significant main effect of time bins ($F_{(5,80)} = 4.64, p < 0.001$), but no significant main effect of drug exposure ($F_{(1,16)} = 0.01, p = 0.92$) or significant time-by-exposure interaction ($F_{(5,80)} = 0.46, p = 0.80$). *Post hoc* analysis collapsed across drug exposure groups showed that cue presentation was sufficient to induce reinstatement of reward seeking, as nosepokes in the 15-min, post-cue time bin was significantly higher than the 10-min, pre-cue time bin ($p < 0.05$). Collectively, these data show that nicotine exposure history had no impact on extinction of reward seeking or reinstatement of responding after re-exposure to reward-associated cues.

DISCUSSION

Epidemiological studies find that initiating nicotine consumption in adolescence correlates with progression to escalating use as well as to the propensity to pursue more illicit substances of abuse (Kandel and Faust, 1975; Kandel et al., 1992). The Gateway Hypothesis of addiction suggests that neurophysiological changes due to nicotine exposure would eventually lead to escalation of drug use due to increased reward valence to substances of abuse (Kandel and Kandel, 2014). Previous findings suggest exposure to nicotine only in adolescence is insufficient to alter adult cocaine self-administration (Pomfrey et al., 2015). Indeed, the escalation of use and progression to stronger drugs may rely on continuous drug exposure throughout adolescence as opposed to priming only (Kandel and Kandel, 2015). Given the propensity of nicotine and ethanol use in adolescence, it is also important to determine if nicotine can be a gateway drug to alcohol use. We hypothesized that animals exposed to daily injections of nicotine beginning in adolescence would be more sensitive to the rewarding and reinforcing properties of sweetened ethanol, and therefore would increase seeking and motivation for ethanol in a self-administration paradigm. However, as discussed below, our findings did not support this hypothesis.

Studies show that co-administration of nicotine increases alcohol seeking (Smith et al., 1999; Lê et al., 2014; Lárraga et al., 2017) and VTA dopamine neuron activity in rodents (Tolu et al., 2017). However, this may be due to nicotine's well-known ability to enhance the reinforcing properties of conditioned cues (Donny et al., 2003; Olausson et al., 2004a,b; Chaudhri et al., 2006; Palmatier et al., 2007, 2013; Caggiula et al., 2009; Guy and Fletcher, 2014a,b; Yager and Robinson, 2015). Indeed, several studies reported that nicotine administered prior to each behavioral session elevated conditioned responding to cues predicting either sucrose (Palmatier et al., 2013; Stringfield et al., 2017) or ethanol (Maddux and Chaudhri, 2017), supporting the contention that nicotine enhances approach behavior. Moreover, presentation of a nicotine-associated context, and not necessarily in the presence of nicotine, can increase ethanol self-administration (Zipori et al., 2017), suggesting the possibility that nicotine-enhancement of contextual cues is what actually drives enhanced ethanol seeking. Therefore, nicotine administered outside of the behavioral context may not alter self-administration, which is somewhat inconsistent with a molecular basis of the Gateway Hypothesis of nicotine (Kandel and Kandel, 2014). To test this, we gave adolescent rats daily injections of nicotine for 5 days prior to the start of behavioral training, and then, every day of behavioral training, animals received nicotine 2 h after the behavioral session. In short, rats received nicotine such that there was no association with the behavioral sessions and minimal pharmacological interaction with the ethanol consumed. We found that this nicotine regimen resulted in no significant impact on self-administration of sweetened ethanol; therefore, these results do not support a strictly "exposure" interpretation of the Gateway Hypothesis of nicotine. However, it should be noted that preclinical studies supporting the Gateway Hypothesis used a continuous exposure model of nicotine in drinking water (Levine et al., 2011), whereas we administered a single bolus of nicotine per day.

NTX is an opioid receptor antagonist that reduces ethanol seeking and the rewarding properties of ethanol (e.g., Kreek et al., 2002; Ripley and Stephens, 2011). We chose a dose range of NTX that has been shown to decrease ethanol seeking with nominal effect on sucrose seeking (Czachowski and Delory, 2009; Hay et al., 2013). NTX is more effective in reducing ethanol use in cigarette smokers compared to nonsmokers (Fucito et al., 2012) and in animals co-administering nicotine and ethanol during self-administration compared to ethanol alone (Lê et al., 2014). However, we found that NTX decreased sweetened ethanol seeking similarly in animals exposed to nicotine and saline. Our study was performed in a peri-adolescent period of development (~P60), whereas most studies showing nicotine promotion of ethanol drinking have been done in adults. However, there is no evidence suggesting that NTX lacks efficacy in curbing ethanol seeking during adolescence. Indeed, NTX has been shown to decrease ethanol seeking in adolescent humans (Deas et al., 2005) and rodents (Sable et al., 2006). Thus, while previous findings show that NTX is a viable tool to decrease ethanol seeking in patients with a history of smoking, our results suggest this is likely due to nicotine-enhanced seeking behavior as opposed to nicotine exposure *per se*. As discussed above, our nicotine administration paradigm was such that animals were not exposed to nicotine in the context of the behavioral paradigm or in tandem with ethanol. As such, the cue reinforcing effects of nicotine (e.g., Caggiula et al., 2009) were likely not contributing factors to the results observed here.

Habit-directed behavior is a form of behavioral inflexibility, in that an animal is less likely to alter habitual behavior following a change in reward value. Ethanol consumption can shift operant behavior from goal- to habit-directed (Dickinson et al., 2002; Corbit et al., 2012; Mangieri et al., 2012). In turn, adolescent ethanol exposure can also lead to reduced behavioral flexibility in adulthood (Coleman et al., 2014; Gass et al., 2014; Madayag et al., 2017). Therefore, it is not surprising that the control animals in our study exhibited heightened habit-directed alcohol seeking in a reward devaluation paradigm, although extended operant training can also be sufficient to induce habit formation (e.g., Ostlund and Balleine, 2008). Repeated use of nicotine leads to habitual nicotine-seeking behavior (Clemens et al., 2014; Loughlin et al., 2017), though this can depend on the number of prior self-administration sessions, as 47 sessions, but not 10 sessions, produced insensitivity to nicotine devaluation (Clemens et al., 2014). Thus, one may expect that rats exposed to nicotine over 40 days would be predisposed to habitual reward seeking, but that is not what we observed in the present study. In fact, animals exposed to nicotine exhibited sensitivity to reward devaluation compared to animals that received saline control. This is not likely due to acute effects of nicotine as the latest injection of nicotine was approximately 22 h prior to the behavioral session. Alternatively, it is possible that the ability of nicotine to maintain goal-directed behavior towards sweetened ethanol seeking was due to long-term exposure, as chronic exposure to nicotine can result in different nicotinic receptor subunit expression. For example, when administered in adolescence, repeated nicotine increases β2 subunit-containing nicotinic receptors (Counotte et al., 2012a). In turn, compounds that selectively target β2 subunit-containing receptors can enhance behavioral flexibility in humans and primates withdrawn from drugs of abuse (Gould et al., 2013; Terry et al., 2016; Lesage et al., 2017). Therefore, the administration of nicotine outside of the behavioral context may have enhanced behavioral flexibility and, therefore, rendered animals in our study resistant to habit-directed behavior.

Contingent nicotine co-administered with ethanol and non-contingent nicotine administered prior to ethanol self-administration sessions increase the motivation for ethanol seeking both in rodents (Bespalov et al., 1999) and humans (Barrett et al., 2006). When administered in conjunction with self-administered ethanol, nicotine enhances the motivation for ethanol in dependent rats (Leão et al., 2015). Consistent with this, administration of nicotine vs. non-nicotine cigarettes in human smokers increased the breakpoint for alcoholic beverages (Barrett et al., 2006). However, we observed no effect on motivation (nosepokes, breakpoint) for sweetened ethanol in animals administered nicotine when the nicotine was given outside of the behavioral context. This indicates that the motivationally enhancing effects of nicotine on ethanol seeking is likely to be highly dependent on the temporal aspect of administration.

Nicotinic receptor agonists including nicotine can be used to enhance cognition and behavioral flexibility (for review see Counotte et al., 2012b). For example, when given after induction of fear conditioning, nicotine has been shown to enhance extinction learning (Elias et al., 2010). Therefore, we expected animals exposed to nicotine to exhibit faster extinction from sweetened ethanol seeking compared to animals exposed to saline. Contrary to this prediction, we observed no significant difference in extinction behavior between the two groups, suggesting that the cognitive-enhancing effects of nicotine did not extend to extinction learning in the present study. Furthermore, when administered during ethanol withdrawal, nicotine can increase reinstatement of ethanol self-administration (López-Moreno et al., 2004). However, we observed no differences in reinstatement behavior after re-exposure to the associated cue. This likely occurred because we avoided acute nicotine effects on the reinstatement session, consistent with previous reports in which a temporally distant exposure had no effect on reinstatement behavior (Hauser et al., 2012).

Synergistic or additive effects on reinforcement circuitry due to co-administration or co-consumption of nicotine and ethanol (Leão et al., 2015; Tolu et al., 2017) are unlikely to contribute to the present results. The half-life of available nicotine in the brain is approximately 52 min (Ghosheh et al., 1999). Therefore, sufficient pharmacologically active nicotine should be available during the behavior session when administered up to 3–4 h prior (Hauser et al., 2012) to render behavioral effects from an acute injection, but not likely when administered approximately 22 h prior to the behavior session as in the present study. On the other hand, Doyon et al. (2013) reported long-term effects of nicotine on ethanol-evoked dopamine levels, lasting up to 40 h. Thus, the lack of effect of nicotine on behavior in the present study is consistent with expected pharmacokinetics, and while it is possible that this nicotine regimen produced persistent effects on the dopamine system, they were evidently insufficient to alter sweetened ethanol self-administration in the present study.

One caveat to the present study is that it used only female rats, as ethanol self-administration extended from mid-adolescence into adulthood, and female rodents are well-known to drink more ethanol than males in adulthood (Becker and Koob, 2016). However, in adolescence the sex difference is less clear, as some studies found that males drank more ethanol than females (e.g., Vetter-O'Hagen et al., 2009) and others found more drinking in females (e.g., Varlinskaya et al., 2015). When administered only during adolescence, nicotine enhanced conditioned reinforcement in both male and female adults, but increased Pavlovian conditioned approach only in adult males (Quick et al., 2014). Thus, it is possible that nicotine would have different effects in males under the current study design, which may be addressed by future studies.

A related issue is that behavioral neuroscience has historically largely used male rodents based on the assumption that females would introduce greater day-to-day variability due to hormonal effects across their estrous cycle (McCarthy, 2015; Guizzetti et al., 2016). Thus, it is possible that the present study "missed" effects of nicotine due to hormone-related variability in female self-administration. However, recent studies analyzing published data found this assumption to be erroneous: in general, female rodents exhibit no different variance in most metrics (physiological, behavioral, histological, etc.) compared to males (Prendergast et al., 2014; Becker et al., 2016). Even for those traits that showed sex differences, female data were not inherently more variable than male data (Becker et al., 2016). In humans, the primary discrepancy between sexes is that women metabolize nicotine faster than men (Benowitz et al., 2006), although menstrual cycle has no impact on the rate of metabolism in human subjects (Hukkanen et al., 2005). Collectively, it appears unlikely that using only females inserted more variability in behavior metrics. However, future studies that directly compare the effects of nicotine on ethanol self-administration in males and females are needed to determine sex differences in day-to-day variability of intake and the potential effects of nicotine.

According to the Gateway Hypothesis of addiction, prior exposure to nicotine leads to an increase in sensitivity to the rewarding properties of other substances of abuse (Kandel and Kandel, 2014). We observed that initiating nicotine administration during adolescence and continuing into adulthood was insufficient to increase ethanol seeking. Therefore, it is likely that nicotine must be self-administered or associative cues must be present while experimenter-administered nicotine is physiologically active for it to produce its reward-amplifying properties. The Gateway Hypothesis should not be discounted, but further investigation should aim to determine in what capacity "gateway drugs" contribute to progression to and escalation of consumption of substances of abuse.

AUTHOR CONTRIBUTIONS

ACM designed the experimental methods and was the primary contributor to authoring the manuscript. KSC performed the experiments and was a secondary contributor to authoring the manuscript. LMW performed the experiments and reviewed the manuscript. DLR helped design the experimental method, reviewed the manuscript and is the principal investigator.

ACKNOWLEDGMENTS

The authors thank Sofia Neira, Hannah Jaggers, Madeline Watson and Brandi Lawrence for valuable technical assistance. Dr. Sierra Stringfield provided valuable discussion and insight. This research was funded by the National Institutes of Health (P60 AA011605). ACM was supported on T32 AA007573 and KSC was supported by the Science and Math Achievement and Resourcefulness Track (SMART) fellowship from the Office of Undergraduate Research at the University of North Carolina, Chapel Hill, NC, USA.

REFERENCES

Bachman, J. G. (2002). *The Decline of Substance Use in Young Adulthood: Changes in Social Activities, Roles, and Beliefs.* Mahwah, NJ: Lawrence Erlbaum Associates.

Barrett, S. P., Tichauer, M., Leyton, M., and Pihl, R. O. (2006). Nicotine increases alcohol self-administration in non-dependent male smokers. *Drug Alcohol Depend.* 81, 197–204. doi: 10.1016/j.drugalcdep.2005.06.009

Becker, J. B., and Koob, G. F. (2016). Sex differenecs in animal models: focus on addiction. *Pharmacol. Rev.* 68, 242–263. doi: 10.1124/pr.115.011163

Becker, J. B., Prendergast, B. J., and Liang, J. W. (2016). Female rats are not more variable than male rats: a meta-analysis of neuroscience studies. *Biol. Sex Differ.* 7:34. doi: 10.1186/s13293-016-0087-5

Benowitz, N. L., Lessov-Schlaggar, C. N., Swan, G. E., and Jacob, P. III (2006). Female sex and oral contraceptive use accelerate nicotine metabolism. *Clin. Pharmacol. Ther.* 79, 480–488. doi: 10.1016/j.clpt.2006.01.008

Bespalov, A., Lebedev, A., Panchenko, G., and Zvartau, E. (1999). Effects of abused drugs on thresholds and breaking points of intracranial self-stimulation in rats. *Eur. Neuropsychopharmacol.* 9, 377–383. doi: 10.1016/s0924-977x(99)00008-5

Bienkowski, P., Koros, E., Kostowski, W., and Bogucka-Bonikowska, A. (2000). Reinstatement of ethanol seeking in rats: behavioral analysis. *Pharmacol. Biochem. Behav.* 66, 123–128. doi: 10.1016/S0091-3057(00)00194-5

Brown, S. A., Tapert, S. F., Tate, S. R., and Abrantes, A. M. (2000). The role of alcohol in adolescent relapse and outcome. *J. Psychoactive Drugs* 32, 107–115. doi: 10.1080/02791072.2000.10400216

Caggiula, A. R., Donny, E. C., Palmatier, M. I., Liu, X., Chaudhri, N., and Sved, A. F. (2009). The role of nicotine in smoking: a dual-reinforcement model. *Nebr. Symp. Motiv.* 55, 91–109. doi: 10.1007/978-0-387-78748-0_6

Chaudhri, N., Caggiula, A. R., Donny, E. C., Booth, S., Gharib, M., Craven, L., et al. (2006). Operant responding for conditioned and unconditioned reinforcers in rats is differentially enhanced by the primary reinforcing and reinforcement-enhancing effects of nicotine. *Psychopharmacology (Berl)* 189, 27–36. doi: 10.1007/s00213-006-0522-0

Chaudhri, N., Caggiula, A. R., Donny, E. C., Booth, S., Gharib, M. A., Craven, L. A., et al. (2005). Sex differences in the contribution of nicotine and nonpharmacological stimuli to nicotine self-administration in rats. *Psychopharmacology (Berl)* 180, 258–266. doi: 10.1007/s00213-005-2152-3

Chaudhri, N., Caggiula, A. R., Donny, E. C., Booth, S., Gharib, M., Craven, L., et al. (2007). Self-administered and noncontingent nicotine enhance reinforced operant responding in rats: impact of nicotine dose and reinforcement schedule. *Psychopharmacology (Berl)* 190, 353–362. doi: 10.1007/s00213-006-0454-8

Clemens, K. J., Castino, M. R., Cornish, J. L., Goodchild, A. K., and Holmes, N. M. (2014). Behavioral and neural substrates of habit formation in rats intravenously self-administering nicotine. *Neuropsychopharmacology* 39, 2584–2593. doi: 10.1038/npp.2014.111

Coleman, L. G. Jr., Liu, W., Oguz, I., Styner, M., and Crews, F. T. (2014). Adolescent binge ethanol treatment alters adult brain regional volumes, cortical extracellular matrix protein and behavioral flexibility. *Pharmacol. Biochem. Behav.* 116, 142–151. doi: 10.1016/j.pbb.2013.11.021

Corbit, L. H., Nie, H., and Janak, P. H. (2012). Habitual alcohol seeking: time course and the contribution of subregions of the dorsal striatum. *Biol. Psychiatry* 72, 389–395. doi: 10.1016/j.biopsych.2012.02.024

Counotte, D. S., Goriounova, N. A., Moretti, M., Smoluch, M. T., Irth, H., Clementi, F., et al. (2012a). Adolescent nicotine exposure transiently increases high-affinity nicotinic receptors and modulates inhibitory synaptic transmission in rat medial prefrontal cortex. *FASEB J.* 26, 1810–1820. doi: 10.1096/fj.11-198994

Counotte, D. S., Smit, A. B., and Spijker, S. (2012b). The yin and yang of nicotine: harmful during development, beneficial in adult patient populations. *Front. Pharmacol.* 3:180. doi: 10.3389/fphar.2012.00180

Czachowski, C. L., and Delory, M. J. (2009). Acamprosate and naltrexone treatment effects on ethanol and sucrose seeking and intake in ethanol-dependent and nondependent rats. *Psychopharmacology (Berl)* 204, 335–348. doi: 10.1007/s00213-009-1465-z

Deas, D., May, M. P., Randall, C., Johnson, N., and Anton, R. (2005). Naltrexone treatment of adolescent alcoholics: an open-label pilot study. *J. Child Adolesc. Psychopharmacol.* 15, 723–728. doi: 10.1089/cap.2005.15.723

Degenhardt, L., Dierker, L., Chiu, W. T., Medina-Mora, M. E., Neumark, Y., Sampson, N., et al. (2010). Evaluating the drug use "gateway" theory using cross-national data: consistency and associations of the order of initiation of drug use among participants in the WHO World Mental Health Surveys. *Drug Alcohol Depend.* 108, 84–97. doi: 10.1016/j.drugalcdep.2009.12.001

Dickinson, A., Wood, N., and Smith, J. W. (2002). Alcohol seeking by rats: action or habit? *Q. J. Exp. Psychol. B* 55, 331–348. doi: 10.1080/0272499024400016

Doherty, J. M., and Gonzales, R. A. (2015). Operant self-administration of sweetened ethanol and time course of blood ethanol levels in adolescent and adult male Long-Evans rats. *Alcohol. Clin. Exp. Res.* 39, 485–495. doi: 10.1111/acer.12630

Donny, E. C., Chaudhri, N., Caggiula, A. R., Evans-Martin, F. F., Booth, S., Gharib, M. A., et al. (2003). Operant responding for a visual reinforcer in rats is enhanced by noncontingent nicotine: implications for nicotine self-administration and reinforcement. *Psychopharmacology (Berl)* 169, 68–76. doi: 10.1007/s00213-003-1473-3

Doyon, W. M., Dong, Y., Ostroumov, A., Thomas, A. M., Zhang, T. A., and Dani, J. A. (2013). Nicotine decreases ethanol-induced dopamine signaling and increases self-administration via stress hormones. *Neuron* 79, 530–540. doi: 10.1016/j.neuron.2013.06.006

Elias, G. A., Gulick, D., Wilkinson, D. S., and Gould, T. J. (2010). Nicotine and extinction of fear conditioning. *Neuroscience* 165, 1063–1073. doi: 10.1016/j.neuroscience.2009.11.022

Fucito, L. M., Park, A., Gulliver, S. B., Mattson, M. E., Gueorguieva, R. V., and O'Malley, S. S. (2012). Cigarette smoking predicts differential benefit from naltrexone for alcohol dependence. *Biol. Psychiatry* 72, 832–838. doi: 10.1016/j.biopsych.2012.03.023

Gass, J. T., Glen, W. B. Jr., McGonigal, J. T., Trantham-Davidson, H., Lopez, M. F., Randall, P. K., et al. (2014). Adolescent alcohol exposure reduces behavioral flexibility, promotes disinhibition and increases resistance to extinction of ethanol self-administration in adulthood. *Neuropsychopharmacology* 39, 2570–2583. doi: 10.1038/npp.2014.109

Ghosheh, O., Dwoskin, L. P., Li, W. K., and Crooks, P. A. (1999). Residence times and half-lives of nicotine metabolites in rat brain after acute peripheral administration of [2′-^{14}C]nicotine. *Drug Metab. Dispos.* 27, 1448–1455.

Gould, R. W., Garg, P. K., Garg, S., and Nader, M. A. (2013). Effects of nicotinic acetylcholine receptor agonists on cognition in rhesus monkeys with a chronic cocaine self-administration history. *Neuropharmacology* 64, 479–488. doi: 10.1016/j.neuropharm.2012.08.004

Guizzetti, M., Davies, D. L., Egli, M., Finn, D. A., Molina, P., Regunathan, S., et al. (2016). Sex and the lab: an alcohol-focused commentary on the NIH initiative to balance sex in cell and animal studies. *Alcohol. Clin. Exp. Res.* 40, 1182–1191. doi: 10.1111/acer.13072

Guy, E. G., and Fletcher, P. J. (2014a). The effects of nicotine exposure during Pavlovian conditioning in rats on several measures of incentive motivation for a conditioned stimulus paired with water. *Psychopharmacology (Berl)* 231, 2261–2271. doi: 10.1007/s00213-013-3375-3

Guy, E. G., and Fletcher, P. J. (2014b). Responding for a conditioned reinforcer, and its enhancement by nicotine, is blocked by dopamine receptor antagonists and a 5-HT_{2C} receptor agonist but not by a 5-HT_{2A} receptor antagonist. *Pharmacol. Biochem. Behav.* 125, 40–47. doi: 10.1016/j.pbb.2014.08.006

Hauser, S. R., Getachew, B., Oster, S. M., Dhaher, R., Ding, Z. M., Bell, R. L., et al. (2012). Nicotine modulates alcohol-seeking and relapse by alcohol-preferring (P) rats in a time-dependent manner. *Alcohol. Clin. Exp. Res.* 36, 43–54. doi: 10.1111/j.1530-0277.2011.01579.x

Hay, R. A., Jennings, J. H., Zitzman, D. L., Hodge, C. W., and Robinson, D. L. (2013). Specific and nonspecific effects of naltrexone on goal-directed and habitual models of alcohol seeking and drinking. *Alcohol. Clin. Exp. Res.* 37, 1100–1110. doi: 10.1111/acer.12081

Hukkanen, J., Gourlay, S. G., Kenkare, S., and Benowitz, N. L. (2005). Influence of menstrual cycle on cytochrome P450 2A6 activity and cardiovascular effects of nicotine. *Clin. Pharmacol. Ther.* 77, 159–169. doi: 10.1016/j.clpt.2004.10.012

Kandel, D., and Faust, R. (1975). Sequence and stages in patterns of adolescent drug use. *Arch. Gen. Psychiatry* 32, 923–932. doi: 10.1001/archpsyc.1975.01760250115013

Kandel, E. R., and Kandel, D. B. (2014). A molecular basis for nicotine as a gateway drug. *N. Eng. J. Med.* 371, 932–943. doi: 10.1056/nejmsa1405092

Kandel, D., and Kandel, E. (2015). The gateway hypothesis of substance abuse: developmental, biological and societal perspectives. *Acta Paediatr.* 104, 130–137. doi: 10.1111/apa.12851

Kandel, D. B., Yamaguchi, K., and Chen, K. (1992). Stages of progression in drug involvement from adolescence to adulthood: further evidence for the gateway theory. *J. Stud. Alcohol* 53, 447–457. doi: 10.15288/jsa.1992.53.447

Kreek, M. J., Laforge, K. S., and Butelman, E. (2002). Pharmacotherapy of addictions. *Nat. Rev. Drug Discov.* 1, 710–726. doi: 10.1038/nrd897

Lárraga, A., Belluzzi, J. D., and Leslie, F. M. (2017). Nicotine increases alcohol intake in adolescent male rats. *Front. Behav. Neurosci.* 11:25. doi: 10.3389/fnbeh.2017.00025

Lê, A. D., Funk, D., Lo, S., and Coen, K. (2014). Operant self-administration of alcohol and nicotine in a preclinical model of co-abuse. *Psychopharmacology (Berl)* 231, 4019–4029. doi: 10.1007/s00213-014-3541-2

Leão, R. M., Cruz, F. C., Vendruscolo, L. F., de Guglielmo, G., Logrip, M. L., Planeta, C. S., et al. (2015). Chronic nicotine activates stress/reward-related brain regions and facilitates the transition to compulsive alcohol drinking. *J. Neurosci.* 35, 6241–6253. doi: 10.1523/JNEUROSCI.3302-14.2015

Lesage, E., Aronson, S. E., Sutherland, M. T., Ross, T. J., Salmeron, B. J., and Stein, E. A. (2017). Neural signatures of cognitive flexibility and reward sensitivity following nicotinic receptor stimulation in dependent smokers: a randomized trial. *JAMA Psychiatry* 74, 632–640. doi: 10.1001/jamapsychiatry.2017.0400

Levine, A., Huang, Y., Drisaldi, B., Griffin, E. A. Jr., Pollak, D. D., Xu, S., et al. (2011). Molecular mechanism for a gateway drug: epigenetic changes initiated by nicotine prime gene expression by cocaine. *Sci. Transl. Med.* 3:107ra109. doi: 10.1126/scitranslmed.3003062

López-Moreno, J. A., Trigo-Díaz, J. M., Rodríguez de Fonseca, F., González Cuevas, G., Gómez de Heras, R., Crespo Galán, I., et al. (2004). Nicotine in alcohol deprivation increases alcohol operant self-administration during reinstatement. *Neuropharmacology* 47, 1036–1044. doi: 10.1016/j.neuropharm.2004.08.002

Loughlin, A., Funk, D., Coen, K., and Lê, A. D. (2017). Habitual nicotine-seeking in rats following limited training. *Psychopharmacology (Berl)* doi: 10.1007/s00213-017-4655-0 [Epub ahead of print].

Madayag, A. C., Stringfield, S. J., Reissner, K. J., Boettiger, C. A., and Robinson, D. L. (2017). Sex and adolescent ethanol exposure influence Pavlovian conditioned approach. *Alcohol. Clin. Exp. Res.* 41, 846–856. doi: 10.1111/acer.13354

Maddux, J. N., and Chaudhri, N. (2017). Nicotine-induced enhancement of Pavlovian alcohol-seeking behavior in rats. *Psychopharmacology (Berl)* 234, 727–738. doi: 10.1007/s00213-016-4508-2

Mangieri, R. A., Cofresi, R. U., and Gonzales, R. A. (2012). Ethanol seeking by Long Evans rats is not always a goal-directed behavior. *PLoS One* 7:e42886. doi: 10.1371/journal.pone.0042886

McCarthy, M. M. (2015). Incorporating sex as a variable in preclinical neuropsychiatric research. *Schizophr. Bull.* 41, 1016–1020. doi: 10.1093/schbul/sbv077

Melendez, R. I. (2011). Intermittent (every-other-day) drinking induces rapid escalation of ethanol intake and preference in adolescent and adult C57BL/6J mice. *Alcohol. Clin. Exp. Res.* 35, 652–658. doi: 10.1111/j.1530-0277.2010.01383.x

Nesil, T., Kanit, L., Collins, A. C., and Pogun, S. (2011). Individual differences in oral nicotine intake in rats. *Neuropharmacology* 61, 189–201. doi: 10.1016/j.neuropharm.2011.03.027

Olausson, P., Jentsch, J. D., and Taylor, J. R. (2004a). Nicotine enhances responding with conditioned reinforcement. *Psychopharmacology (Berl)* 171, 173–178. doi: 10.1007/s00213-003-1575-y

Olausson, P., Jentsch, J. D., and Taylor, J. R. (2004b). Repeated nicotine exposure enhances responding with conditioned reinforcement. *Psychopharmacology (Berl)* 173, 98–104. doi: 10.1007/s00213-003-1702-9

Ostlund, S. B., and Balleine, B. W. (2008). On habits and addiction: an associative analysis of compulsive drug seeking. *Drug Discov. Today Dis. Models* 5, 235–245. doi: 10.1016/j.ddmod.2009.07.004

Palmatier, M. I., Liu, X., Matteson, G. L., Donny, E. C., Caggiula, A. R., and Sved, A. F. (2007). Conditioned reinforcement in rats established with self-administered nicotine and enhanced by noncontingent nicotine. *Psychopharmacology (Berl)* 195, 235–243. doi: 10.1007/s00213-007-0897-6

Palmatier, M. I., Marks, K. R., Jones, S. A., Freeman, K. S., Wissman, K. M., and Sheppard, A. B. (2013). The effect of nicotine on sign-tracking and goal-tracking in a Pavlovian conditioned approach paradigm in rats. *Psychopharmacology (Berl)* 226, 247–259. doi: 10.1007/s00213-012-2892-9

Palmer, R. H., Button, T. M., Rhee, S. H., Corley, R. P., Young, S. E., Stallings, M. C., et al. (2012). Genetic etiology of the common liability to drug dependence: evidence of common and specific mechanisms for DSM-IV dependence symptoms. *Drug Alcohol Depend.* 123, S24–S32. doi: 10.1016/j.drugalcdep.2011.12.015

Pomfrey, R. L., Bostwick, T. A., Wetzell, B. B., and Riley, A. L. (2015). Adolescent nicotine exposure fails to impact cocaine reward, aversion and self-administration in adult male rats. *Pharmacol. Biochem. Behav.* 137, 30–37. doi: 10.1016/j.pbb.2015.08.004

Prendergast, B. J., Onishi, K. G., and Zucker, I. (2014). Female mice liberated for inclusion in neuroscience and biomedical research. *Neurosci. Biobehav. Rev.* 40, 1–5. doi: 10.1016/j.neubiorev.2014.01.001

Quick, S. L., Olausson, P., Addy, N. A., and Taylor, J. R. (2014). Repeated nicotine exposure during adolescence alters reward-related learning in male and female rats. *Behav. Brain Res.* 261, 171–176. doi: 10.1016/j.bbr.2013.12.001

Ripley, T. L., and Stephens, D. N. (2011). Critical thoughts on current rodent models for evaluating potential treatments of alcohol addiction and withdrawal. *Br. J. Pharmacol.* 164, 1335–1356. doi: 10.1111/j.1476-5381.2011.01406.x

Sable, H. J., Bell, R. L., Rodd, Z. A., and Mcbride, W. J. (2006). Effects of naltrexone on the acquisition of alcohol intake in male and female periadolescent and adult alcohol-preferring (P) rats. *Int. J. Adolesc. Med. Health* 18, 139–149. doi: 10.1515/ijamh.2006.18.1.139

Schassburger, R. L., Pitzer, E. M., Smith, T. T., Rupprecht, L. E., Thiels, E., Donny, E. C., et al. (2016). Adolescent rats self-administer less nicotine than adults at low doses. *Nicotine Tob. Res.* 18, 1861–1868. doi: 10.1093/ntr/ntw006

Serlin, H., and Torregrossa, M. M. (2015). Adolescent rats are resistant to forming ethanol seeking habits. *Dev. Cogn. Neurosci.* 16, 183–190. doi: 10.1016/j.dcn.2014.12.002

Shillinglaw, J. E., Everitt, I. K., and Robinson, D. L. (2014). Assessing behavioral control across reinforcer solutions on a fixed-ratio schedule of reinforcement in rats. *Alcohol* 48, 337–344. doi: 10.1016/j.alcohol.2013.12.006

Shnitko, T. A., and Robinson, D. L. (2015). Regional variation in phasic dopamine encoding of alcohol self-administration in rats. *ACS Chem. Neurosci.* 6, 147–154. doi: 10.1021/cn500251j

Shram, M. J., Funk, D., Li, Z., and Lê, A. D. (2008). Nicotine self-administration, extinction responding and reinstatement in adolescent and adult male rats: evidence against a biological vulnerability to nicotine addiction during adolescence. *Neuropsychopharmacology* 33, 739–748. doi: 10.1038/sj.npp.1301454

Shram, M. J., and Lê, A. D. (2010). Adolescent male Wistar rats are more responsive than adult rats to the conditioned rewarding effects of intravenously administered nicotine in the place conditioning procedure. *Behav. Brain Res.* 206, 240–244. doi: 10.1016/j.bbr.2009.09.018

Smith, B. R., Horan, J. T., Gaskin, S., and Amit, Z. (1999). Exposure to nicotine enhances acquisition of ethanol drinking by laboratory rats in a limited access paradigm. *Psychopharmacology (Berl)* 142, 408–412. doi: 10.1007/s002130050906

Stringfield, S. J., Palmatier, M. I., Boettiger, C. A., and Robinson, D. L. (2017). Orbitofrontal participation in sign- and goal-tracking conditioned responses: effects of nicotine. *Neuropharmacology* 116, 208–223. doi: 10.1016/j.neuropharm.2016.12.020

Tambour, S., Brown, L. L., and Crabbe, J. C. (2008). Gender and age at drinking onset affect voluntary alcohol consumption but neither the alcohol deprivation effect nor the response to stress in mice. *Alcohol. Clin. Exp. Res.* 32, 2100–2106. doi: 10.1111/j.1530-0277.2008.00798.x

Terry, A. V. Jr., Plagenhoef, M., and Callahan, P. M. (2016). Effects of the nicotinic agonist varenicline on the performance of tasks of cognition in aged and middle-aged rhesus and pigtail monkeys. *Psychopharmacology (Berl)* 233, 761–771. doi: 10.1007/s00213-015-4154-0

Tolu, S., Marti, F., Morel, C., Perrier, C., Torquet, N., Pons, S., et al. (2017). Nicotine enhances alcohol intake and dopaminergic responses through β2* and β4* nicotinic acetylcholine receptors. *Sci. Rep.* 7:45116. doi: 10.1038/srep45116

Torres, O. V., Natividad, L. A., Tejeda, H. A., Van Weelden, S. A., and O'Dell, L. E. (2009). Female rats display dose-dependent differences to the rewarding and aversive effects of nicotine in an age-, hormone-, and sex-dependent manner. *Psychopharmacology (Berl)* 206, 303–312. doi: 10.1007/s00213-009-1607-3

Truxell, E. M., Molina, J. C., and Spear, N. E. (2007). Ethanol intake in the juvenile, adolescent, and adult rat: effects of age and prior exposure to ethanol. *Alcohol. Clin. Exp. Res.* 31, 755–765. doi: 10.1111/j.1530-0277.2007.00358.x

Varlinskaya, E. I., Truxell, E. M., and Spear, L. P. (2015). Ethanol intake under social circumstances or alone in Sprague-Dawley rats: impact of age, sex, social activity, and social anxiety-like behavior. *Alcohol. Clin. Exp. Res.* 39, 117–125. doi: 10.1111/acer.12604

Vetter-O'Hagen, C., Varlinskaya, E., and Spear, L. (2009). Sex differences in ethanol intake and sensitivity to aversive effects during adolescence and adulthood. *Alcohol Alcohol.* 44, 547–554. doi: 10.1093/alcalc/agp048

Walker, B. M., and Ehlers, C. L. (2009). Age-related differences in the blood alcohol levels of Wistar rats. *Pharmacol. Biochem. Behav.* 91, 560–565. doi: 10.1016/j.pbb.2008.09.017

Walker, B. M., and Koob, G. F. (2007). The γ-aminobutyric acid-B receptor agonist baclofen attenuates responding for ethanol in ethanol-dependent rats. *Alcohol. Clin. Exp. Res.* 31, 11–18. doi: 10.1111/j.1530-0277.2006.00259.x

Yager, L. M., and Robinson, T. E. (2015). Individual variation in the motivational properties of a nicotine cue: sign-trackers vs. goal-trackers. *Psychopharmacology (Berl)* 232, 3149–3160. doi: 10.1007/s00213-015-3962-6

Zipori, D., Sadot-Sogrin, Y., Goltseker, K., Even-Chen, O., Rahamim, N., Shaham, O., et al. (2017). Re-exposure to nicotine-associated context from adolescence enhances alcohol intake in adulthood. *Sci. Rep.* 7:2479. doi: 10.1038/s41598-017-02177-2

Permissions

All chapters in this book were first published in LTCADUEPCCM, by Frontiers; hereby published with permission under the Creative Commons Attribution License or equivalent. Every chapter published in this book has been scrutinized by our experts. Their significance has been extensively debated. The topics covered herein carry significant findings which will fuel the growth of the discipline. They may even be implemented as practical applications or may be referred to as a beginning point for another development.

The contributors of this book come from diverse backgrounds, making this book a truly international effort. This book will bring forth new frontiers with its revolutionizing research information and detailed analysis of the nascent developments around the world.

We would like to thank all the contributing authors for lending their expertise to make the book truly unique. They have played a crucial role in the development of this book. Without their invaluable contributions this book wouldn't have been possible. They have made vital efforts to compile up to date information on the varied aspects of this subject to make this book a valuable addition to the collection of many professionals and students.

This book was conceptualized with the vision of imparting up-to-date information and advanced data in this field. To ensure the same, a matchless editorial board was set up. Every individual on the board went through rigorous rounds of assessment to prove their worth. After which they invested a large part of their time researching and compiling the most relevant data for our readers.

The editorial board has been involved in producing this book since its inception. They have spent rigorous hours researching and exploring the diverse topics which have resulted in the successful publishing of this book. They have passed on their knowledge of decades through this book. To expedite this challenging task, the publisher supported the team at every step. A small team of assistant editors was also appointed to further simplify the editing procedure and attain best results for the readers.

Apart from the editorial board, the designing team has also invested a significant amount of their time in understanding the subject and creating the most relevant covers. They scrutinized every image to scout for the most suitable representation of the subject and create an appropriate cover for the book.

The publishing team has been an ardent support to the editorial, designing and production team. Their endless efforts to recruit the best for this project, has resulted in the accomplishment of this book. They are a veteran in the field of academics and their pool of knowledge is as vast as their experience in printing. Their expertise and guidance has proved useful at every step. Their uncompromising quality standards have made this book an exceptional effort. Their encouragement from time to time has been an inspiration for everyone.

The publisher and the editorial board hope that this book will prove to be a valuable piece of knowledge for researchers, students, practitioners and scholars across the globe.

List of Contributors

Lisa D. Goldberg-Looney and Paul B. Perrin
Department of Psychology, Virginia Commonwealth University, Richmond, Virginia, USA

Miriam Sánchez-SanSegundo, Rosario Ferrer-Cascales and Natalia Albaladejo-Blazquez
Department of Health Psychology, University of Alicante, Alicante, Spain

Shashwath A. Meda
Olin Neuropsychiatry Research Center, Hartford HealthCare Corporation, Hartford, CT, United States

Keith A. Hawkins
Department of Psychiatry, Yale University, New Haven, CT, United States

Alecia D. Dager
Olin Neuropsychiatry Research Center, Hartford HealthCare Corporation, Hartford, CT, United States, Department of Psychiatry, Yale University, New Haven, CT, United States

Howard Tennen
Department of Community Medicine, University of Connecticut School of Medicine, Farmington, CT, United States

Sarah Raskin
Department of Psychology and Neurosciences, Trinity College, Hartford, CT, United States

Rebecca M. Wood, Carol S. Austad and Carolyn R. Fallahi
Department of Psychology, Central Connecticut State University, New Britain, CT, United States

Godfrey D. Pearlson
Olin Neuropsychiatry Research Center, Hartford HealthCare Corporation, Hartford, CT, United States Department of Psychiatry, Yale University, New Haven, CT, United States Department of Neuroscience, Yale University, New Haven, CT, United States

Ove Heradstveit
Center for Alcohol and Drug Research, Stavanger University Hospital, Stavanger, Norway Regional Centre for Child and Youth Mental Health and Child Welfare, Norwegian Research Centre Bergen, Norway

Mari Hysing
Regional Centre for Child and Youth Mental Health and Child Welfare, Norwegian Research Centre, Bergen, Norway Department of Psychosocial Science, Faculty of Psychology, University of Bergen, Bergen, Norway

Jens Christoffer Skogen
Center for Alcohol and Drug Research, Stavanger University Hospital, Stavanger, Norway Department of Health Promotion, Norwegian Institute of Public Health, Bergen, Norway

Jørn Hetland
Department of Psychosocial Science, Faculty of Psychology, University of Bergen, Bergen, Norway

Robert Stewart
Institute of Psychiatry, Psychology and Neuroscience, King's College London, London, United Kingdom, South London and Maudsley NHS Foundation Trust, London, United Kingdom

Víctor De la Peña-Arteaga and Sarah O. Nogueira
Bellvitge Biomedical Research Institute, Barcelona, Spain Faculty of Medicine and Health Sciences, University of Barcelona, Barcelona, Spain

Michael Lynskey
Addictions Department, Institute of Psychiatry, Psychology & Neuroscience (IoPPN), King's College London, London, United Kingdom

Lindsey A. Hines
Centre for Academic Mental Health, Population Health Sciences, University of Bristol, Bristol, United Kingdom

Maaike Labots, Linda A. Jolink, Louk J. M. J. Vanderschuren and Heidi M. B. Lesscher
Department of Animals in Science and Society, Division of Behavioural Neuroscience, Faculty of Veterinary Medicine, Utrecht University, Utrecht, Netherlands

Janna Cousijn
ADAPT-Lab, Department of Psychology, University of Amsterdam, Amsterdam, Netherlands Amsterdam Brain and Cognition (ABC), University of Amsterdam, Amsterdam, Netherlands

J. Leon Kenemans
Department of Experimental Psychology, Helmholtz Research Institute, Utrecht University, Utrecht, Netherlands

Alina Quach
1 Department of Psychology, University of Pittsburgh, Pittsburgh, PA, United States

Brenden Tervo-Clemmens
Department of Psychology, University of Pittsburgh, Pittsburgh, PA, United States Center for the Neural Basis of Cognition, University of Pittsburgh, Pittsburgh, PA, United States

Beatriz Luna
Department of Psychology, University of Pittsburgh, Pittsburgh, PA, United States Center for the Neural Basis of Cognition, University of Pittsburgh, Pittsburgh, PA, United States Department of Psychiatry, University of Pittsburgh, Pittsburgh, PA, United States

William Foran, Tammy Chung and Duncan B. Clark
Department of Psychiatry, University of Pittsburgh, Pittsburgh, PA, United States

Michael D. De Bellis
Department of Psychiatry and Behavioral Sciences, Duke University Medical Center, Durham, NC, United States

Erin K. Kirschmann and Daniel M. McCalley
Department of Psychiatry, Translational Neuroscience Program, University of Pittsburgh, Pittsburgh, PA, United States

Caitlyn M. Edwards and Mary M. Torregrossa
Department of Psychiatry, Translational Neuroscience Program, University of Pittsburgh, Pittsburgh, PA, United States Center for Neuroscience, University of Pittsburgh, Pittsburgh, PA, United States

Aurélie Vilenne and Etienne Quertemont
Dépertement Psychologie, Cognition et Comportement, Université de Liège, Liège, Belgium

Lauren C. Kruse, Sophia J. Weber and Jeremy J. Clark
Department of Psychiatry and Behavioral Sciences, University of Washington, Seattle, WA, United States

Abigail G. Schindler
Department of Psychiatry and Behavioral Sciences, University of Washington, Seattle, WA, United States Geriatric Research Education and Clinical Center, VA Puget Sound Health Care System, Seattle, WA, United States

Rapheal G. Williams
Graduate Program in Neuroscience, University of Washington, Seattle, WA, United State

Zachary M. Weil and Kate Karelina
Behavioral Neuroendocrinology Group, Department of Neuroscience, Center for Brain and Spinal Cord Repair, Ohio State University Wexner Medical Center, Columbus, OH, United States

Qi Li
Department of Psychiatry, The University of Hong Kong, Hong Kong, Hong Kong State Key Laboratory for Cognitive and Brain Sciences, The University of Hong Kong, Hong Kong, Hong Kong The University of Hong Kong Shenzhen Institute of Research and Innovation (HKU-SIRI), The University of Hong Kong, Hong Kong, Hong Kong

Lin Shi
Department of Medicine and Therapeutics, Chinese University of Hong Kong, Hong Kong, Hong Kong Chow Yuk Ho Center of Innovative Technology for Medicine, Chinese University of Hong Kong, Hong Kong, Hong Kong

Gang Lu
School of Biomedical Sciences, Chinese University of Hong Kong, Hong Kong, Hong Kong

Hong-Luan Yu
Department of Psychology, Qilu Hospital of Shandong University, Jinan, China

Fu-Ki Yeung, Kai Liu and De-Feng Wang
Research Center for Medical Image Computing, Department of Imaging and Interventional Radiology, Chinese University of Hong Kong, Hong Kong, Hong Kong

Nai-Kei Wong
Chemical Biology Laboratory for Infectious Diseases, Shenzhen Institute of Hepatology, The Third People's Hospital of Shenzhen, Shenzhen, China

Lin Sun
Department of Psychology, Weifang Medical University, Weifang, China

David Yew
School of Chinese Medicine, Chinese University of Hong Kong, Hong Kong, Hong Kong

Fang Pan
Department of Medical Psychology, Shandong University School of Medicine, Jinan, China

Pak C. Sham
Department of Psychiatry, The University of Hong Kong, Hong Kong, Hong Kong State Key Laboratory for Cognitive and Brain Sciences, The University of Hong Kong, Hong Kong, Hong Kong Genome Research Centre, The University of Hong Kong, Hong Kong, Hong Kong

Andrew S. Vore, Anny Gano and Terrence Deak
Behavioral Neuroscience Program, Department of Psychology, Binghamton University, Binghamton, NY, USA

Tamara Doremus-Fitzwater
Department of Psychology, Ithaca College, Ithaca, NY, USA

Wen Liu and Fulton T. Crews
Bowles Center for Alcohol Studies, University of North Carolina at Chapel Hill, Chapel Hill, NC, United States

Emily J. Jaehne, Dzeneta Ameti and Tehani Paiva
Department Psychology and Counselling, School of Psychology and Public Health, La Trobe University, Melbourne, VIC, Australia

Maarten van den Buuse
Department Psychology and Counselling, School of Psychology and Public Health, La Trobe University, Melbourne, VIC, Australia Department of Pharmacology, University of Melbourne, Melbourne, VIC, Australia The College of Public Health, Medical and Veterinary Sciences, James Cook University, Townsville, QLD, Australia

Jacqueline M. Barker, Kathleen G. Bryant, Jennifer I. Osborne and L. J. Chandler
Department of Neuroscience, Medical University of South Carolina, Charleston, SC, United States

Duncan B. Clark, Tammy Chung, Christopher S. Martin, Brant P. Hasler , Douglas H. Fitzgerald and Beatriz Luna
Department of Psychiatry, University of Pittsburgh, Pittsburgh, PA, United States

Sandra A. Brown, Susan F. Tapert, Ty Brumback and Kevin Cummins
Department of Psychology and Psychiatry, University of California, San Diego, La Jolla, CA, United States,

Kilian M. Pohl , Ian M. Colrain and Fiona C. Baker
Center for Health Sciences, SRI International, Menlo Park, CA, United States

Edith V. Sullivan
Department of Psychiatry and Behavioral Sciences, School of Medicine, Stanford University, Palo Alto, CA, United States

Adolf Pfefferbaum
Center for Health Sciences, SRI International, Menlo Park, CA, United States Department of Psychiatry and Behavioral Sciences, School of Medicine, Stanford University, Palo Alto, CA, United States

Michael D. De Bellis
Department of Psychiatry, Duke University, Durham, NC, United States

Kate B. Nooner
Department of Psychology, University of North Carolina Wilmington, Wilmington, NC, United States

Bonnie J. Nagel
Department of Psychiatry, Oregon Health and Science University, Portland, OR, United States

Laura Sanchez-Marin, Francisco J. Pavon, Juan Decara, Juan Suarez, Ana Gavito, Estela Castilla-Ortega, Fernando Rodriguez de Fonseca and Antonia Serrano
Unidad de Gestion Clinica de Salud Mental, Instituto de Investigacion Biomedica de Malaga, Hospital Regional Universitario de Malaga, Universidad de Malaga, Malaga, Spain

Teuku Tahlil
Department of Community Health Nursing, Nursing Faculty, Universitas Syiah Kuala, Banda Aceh, Indonesia

Aiyub Aiyub
Department of Psychiatry, Nursing Faculty, Universitas Syiah Kuala, Banda Aceh, Indonesia

Kyle S. Czarnecki and Lynde M. Wangler
Bowles Center for Alcohol Studies, University of North Carolina, Chapel Hill, NC, United States

Aric C. Madayag
Bowles Center for Alcohol Studies, University of North Carolina, Chapel Hill, NC, United States Department of Pharmacology, University of North Carolina, Chapel Hill, NC, United States

Donita L. Robinson
Bowles Center for Alcohol Studies, University of North Carolina, Chapel Hill, NC, United States Department of Psychiatry, University of North Carolina, Chapel Hill, NC, United States

Index

P

R

S

T

W

www.ingramcontent.com/pod-product-compliance
Lightning Source LLC
LaVergne TN
LVHW060515210926
848485LV00005B/1083
* 9 7 8 1 6 3 9 8 9 0 1 6 3 *